Stunned Myocardium

FUNDAMENTAL AND CLINICAL CARDIOLOGY

Editor-in-Chief

Samuel Z. Goldhaber, M.D.

Harvard Medical School
and Brigham and Women's Hospital
Boston, Massachusetts

Associate Editor, Europe

Henri Bounameaux, M.D.

University Hospital of Geneva
Geneva, Switzerland

1. *Drug Treatment of Hyperlipidemia*, edited by Basil M. Rifkind
2. *Cardiotonic Drugs: A Clinical Review. Second Edition, Revised and Expanded*, edited by Carl V. Leier
3. *Complications of Coronary Angioplasty*, edited by Alexander J. R. Black, H. Vernon Anderson, and Stephen G. Ellis
4. *Unstable Angina*, edited by John D. Rutherford
5. *Beta-Blockers and Cardiac Arrhythmias*, edited by Prakash C. Deedwania
6. *Exercise and the Heart in Health and Disease*, edited by Roy J. Shephard and Henry S. Miller, Jr.
7. *Cardiopulmonary Physiology in Critical Care*, edited by Steven M. Scharf
8. *Atherosclerotic Cardiovascular Disease, Hemostasis, and Endothelial Function*, edited by Robert Boyer Francis, Jr.
9. *Coronary Heart Disease Prevention*, edited by Frank G. Yanowitz
10. *Thrombolysis and Adjunctive Therapy for Acute Myocardial Infarction*, edited by Eric R. Bates
11. *Stunned Myocardium: Properties, Mechanisms, and Clinical Manifestations*, edited by Robert A. Kloner and Karin Przyklenk

Additional Volumes in Preparation

Prevention of Venous Thromboembolism, edited by Samuel Z. Goldhaber

Heart Failure: Basic Science and Clinical Aspects, edited by Judith K. Gwathmey, Gordon M. Briggs, and Paul Allen

Stunned Myocardium

Properties, Mechanisms, and Clinical Manifestations

edited by

Robert A. Kloner
Karin Przyklenk

Hospital of the Good Samaritan and
University of Southern California
Los Angeles, California

Marcel Dekker, Inc. **New York • Basel • Hong Kong**

Library of Congress Cataloging-in-Publication Data

Stunned myocardium : properties, mechanisms, and clinical
manifestations / edited by Robert A. Kloner and Karin Przyklenk.
p. cm. -- (Fundamental and clinical cardiology ; v. 11)
Includes bibliographical references and index.
ISBN 0-8247-8722-6
1. Myocardial stunning. I. Kloner, Robert A. II. Przyklenk,
Karin. III. Series.
[DNLM: 1. Coronary Disease--complications. 2. Coronary Disease-physiopathology. 3. Myocardial Reperfusion Injury--drug therapy.
4. Myocardial Reperfusion Injury--physiopathology. W1 FU538TD v.
11 / WG 280 S934]
RC682.9.S775 1993
616.1'23--dc20 92-49722
DNLM/DLC CIP

This book is printed on acid-free paper.

MARCEL DEKKER, INC.
270 Madison Avenue, New York, New York 10016

Current printing (last digit):
10 9 8 7 6 5 4 3 2 1

PRINTED IN THE UNITED STATES OF AMERICA

We thank our families for their patience and unfailing support throughout the preparation of this book.

Series Introduction

Marcel Dekker, Inc., has focused on the development of various series of beautifully produced books in different branches of medicine. These series have facilitated the integration of rapidly advancing information for both the clinical specialist and the researcher.

My goal as editor of the Fundamental and Clinical Cardiology series is to assemble the talents of world-renowned authorities to discuss virtually every area of cardiovascular medicine. In the current monograph, *Stunned Myocardium: Properties, Mechanisms, and Clinical Manifestations*, Robert A. Kloner and Karin Przyklenk have edited a much needed and timely book. Future contributions to this series will include books on molecular biology, interventional cardiology, and clinical management of such problems as coronary artery disease and ventricular arrhythmias.

Samuel Z. Goldhaber

Preface

Less than 20 years ago, left ventricular contractile dysfunction was considered a good indication that the abnormally contracting segment was necrotic, with no hope of recovery. However, in 1975 Heyndrickx and colleagues made an observation that profoundly altered our perception of contractile dysfunction: using the experimental canine model, they observed persistent hypokinesis of *viable myocardium* during the initial hours following relief of a brief ischemic insult.

An example of this apparent anomaly is shown in Figure 1, which illustrates segment shortening (an index of regional systolic function) measured prior to, during, and following 15 minutes of coronary artery occlusion in the canine model. Although all of the myocardium at risk in this brief occlusion model was salvaged by reperfusion, segment shortening remained markedly depressed following restoration of blood flow (Przyklenk and Kloner, 1986; Kloner and Przyklenk, 1990). It is this prolonged postischemic dysfunction of viable tissue salvaged by reperfusion that has been termed the "stunned myocardium" (Braunwald and Kloner, 1982).

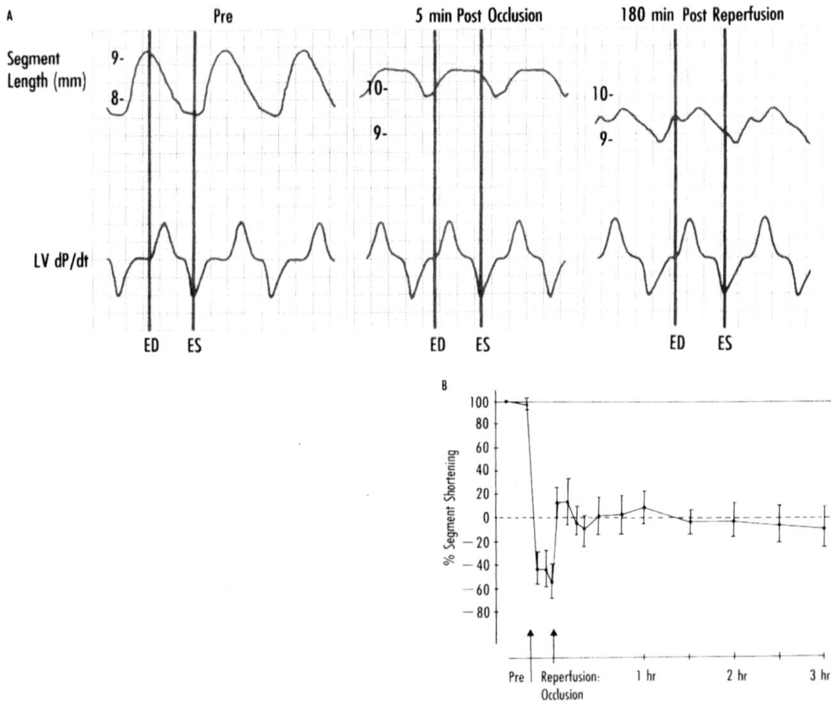

Figure 1 (A) Actual tracings of segment shortening (measured using sonomicrometry) in an anesthetized, open-chest canine preparation. During normal, active contraction (i.e., preocclusion), the ultrasonic crystals move together between end diastole (ED) and end systole (ES), indicated by the strong downward deflection of the preocclusion tracing. During a 15-minute period of coronary occlusion, active contraction is replaced by passive bulging: i.e., the crystals move apart during systole, indicated by the net upward deflection of the tracing. At 180 minutes postreperfusion, active contraction had been restored in this animal (indicated by the net downward deflection of the tracing); however, the previously ischemic tissue is only contracting at approximately 20% of its normal preocclusion value. (B) Mean values of segment shortening, normalized and expressed as a percentage of baseline, preocclusion values, obtained from 12 dogs that underwent 15 minutes of coronary occlusion followed by 3 hours of reperfusion. Note that segment shortening only recovered to 10% of baseline values during the 3 hours of reflow. (Data from Przyklenk and Kloner, 1986. Reprinted with permission from Kloner and Przyklenk, 1990.)

There is no doubt that stunned myocardium has sparked the curiosity of basic scientists and clinicians worldwide. What causes stunned myocardium? How can it be identified? Does it occur in patients? Can (and should) it be treated? With these questions in mind, our objective is to provide a broad overview of the concept of the stunned myocardium, including a review of both its basic characteristics and its relevance to clinical medicine. The book is divided into four sections: Part I summarizes the early experimental evidence that characterized the properties of stunned myocardium and describes postischemic dysfunction in a variety of ischemia/reperfusion scenarios including single coronary artery occlusion, repeated coronary occlusion, partial coronary stenosis, and global ischemia models. Part II describes the current theories regarding the mechanism(s) of stunned myocardium, with particular emphasis on the roles of (and interrelationships among) oxygen radicals, altered calcium homeostasis, and the cyclooxygenose pathway. Part III reviews potential pharmacological therapies for stunned myocardium as identified from experimental models of ischemia/reperfusion, including angiotensin converting enzyme inhibitors, inotropic agents, calcium antagonists, and beta blockers. Part IV describes clinical situations in which stunned myocardium has been documented and includes evidence of postischemic dysfunction following thrombolysis for acute myocardial infarction, following angioplasty, after exercise-induced ischemia, and after cardiac surgery. Finally, the book concludes with a discussion of whether stunned myocardium is important from a clinical standpoint. Our hope is that this text will help clarify the concept of the stunned myocardium; we also share with our readers the many unknowns regarding this phenomenon, which remain to be solved.

In organizing this book we requested the input of authors who have made—and continue to make—important contributions to our understanding of the stunned myocardium. Pathologists, physiologists, cellular biologists, and clinicians have all contributed their scientific data and personal opinions to this text, and we are grateful for the contributions of such experts. In addition, we appreciate the excellent typing skills of Cathy Davisson in the preparation of this text. Finally, we thank Charles T. Munger, Mirion P. Bowers, Roxane Spitzer-Lehmann, John H. Westerman, David Cannom, Barbara Fordyce, James Schoeck, and the members of the board of directors and the administration of the Heart Institute of the Hospital of the Good Samaritan for allowing us to pursue our research and educational endeavors.

Robert A. Kloner
Karin Przyklenk

REFERENCES

Braunwald, E., and Kloner, R. A. (1982). The stunned myocardium: Prolonged, postischemic ventricular dysfunction. *Circulation 66*: 1146.

Heyndrickx, G. R., Millard, R. W., McRitchie, R. J., Maroko, P. R., and Vatner, S. F. (1975). Regional myocardial function and electrophysiological alterations after brief coronary artery occlusion in conscious dogs. *J. Clin. Invest. 56*: 978.

Kloner, R. A., and Przyklenk, K. (1990). Recent advances in stunned myocardium. *Cardiovasc. Rev. Rep. 11*: 68.

Przyklenk, K., and Kloner, R. A. (1986). Superoxide dismutase plus catalase improve contractile function in the canine model of the "stunned myocardium." *Circ. Res. 58*: 148.

Contents

Contributors

John W. Allen, M.D. Clinical Associate Professor of Medicine, Department of Internal Medicine, Hospital of the Good Samaritan, and University of Southern California, Los Angeles, California

Atsushi Aoki, M.D. Cardiovascular Surgery Fellow, Heart Institute, Hospital of the Good Samaritan, Los Angeles, California

Carl S. Apstein, M.D. Professor of Medicine and Director, Cardiac Muscle Research Laboratory, Boston University School of Medicine, and Chief of Cardiology, Department of Cardiology, Boston City Hospital, Boston, Massachusetts

Robert J. Bache, M.D. Professor of Medicine, Departments of Cardiology and Internal Medicine, University of Minnesota, Minneapolis, Minnesota

Lewis C. Becker, M.D. Professor of Medicine, Division of Cardiology, Department of Medicine, Johns Hopkins University School of Medicine, Baltimore, Maryland

Roberto Bolli, M.D. Associate Professor of Medicine and Director, Experimental Animal Laboratory, Section of Cardiology, Department of Medicine, Baylor College of Medicine, Houston, Texas

Eugene Braunwald, M.D. Hersey Professor of the Theory and Practice of Medicine, Harvard Medical School, and Chairman, Department of Medicine, Brigham and Women's Hospital, Boston, Massachusetts

Denis B. Buxton, M.D. Associate Professor, Department of Radiological Sciences, UCLA School of Medicine, Los Angeles, California

Calvin Eng, M.D. Associate Professor of Medicine, Physiology, and Biophysics, Division of Cardiology, Departments of Medicine, Physiology, and Biophysics, Albert Einstein College of Medicine, Bronx, New York

Stephen M. Factor, M.D. Professor of Pathology and Medicine, Departments of Pathology and Medicine, Albert Einstein College of Medicine, Bronx, New York

Neil E. Farber, M.D., Ph.D. Adjunct Assistant Professor, Departments of Pharmacology, Toxicology, and Anesthesiology, Medical College of Wisconsin, Milwaukee, Wisconsin

Timothy J. Gardner, M.D. Professor of Surgery, Department of Cardiac Surgery, Johns Hopkins University School of Medicine, Baltimore, Maryland

Garrett J. Gross, Ph.D. Professor of Pharmacology and Toxicology, Departments of Pharmacology and Toxicology, Medical College of Wisconsin, Milwaukee, Wisconsin

Guy R. Heyndrickx, M.D., Ph.D. Associate Director, Cardiovascular Center, O.L.V. Ziekenhuis, Aalst, Belgium, and the Department of Physiology, University of Gent, Gent, Belgium

David C. Homans, M.D. Associate Professor of Medicine, Department of Internal Medicine, University of Minnesota, Minneapolis, Minnesota

Robert B. Jennings, M.D. James B. Duke Professor of Pathology, Department of Pathology, Duke University Medical Center, Durham, North Carolina

Gregory Louis Kay, M.D. Attending Cardiothoracic Surgeon, Heart Institute, Hospital of the Good Samaritan, Los Angeles, California

Robert A. Kloner, M.D., Ph.D. Director of Research, Heart Institute, Hospital of the Good Samaritan, and Professor of Medicine, Section of Cardiology, University of Southern California, Los Angeles, California

Hideo Kusuoka, M.D., Ph.D.* Assistant Professor of Medicine, Division of Cardiology, Department of Medicine, Johns Hopkins University School of Medicine, Baltimore, Maryland

Eduardo Marban, M.D., Ph.D. Professor of Medicine, Division of Cardiology, Department of Medicine, Johns Hopkins University School of Medicine, Baltimore, Maryland

Edward S. Murphy, M.D. Professor of Medicine, Division of Cardiology, Department of Medicine, Oregon Health Sciences University, and Veterans Administration Hospital, Portland, Oregon

Winifred G. Nayler, M.Sc., D.Sc. Department of Medicine, Austin Hospital, University of Melbourne, Heidelberg, Victoria, Australia

Curtis Anthony Prejean, Jr., M.D. Cardiothoracic Surgeon, Heart Institute, Hospital of the Good Samaritan, Los Angeles, California

Karin Przyklenk, Ph.D. Assistant Director of Research and Director of Cardiac Function, Heart Institute, Hospital of the Good Samaritan, and Associate Professor of Research Medicine, Department of Medicine, University of Southern California, Los Angeles, California

Keith A. Reimer, M.D., Ph.D. Professor of Pathology and Head of Cardiovascular Pathology, Department of Pathology, Duke University Medical Center, Durham, North Carolina

Heinrich R. Schelbert, M.D. Professor of Radiological Science and Chief, Cardiovascular Nuclear Medicine Section, Division of Nuclear Medicine and Biophysics, Department of Radiological Sciences, and the Laboratory of Nuclear Medicine, UCLA School of Medicine, Los Angeles, California

Patrick W. Serruys, M.D., Ph.D. Professor of Interventional Cardiology, Department of Cardiology, Erasmus University, Rotterdam, The Netherlands

Stephen F. Vatner, M.D. Professor of Medicine, Department of Medicine, Harvard Medical School, Boston, Massachusetts, and Chairman, Cardiovascular Medicine, New England Regional Primate Research Center, Southborough, Massachusetts

Peter Whittaker, Ph.D. Director of Microscopy, Heart Institute, Hospital of the Good Samaritan, and Assistant Professor of Research Medicine, Department of Medicine, University of Southern California, Los Angeles, California

---

**Current affiliation*: Biomedical Research Center, Osaka University, Osaka, Japan

William Wijns, M.D. Associate Professor of Medicine, Division of Cardiology, University of Louvain Medical School, Brussels, Belgium

Ian C. Wilson, M.B., Ch.B. Research Fellow, Division of Cardiac Surgery, Johns Hopkins University School of Medicine, Baltimore, Maryland

Mengjia Zhao, M.D., Ph.D. Assistant Professor, Division of Cardiology, Departments of Medicine, Physiology, and Biophysics, Albert Einstein College of Medicine, Bronx, New York

Stevan D. Zimmer, M.D. Assistant Professor, Cardiovascular Division, Department of Medicine, University of Minnesota, Minneapolis, Minnesota

Pablo Zubiate, M.D. Cardiothoracic Surgeon, Heart Institute, Hospital of the Good Samaritan, Los Angeles, California

Stunned Myocardium

Part I

What Is Stunned Myocardium?

The following section reviews the definition and characteristics of the stunned myocardium as it was first defined in experimental animal studies. In Chapter 1, Drs. Heyndrickx and Vatner describe their seminal findings of postischemic dysfunction in canine myocardium subjected to a brief episode of ischemia followed by reperfusion. Chapter 2 reviews several of the early experimental studies demonstrating that stunning occurs not only following brief periods of ischemia and reperfusion, but also in models of prolonged coronary occlusion (resulting in necrosis) followed by reflow. In addition to the depression in systolic function that has been the hallmark of the stunned myocardium, associated abnormalities in diastolic relaxation, high energy phosphate metabolism, ultrastructure, and microvascular vasodilator reserve are also described. Drs. Zimmer and Bache discuss in Chapter 3 various metabolic correlates of stunned myocardium including the status of myocardial oxygen consumption and carbon substrate metabolism of the stunned, postischemic tissue.

Chapters 4 through 6 focus on experimental models of stunned myocardium other than the classic in vivo model of a single coronary artery occlusion followed by reperfusion. Drs. Zhao, Factor, and Eng review in Chapter 4 the effects of repeated coronary occlusions on postischemic function and cardiac morphology. In Chapter 5, Dr. Homans describes stunned myocardium in models of exercise in the setting of partial coronary artery stenosis. Drs. Przyklenk and Apstein explore in Chapter 6 the phenomenon of stunning in isolated perfused heart preparations following episodes of hypoxia or ischemia. Finally, the section concludes with a chapter by Drs. Reimer and Jennings, who discuss whether they believe the phenomenon of stunned myocardium is a protective mechanism.

1

Stunned Myocardium

Historical Perspective

Guy R. Heyndrickx

Cardiovascular Center, O.L.V. Ziekenhuis, Aalst, Belgium, and University of Gent, Gent, Belgium

Stephen F. Vatner

Harvard Medical School, Boston, Massachusetts, and the New England Regional Primate Research Center, Southborough, Massachusetts

I. INTRODUCTION

In 1973 we studied the effects of brief periods of myocardial ischemia followed by prolonged reperfusion in a conscious animal model. The results of this study, published in 1975, described for the first time an unexpected observation of severely depressed regional myocardial function, occurring subsequent to a short episode of ischemia of less than 20 minutes duration, in spite of normal perfusion and absence of cell necrosis (Heyndrickx et al., 1975, 1978). At that time the extent to which this observation was to stimulate future experimental and clinical research could not have been predicted. However, the last 10 years have witnessed an explosive growth of research effort both experimentally as well as clinically in order to learn more about this phenomenon and to assess its full impact in clinical practice. Widespread attention to this observation was catalyzed by the editorial in *Circulation* in which Braunwald and Kloner (1982) proposed naming this state of postischemic left ventricular dysfunction "stunned myocardium." With the subsequent introduction of thrombolytic therapy for the treatment of acute myocardial infarction, a clinical corollary of postischemic myocardial dysfunction was soon appreciated, and the term stunned myocardium was added permanently to our medical jargon.

II. BACKGROUND

At the time that a research fellowship was established at the Harvard Medical School in 1973, a great deal of cardiological research was focused on the concept of infarct size limitation. The hypothesis that the extent of infarction could be modulated during the evolution of the ischemic process stimulated the search for noninvasive clinical tools to accurately quantify the extension of the infarct area. A widely used experimental model at that time was the recording of ST segment elevation from multiple epicardial electrodes in open chest anesthetized animals and from serial precordial ECG mapping in patients. ST-segment elevation during the initial phase of acute myocardial infarction was correlated with several parameters related to infarct size, such as depletion in myocardial creatine-kinase and pathological evidence of tissue necrosis. ECG mapping has been extensively used to evaluate a large number of hemodynamic and pharmacological interventions aimed at reducing infarct size, both in the animal laboratory and in the clinical setting (Maroko et al., 1971). These experiments were most frequently carried out in open chest anesthetized dogs. The latter experimental model is limited due to the surgical manipulation, the artificial ventilation, and the myocardial depressant effects of the anesthesia, which not only exert direct effects on the coronary circulation and the myocardium, but also induce instability in baseline conditions. It is therefore not surprising that small hemodynamic variations and subtle ECG changes could be blurred by spontaneous alterations induced by this less than optimal experimental model.

In the research environment at Harvard Medical School, the author was introduced to a different field of cardiovascular experimentation being developed under the leadership of the coauthor, i.e., the study of cardiovascular dynamics in conscious animals, chronically instrumented with miniaturized transducers, allowing simultaneous and continuous measurements of indices of overall and regional left ventricular function, myocardial blood flow, and pressures. The study of regional ventricular function by means of online measurements of segment length and wall thickness was made possible by adapting the ultrasonic electronic circuitry for short distance measurements, and by miniaturizing the ultrasonic piezoelectric crystals so that the embedding in the free wall of the left ventricle would cause minimal constraint and damage (Bugge-Asperheim, 1969; Theroux et al., 1974). One of our primary goals at that time was to extend these techniques to the conscious animal (Heyndrickx et al., 1975, 1978; Patrick and Vatner, 1984). Using these techniques, multiple pairs of crystals are implanted in different zones of the left ventricle and are interrogated simultaneously to provide regional measurements of ventricular dimensions (Fig. 1). It was clear that such a chronically instrumented conscious animal model could yield exciting new perspectives for repeated measurements of regional left ventricular function, particularly since recording on sequential days in the baseline situation yielded almost identical hemodynamic measurements. We felt that this model would allow us to make another step forward in the integrated analysis of cardiovascular dynamics by combining the information of regional mechanical function with the information of regional blood flow measured with radioactive micropheres and the intramyocardial electrophysiological activity.

The extension of these instrumentation techniques to conscious animals or to experiments necessitating unrestrained animals (such as during exercise) made the development of telemetry systems for the transmission of data from the animal to the recording station mandatory (Patrick et al., 1974). In addition, such a chronic animal model would be ideal to compare, in the same animal, the results of several therapeutic interventions aimed at modulating the effect of short-term myocardial ischemia.

III. INITIAL OBSERVATIONS

Taking advantage of this new technology, we designed experiments to assess the acute effects of a short episode of myocardial ischemia induced by coronary artery occlusion followed by reperfusion on regional left ventricular function integrated with measurements of regional myocardial blood flow and electrograms. The time course of the ischemic result was arbitrarily set to less than 20 minutes duration based on the fundamental observation made by Jennings et al. in 1960 that this ischemic burden did not result in irreversible and permanent cellular damage (Jennings et al., 1969). From these experiments several conclusions were drawn.

A. Effects of Coronary Artery Occlusion

These experiments clearly demonstrated that segmental contraction expressed as segment length shortening and wall thickening in the ischemic area ceased almost immediately upon occlusion of the coronary artery and displayed a paradoxical motion in a matter of 30 seconds, confirming what Tennant and Wiggers (1935) had shown years ago, i.e., that mechanical function is highly sensitive to O_2 deprivation. In contrast, changes in the intramyocardial ECG, recorded at the same sites where regional function was measured, were considerably slower in onset (Fig. 2).

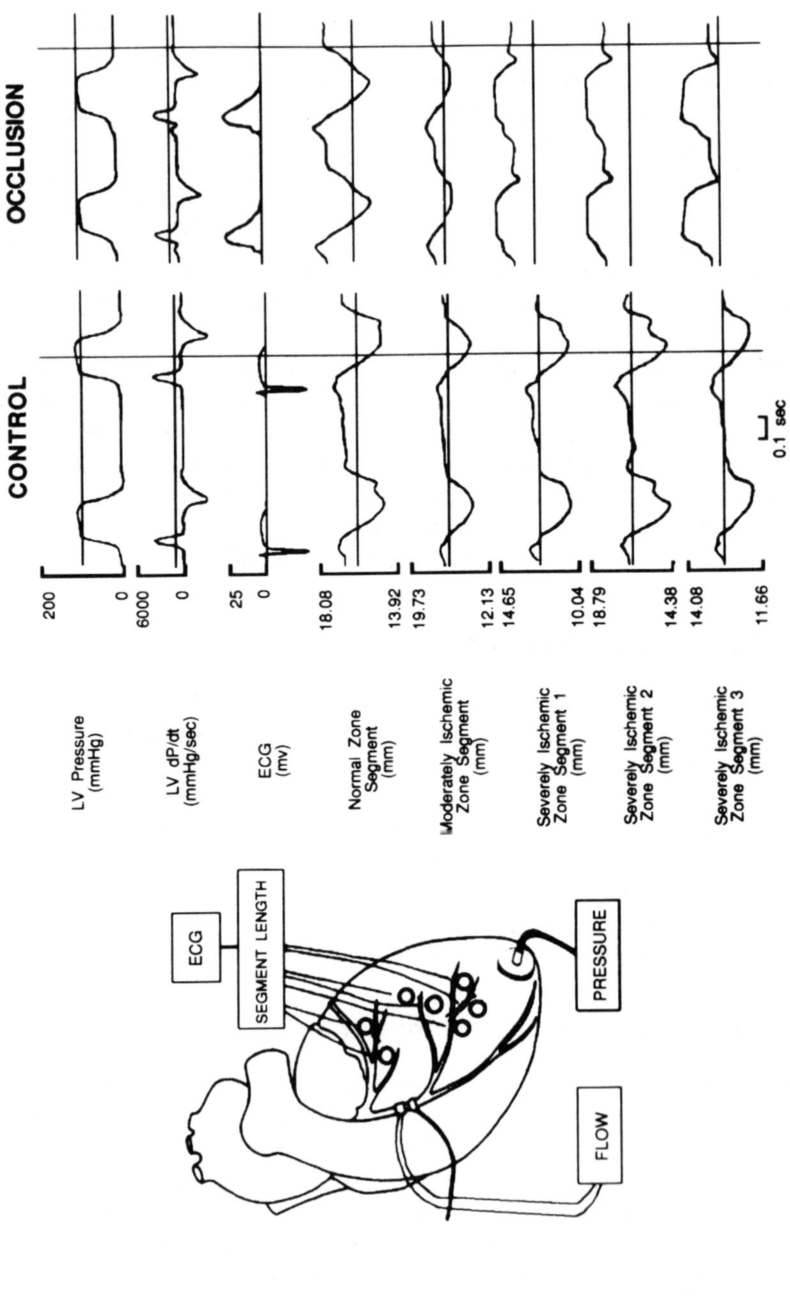
CONTROL
OCCLUSION
0.1 sec
LV Pressure (mmHg)
200
0
LV dP/dt (mmHg/sec)
6000
0
ECG (mv)
25
0
Normal Zone Segment (mm)
18.08
13.92
Moderately Ischemic Zone Segment (mm)
19.73
12.13
Severely Ischemic Zone Segment 1 (mm)
14.65
10.04
Severely Ischemic Zone Segment 2 (mm)
18.79
14.38
Severely Ischemic Zone Segment 3 (mm)
14.08
11.66
ECG
SEGMENT LENGTH
PRESSURE
FLOW

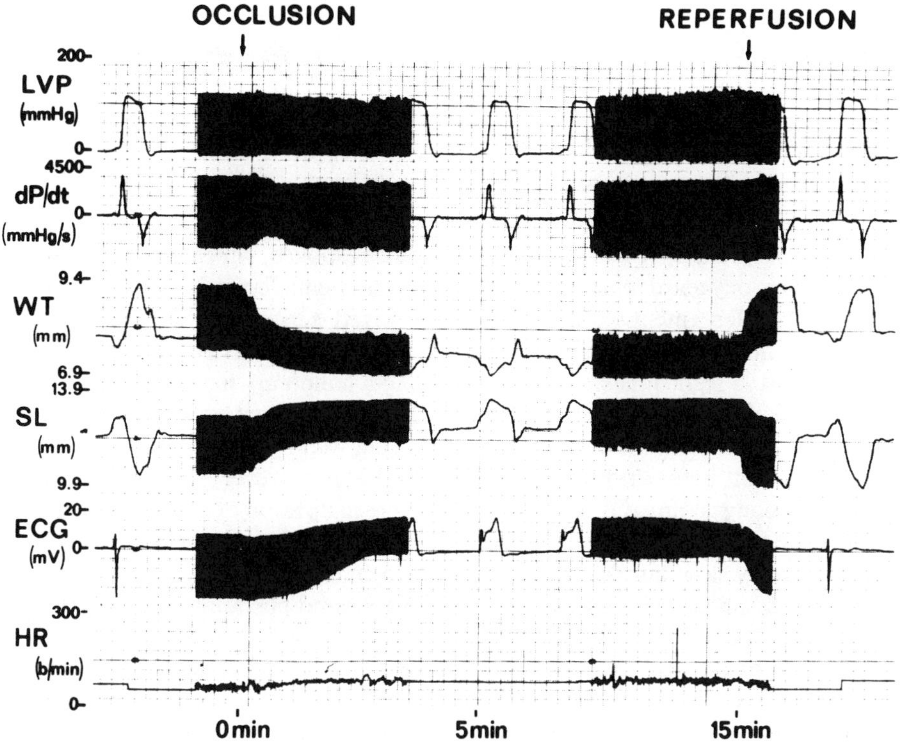

Figure 2 A continuous tracing of effects of coronary occlusion and reperfusion on simultaneous measurements of left ventricular pressure (LVP) and dP/dt, wall thickness (WT), segment-length (SL) shortening, and electrogram (ECG) in the ischemic zone and heart rate (HR) in a conscious dog. Phasic waveforms at rapid paper speed are shown during control, occlusion, and immediately after reperfusion. Note prolonged wall thickening and segment shortening that occurred after reperfusion. (Reproduced from Heyndrickx et al. (1978) by permission of the authors and the American Physiology Society.)

Figure 1 Techniques for measuring regional myocardial function, flow, and electrograms in conscious dogs with regional myocardial ischemia. A miniature pressure gauge is implanted in the left ventricle to measure pressure and dP/dt. A coronary flow probe and hydraulic occluder are implanted on the coronary artery to occlude the vessel and to confirm the occlusion. Multiple pairs of miniature piezoelectric crystals are implanted in the potentially ischemic zone and normal zone to measure regional segment length shortening and electrograms from the same transducers. The panels at the right show typical phasic waveforms prior to occlusion (left panel) and then after coronary occlusion (right panel). Note that coronary occlusion induced only mild changes in left ventricular pressure and dP/dt, but caused striking ST-segment elevation and reversal of normal systolic shortening to paradoxical bulging in the severely ischemic zones. (Reproduced from Vatner and Baig (1979) by permission of the authors and the Transactions of Association of American Physicians.)

B. Effects of Reperfusion

1. Reactive Hyperemic Phase

Upon reperfusion, coronary flow (measured with a Doppler flow transducer) displayed the typical reactive hyperemic response, which more than repayed the oxygen debt incurred during the ischemic episode. At the same time, the ST-segment elevation, which occurred during coronary artery occlusion, normalized rapidly. The reactive hyperemia was accompanied by a rebound in segmental shortening displaying a temporary increase in regional function above baseline conditions (Fig. 2). As in many other circulatory systems, short-term disturbances are often followed by a temporary rebound phenomenon before normalization. In this case, however, the initial overshoot in contractility did not presage rapid normalization of segmental shortening but, in contrast, was replaced by a depression in regional function, followed by slow but full recovery of segment shortening.

Several conceivable mechanisms for this rebound phenomenon have been considered: (1) major determinants of myocardial performance (such as preload, afterload, and heart rate) were unchanged at the time of hypercontractility and could therefore not be held responsible for this phenomenon; (2) reflexly increased beta-adrenergic stimulation, although present, did not influence this phenomenon since the overshoot was still present after beta receptor blockade; and (3) only the prevention of the reactive hyperemic response, by restricting coronary perfusion at the time of reperfusion to the preocclusion levels, was able to completely prevent the overshoot, pointing towards a "garden-hose effect" as a potential mechanism for this rebound reaction (Pagani et al., 1978).

2. Delayed Functional Recovery

In contrast to the rapid normalization of intramyocardial ECG, regional segment length and wall thickening did not return immediately to preocclusion levels but remained depressed for many hours. For example, a 15-minute coronary artery occlusion resulted in more than 12 hours of postischemic dysfunction. This prolonged depression in LV function was an unexpected finding and evolved into the description of a new and what would later appear to be an important pathophysiological condition, i.e., the sustained postischemic regional LV dysfunction subsequent to a temporary ischemic injury (Figs. 3,4).

This condition of temporary prolonged contractile dysfunction differs in many ways from the more common condition of ischemic contractile dysfunction. Three essential features were characteristic of stunned myocardium: (1) the absence of necrosis during a relatively short episode of intense myocardial ischemia, (2) presence of full reperfusion without evidence of

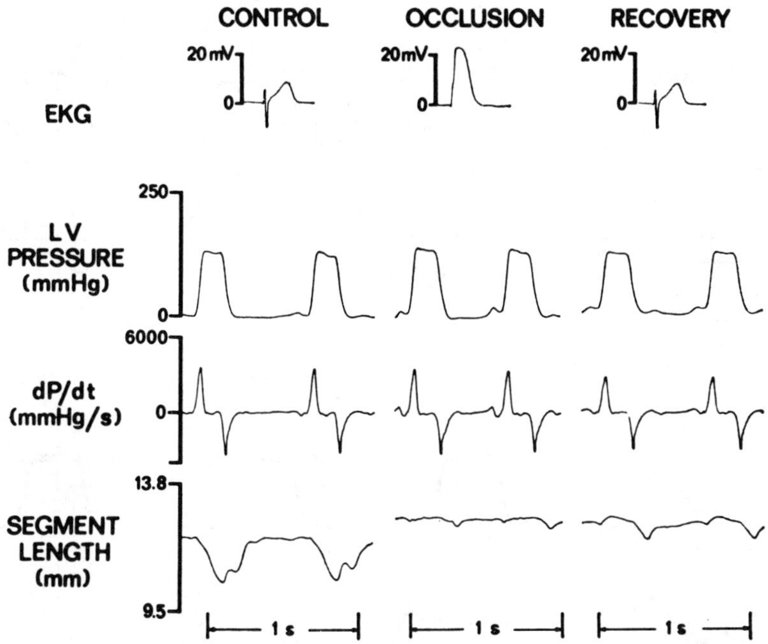

Figure 3 Effects of a 5-minute left circumflex coronary occlusion on LV pressure, dP/dt, and segment length in the ischemic zone along with the electrogram from the ischemic zone (top). During coronary occlusion (middle panel) intense ischemia reflected by substantial ST-segment elevation correlates well with impaired function in the ischemic zone. Five minutes after release of occlusion, reperfusion, and repayment of coronary flow debt (right panel), the electrogram is again completely normal, but regional function is still markedly deranged, i.e., the ischemic segment is expanding paradoxically during systole. (Reproduced from Heyndrickx et al. (1975) by permission of the authors and the *Journal of Clinical Investigation*.)

residual chronic ischemia, and (3) documentation of eventual complete functional recovery (Table 1). It is important to realize that this last point of the definition is often absent in many experiments performed in acute and/or isolated preparations, where the ultimate functional recovery is not always documented.

IV. SUBSEQUENT STUDIES

Confirmation of our findings was reported soon after the *publicatio princeps*. Stunned myocardium was observed in different types and modalities of myocardial ischemia/reperfusion, in different experimental models, in

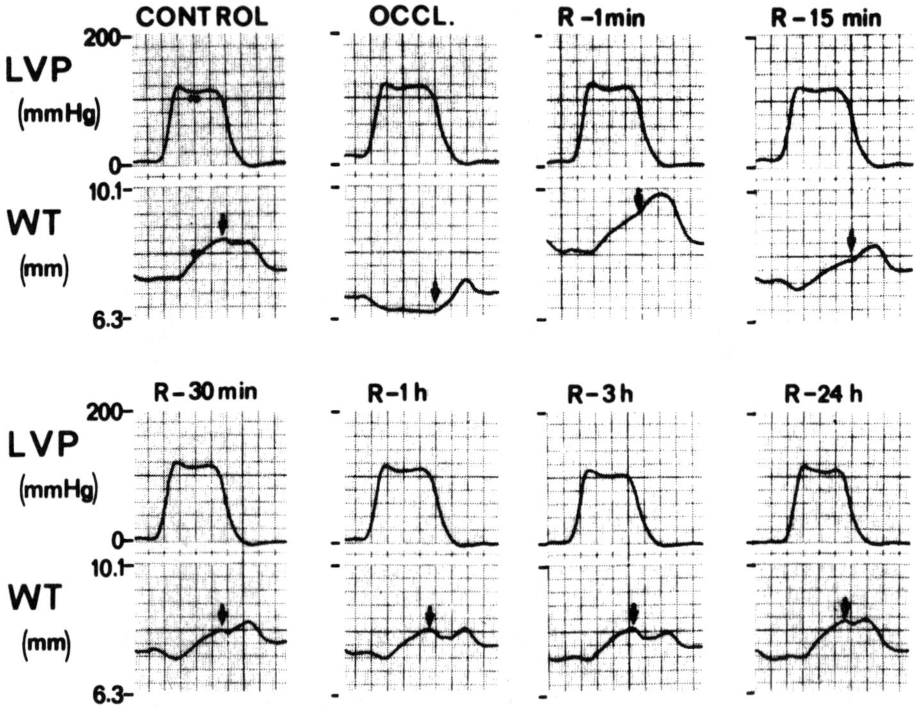

Figure 4 Tracings of left ventricular pressure (LVP) and wall thickness (WT) during control, during a 15-minute coronary occlusion, and at 1 minute, 15 minutes, 30 minutes, 1 hour, 3 hours, and 24 hours after reperfusion. Arrows denote end-systole. Peak systolic wall thickening was absent during occlusion, significantly prolonged early during reperfusion, and significantly diminished up to the 24-hour recording. Complete return to normal for the wall-thickness phasic waveform indicates the stability of the measurement and that no permanent damage had occurred. (Reproduced from Heyndrickx et al. (1978) by permission of the authors and the American Physiology Society.)

Table 1 Definition of Stunned Myocardium

Postischemic LV dysfunction with:
normal myocardial perfusion
preserved contractile reserve
enzyme release
delayed but full recovery of function

different species, as well as in isolated hearts. Multiple short (2-10 minutes) episodes of coronary artery occlusion (Nicklas et al., 1985), coronary stenosis with less intense ischemia but over a prolonged period (several hours) (Matsuzaki et al., 1988), stress-induced ischemia in normal myocardium subtended by a coronary stenosis (Homans et al., 1986) as well as in hypertrophied myocardium with normal coronary arteries (Hittinger et al., 1990) have all shown different expression of myocardial stunning. In addition, peri-infarcted tissue, which recovers after either permanent coronary artery occlusion or following coronary artery reperfusion, exhibits prolonged dysfunction, gradually disappearing over a period of weeks (Lavallee et al., 1983; Heyndrickx et al., 1985a). All of these conditions have in common the occurrence of an episode of myocardial ischemia, either severe and of short duration or less severe but more prolonged. The ischemia can be global, transmural, in one region, or even selective to the subendocardium followed by full reperfusion and without evidence of permanent cellular injury. The degree of severity of stunning, however, may vary considerably. For example, an identical period of ischemia induced by brief coronary artery occlusion in an acute open chest animal will produce a much greater degree of myocardial stunning than observed in the conscious animal, indicating that factors other than ischemia per se, i.e., the baseline level of myocardial contractility prior to the ischemic insult, may amplify this phenomenon. It is also of interest to note that brief episodes of ischemia not long enough to result in myocardial necrosis may be associated with a significant increase in plasma CK as well as in CK-MB. This suggests that creatine kinase release is not necessarily a hallmark for cell death, but may indicate that severe ischemia reversibly alters cell membrane permeability sufficiently to lose all cell constituents with a molecular weight up to 80,000 (Heyndrickx et al., 1985b).

Another matter of debate concerns the myocardial oxygen consumption of stunned myocardium. One would anticipate that, with decreased regional contractility, a major determinant of oxygen consumption, stunned myocardium will be associated with a decreased myocardial oxygen consumption. Although reduced oxygen consumption in stunned myocardium was documented by several groups using both the Fick principle and positron emission tomography techniques, (Schaper et al., 1990; Armbrecht et al., 1990) others have found either no reduction or even an increase in oxygen consumption in this situation (Laxon et al., 1989). Part of this discrepancy can be explained by the fact that in certain conditions oxygen wasting may occur as a result of paradoxically high oxygen consumption in severely dysfunctioning segments subjected to passive stretch. Additional studies will be needed to further elucidate the oxidative metabolism of stunned myocardium.

V. NEW CONCEPTS REGARDING THE INTRINSIC ADAPTATION OF ISCHEMIC MYOCARDIUM

Not only have our initial studies on postischemic myocardial dysfunction fostered further research directed at elucidating the underlying pathophysiological mechanisms of stunned myocardium, but other concepts have evolved to explain the paradox that repetitive episodes of ischemia do not uniformly result in cumulative injury leading unequivocally towards cell death. Swain et al. (1984), have shown the absence of cumulative injury in a model of repetitive short episodes of myocardial ischemia, suggesting that cardiac myocytes seem to adapt and tolerate a second ischemic period better than the first. In this respect a possible link between stunned myocardium and hibernating myocardium has recently been suggested (Rahimtoola 1989; Schaper 1991). Could it be possible that cardiac cells have the inborn faculty to achieve a state of endogenous downregulation of its contractile function as well as its metabolic system in response to an ischemic insult? This concept was advanced further when Reimer et al. (1986) and Murry et al. (1986) discovered that short episodes of myocardial ischemia had a marked protective effect against a subsequent more severe ischemic insult. This phenomenon was termed "preconditioning." Thus, an episode of myocardial stunning can be responsible for much more than simply prolonged postischemic dysfunction. Conceivably those biochemical pathways altered during stunning could play a role in mediating preconditioning.

VI. CLINICAL IMPLICATIONS

With the advent of thrombolytic therapy and interventional cardiology in patients with acute myocardial infarction, a clinical correlate for the experimental model of coronary artery occlusion and reperfusion was introduced in clinical practice. As described in detail in Part IV of this book, several studies have shown that upon successful reperfusion regional function in the infarct related territory did improve gradually with time comparable to the time frame observed in the experimental model (Reduto et al., 1981). Similar findings of regional dysfunction in the absence of myocardial infarction displaying slow normalization occur in patients with unstable angina as well as in patients with exercise-induced ischemia (Nixon et al., 1982). The finding that akinetic segments could potentially recover depending on the pathophysiological substrate adds a new diagnostic and therapeutic challenge in clinical practice. The search for signs of viable myocardium in dyskinetic areas is particularly important in light of guiding therapeutic decisions.

VII. SUMMARY

The observation of a state of prolonged depressed regional function during the reperfusion phase following myocardial ischemia of short duration aroused considerable interest when thrombolytic therapy and interventional cardiology was introduced in clinical practice for the treatment of acute myocardial infarction. Stunned myocardium after reperfusion has become a clinical diagnostic and therapeutic challenge. This observation has also led to further investigations, which have illuminated some of the adaptive changes of the myocardium to ischemia, and led to provocative concepts of a possible downregulation of myocardial performance. Further research at the molecular level will eventually reveal the fundamental mechanisms whereby survival of cardiac cells requires adaptation to the most common clinical disorder, i.e., transient ischemia.

ACKNOWLEDGMENT

This work was supported in part by U.S. Public Health Service grants HL-38070 and HL-33065.

REFERENCES

Armbrecht, J. J., Buxton, B. B., and Schelbert, H. R. (1990). Validation of [1-C-11] acetate as a tracer for noninvasive assessment of oxidative metabolism with Positron Emission Tomography in normal, ischemic, postischemic and hyperemic canine myocardium. *Circulation 81*: 1594.

Braunwald, E., and Kloner, R. A. (1982). The stunned myocardium: Prolonged, postischemic ventricular dysfunction. *Circulation 66*: 1146.

Bugge-Asperheim, B., Leraand, S., and Kiil, F. (1969). Local dimensional changes of the myocardium measured by ultrasonic technique. *Scand. J. Clin. Lab. Invest. 24*: 361.

Heyndrickx, G. R., Millard, R. W., McRitchie, R. J., Maroko, P. R., and Vatner, S. F. (1975). Regional myocardial functional and electrophysiological alterations after brief coronary artery occlusion in conscious dogs. *J. Clin. Invest. 56*: 978.

Heyndrickx, G. R., Baig, H., Nellens, P., Leusen, I., Fishbein, M. C., and Vatner, S. F. (1978). Depression of regional blood flow and wall thickening after brief coronary occlusions. *Am. J. Physiol. 234*: H653.

Heyndrickx, G. R., Amano, J., Patrick, T. A., Manders, W. T., Rogers, G. G., Rosendorff, C., and Vatner, S. F. (1985a). Effects of coronary artery reperfusion on regional blood flow and function in conscious baboons. *Circulation 71*: 1029.

Heyndrickx, G. R., Amano J., Kenna, T., Fallon, J. T., Patrick, T. A., Manders, T. W., Rogers, G. G., Rosendorff, C., and Vatner, S. F. (1985b). Creatine kinase release not associated with myocardial necrosis after short periods of coronary artery occlusion in conscious baboons. *J. Am. Coll Cardiol. 6*: 1299.

Hittinger, L., Shannon, R. P., Kohin S., Manders, W. T., Kelly P., and Vatner, S. F. (1990). Exercise induced subendocardial dysfunction in dogs with left ventricular hypertrophy. *Circ. Res. 46*: 329.

Homans, D. C., Sublett E., Dai, X. Z., and Bache, R. J. (1986). Persistence of regional left ventricular dysfunction after exercise-induced myocardial ischemia. *J. Clin. Invest. 77*: 66.

Jennings, R. B., Sommers, H. M., Herdson, P. B., and Kaltenbach, J. P. (1969). Ischemic injury of myocardium. *Ann. N.Y. Acad. Sci. 156*: 61.

Lavallee, M., Cox, D., Patrick, T. A., and Vatner, S. F. (1983). Salvage of myocardial function by coronary artery reperfusion 1, 2 and 3 hours after occlusion in conscious dogs. *Circ. Res. 53*: 235.

Laxon, D. D., Homans, D. C., Dai, X., Sublett, E., and Bache, R. J. (1989). Oxygen consumption and coronary reactivity in postischemic myocardium. *Circ. Res. 64*: 9.

Maroko, P. R., Kjekhus, J. K., Sobel, B. E., Watanabe, T., Covell, J. W., Ross, J., Jr., and Braunwald, E. (1971). Factors influencing infarct size following coronary artery occlusion. *Circulation 43*: 67.

Matsuzaki, M., Gallagher, K. P., Kemper, W. S., White, F., and Ross, J., Jr. (1983). Sustained regional dysfunction produced by prolonged coronary stenosis: Gradual recovery after reperfusion. *Circulation 68*: 170.

Murry, C. E., Jennings, R. B., and Reimer, K. A. (1986). A delay of lethal cell injury in ischemic myocardium. *Circulation 74*: 1124.

Nicklas, J. M., Becker, L. C., and Bulkley, B. H. (1985). Effects of repeated brief coronary occlusion on regional left ventricular function and dimension in dogs. *Am. J. Cardiol. 56*: 473.

Nixon, J. V., Brown, C. N., and Smitherman, T. C. (1982). Identification of transient and persistent segmental wall motion abnormalities in patients with unstable angina by two-dimensional echocardiography. *Circulation 65*: 1497.

Pagani, M., Vatner, S. F., Baig, H., and Braunwald, E. (1978). Initial myocardial adjustments to brief periods of ischemia and reperfusion in the conscious dogs. *Circ. Res. 43*: 83.

Patrick, T. A., and Vatner, S. F. (1984). Instrumentation techniques for cardiovascular research in conscious dogs. In *Physiology,* Vol. II, Elsevier Scientific Publishers, County Clare, Ireland Ltd.

Patrick, T. A., Vatner, S. F., Kemper, W. S., and Franklin, D. (1974). Telemetry of left ventricular diameter and pressure measurements from unrestrained animals. *J. Appl. Physiol. 37*: 276.

Rahimtoola, S. H. (1989). The hibernating myocardium. *Am. Heart J. 117*: 211.

Reduto, L. A., Freund, G. C., Gaeta, J. M., Smalling, R. W., Lewis, B., and Gould, K. L. (1981). Coronary artery reperfusion in acute myocardial infarction: Beneficial effects of intracoronary streptokinase on left ventricular salvage and performance. *Am. Heart J. 102*: 1168.

Reimer, K. A., Murry, C. E., Yamasawa, I., and Jennings, R. B. (1986). Four brief periods of myocardial ischemia cause no cumulative ATP loss or necrosis. *Am. J. Physiol. 251*: H1306.

Schaper, W., Schott, R. J., and Kobayashi M. (1990). Reperfused myocardium: stunning, preconditioning and reperfusion injury. In *Pathophysiology and Rational Pharmaco-therapy of Myocardial Ischemia* (G. Heusch, ed.), Verlag, Darmstadt, p. 175.

Schaper, W. (1991). Molecular Mechanisms in "Stunned" Myocardium. *Cardiovasc. Drugs Ther. 5*: 925.

Swain, J. L., Sabina, R. L., Hines, J. J., Greenfield, J. C. Jr., and Holmes, E. W. (1984). Repetitive episodes of brief ischaemia (12 min) do not produce a cumulative depletion of high energy phosphate compounds. *Cardiovas Res. 18*: 264.

Tennant, R., and Wiggers, C. J. (1935). The effect of coronary occlusion on myocardial contraction. *Am. J. Physiol. 112*: 351.

Theroux, P., Franklin, D., Ross, J., Jr., and Kemper, W. S. (1974). Regional myocardial function during acute coronary artery occlusion and its modification by pharmacologic agents in the dog. *Circ. Res. 35*: 896.

Vatner, S. F., and Baig, H. (1979). The effects of inotropic stimulation on ischemic myocardium in conscious dogs. *Trans. Assoc. Am. Phys. 91*: 282.

2

First Evidence

Postischemic Dysfunction of Viable Myocardium

Robert A. Kloner and Karin Przyklenk

Hospital of the Good Samaritan and University of Southern California, Los Angeles, California

I. INTRODUCTION

The primary objective of this chapter is to describe the fundamental properties of stunned myocardium that have been observed in experimental models of coronary artery occlusion followed by reperfusion. Specifically, we review the characteristic abnormalities in both systolic contraction and diastolic relaxation that have become the hallmark of stunned myocardium, and discuss the factors that determine or predict the severity of postischemic dysfunction. Associated abnormalities in cardiac ultrastructure, high energy phosphate metabolism, electrophysiological properties, and coronary vasculature are also reviewed. Finally, we compare and contrast the characteristics of the stunned myocardium to the concept of hibernating myocardium in an effort to resolve the confusion surrounding these two very different phenomena.

II. CHARACTERISTICS OF STUNNED MYOCARDIUM

A. Postischemic Dysfunction Following Brief Ischemia

1. Systolic Dysfunction

In the mid-1970s, Heyndrickx and collegues (1975, 1985) published two seminal papers which provided the scientific community with the earliest descriptions of what later would be called stunned myocardium. In their initial study (Heyndrickx et al., 1975), conscious dogs were instrumented with left ventricular (LV) pressure transducers and pairs of miniature ultrasonic segment length transducers in order to assess global and regional contractile function. The animals then underwent either 5 or 15 minutes of left anterior descending or circumflex coronary occlusion followed by up to 24 hours of reperfusion. Regional electrocardiograms as well as coronary flow were also measured.

Global indices of systolic left ventricular function (LV pressure and its first derivative, dP/dt) did not change significantly during coronary occlusion or following reperfusion. In contrast, these investigators did observe profound changes in *regional* contractile function. As expected, during occlusion there was an increase in both end-diastolic and end-systolic segment lengths, and there was zero stroke shortening within the myocardial segment supplied by the occluded coronary artery. Reperfusion did not, however, resolve these abnormalities in regional function. When blood flow was restored following a 5-minute coronary artery occlusion, regional function remained significantly depressed after 2 hours of reperfusion, but returned to normal by 6 hours of reperfusion. When the duration of transient ischemia was increased to 15 minutes, end-diastolic segment length remained elevated and velocity of shortening and end-systolic segment length remained depressed at 6 hours following reflow. Normal function was, however, restored when measured at 24 hours after reperfusion. Electrocardiographic abnormalities included ST segment elevation during coronary occlusion, which rapidly reversed upon reperfusion. Coronary blood flow, although elevated for the initial 7-10 minutes following reflow, also showed a rapid return to normal values.

These initial results of Heyndrickx et al. were confirmed in their second study (Heyndrickx et al., 1978) in which conscious dogs were subjected to a 15-minute coronary occlusion followed by 24 hours of reperfusion. In this second protocol, wall thickening was measured with ultrasonic crystals, and regional myocardial blood flow was assessed using radioactive microspheres. Not surprisingly, wall thickening was reduced to zero during coronary occlusion. Reperfusion was accompanied by an acute trend toward recovery of thickening, which corresponded temporally to the acute hyperemia following reflow, but systolic thickening then rapidly deteriorated and remained depressed for at least the initial 3 hours postreperfusion. This abnormality in wall motion proved, however, to be transient: wall thickening was restored to baseline values at 24 hours after reflow. Heyndrickx et al. further noted that this depressed contractile function of the previously ischemic tissue could not be explained by either persistent ischemia or irreversible myocyte injury. Only mild depressions in regional myocardial blood flow (11-20% of normal) were observed at 15-60 minutes postreperfusion. Furthermore, both macroscopic staining of tissue slices with triphenyltetrazolium chloride and evaluation of histological sections revealed no evidence of irreversible tissue damage.

We subsequently reported a series of studies (Kloner et al., 1983a) that compared return of regional contractile function in anesthetized dogs subjected to 1 minute, 5 minutes, 15 minutes, or 3 hours of coronary occlusion followed by reperfusion. In these studies, contractile function was assessed by sonomicrometry: ultrasonic crystals were placed in a circumferential fashion in the soon-to-be ischemic left anterior descending coronary artery bed to assess fractional systolic shortening, expressed as a percentage of end-diastolic myocardial segment length. During coronary artery occlusion, active shortening of the ischemic segments was replaced by passive systolic lengthening (paradoxical systolic bulging) and accompanied by a net increase in end-diastolic segment length. Upon reperfusion, end-diastolic length returned to normal. However, the recovery of systolic function after reperfusion was dependent upon the occlusion time. With a 1-minute period of transient ischemia, abnormalities in systolic function were rapidly resolved and, by 30 minutes of reperfusion, did not differ from control values. Five minutes of transient ischemia resulted in hypokinesis following reflow: at 30 minutes postreperfusion, systolic shortening averaged only 67% of baseline values, and remained depressed after 60 minutes of reperfusion. Postischemic dysfunction was further exacerbated as the duration of ischemia was increased. Reperfusion following a 15-minute or 3-hour occlusion was associated with persistent paradoxical systolic bulging. Thus, although we did not observe evidence of postischemic dysfunction following a 1-minute period of coronary occlusion, persistent abnormalities in systolic function were evident following episodes of ischemia ≥5 minutes in duration.

There is no doubt that, while the stunned myocardium is a transient phenomenon, the severity and duration of postischemic dysfunction increases with increasing duration of coronary occlusion. However, for a given ischemic insult (e.g., 15 minutes) there have been differences among various laboratories regarding the rate of return of systolic function. In the anesthetized canine preparation, Przyklenk and Kloner (1989a) observed persistent regional wall motion abnormalities by two-dimensional echocardiography for at least 30 hours following reperfusion (Fig. 1). Heyndrickx et al. (1975, 1978) reported restoration of normal function by 24 hours of reflow in the conscious canine model. These findings differ from those of a more recent study by Charlat et al. (1989) in a similar conscious model, in which 48 hours of reperfusion was necessary for postischemic dysfunction to resolve (Fig. 2). While the reason for these differences in duration of dysfunction is not known, one possibility may involve the differences in the techniques utilized

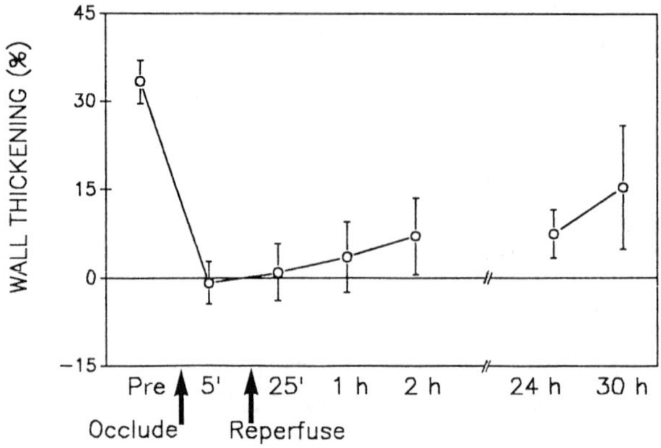

Figure 1 Mean values of regional wall thickening in the central ischemic zone (assessed by two-dimensional echocardiography) obtained from six anesthetized dogs that underwent 15 minutes of coronary artery occlusion and 30 hours of reperfusion. (Adapted from Przyklenk and Kloner, 1989a, and reprinted from Przyklenk and Kloner, 1989c.)

to measure regional wall motion (i.e., sonomicrometry vs. echocardiography vs. doppler ultrasound). In addition, it has been suggested that stunning may be less prominent in conscious versus anesthetized preparations. However, at least one laboratory has found no difference in recovery of function between the conscious and anesthetized canine models (Preuss et al., 1987).

2. Diastolic Dysfunction

While initial reports of stunned myocardium focused exclusively on the systolic abnormalities of the previously ischemic tissue, more recent studies have also described diastolic dysfunction following a brief episode of transient occlusion. For example, Przyklenk et al. (1987) analyzed data from nine anesthetized open chest dogs subjected to 15 minutes of coronary artery occlusion followed by 3 hours of reperfusion. Regional contractile function throughout the cardiac cycle was assessed by plotting global LV pressure versus segment length (i.e., separation between ultrasonic crystals), and diastolic relaxation time (a global index of LV diastolic function) was measured using the method of Weiss et al. (1976). We observed that, in myocardium stunned by a 15-minute period of ischemia, shortening of the previously ischemic segment continued into what should have been isovolumic diastole. Whether this postsystolic contraction is active or passive remains unknown, but, by continuing to contract during diastole, the stunned segment may have impaired ventricular filling. In addition, diastolic relaxation times were prolonged at approximately 125-150% of baseline values throughout the

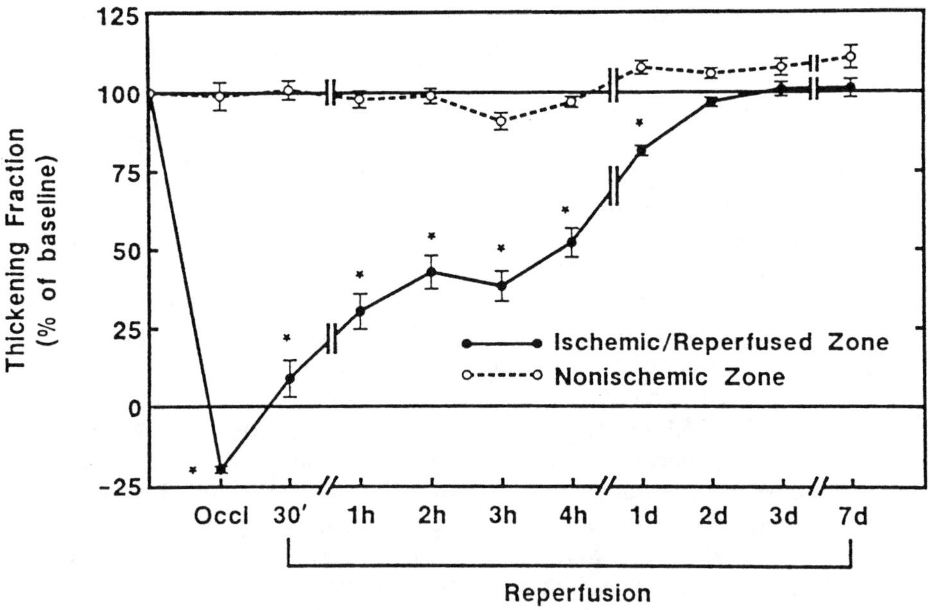

Figure 2 Changes in systolic thickening fraction during coronary occlusion (Occl) and at selected times after reperfusion in the nonischemic region and in the ischemic-reperfused region. Thickening fraction is expressed as percent of preocclusion (baseline) values. Data are mean values ± SEM ($n = 10$). Systolic function in the re reperfused myocardium recovered slowly; on the average, thickening fraction was still significantly depressed at 24 h and returned to baseline at 48 h after reflow. $^*p < 0.001$ versus baseline. (Reprinted from Charlat et al., 1989 with permission of the American College of Cardiology.)

initial 3 hours of reflow. More recently, Charlat et al. (1989) confirmed these findings in conscious dogs subjected to 15 minutes of transient ischemia. Specifically, they observed abnormalities in mean rate to achieve half end-diastolic thinning and late diastolic thinning fraction during the first 4 hours following reperfusion. This diastolic dysfunction was resolved, however, at 24 hours postreflow.

B. Evidence for Stunned Myocardium Following Prolonged but Transient Coronary Occlusion

Experimental canine studies have clearly shown that reperfusion within 1-3 hours after the onset of coronary occlusion can salvage ischemic tissue in the mid to outer left ventricular wall (Reimer et al., 1977; Reimer and Jennings, 1979; Przyklenk et al., 1986). That is, a 40-minute period of ischemia in the anesthetized canine preparation results in a small subendocardial infarction, with salvage of tissue in the overlying midmyocardium and subepicardium. Reperfusion after 40 minutes to 3 hours results in a progressively larger infarct involving the subendocardium to midmyocardium, with sparing of tissue in the subepicardium (Reimer and Jennings, 1979) (Fig. 3). While contractile function will obviously never be restored in the necrotic subendocardium, the salvaged peri-infarct tissue remains viable and eventually will contract. However, as in the brief occlusion models, the salvaged subepicardium remains stunned following reflow.

Postischemic dysfunction following prolonged but transient ischemia is especially relevant given the current use of thrombolytic agents in the treatment of acute myocardial infarction. This issue will be addressed in detail in Part IV of this book. As might be expected, however, experimental results indicate that recovery of function following prolonged coronary occlusion is much slower than recovery following short periods of ischemia. For example, Ellis et al. (1983) utilized two-dimensional echocardiography to monitor the return of function in the central ischemic zone of dogs that underwent 2 hours of occlusion and 14 days of reflow and compared the results to those obtained with 2 weeks of permanent coronary artery occlusion without reperfusion (Fig. 4A). Myocardial necrosis in the reperfused group was confined to the subendocardium, with salvage of tissue in the overlying subepicardium and portions of the midmyocardium. In contrast, permanent coronary artery occlusions resulted in myocardial infarcts, which were for the most part transmural. In the early hours following reperfusion, paradoxical LV wall thinning was modestly attenuated in the reperfused group compared to the permanently occluded group, but active wall thickening was not restored. Recovery of function following reflow was slow; it was not until 48 hours after reperfusion that active wall thickening became evident in the previously ischemic zone. Further gradual improvement in function occurred during the 2 weeks following reflow, but, due to the presence of the subendocardial infarct, wall motion did not recover to normal, preocclusion values. In the peripheral ischemic zone, return of function also was gradual following reperfusion (Fig. 4B). In contrast, animals subjected to permanent coronary artery occlusion showed no evidence of active contraction in the central ischemic zone, and only mild recovery of function in the peripheral ischemic zones at 14 days postinfarction. Thus, stunned myocardium clearly occurs both following brief periods of ischemia not associated with myocyte death, and following longer periods of ischemia in which reperfusion spares peri-infarct tissue overlying a nontransmural infarction.

C. Determinants of Stunned Myocardium

Whether postischemic dysfunction occurs following a transient episode of coronary occlusion depends on several factors. One major factor is the degree or severity of ischemia. In our experimental canine studies, we observed stunning

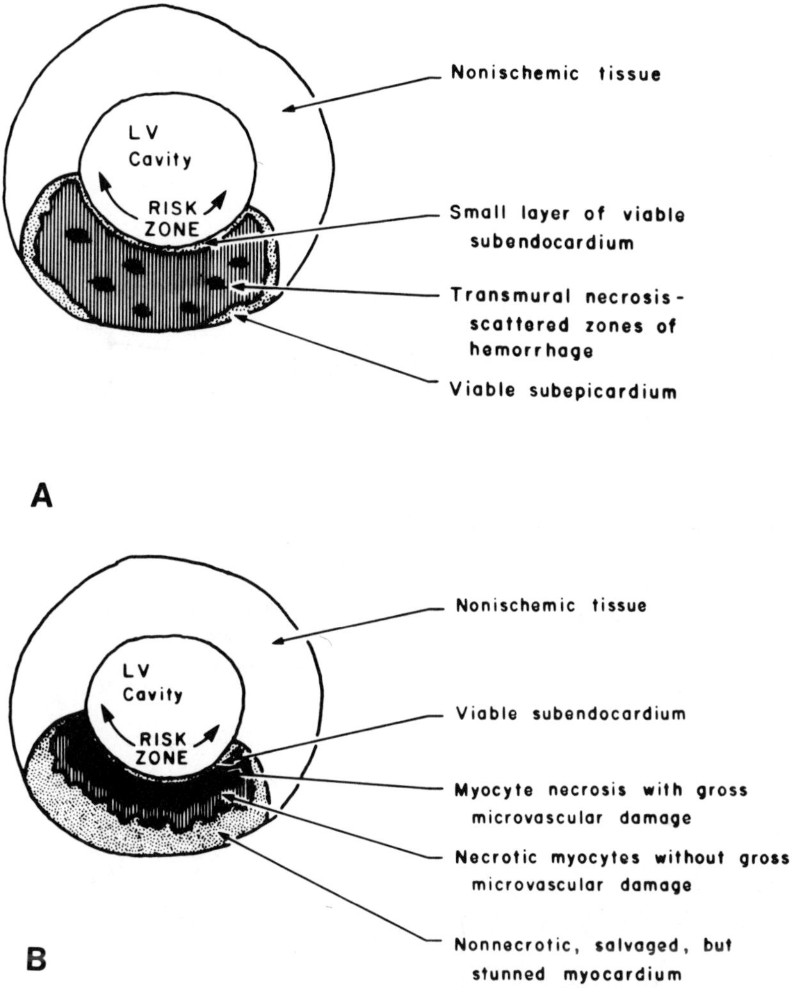

Figure 3 Schematic diagram showing a transverse section through a canine left ventricle. (A) Subjected to permanent coronary occlusion without reperfusion. The white area represents nonischemic myocardium supplied by the nonoccluded vessel. The infarct (hatched area) is transmural or near-transmural. There are scattered zones of hemorrhage (solid black). A small layer of viable subendocardium is present, which derives its oxygen directly from the ventricular cavity. Where collateral flow is high, there may be a small rim of surviving subepicardium (stippled areas). (B) Subjected to 1-2 hours of coronary occlusion followed by coronary reperfusion. The hatched and solid black areas represent the infarct, which is confined to the inner half of the myocardium. The solid black area represents the zone of gross microvascular damage, including the zones of no reflow and hemorrhage. The remainder of the infarct without severe microvascular damage is represented by the hatched area and is located in the midmyocardium. The epicardial portion of the ischemic zone (stippled area) has been salvaged by coronary reperfusion, but remains stunned for hours or days following reflow. (Reprinted from Braunwald and Kloner, 1985.)

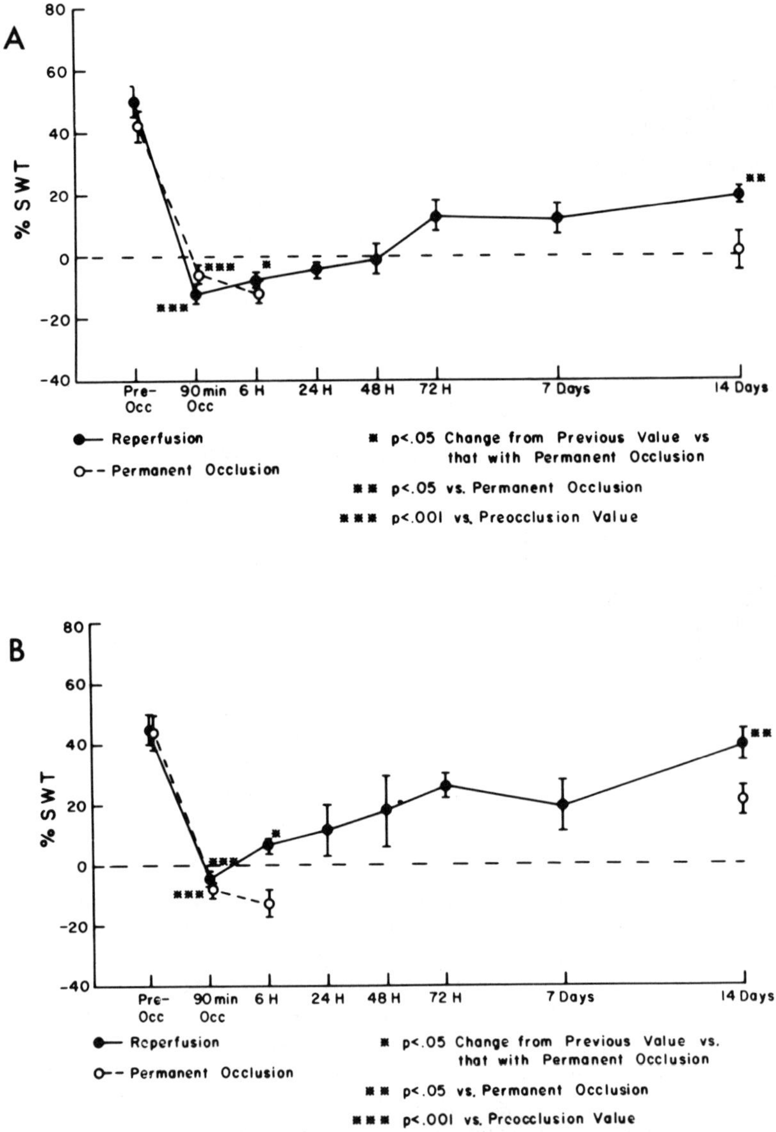

Figure 4 Contractile function in the central ischemic zone (A) and peripheral ischemic zone (B). Shown on the abscissa is time after coronary occlusion and on the ordinate, percent systolic wall thickening (% SWT). No values were obtained for dogs with permanent occlusion between 6 hours and 14 days. Occ = occlusion; p = probability; Pre-Occ = preocclusion measurement. (Reprinted from Ellis et al., 1987 with permission from the American College of Cardiology.)

only if the ischemic epidose is severe (i.e., subendocardial blood flow reduced to <20% of baseline values): if collateral flow is high and ischemia is mild, postischemic dysfunction is rapidly resolved (Przyklenk and Kloner, 1989b). Bolli et al. (1988) further concluded that stunning is most severe in myocardial segments that have the lowest myocardial blood flow during occlusion. However, data from our laboratory suggests that the best predictor of postischemic dysfunction is the degree of dyskinesis and exhibited during coronary artery occlusion. That is, segments with the most severe paradoxical systolic bulging during ischemia tend to be the segments with the most severe dysfunction following reflow (Fig. 5) (Przyklenk and Kloner, 1989b).

The duration of ischemia is another critical determinant of the degree of stunning. As described previously, 1 minute of coronary artery occlusion in the canine model is unlikely to result in stunning, a 5-minute period of ischemia may cause only mild postischemic dysfunction, while a 15-minute episode of ischemia is associated with more severe stunning (Kloner et al., 1983a). Another mode by which the net duration of ischemia may be increased is by repetitive episodes of brief ischemia. We did not observe a progressive worsening of postischemic function with three repeated 5- or 15-minute episodes of ischemia (Lange et al., 1984). In fact, segment shortening following repeated ischemia was similar to that observed following a single ischemic insult (Fig. 6). However, other investigators have suggested that 12

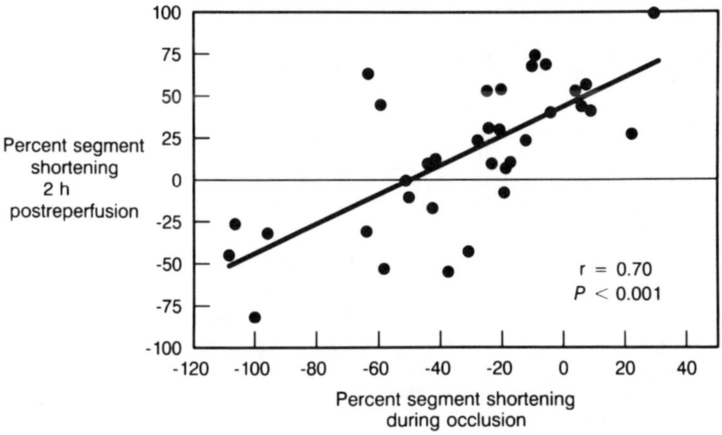

Figure 5 Effect of segment shortening measured during coronary occlusion on segment shortening measured after reperfusion. The degree of hypokinesia/dyskinesia observed during the period of ischemia reliably predicted acute recovery of contractile function ($r = 0.70$ and $p < 0.001$). (Reprinted from Przyklenk and Kloner, 1989b.)

A

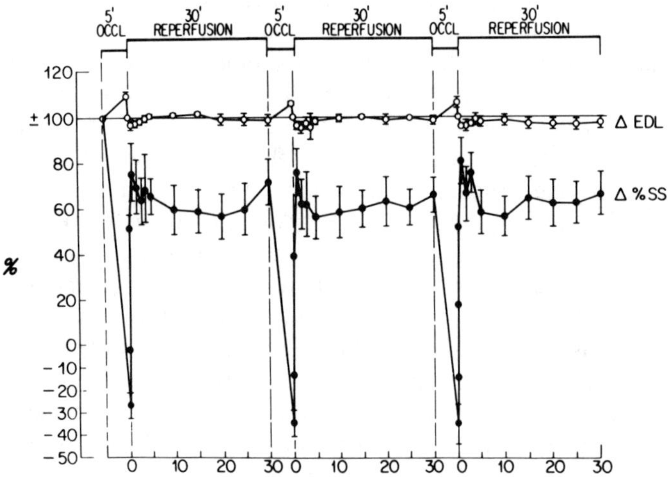

B

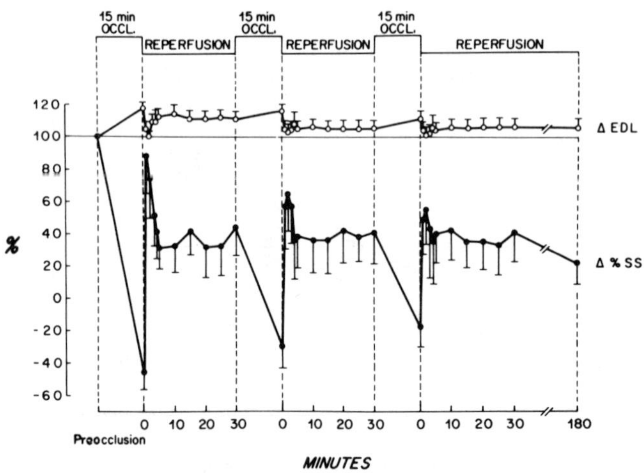

Figure 6 The effect of three repeated episodes of ischemia of regional wall motion. The end-diastolic length (EDL) increased upon each occlusion, and %SS showed paradoxical systolic bulging. Recovery was incomplete but almost identical during the three reperfusion periods (mean ± SEM). (A) Five-minute occlusion group. (B) Fifteen-minute occlusion group. (Reprinted from Lange et al., 1984 with permission from the American Heart Association.)

or more repeated 5-minute occlusions interrupted by reflow cause a progressive deterioration in function observed during the reperfusion phases (Zhao et al., 1987; Geft et al., 1982). Whether ultimate recovery of normal function is impaired or delayed following repeated ischemia versus a single ischemic insult remains, however, to be determined.

Another determinant of the severity of stunning is the site of ischemia. For example, it appears that stunning is most severe in the previously ischemic subendocardium. Myocardium subjected to 15 minutes of ischemia and reperfusion continues to exhibit postischemic dysfunction in the subendocardium at 24 hours after reperfusion, whereas subepicardial function is recovered at this time (Bolli et al., 1989). In addition, one study in the canine model has suggested that stunned myocardium is more severe and more reproducible following left anterior descending occlusion than following circumflex occlusion (Farber et al., 1987). The fact that postischemic dysfunction is most prominent in the subendocaridum is not surprising as, in the canine model, ischemia is most severe (with lower coronary collateral flow) in the inner ventricular wall. However, the reason why stunning is less severe in myocardium supplied by the circumflex artery remains unresolved (Farber et al., 1987).

In addition to the severity of ischemia, the degree of paradoxical bulging, the duration of ischemia, and the region of the heart under study, the mode by which reperfusion occurs may also mediate the degree of postischemic dysfunction. Recovery of function of stunned myocardium was inhibited when reperfusion occurred through a coronary stenosis, when compared with reperfusion into a fully patent coronary artery (Farber et al., 1988).

D. Other Properties Associated with Stunned Myocardium

1. Abnormalities in High Energy Phosphates

In addition to the profound but transient abnormalities in systolic and diastolic function of viable tissue salvaged by reflow, the stunned myocardium is also characterized by abnormalities in high energy phosphate stores. For example, DeBoer et al. (1980) described abnormalities in myocardial purine metabolism in anesthetized dogs subjected to 15 minutes of coronary artery occlusion and 72 hours of reperfusion. During the ischemic episode, subendocardial adenosine triphosphate (ATP) concentrations were depressed within the ischemic zone, averaging approximately 50% of values measured in normal, nonischemic tissue. Following 90 minutes of reperfusion, subendocardial ATP concentrations were significantly depressed at 70% of normal values, and remained depressed at 80% of normal even after 72 hours of reflow. Subepicardial ATP levels were also mildly depleted.

Total purine content (the sum of nucleotides, nucleosides, and bases) did not change during ischemia. However, purine content was depressed at 90 minutes after reperfusion and remained depleted at 72 hours of reflow. In contrast, creatine phosphate (CP) concentrations, although markedly depressed during ischemia, rapidly rebounded following restoration of blood flow.

The prolonged depression in ATP concentration following reperfusion is due to the fact that the nucleoside precursors adenosine, inosine, and hypoxanthine are washed out of the ischemic myocytes upon restoration of blood flow. As resynthesis of ATP in the myocardium preferentially occurs by the "salvage pathway" (i.e., preformed purines are utilized to reconstruct ATP), the loss of these precursors makes it difficult for the salvage pathway to be effective. The denovo purine nucleotide synthesis pathway for ATP repletion is a much slower process than the salvage pathway. Our data indicate that even 3 days of reperfusion was inadequate for purine resynthesis to fully replete ATP concentrations.

Other investigators have confirmed that repletion of ATP concentrations following a brief episode of ischemia and reperfusion is a slow process (Reimer et al., 1981; Swain et al., 1982). For example, Reimer et al. (1981) observed residual reduction in ATP levels even at 4 days after a 15-minute period of ischemia. As in our studies, CP concentrations were rapidly restored following reperfusion.

Abnormalities in ATP concentrations also occur in salvaged postischemic subepicardium overlying a subendocardial infarct. Ellis et al. (1983) studied ATP and CP levels in this zone in dogs subjected to 2 hours of transient coronary artery occlusion. Subepicardial ATP levels were depleted to 25% of normal after 90 minutes of coronary occlusion. At 4 hours of reperfusion, ATP remained depressed at 40% of nonischemic values, but, after 7 days of reperfusion, ATP levels had recovered to normal. As in the brief occlusion models, recovery of CP stores was rapid: subepicardial CP content was restored to normal by 4 hours postreflow.

2. Ultrastructural Findings in Stunned Myocardium

Despite the profound postischemic depression in contractile function, myocardium subjected to a 15-minute coronary artery occlusion plus reperfusion for 72 hours appeared normal by routine light microscopy (DeBoer et al., 1980). Furthermore, electron microscopy of this tissue revealed only subtle and fully reversible injury. Mild ultrastructural abnormalities that had been present at the end of 15 minutes of ischemia (i.e., relaxation of myofibrils as manifest by wide I bands, glycogen depletion, mild intermyofibrillar edema, rare cytoplasmic vacuoles, and chromatin clumping of the nuclei) had resolved. Vacuoles (perhaps containing lipids) were often observed (Fig. 7) (Kloner et al., 1983a), and mitochondrial cristae sometimes demonstrated a twisted or "unfolded" configuration. These mild postischemic abnormalities had disappeared, however, by 7 days following reflow.

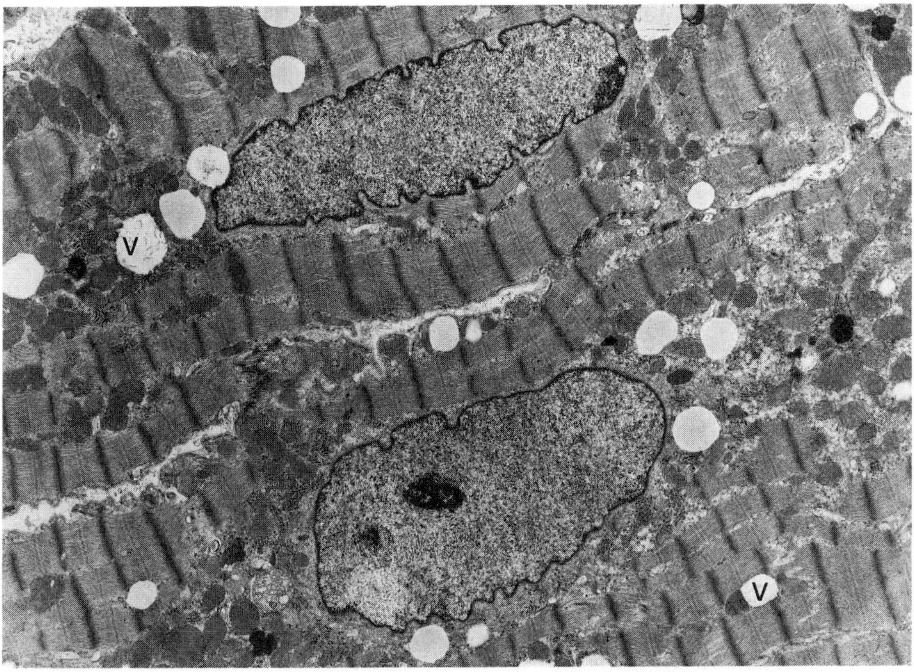

Figure 7 Electron micrograph of canine myocardium subjected to 15 minutes of ischemia and 72 hours of reperfusion. The nucleus appears normal. Glycogen is present and I bands are absent. Intermyofibrillar edema is absent. However, there are numerous vacuoles (v) throughout the cytoplasm. Original magnification ×7200. (Reprinted from Kloner et al., 1983a with permission from the American Heart Association.)

Similar electron-microscopic abnormalities have also been observed in salvaged, reperfused subepicardium overlying subendocardial infarcts (Kloner et al., 1983b). In canine myocardium subjected to 2 hours of coronary artery occlusion and by 4 hours of reperfusion, the viable subepicardium again exhibited small discrete vacuolelike structures adjacent to mitochondria, some of which contained what appeared to be remnants of lipid. These vacuoles were still present in some cells after 2 weeks of reperfusion. Other cells in the salvaged reperfused subepicardium demonstrated a moth-eaten appearance, suggestive of mild sarcoplasmic reticular edema. As with myocardium subjected to 15 minutes of transient occlusion, tissue salvaged following prolonged ischemia did not demonstrate any evidence of irreversible damage.

Scanning electron-microscopic abnormalities have been described in models of stunning induced by repeated brief episodes of ischemia. For example, both Zhao et al. (1987) and Whittaker et al. (1991) have reported a deterioration of the interstitial collagen substructure following repeated coronary occlusion. However, we found no evidence of collagen degradation (assessed by polarized light microscopy) with a single 15-minute period of transient coronary occlusion (Whittaker et al., 1991). Additional discussion of collagen damage in stunned myocardium is presented in Chapter 11.

3. Electrophysiological Abnormalities of the Stunned Myocardium

In myocardium stunned by 15 minutes of coronary artery occlusion, electrocardiographic (ECG) abnormalities during ischemia, such as ST segment shifts, resolve within minutes of reperfusion (Heyndrickx et al., 1975, 1978). However, Levine et al. (1987) reported a reduction in conduction velocity, resting membrane potential, and action potential amplitude in isolated canine epicardial preparations that had undergone 15 minutes of ischemia and 20 minutes of reflow. The authors postulated that these electrophysiological abnormalities within the stunned myocardium might contribute to reperfusion arrhythmias and postischemic contractile dysfunction. Clinical cases (Gensini et al., 1980) reported reversion of electrocardiographic changes of myocardial infarction, which were attributed to stunned myocardium.

4. Vascular Stunning

While the term stunned myocardium specifically refers to an abnormality in contraction of salvaged *myocytes*, there is increasing evidence that stunned myocardium may also be associated with functional abnormalities in the previously ischemic vasculature. For example, some investigators (Heyndrickx et al., 1978; Bolli et al., 1990) have described a mild depression in regional myocardial blood flow following a brief, 15-minute episode of ischemia and reperfusion. However, flow was only reduced to 60-80% of that observed in normal, nonischemic tissue—values too high to explain the severe depression of function seen in the early hours postreperfusion (Heyndrickx et al., 1978; Bolli et al., 1990). Furthermore, this "low reflow" following brief ischemia may worsen over time (Vanhaecke et al., 1990). For example, retrospective analysis from our laboratory revealed that regional flow was lower at 2.5 hours after reflow than at 1.5 hours after reperfusion (Kloner and Przyklenk, 1992). In contrast, other investigators (Stahl et al., 1986; Jeremy et al., 1989) found no evidence of depressed blood flow following a brief period of ischemia.

Low reflow has also been described in viable subepicardium overlying a subendocardial infarct (Kloner and Alker, 1984; Kloner et al., 1989a). Again, the degree of flow reduction in the previously ischemic tissue is mild, averaging 60-80% of normal values (Kloner and Alker, 1984; Kloner et al., 1989a).

Why low reflow occurs is unclear. This mild depression in blood flow is not accompanied by obvious morphological damage to the endothelial cells.

Low reflow may, however, be due to transient and mild myocyte and/or interstitial edema associated with brief reversible ischemia followed by reperfusion, which may be sufficient to increase resistance within the microvasculature. Another explanation for this low reflow phenomenon may involve the fact that the stunned myocardium is hypokinetic and therefore may have a low oxygen demand. However, as will be discussed in later chapters, some evidence suggests that myocardial oxygen demand within the stunned myocardium is either normal or actually increased (Stahl et al., 1988). Thus, it is unlikely that low reflow represents an autoregulatory phenomenon.

Another manifestation of microvascular abnormalities in the stunned myocardium is the apparent reduction in coronary vasodilator reserve following ischemia/reperfusion. Nicklas and Gips (1989) studied vascular stunning in dogs subjected to 15 minutes of coronary occlusion followed by reperfusion. Hyperemia following either a brief 30-second occlusion or after intracoronary injection of adenosine remained depressed with respect to normal baseline values for at least 1 hour after reperfusion, and coronary vascular resistances remained elevated. Similar results have also been reported by Bolli et al. (1990) and Vanhaecke et al. (1990).

Not all studies however, have observed abnormalities in coronary vascular reserve following brief periods of ischemia/reperfusion. Jeremy et al. (1989) studied both the changes in blood flow following administration of adenosine and peak hyperemia after 100 seconds of coronary artery occlusions in dogs that had undergone 10 minutes of regional ischemia. No change in vascular reserve was reported. Stahl et al. (1986) investigated the effect of 12 repeated 5-minute coronary occlusions on vasodilator reserve using dipyridamole, papaverine, and nitroglycerin. No change in vascular reserve was detected following ischemia with these vasodilators. Reasons for the discrepancy between these two studies and the previous reports may be related to the shorter duration of single occlusions or the use of a repetitive occlusion model.

Another form of microvascular dysfunction that has been described in viable postischemic myocardium is an increase in vascular permeability. Studies by Tillmanns et al. (1990) support the concept that even brief periods of ischemia and reperfusion may be associated with "leaky" capillaries: rats subjected to 6-10 minutes of ischemia exhibited leakage of fluorescent dextran from the microvasculature into the interstitium.

Finally, abnormalities in large vessel function have been also described following transient ischemia. Isolated coronary artery rings that had been subjected to occlusion and reperfusion demonstrated a reduced response to the endothelium-dependent vasodilator acetylcholine (Van Benthuysen et al., 1987). These data raise the possibility that the vasoconstrictor endothelin may play a role in altering postreperfusion blood flow.

III. STUNNED MYOCARDIUM IN OTHER MODELS OF TRANSIENT ISCHEMIA

While stunned myocardium was initially described in models of total coronary artery occlusion followed by reperfusion, it is now clear that a total coronary artery occlusion is not a prerequisite for stunning to occur. Ischemia due to any cause can lead to subsequent postischemic dysfunction. For example, a transient increase in oxygen demand caused by exercise in the setting of a partial coronary artery stenosis has been shown to cause postischemic stunning in both animals (Homans et al., 1989) and humans (Patel et al., 1988). In addition, Hittinger et al. (1990) observed subendocardial dysfunction in dogs with left ventricular hypertrophy following recovery from exercise. Presumably, hypertrophied ventricles have a mismatch of oxygen supply/demand during exercise stress, which may lead to subendocardial ischemia sufficient to result in subsequent stunning. This concept is supported by clinical case reports (Fine et al., 1989; Yasutomi et al., 1989), which demonstrate that stunning may occur in hypertrophied hearts without coronary artery disease. Thus, stunned myocardium may occur in a variety of clinical situations, which may or may not involve total occlusion or atherosclerotic narrowing of an epicardial coronary artery.

IV. STUNNED MYOCARDIUM VERSUS HIBERNATING MYOCARDIUM

Although this book focuses specifically on stunned myocardium, it must be stressed that that is not the only phenomenon characterized by contractile dysfunction of viable tissue. Another example is the concept of "hibernating myocardium." Hibernating myocardium is a term commonly found in the cardiac literature and has been defined by Rahimtoola (1985, 1989) as the persistent impairment of ventricular function at rest due to diminished coronary flow, which can be resolved by either increasing coronary blood flow or reducing myocardial oxygen demand. Stunned myocardium and hibernating myocardium are similar in that they both refer to an abnormality in contraction of viable myocytes. These two concepts differ, however, in terms of the blood flow status of the tissue. Hibernating myocardium is a chronic phenomenon in which *ischemia is ongoing* (Braunwald and Rutherford, 1986). That is, persistent wall motion abnormalities may be present for months to years in regions supplied by severely narrowed coronary vessels (Fig. 8). In contrast, stunning represents an acute or subacute phenomenon in which *ischemia has been relieved* but recovery of function takes hours to days (Fig. 9).

The concept of stunned myocardium originated in the experimental animal laboratory and has only recently been recognized as a true clinical entity. The concept of hibernating myocardium, on the other hand, originated

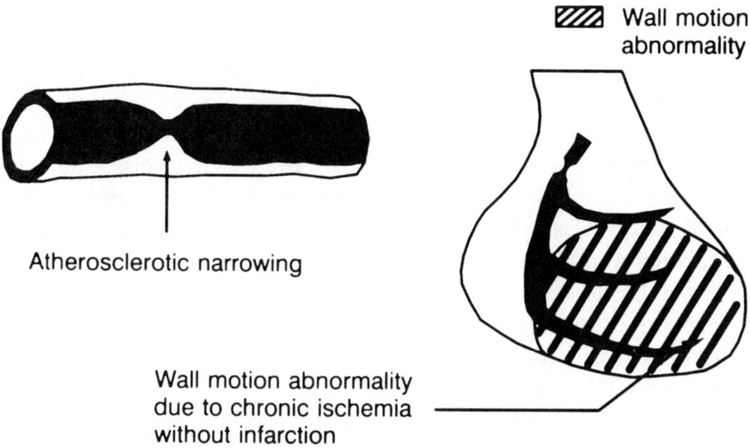

Figure 8 Schematic diagram of hibernating myocardium. Chronic ischemia without infarction results in a persistent regional wall motion abnormality. There is enough blood flow through the severe stenosis to allow for myocyte viability, but not enough to allow for normal contraction. The wall motion abnormality may be a protective mechanism whereby the left ventricle tries to reduce its oxygen demand in the setting of reduced oxygen supply. (Reprinted from Kloner et al., 1989b.)

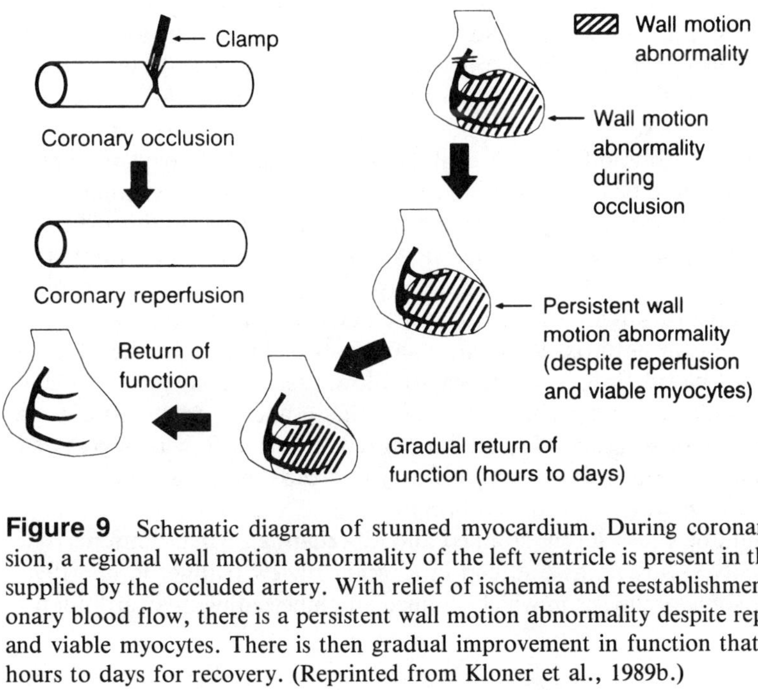

Figure 9 Schematic diagram of stunned myocardium. During coronary occlusion, a regional wall motion abnormality of the left ventricle is present in the region supplied by the occluded artery. With relief of ischemia and reestablishment of coronary blood flow, there is a persistent wall motion abnormality despite reperfusion and viable myocytes. There is then gradual improvement in function that requires hours to days for recovery. (Reprinted from Kloner et al., 1989b.)

from clinical observations made in the 1970s and has only recently been explored in the experimental laboratory (Kloner et al., 1990). In the 1970s, it was observed that some patients with chronic wall motion abnormalities in myocardium supplied by severely narrowed atherosclerotic coronary arteries had sustained improvement in regional function following coronary artery bypass surgery (Rahimtoola, 1985, 1989). In some cases, improvement in function was very rapid. Immediate recovery in regional function has also been described following angioplasty (Topol et al., 1984). Positron emission tomography, brief stimulation of hibernating myocardium by agents (such as nitroglycerin) that lower myocardial oxygen demand, and thallium reinjection studies are all techniques that have been employed to differentiate viable hibernating myocardium from nonviable scar tissue (Kloner et al., 1990). Such identification is important, as viable, poorly contracting hibernating myocardium would be expected to contract following revascularization, while infarcted or scarred myocardium obviously will not recover.

The term hibernating myocardium implies that the chronically ischemic tissue downregulates its function and oxygen demand in the setting of reduced oxygen supply in order to survive. Recent experimental evidence obtained from the porcine model supports this concept of a time-dependent adjustment in cardiac metabolism that develops fairly rapidly after placement of a partial coronary artery stenosis. Specifically, Fedele et al. (1988) observed an initial decline in myocardial pH at 5 minutes poststenosis, which then returned to baseline by 1 hour after the onset of ischemia. Furthermore, lactate consumption prior to stenosis changed to lactate production following stenosis, but lactate consumption was again restored by 3 hours after ischemia. Regional wall motion deteriorated during the initial 40 minutes after placement of the stenosis, and hypokinesis persisted throughout the 3 hours of ischemia. In addition, Pantely et al. (1990) observed that myocardial phosphocreatine could be regenerated in the setting of moderate ischemia. These observations appear to support the concept of a metabolic readjustment during partial coronary artery stenosis. Alternatively, however, hibernating myocardium may simply represent a threshold phenomenon. That is, blood flow supplied through an atherosclerotic narrowing may initially be sufficient to preserve both tissue viability and contractility. As further narrowing occurs, blood flow is sufficient to allow tissue viability but not high enough to allow normal contractility. At this point the myocardium may appear to be hibernating. Any additional reductions in flow or increases in myocardial oxygen demand could then jeopardize the tissue and result in myocyte death.

It should be stressed that stunned and hibernating myocardium need not be mutually exclusive: as outlined in a recent review (Kloner et al., 1990), there are some situations in which stunned and hibernating myocardium may coexist. In addition, the hibernating myocardium may go through a phase of stunning once ischemia is relieved. In fact, recent work by Przyklenk et al. (1990) has confirmed this in an experimental model. Finally, the syndrome of ischemic cardiomyopathy may be due to hibernating myocardium, stunned myocardium, or some combination of both (Kloner, 1991).

V. SUMMARY

Stunned myocardium is viable previously ischemic tissue, which exhibits prolonged but transient postischemic contractile dysfunction. This phenomenon occurs both following brief episodes of ischemia (as might occur in experimental models that mimic angina) and following more prolonged episodes of ischemia as would occur following reperfusion of an acute myocardial infarction. Stunning has been reported to last for hours to days following reflow, but the duration of dysfunction is dependent upon the experimental model being used. Determinants of stunning include the severity and duration of ischemia, the degree of paradoxical systolic bulging of the ischemic segment, the region of the heart under study, and the mode by which reperfusion is induced. Stunned myocardium is also characterized by a decrease in myocardial ATP and purine content, subtle ultrastructural abnormalities (i.e., vacuoles adjacent to mitochondria), electrophysiological abnormalities, "low reflow," and reduced coronary vasodilator reserve. It should be noted that total coronary artery occlusion is not a prerequisite for stunning: postischemic dysfunction has been documented following exercise-induced ischemia, in models of partial coronary artery stenosis, and in hypertrophied ventricles without coronary stenosis.

REFERENCES

Bolli, R., Zhu, W. X., Thornby, J. I., O'Neill, P. G., and Roberts, R. (1988). Timecourse and determinants of recovery of function after reversible ischemia in conscious dogs. *Am. J. Physiol. 254*: H102.

Bolli, R., Patel, B. S., Hartley, C. J., Thornby, J. I., Jeroudi, M. O., and Roberts, R. (1989). Nonuniform transmural recovery of contractile function in stunned myocardium. *Am. J. Physiol. 257*: H375.

Bolli, R., Triani, J. F., and Jeroudi, M. O. (1990). Prolonged impairment of coronary vasodilation after reversible ischemia. Evidence for microvascular stunning. *Circ. Res. 67*: 332.

Braunwald E., and Kloner, R. A. (1982). The stunned myocardium: Prolonged, postischemic ventricular dysfunction. *Circulation 66*: 1146.

Braunwald, E., and Kloner, R. A. (1985). Myocardial reperfusion: A double-edged sword? *J. Clin. Invest. 76*: 1713.

Braunwald, E., and Rutherford, J. D. (1986). Reversible ischemic left ventricular dysfunction: Evidence for the "hibernating myocardium." *J. Am. Coll. Cardiol.* *8*: 1467.

Charlat, J. L., O'Neill, R. G., Hartley, C. J., Roberts, R., and Bolli, R. (1989). Prolonged abnormalities of left ventricular diastolic wall thinning in the "stunned" myocardium in conscious dogs: Time course and relation to systolic function. *J. Am. Coll. Cardiol.* *13*: 185.

DeBoer, L. W. V., Ingwall, J. S., Kloner, R. A., and Braunwald, E. (1980). Prolonged derangements of canine myocardial purine metabolism after a brief coronary artery occlusion not associated with anatomic evidence of necrosis. *Proc. Natl. Acad. Sci.* *77*: 5471.

Ellis, S. G., Henschke, C. I., Sandor, T., Wynne, J., Braunwald, E., and Kloner, R. A. (1983). Time course of functional and biochemical recovery of myocardium salvaged by reperfusion. *J. Am. Coll. Cardiol.* *1*: 1047.

Farber, N. E., Pieper, G. M., and Gross, G. J. (1987). Regional differences in postischemic recovery in the stunned myocardium. *Am. Heart J.* *114*: 1086.

Farber, N. E., Pieper, G. M., and Gross, G. J. (1988). Postischemic recovery in the stunned myocardium after reperfusion in the presence or absence of a flow-limiting coronary artery stenosis. *Am. Heart J.* *116*: 407.

Fedele, F. A., Gerwitz, H., Capone, R. J., Sharaf, B., and Most, A. S., (1988). Metabolic response to prolonged reduction of myocardial blood flow distal to a severe coronary artery stenosis. *Circulation* *78*: 729.

Fine, D. G., Clements, I. D., and Callahan, M. J. (1989). Myocardial stunning in hypertrophic cardiomyopathy. Recovery predicted by single photon emission computed tomographic thallium-201 scintigraphy. *J. Am. Coll. Cardiol.* *13*: 1415.

Geft, I. L., Fishbein, M. C., Ninomiya, K., Hashida, J., Chanx, E., Yano, J., Y-Rit, J., Genov, T., Shell, W., and Ganz, W. (1982). Intermittent brief periods of ischemia have a cumulative effect and may cause myocardial necrosis. *Circulation* *66*: 1150.

Gensini, G. G., Esente, P., Marmor, B., Black, A., Black M., Giambartolome, A., and Effler, D. B. (1980). "Stunned" myocardium or myocardial infarction?: Diagnosis and treatment. In *Quantification of Myocardial Ischemia* (Kreuzer H., Parmley, W. W., Rentrop, P., Heiss, H. W., eds.), Gerhard Witzstrock Publishing, New York, p. 593.

Heyndrickx, G. R., Millard, R. W., McRitchie, R. J., Maroko, P. R., and Vatner, S. F. (1975). Regional myocardial function and electrophysiological alterations after brief coronary artery occlusion in conscious dogs. *J. Clin Invest.* *56*: 978.

Heyndrickx, G. R., Baig, H., Nellens, P., Leusen, I., Fishbein, M. C., and Vatner, S. F., (1978). Depression of regional blood flow and wall thickening after brief coronary occlusions, *Am. J. Physiol.* *234*: H653.

Hittinger, L., Shannon, R., Kohin, S., Manders, T., Kelly, P., and Vatner, S. (1990). Exercise-induced subendocardial dysfunction in dogs with left ventricular hypertrophy. *Circ. Res.* *66*: 329.

Homans, D. L., Laxson, D. D., Sublett, E., Lindstrom, P., and Bache, R. J. (1989). Cumulative deterioration of myocardial function after repeated episodes of exercise-induced ischemia. *Am. J. Physiol.* *256*: H1462.

Jeremy, R. W., Stahl, L., Gillinvov, M., Litt, M., Aversano, T. R., and Becker, L. C. (1989). Preservation of coronary flow reserve in stunned myocardium. *Am. J. Physiol. 256*: H1303.

Kloner, R. A., Ellis, S. G., Lange, L., and Braunwald E. (1983a). Studies of experimental coronary artery reperfusion. Effects on infarct size, myocardial function, biochemistry, ultrastructure, and microvascular damage. *Circulation 68 (Suppl 1)*: 1-8.

Kloner, R. A., Ellis, S. G., Carlson, N. V., and Braunwald, E. (1983b). Coronary reperfusion for the treatment of acute myocardial infarction: postischemic ventricular dysfunction. *Cardiology 70*: 233.

Kloner, R. A., and Alker K. J. (1984). The effect of streptokinase on intramyocardial hemorrhage, infarct size, and the no-reflow phenomenon during coronary reperfusion. *Circulation 70*: 513.

Kloner, R. A., Alker, K. J., Campbell, C., Figures, G., Eisenhauer, A., and Hale, S. (1989a). Does tissue-type plasminogen activator have direct beneficial effects on the myocardium independent on its ability to lyse intracoronary thrombi? *Circulation 79*: 1125.

Kloner, R. A., Przyklenk, K., and Patel, B. (1989b). Altered myocardial states: The stunned and hibernating myocardium. *Am. J. Med. 86 (Suppl 1A)*: 14.

Kloner, R. A., Przyklenk, K., Rahimtoola, S. H., and Braunwald, E. (1990). Myocardial stunning and hibernation: Mechanisms and clinical implications. In *Heart Disease Update* (E. Braunwald, ed.), Saunders Co., Philadelphia, p. 241.

Kloner R. A. (1991). Ischemic cardiomyopathy: A manifestation of stunned myocardium? *Heart Failure 7*: 5.

Kloner, R. A., and Przyklenk, K. (1992). Consequences of ischemia/reperfusion on the coronary microvasculature. In *The Pathophysiology of Reperfusion and Reperfusion Injury* (D. Yellon, R. B. Jennings, eds.), Raven Press, New York, p. 85.

Lange, R., Ware, J., and Kloner, R. A. (1984). Absence of a cumulative deterioration of regional function during three repeated 5 or 15 minute coronary occlusions. *Circulation 69*: 400.

Levine, J. H., Moore, E. N., Weisman, H. F., Kadish, A. H., Becker, L. C., and Spear, J. F. (1987). Depression of action potential characteristics and a decreased space constant are present in postischemic, reperfused myocardium. *J. Clin. Invest. 79*: 107.

Nicklas, J. M., and Gips, S. J. (1989). Decreased coronary flow reserve after transient myocardial ischemia in dogs. *J. Am. Coll. Cardiol. 13*: 195.

Pantely, G. A., Malone, S. A., Rhen, W. S., Anselone, C. G., Arai, A., and Bristow, J., Bristow, J. D. (1990). Regeneration of myocardial phosphocreatine in pigs despite continued moderate ischemia. *Circ. Res. 67*: 1481.

Patel, B., Kloner, R. A., Przyklenk, K., and Braunwald, E. (1988). Postischemic myocardial "stunning": A clinically relevant phenomenon. *Ann. Int. Med. 108*: 626.

Preuss, K. C., Gross, G. J., Brooks, H. L., and Warltier, D. C. (1987). Time course of recovery of "stunned" myocardium following variable periods of ischemia in conscious and anesthetized dogs. *Am. Heart J. 114*: 696.

Przyklenk, K., Vivaldi, M. T., Schoen, F. J., Arnold, J. M. O., and Kloner, R. A. (1986). Salvage of ischemia myocardium by reperfusion: Importance of collateral blood flow and myocardial oxygen demand during occlusion, *Cardiovasc. Res. 20*: 403.

Przyklenk, K., Patel, B., and Kloner, R. A. (1987). Diastolic abnormalities of postischemic "stunned" myocardium. *Am. J. Cardiol. 60*: 1211.

Przyklenk, K., and Kloner, R.A. (1989a). Is "stunned myocardium" a protective mechanism? Effect of acute recruitment and acute beta blockade in recovery of contractile function and high energy phosphate stores at one day post reperfusion. *Am. Heart J. 118*: 480.

Przyklenk, K., and Kloner, R. A. (1989b). What factors predict recovery of contractile function in the canine model of the "stunned" myocardium? *Am. J. Cardiol. 64 (Suppl)*: 18F.

Przyklenk, K., and Kloner, R. A. (1989c). The "stunned myocardium:" Characteristics, causes and clinical implications. *Cardio* (April 1989): 130.

Przyklenk, K., Bauer, B., and Kloner, R. A. (1990). Contractile function of hibernating myocardium. Effect of collateral vs. stenotic perfusion. *Circulation 82 (Suppl III)*: 273.

Rahimtoola, S. H. (1985). A perspective on the three large multicenter randomized clinical trials of coronary bypass surgery for chronic stable angina. *Circulation 72 (Suppl V)*: 123.

Rahimtoola, S. H. (1989). The hibernating myocardium. *Am. Heart J. 117*: 211.

Reimer, K. A., Lowe, J. E., Rasmussen, M. M., and Jennings, R. B. (1977). The wavefront phenomenon of ischemic cell death: myocardial infarct size vs. duration of coronary occlusion in dogs. *Circulation 56*: 786.

Reimer, K. A., and Jennings, R. B. (1979). The "wavefront phenomenon" of myocardial ischemic cell death. II. Transmural progression of necrosis within the framework of ischemic bed size (myocardium at risk) and collateral flow. *Lab. Invest. 40*: 633.

Reimer, K. A., Hill, M. L., and Jennings, R. B. (1981). Prolonged depletion of ATP and of the adenine nucleotide pool due to delayed resynthesis of adenine nucleotide following reversible myocardial ischemia in dogs. *J. Mol. Cell. Cardiol. 13*: 229.

Stahl, L. D., Aversano, T. R., and Becker, L. C. (1986). Selective enhancement of function of stunned myocardium by increased flow. *Circulation 74*: 843.

Stahl, L. D., Weiss, H., and Becker, L. C. (1988). Myocardial oxygen consumption, oxygen supply/demand heterogeneity, and microvascular patency in regionally stunned myocardium. *Circulation 77*: 865.

Swain, J. L., Sabina, R. L., McHale, P. A., Greenfield, J. C., and Holmes, E. W. (1982). Prolonged myocardial nucleotide depletion after brief ischemia the openchest dogs. *Am. J. Physiol. 242*: H818.

Tillmanns, H., Neumann, F. J., Parekh, N., Zimmermann, R., Tiefenbacher, C., Dorigo, O., Steinhausen, M., and Kubler, W. (1990). Microcirculation in the hypertrophied and ischemic heart. *Eur. J. Clin. Pharmacol. 39 (Suppl 1)*: S9.

Topol, E. J., Weiss, J. L., Guzman, P. A., Dorsey-Lima, S., Blanck, T. J. J., Humphrey, L. S., Baumgartner, W. A., Flaherty, J. T., and Reitz, B. A. (1984). Immediate improvement of dysfunctional myocardial segments after coronary revascularization: Detection by intraoperative transesophageal echocardiography. *J. Am. Coll. Cardiol. 4*: 1123.

Van Benthuysen, K. M., McMurty, I. F., and Horwitz, L. D. (1987). Reperfusion after acute coronary occlusion in dogs impairs endothelium-dependent relaxation to acetylcholine and augments contractile reactivity in vitro. *J. Clin. Invest. 79*: 265.

Vanhaecke, J., Flameng, W., Borgens, M., Jang, I-K., Van-de-Werf, F., and De-Geest, H. (1990). Evidence for decreased coronary flow reserve in viable postischemic myocardium. *Circ. Res. 67*: 1201.

Weiss, J. L., Frederiksen, J. W., and Weisfeldt, M. L., (1976). Hemodynamic determinants of the time course of fall in canine left ventricular pressure. *J. Clin. Invest. 58*: 751.

Whittaker, P., Boughner, D. R., Kloner, R. A., and Przyklenk, K. (1991). Stunned myocardium and myocardial collagen damage. Differential effects of a single and repeated occlusions. *Am. Heart J. 121*: 434.

Yasutomi, N., Kogame, T., Kawakami, K., Komasa, N., and Iwasaki, T. (1989). Stunned myocardium in hypertrophic cardiomyopathy with normal coronary arteries. *Am. Heart J. 118*: 1069.

Zhao, M., Zhang, H., Robinson, T. F., Factor, S. M., Sonnenblick, E. H., and Eng, C. (1987). Profound structural alterations of the extracellular collagen matrix in postischemic dysfunctional ("stunned") but viable myocardium. *J. Am. Coll. Cardiol. 10*: 1322.

3

Metabolic Correlates of Reversibly Injured Myocardium

Myocardial Oxygen Consumption and Carbon Substrate Utilization

Stevan D. Zimmer and Robert J. Bache

University of Minnesota, Minneapolis, Minnesota

In addition to the well-described mechanical dysfunction accompanying non-lethal ischemic-reperfusion injury, there are significant changes in myocardial oxygen consumption (MVO_2), oxidative phosphorylation, and carbon substrate metabolism (glucose, lipid, and glycolytic intermediate utilization). These changes are indicative of the complex nature of the cellular insult caused by the ischemia-reperfusion process and describe the metabolic limitations of the injured system. Analysis of these changes has potential for separating mechanically depressed but viable myocardium from lethally injured myocardium. The results of continuing investigation of the metabolic aspects of stunned myocardium will further identify the nature of the insult and thereby assist in developing strategies to minimize the insult and to improve myocardial performance after the injury has occurred.

I. MYOCARDIAL OXYGEN CONSUMPTION

In a variety of experimental models of ischemic-reperfusion injury, MVO_2 appears to be paradoxically increased relative to developed mechanical force. This phenomenon has been seen in isolated, crystalloid perfused heart preparations (Laster et al., 1989; Zimmer et al., 1989), in globally and regionally stunned in vivo models (Stahl et al., 1988; Laxson et al., 1989; Finney et al., 1990; Dean et al., 1990) (Fig. 1), and in hearts subjected to hypothermic, cardioplegic ischemia (Krukenkamp et al., 1986). The occurrence of increased MVO_2 in crystalloid perfused preparations indicates that a contribution from blood components (e.g., oxidant injury due to neutrophil infiltration) is not necessary to produce increased MVO_2. Moreover, the observation of increased MVO_2 in a wide variety of experimental preparations indicates that this is a fundamental consequence of the ischemic-reperfusion process.

A. Conditions for Elevated MVO_2

To validly conclude that MVO_2 is elevated after an ischemic-reperfusion injury, three conditions in addition to the measurement of MVO_2 must be met. First, a sufficient period of ischemia must have occurred to elicit the

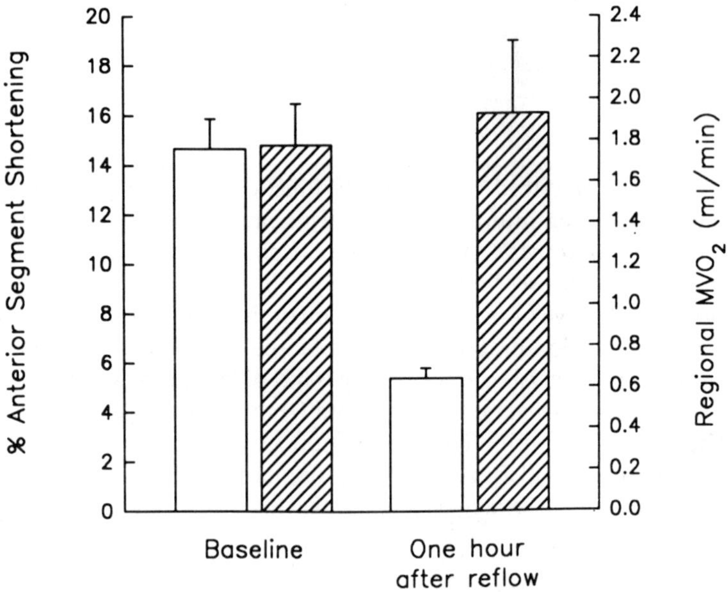

Figure 1 Percent segment shortening (open bars) and MVO_2 (hatched bars) in the anterior left ventricular wall before and one hour after a 15-minute occlusion of the left anterior descending coronary artery of open-chest dogs. Despite persistent contractile dysfunction after reperfusion, regional MVO_2 was not decreased. (Adapted from Laxson et al., 1988.)

abnormality; second, MVO_2 measurements need to be related to some measure of postischemic mechanical function to observe the effect; and third, adequate oxygen delivery must be restored to the postischemic tissue over the range of observed mechanical activity.

1. Duration of Ischemia

The first condition has usually been satisfied in canine or porcine preparations exposed to repeated coronary occlusions and in global models where ischemia has been sufficient to produce mechanical dysfunction or substantial (> 30%) depletion of high-energy phosphates. In an isolated rat heart model, we observed that with several carbon substrates (glucose-insulin and pyruvate-glucose), ischemic durations sufficient to produce ischemic contracture (10–12 minutes of normothermic no-flow ischemia for glucose-insulin and 17–18 minutes for pyruvate-glucose-perfused hearts) were associated with elevations in MVO_2 in the postischemic period after steady-state mechanical function was achieved (Zimmer, 1989) (Fig. 2). When the duration of ischemia was shorter than that required to produce ischemic contracture, elevated MVO_2 was not observed. In addition, in glucose-insulin-perfused hearts, some subtle mechanical dysfunction could be observed without a relative increase in MVO_2 when the duration of ischemia was slightly less than that required to produce ischemic contracture. Thus, the presence of mechanical dysfunction is generally associated with increased postischemic MVO_2, although data obtained in the isolated heart suggest that there is a threshold of ischemic injury that is necessary to produce the increased MVO_2.

It is unclear whether a predictable relationship exists between the duration of ischemic injury and the subsequent magnitude of mismatch between MVO_2 and postischemic mechanical function. In the isolated perfused rat heart system, a greater mismatch of MVO_2 to mechanical activity was observed when normothermic no-flow ischemia was increased from 11–12 minutes (Zimmer et al., 1989) to 17–18 minutes (Sako et al., 1988). This occurred primarily because mechanical function was more depressed as ischemia was increased, with only a modest further increase in MVO_2. This finding suggests that increasing ischemia may worsen the disparity between MVO_2 and mechanical activity and that this occurs because of a greater depression of contractile function rather than a further increase in the absolute level of MVO_2. This conclusion is further supported by the observations in regionally stunned models: while mechanical dysfunction is more pronounced in the subendocardium than in the subepicardium (Bolli et al., 1989), MVO_2 values are similar (Stahl et al., 1988; Acad and Weiss, 1989). One study did identify a decrease in MVO_2 after 4 hours versus 15 minutes of regional ischemia (Dean et al., 1990). Clearly, however, the upper limit for experimental studies is defined by the occurrence of irreversible myocardial injury as

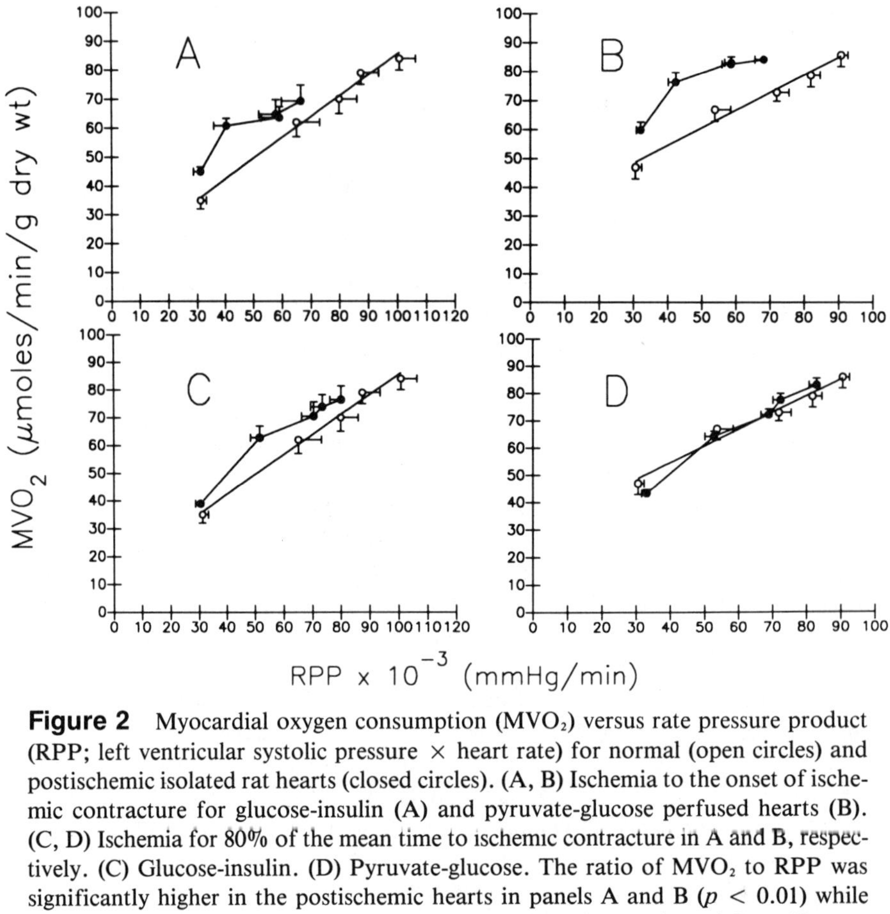

Figure 2 Myocardial oxygen consumption (MVO_2) versus rate pressure product (RPP; left ventricular systolic pressure × heart rate) for normal (open circles) and postischemic isolated rat hearts (closed circles). (A, B) Ischemia to the onset of ischemic contracture for glucose-insulin (A) and pyruvate-glucose perfused hearts (B). (C, D) Ischemia for 80% of the mean time to ischemic contracture in A and B, respectively. (C) Glucose-insulin. (D) Pyruvate-glucose. The ratio of MVO_2 to RPP was significantly higher in the postischemic hearts in panels A and B ($p < 0.01$) while not significant ($p > 0.05$) in the hearts in panels C and D. (Adapted from Zimmer et al., 1990.)

the duration of ischemia is extended. It is apparent that the relative increase of MVO_2 persists for at least 4 hours after reperfusion (Upsher et al., 1988). MVO_2 may be elevated even in reperfused preparations with ultrastructural evidence of irreversible damage (Görge et al., 1991).

2. Increased MVO_2 Relative to Mechanical Performance

The second condition is that measured MVO_2 must be referenced not only to postischemic mechanical function but also to preischemic MVO_2 relative to preischemic mechanical performance. While the observation of increased postischemic MVO_2 is in relation to postischemic mechanical performance, the absolute value of postischemic MVO_2 typically is within the range observed in normal myocardium. Since contractile activity is the major determinant of MVO_2 in normal and reversibly injured myocardium, it is necessary to compare pre- and postischemic states at either similar levels of mechanical performance or at similar MVO_2 values (Zimmer et al., 1990).

In several studies, the increase in MVO_2 appeared to be relatively constant over a moderate range of postischemic mechanical performance (Ohgoshi et al., 1991; Krukenkamp et al., 1986). The absolute increase in MVO_2 is not influenced by changes in ventricular loading conditions (Ohgoshi et al., 1991). When postischemic mechanical dysfunction is relatively mild, an increase in MVO_2 may not be apparent (Krukenkamp et al., 1986; Zimmer et al., 1990) or may be less than that observed with longer ischemic durations (Sako et al., 1988; Upsher et al., 1988).

Several investigators have examined the response of mechanical performance and MVO_2 during administration of inotropic agents in the postischemic period (Lekven et al., 1988; Acad and Weiss, 1989; Ohgoshi et al., 1991; Zimmer et al., 1990). Most of these studies have demonstrated that contractile performance remains responsive to inotropic intervention, and that the increased contractility is associated with significant increases in MVO_2 at a given level of mechanical function. In a model of global ischemia, infusion of epinephrine was associated with a significant increase in postischemic MVO_2 without a concomitant increase in mechanical performance under identical loading conditions (Lekven et al., 1988). In a similar model of global ischemia, when depressed postischemic mechanical function was returned to preischemic control levels with calcium infusion, postischemic MVO_2 was increased relative to preischemic values (Ohgoshi et al., 1991) (Fig. 3). In both of these studies, MVO_2 and mechanical performance were not evaluated over the range of obtainable values. It is clear from reviewing the studies using inotropic agents that MVO_2 increases out of proportion to the increase obtained in mechanical performance with the administration of these agents.

In an isolated heart model, we observed that when postischemic mechanical performance was progressively increased to maximal levels with dobutamine, the relationship was curvilinear with the largest increase in MVO_2 occurring with the initial addition of dobutamine (Zimmer, 1989) (see Fig. 2). As dobutamine concentrations were increased, MVO_2 plateaued while mechanical performance continued to increase by 50–75%. These data suggest that higher concentrations of inotropic agents may promote better coupling of mechanical performance to MVO_2.

3. Oxygen Availability

a. Coronary Flow Reserve. The third condition required to observe increased postischemic MVO_2 is axiomatic. Increased oxygen consumption implies adequate oxygen delivery and oxidative capacity of the mitochon-

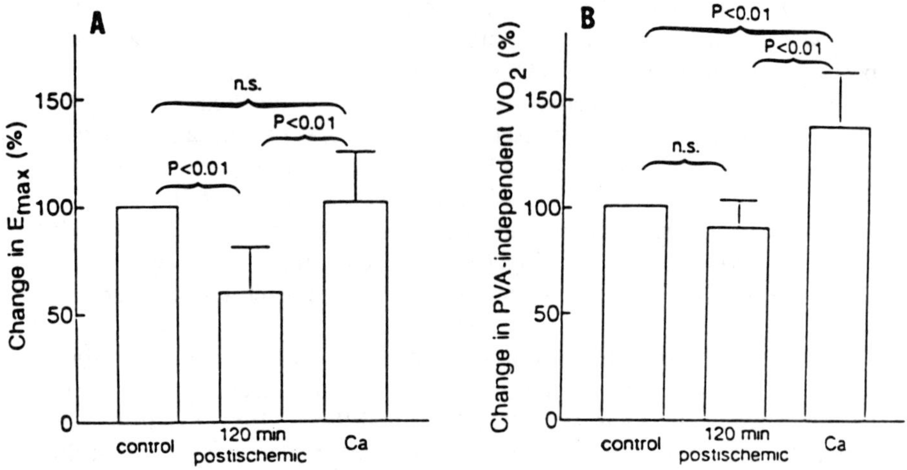

Figure 3 (A) Change in E_{max} (load-independent contractility) during control conditions, 2 hours postischemia and 2 hours postischemic with Ca^{2+} infusion. Ca^{2+} infusion restored E_{max} to control levels. (B) Change in pressure-volume area (PVA)-independent MVO_2 during conditions in A. PVA-independent MVO_2 was similar in control and 2 hours postischemic hearts despite the decrease in systolic mechanical function (E_{max}). Ca^{2+} infusion significantly increased PVA-independent MVO_2 relative to the control MVO_2. (With permission of Ohgoshi et al., 1991).

dria. While the effects of ischemia-reperfusion injury on coronary flow are discussed in detail elsewhere, several regional ischemia models have identified no substantial reductions of coronary vasodilator capacity in the post ischemic period (after reperfusion and resumption of steady-state coronary flow and mechanical activity) (Laxson et al., 1989; Jeremy et al., 1989).

b. Mitochondrial Oxidative Capacity. Both normal function and decreased maximal oxidative capacity (maximal State 3 activity, decreased respiratory control ratio) have been observed in mitochondria isolated from postischemic myocardium after nonlethal injury (Dean et al., 1990; Mukherjee et al., 1982; Murphy et al., 1982; Edoute et al., 1983; Peng et al., 1986; Weinstein et al., 1986; Nakahara et al., 1986). Although isolated mitochondrial preparations allow detailed examination of specific aspects of organelle function, there are several limitations to this methodology. First, isolation techniques may inadvertently bias either for or against specific subpopulations of mitochondria (Schafer et al., 1981; Edoute et al., 1983). Second, evaluation of function in isolated mitochondria depends on the particular set of conditions chosen for the in vitro assays. These conditions may not accurately reproduce the in vivo situation, especially after the profound alterations in the intracellular milieu that may occur subsequent to ischemia and reperfusion.

In an isolated perfused rat heart model, maximal MVO_2 during intense inotropic and chronotropic stimulation was decreased after an ischemic insult equal in duration to the onset of ischemic contracture (Zimmer et al., 1989) (see Fig. 2). This might be expected solely on the basis of the reduction in maximal postischemic contractile performance. However, when the factors responsible for regulation of oxidative-phosphorylation, and hence MVO_2, were examined under a variety of substrate conditions, we observed that after an ischemic duration equal to the onset of ischemic contracture, oxidative phosphorylation was apparently regulated by adenosine diphosphate (ADP) concentration (Fig. 4). Since postischemic ADP concentration and MVO_2 exhibited a Michaelis-Menten relationship, it was possible to calculate the maximal oxidative capacity (maximal MVO_2) of the mitochondria. The computed values for the maximal oxidative capacity (V_{max}) of the isolated heart system was significantly reduced and in agreement with the observed maximal values for MVO_2. While these observations need to be replicated in an in vivo system, they suggest that not only is MVO_2 in the postischemic heart elevated out of proportion to postischemic mechanical activity, but also that maximal MVO_2 is reduced. This reduction in maximal oxidative capacity would not be responsible for the postischemic contractile dysfunction seen during basal conditions, but might contribute to the limitation of maximal mechanical performance.

B. Sources of Elevated Postischemic MVO_2

In normal myocardium, MVO_2 is closely coupled to the production of adenosine triphosphate (ATP). In postischemic myocardium where MVO_2 is increased relative to mechanical performance, the source of elevated MVO_2 may be due either to oxygen consumption that no longer results in the same production of ATP per mole of O_2 consumed ("uncoupling") or to inefficient use of ATP in relation to mechanical performance. More specifically, the inefficient use of ATP can be further examined with respect to the various consumptive myocardial ATPases. The three predominant consumptive ATPases are the Na^+, K^+-ATPase, the sarcoplasmic reticulum Ca^{2+}-ATPase, and the myosin ATPase, with the latter being dominant with regard to ATP utilization in contracting myocardium. Figure 5 illustrates the potential cellular sources of increased postischemic MVO_2.

1. Uncoupling of MVO_2 from ATP Synthesis

In classic mitochondrial studies, uncoupling of MVO_2 from ATP synthesis is induced with agents such as dinitrophenol, which disrupt mitochondrial membrane integrity and dissipate the transmembrane proton gradient. The

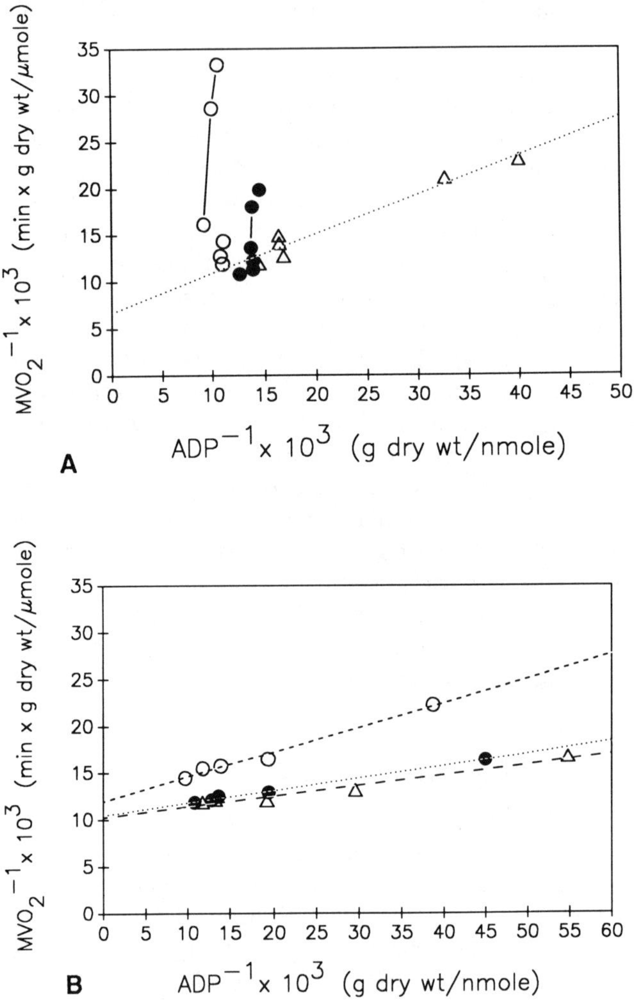

Figure 4 Double-reciprocal (Lineweaver-Burke) plot of ADP concentrations versus MVO_2 for three exogenous carbon sources: glucose-insulin (GI; open circles), palmitate-glucose (Palm G; closed circles), and pyruvate-glucose (PyrG; open triangles) in normal perfused rat hearts (A) and in reperfused hearts after an ischemic duration to the onset of ischemic contracture (B). (From Zimmer et al., 1989.)

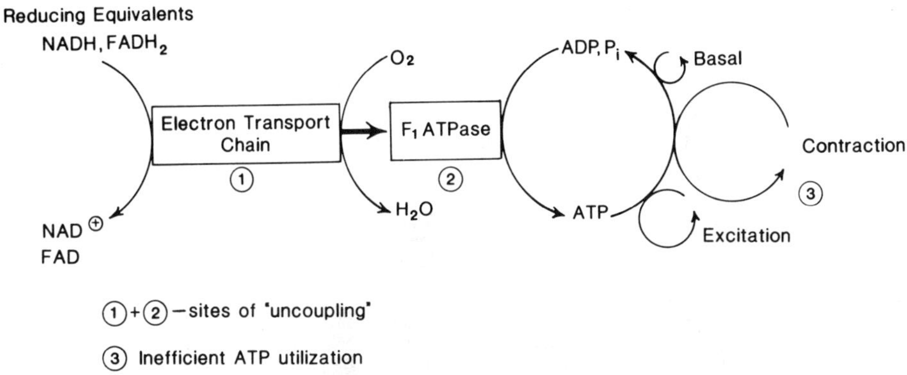

Figure 5 Schematic outline of oxidative-phosphorylation and the potential sources of increased MVO_2 in the postischemic heart. (1) The electron transport chain where classical uncouplers such as dinitrophenol exert their effect. (2) ATP synthetase (F_1 ATPase) where changes resulting in inefficient use of the transmitochondrial proton gradient per mole of ATP could produce uncoupling. (3) The partitioning of ATP utilization between basal, excitation, and contraction processes. An increase in ATP consumption at any of these sites would cause increased MVO_2 relative to mechanical activity.

proton gradient provides the coupling between the electron transport chain and the F_1 ATPase (ATP synthetase). To date, the only evidence for uncoupling of this nature after an ischemic-reperfusion injury is the observation of increased MVO_2. Most studies of isolated mitochondria from myocardium subjected to an ischemic-reperfusion insult have not shown significant uncoupling. The observation that MVO_2 was not different from normal in postischemic myocardium during KCL arrest argues against a fixed degree of uncoupling as the explanation for increased postischemic MVO_2 (Laster et al., 1989). However, the possibility that uncoupling may be proportional to MVO_2 and therefore not evident at lower MVO_2 values cannot be excluded from the above observations.

Using the nuclear magnetic resonance (NMR) spectroscopic method termed saturation transfer, it is possible to determine the unidirectional rate of oxidative ATP synthesis (Pi to ATP) over the range of MVO_2 obtained in the beating heart (Kingsley-Hickman et al., 1990; Sako et al., 1988). When the portion of the observed rate due to other Pi $\rightarrow$ ATP exchanges was taken into account (Sako et al., 1988) (Fig. 6), the P:O ratio (moles of ATP produced to moles of oxygen consumed) was unchanged after 18 minutes of no-flow, normothermic ischemia. These hearts exhibited significant contractile dysfunction as well as increased MVO_2 relative to mechanical performance. Increases

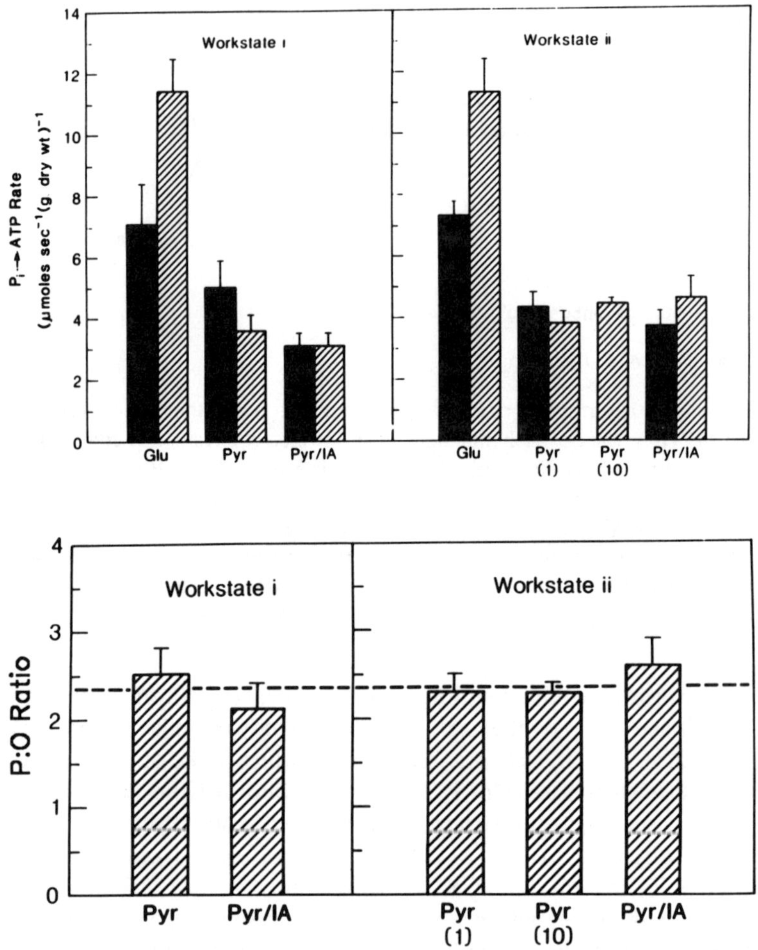

Figure 6 Upper panel: NMR-determined Pi to ATP exchange for glucose (Glu), pyruvate (Pyr), and pyruvate + iodoacetate (Pyr/IA). Solid and hatched bars represent control and postischemic data, respectively. Note the large contribution to the NMR-determined Pi to ATP rate in glucose perfused hearts, especially in the postischemic hearts. This is due to rapid exchange via glyceraldelyde 3-phosphate dehydrogenase and phosphoglycerate kinase. When this is eliminated with pyruvate perfusion or low-dose iodoacetate, a true estimate of the net forward rate of ATP synthesis is possible. Lower panel: NMR-derived P:O ratio in intact postischemic hearts. The dashed line represents the mean P:O ratio (Pi to ATP rate/MVO) observed for nonischemic hearts over a wide range of MVO_2. The mean postischemic P:O ratio was unchanged from nonischemic hearts. (With permission of Sako et al., 1988.)

in mechanical function and MVO_2 produced by inotropic stimulation with dobutamine in the postischemic hearts caused no change in the observed P:O ratio. These data indicate that uncoupling of MVO_2 from ATP synthesis is unlikely to contribute significantly to the increased MVO_2 in postischemic myocardium. In addition, augmentation of MVO_2 associated with beta-adrenergic inotropic agents in the postischemic myocardium is not the result of uncoupling.

2. Inefficient ATP Utilization by the Postischemic Myocardium

a. Alterations in Basal MVO_2. As uncoupling is not the mechanism for increased postischemic MVO_2, inappropriately high ATP utilization for a given level of mechanical function appears to be the proximate cause of relative elevation of MVO_2. As mentioned previously, although MVO_2 was inappropriately increased in the working postischemic heart, MVO_2 during KCL arrest was not different from normal hearts (Laster et al., 1989). MVO_2 during KCL arrest is accounted for primarily through ATP utilization in various basal metabolic processes, including fatty acid activation, protein synthesis, and basal transmembrane ionic transport activity. Although a small amount of Ca^{2+} cycling continues (Burkhoff et al., 1990), Na^+, K^+-ATPase, Ca^{2+}-ATPase, and myosin ATPase activities are markedly reduced. This observation indicates that increased postischemic MVO_2 is not due to increased basal metabolic needs or reparative processes.

b. Alterations in Ca^{2+} Homeostasis. The well-described abnormalities in intracellular Ca^{2+} dynamics after an ischemic-reperfusion injury are a potential source of increased MVO_2. In particular, increased diastolic calcium (Steenbergen et al., 1987; Stern et al., 1989; Weiss et al., 1990), increased activator calcium (Kusuoka et al., 1987), and decreased Ca^{2+} sensitivity of the contractile apparatus (Kusouka et al., 1990) may potentially make ATP utilization more inefficient by increasing sarcoplasmic reticulum Ca^{2+}-ATPase activity. In isolated postischemic hearts, low extracellular $[Na^+]$ during ischemia or low extracellular $[Ca^+]$ during reperfusion lessen the ischemic reperfusion injury presumably by decreasing reperfusion Ca^{2+} entry (Koomen et al., 1983; Renlund et al., 1984; Kusuoka et al., 1987; Weiss et al., 1990). However, the relationship between interventions that lessen Ca^{2+} entry in the postischemic myocardium and potential alterations in MVO_2 remains unexplored. The presence of unchanged pressure volume area independent MVO_2, despite a decrease in contractile force in the postischemic canine heart, has also been used to support the concept of altered Ca^{2+} dynamics as a source of increased MVO_2 (Ohgshi et al., 1991) (see Fig. 3). When isolated, nonischemic hearts are perfused at low sodium concentrations, diastolic pressure rises while developed pressure and high-energy phosphate levels fall; surprisingly, MVO_2 remains near baseline levels (Renlund et al., 1985). These effects are significantly blunted if extracellular Ca^{2+} is reduced or release of calcium from the sarcoplasmic reticulum is inhibited with ryanodine.

These observations suggest that alterations in intracellular calcium dynamics may be a source of the increased MVO_2 in postischemic hearts. It remains unclear, however, whether the presumed increase in the sarcoplasmic reticulum Ca^{2+}-ATPase activity in postischemic myocardium accounts for a significant portion of the observed increase in MVO_2. Since Ca^{2+}-ATPase activity cannot be measured in vivo, it is difficult to estimate its contribution to increased MVO_2. The importance of perturbations of calcium dynamics would be supported by demonstrating that the time course of the altered intracellular Ca^{2+} dynamics parallels the time course of inefficient ATP (MVO_2) utilization. In general, most observations of altered calcium dynamics have been continued for approximately 1–2 hours following reperfusion. Thus, there is a correlation between early postischemic contractile dysfunction, elevated MVO_2, and altered calcium dynamics. However, one index of altered intracellular Ca^{2+} dynamics, SLIF (scattered light intensity fluctuations, a measure of diastolic calcium cycling), appears to return to normal levels 30 minutes after reperfusion (Weiss et al., 1990), at a time when contractile function and MVO_2 remain abnormal. Despite the appealing hypothesis of altered calcium dynamics as a source of increased MVO_2, there is a paucity of data past the immediate postreperfusion period correlating the time course of recovery of calcium dynamics with more efficient MVO_2. The increased mismatch between load-independent postischemic MVO_2 and contractile function observed in the canine heart attributed to altered calcium dynamics (Ohgoshi et al., 1991) (see Fig. 3) can also potentially arise from inefficiencies in cross-bridge ATP utilization, since the cross-bridges are actively cycling in the unloaded ventricle.

Using butanedione monoxime (BDM) as a negative inotropic agent, we observed no difference in MVO_2 between normal and postischemic hearts when contractile activity was inhibited (Zimmer et al., 1988b). Prior to the administration of BDM, postischemic hearts exhibited increased MVO_2 relative to normal hearts. Figure 7 shows the relationship between normal and postischemic MVO_2 at several workstates (heart rate, end-diastolic pressure, and dobutamine concentration) during BDM infusion and compares these values with values obtained during KCL arrest in a different group of hearts. There was no significant difference in MVO_2 when contraction was inhibited with BDM over a wide range of workstates. During BDM infusion, the absolute values of MVO_2 for both normal and postischemic hearts were significantly higher than those observed during KCL arrest. With increasing workstate, MVO_2 values for normal and postischemic hearts remained similar.

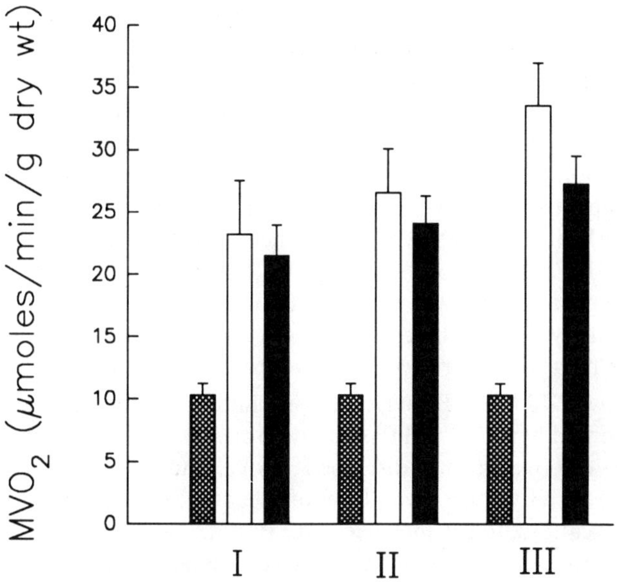

Figure 7 MVO_2 for normal (open bar) and postischemic (solid bar) hearts during infusion of BDM sufficient to reduce LV-developed pressure to less than 4 mmHg. I, II, and III refer to a series of progressively increasing workstates defined by pacing rate (300–600), EDP (8–16) and dobutamine (40–80 mg/ml perfusate). MVO_2 during KC1 arrest is included for reference (cross-hatched bar). MVO_2 at all workstates was not significantly different between normal and postischemic hearts. (From Zimmer et al., 1988b.)

In addition, less BDM was required to inhibit contraction in postischemic hearts than in normal hearts.

MVO_2 values are higher in BDM-perfused hearts than in KCL-arrested hearts despite the lack of contractile activity in both preparations. This occurs because BDM does not interfere with the action potential (Li et al., 1985; Blanchard et al., 1987). Rather, the major effect of BDM is the apparent desensitization of the contractile apparatus to Ca^{2+} (Ohkusa and Gwathmey, 1989; Gwathmey and Solaro, 1990; Blanchard et al., 1990; Marijic et al., 1991). In isolated papillary muscle, BDM has a variable effect on the calcium transient, which is in part dose dependent. At doses equivalent to those used in our study, an increase in the calcium transient was observed (Marijic et al., 1991).

These results indicate that increased Na^+, K^+-ATPase activity is unlikely to be the source of increased postischemic MVO_2. In addition, assuming that BDM has a similar effect in normal and postischemic myocardium and that the calcium transient is elevated in postischemic myocardium, these results also suggest that altered calcium dynamics are not the major source of inefficient ATP utilization in the postischemic myocardium. If altered Ca^{2+} dynamics and, hence, increased Ca^{2+}-ATPase activity were the major source of increased MVO_2, then MVO_2 values should have been higher than normal during BDM infusion in postischemic hearts. The observation that less BDM was required in postischemic hearts than in normal hearts to suppress contraction, particularly at the lowest workstate where mechanical function was similar, supports this conclusion and indicates that a substantial differential effect of BDM on the calcium transient between normal and postischemic hearts is unlikely. Thus, the results do not support alterations in Ca^{2+} dynamics as the principal source of increased postischemic MVO_2.

c. Alterations in Myosin ATPase Activity. After eliminating increases of basal MVO_2 and increased Na^+, K^+-ATPase activity as sources, and taking into account the BDM observations discussed above, increased myosin ATPase (cross-bridge) activity for a given level of mechanical performance becomes a more likely candidate for inefficient ATP utilization in the postischemic heart. No direct evidence exists to implicate this potential source. However, the increased MVO_2 in postischemic hearts is similar to findings in hyperthyroid rats (Wikman-Coffelt et al., 1985; Kissling and Rupp, 1986). In these animals, thyroid hormone causes transcription of a different myosin isozyme (V_1). This isozyme has a faster velocity; however, at a given level of force development, it consumes more oxygen. This presumably occurs because of increased cross-bridge turnover rate. The effect of inotropic stimulation on MVO_2 of the V_1 myosin isozyme is also similar to the effect of inotropic stimulation on postischemic MVO_2, i.e., MVO_2 is proportionally greater for a given level of mechanical performance. In postischemic hearts, transcription of a different myosin isozyme is unlikely to occur within the time frame of the observations of increased postischemic MVO_2. However, it is possible that alterations of the cross-bridges and the troponin-tropomyosin regulatory system result in increased cross-bridge cycling rates (and consequently ATP utilization) for a given level of tension development. A similar disassociation of ATP utilization from tension development has been observed in cardiac muscle during acidosis (Takayasu et al., 1990). While the intracellular pH in reperfused, reversibly injured hearts promptly normalizes (Zimmer et al., 1990), this phenomenon supports the possibility of a contractile apparatus origin for elevated postischemic MVO_2.

C. Summary

Increased MVO_2 relative to mechanical function is a distinct and predictable result of ischemic-reperfusion injury to the myocardium. Longer durations of reversible ischemic reperfusion injury increase the disparity between MVO_2 and mechanical function. Under normothermic conditions, there is a close association between the presence of mechanical dysfunction and increased MVO_2. The degree of disparity is also influenced by the inotropic state; the administration of inotropic agents causes an initial increase in MVO_2 out of proportion to the increase in mechanical function. Higher concentrations of inotropic agents may improve the coupling between MVO_2 and mechanical function. In the range where increased MVO_2 has been observed, this observation implies that adequate oxygen delivery is preserved. However, maximal MVO_2 in postischemic hearts is limited by a reduction in maximal oxidative capacity by the mitochondria. This injury, along with altered Ca^{2+} sensitivity of the contractile apparatus, determines the degree of maximal postischemic mechanical function.

The mechanisms responsible for the elevated MVO_2 in myocardial ischemic-reperfusion injury are unknown. It is not secondary to mitochondrial uncoupling or increased ATP utilization by noncontractile, nonionic processes. While calcium dynamics are altered in the postischemic myocardium and calcium overload in nonischemic hearts can produce increased MVO_2, observations with the negative inotropic agent, butadione monoxime, indicate that the alterations of sarcoplasmic reticulum Ca^{2+}-ATPase activity are unlikely to be the important source of increased MVO_2. Rather, inefficient ATP utilization by the contractile apparatus is the most likely candidate responsible for increased MVO_2 in the postischemic myocardium.

A unifying hypothesis regarding these observations is that the ischemic-reperfusion insult alters the Ca^{2+} sensitivity of the contractile regulatory proteins and may also affect myosin ATPase activity such that there is an increased ratio of MVO_2 to force generation in the postischemic myocardium as well as reduced force development. Further investigation is needed to clarify the relationship between the time course of altered calcium dynamics and elevated MVO_2 and to examine the possibility that myosin ATPase activity relative to tension development may be altered in the postischemic heart. Finally, the mechanisms responsible for production of the injury leading to elevated MVO_2 need to be more throughly characterized.

II. CARBON SUBSTRATE METABOLISM

A. Metabolism in the Normal and Ischemic Myocardium

Carbon substrate metabolism refers to the series of biochemical pathways from membrane transport to the production of ATP by glycolytic or oxidative means utilizing the carbon skeleton of long-chain fatty acids, glucose, and glycolytic intermediates such as lactate. In the normal heart, substrate preference is observed; nonesterified fatty acids (NEFA) (e.g., palmitate) are the predominant source of acetyl coenzyme A (CoA) entering the tricarboxylic acid (TCA) cycle (Neely et al., 1974). Under conditions of high arterial lactate concentrations as during strenuous exercise, the myocardium will preferentially utilize lactate at the expense of NEFA (Drake-Holland, 1983). Glycolytic activity under normal in vivo perfusion conditions is minimal and not a major source of ATP synthesis.

During ischemia, characteristic changes occur in glucose and NEFA metabolism with concomitant changes in the relative contributions of oxidative phosphorylation and glycolysis to ATP synthesis. With a mild reduction of coronary flow (20–25%), oxidative phosphorylation and, presumably, NEFA utilization continue, but the rate of both is limited by the absolute rate of oxygen delivery (Whitmer et al., 1978; Owen et al., 1990). High energy phosphates [creatine phosphate (CP) and ATP] decline to 40–50% of normal values, with CP showing delayed recovery (Pantley et al., 1990). Glycolytic activity is roughly proportional to the degree of flow reduction and, given sufficient perfusate glucose concentration, is derived not from glycogenolysis but from membrane transport (Owen et al., 1990). Little, if any, glucose enters the TCA cycle, so that ATP production from glucose is anaerobic. Mechanical function in this domain of mild ischemia is reduced, but net transmural systolic shortening continues to occur (Pantley et al., 1991).

With progressive reductions in flow (>50–60%) or oxygen delivery (i.e., hypoxia), oxidative phosphorylation and mechanical activity cease. Activated long-chain NEFA intermediates (acyl CoA and acyl carnitine CoA) accumulate via inhibition of beta-oxidation. There is concomitant breakdown and reesterification of intracellular triglycerides, which accelerates the hydrolysis of ATP and contributes to the increasing intracellular acidosis (Trach et al., 1986). The consequences of accumulation of NEFA metabolites prior to beta-oxidation include increased arrhythmogenesis (Corr et al., 1982), membrane injury secondary to detergent effects (Corr et al., 1984), relative inhibition of important intracellular enzymes (Devaux et al., 1975; Adams et al., 1979), and possible amplification of free radical-associated reperfusion injury via lipid peroxidation (Grisham and McCord, 1986). Inhibition of carnitine palmitoyl transferase I (CPT I) with oxyfenicine reduces the accumulation of NEFA intermediates and improves mechanical function during low-flow ischemia (Liedtke et al., 1987; Molaparast-Saless et al., 1987). The improvement seen in mechanical function with oxyfenicine may also be related to increased activation of pyruvate dehydrogenase with consequent increased formation of acetyl CoA from glycolysis (Liedtke et al., 1987).

During severe ischemia, high energy phosphates progressively decline despite ongoing glycolysis. The source of glucose is entirely from glycogenolysis (Owen et al., 1990). The cessation of glycolysis occurs when sufficient lactate is accumulated and is associated with the onset of ischemic contracture (Zimmer et al., 1989; Kingsley-Hickman et al., 1990). Glycolytic activity during moderate to severe ischemia is not sufficient to maintain contractile function in the absence of oxidative phosphorylation. However, the proximity of glycolytic enzymes to the sarcolemma and cross-bridges likely facilitates ATP delivery to prevent rigor bond formation leading to contracture and maintain cellular ionic homeostasis via continued membrane ATPase activity (Weiss and Hiltbrand, 1985). In general during ischemia, contractile activity is preferentially supplied by residual oxidative phosphorylation while glycolysis preferentially supports ATP utilization by the membrane ATPases.

B. Metabolism in the Postischemic Myocardium

When flow is restored to the ischemic myocardium, there is a brief initial period when ATP synthesis is dependent on anaerobic glycolysis. Within 1–2 minutes, oxidative phosphorylation becomes the major source of ATP synthesis (Görge et al., 1991). With more severe ischemia, the delay in resumption of oxidative phosphorylation may be substantially longer (Görge et al., 1991). Ultimately, the metabolic hallmark of reversibly injured myocardium is the ability to resume oxidative phosphorylation. In areas of the myocardium in which flow is only restored to a limited degree, glycolysis may maintain viability without restoration of mechanical activity (“hibernating myocardium”).

1. Postischemic Fatty Acid Metabolism

There is general agreement from traditional biochemical methods and positron emission tomography (PET) that NEFA are the preferred substrate in postischemic myocardium (Mickle et al., 1986; Myears et al., 1987; Liedtke et al., 1988). In contrast to normal myocardium, the preference for NEFA in the postischemic myocardium may continue in spite of high arterial lactate concentrations (Mickle et al., 1986). The reduced clearance in reperfused myocardium of positron-labeled palmitate is not necessarily indicative of impaired utilization but may reflect increased turnover of the endogenous lipid pool and preferential incorporation of exogenous lipid substrate into triglyceride in the reperfused heart (Lopaschuk et al., 1990; Görge et al., 1991). In addition, certain methodological restraints such as incorporation of label into non-NEFA pathways or an increased back diffusion of unlabeled substrate may accentuate the persistence of $1\text{-}^{11}C$ palmitate in reperfused myocardium (Fox et al., 1985; Rosamond et al., 1987).

The NEFA metabolites accumulated in the myocardium during ischemia are preferentially utilized upon reperfusion (Lopashuk et al., 1990). Triglycerides are unchanged from the preischemic state (Lopashuk et al., 1990).

The level of fatty acid intermediates shortly after reperfusion is variable; in one study the absence of elevated fatty acid intermediates after one hour of reperfusion did not alleviate mechanical dysfunction (Liedtke et al., 1988). Conversely, increasing the concentration of fatty acid perfusing the myocardium above nominal physiological concentrations did not worsen mechanical dysfunction during ischemia or after reperfusion, but did reduce function during aerobic perfusion (Liedtke et al., 1988).

An inhibitor of CPT 1, sodium 2-[5-(4-chlorophenyl)-pentyl] oxirane-2-carboxylate (POCA), given before the onset of ischemia, was shown to reduce mechanical dysfunction during ischemia and also reduced postischemic mechanical dysfunction in parallel with reductions in accumulated fatty acid intermediates (Paulson et al., 1986). Another inhibitor of CPT I, etomoxir, given in low concentrations (10^{-9} M) during reperfusion, was shown to decrease postischemic fatty acid intermediates without improving mechanical function (Lopaschuk et al., 1988). In a higher concentration (10^{-6} M) given during reperfusion, etomoxir caused an increase in fatty acid intermediates but a significant improvement in mechanical performance (Lopashuk et al., 1990). It should be noted that the higher concentration of etomoxir (10^{-6} M) is much greater than the concentration necessary to inhibit CPT I. Its effects on postischemic mechanical function at this concentration may be related to other properties of the agent unrelated to its effects on lipid metabolism.

It is apparent from the above observations that the accumulation of fatty acid intermediates during ischemia reduces mechanical function during ischemia and that these accumulations may participate in the injury of reperfusion as well. It is less clear that residual accumulations of these intermediates early after reperfusion affect postischemic mechanical function. In fact, inhibitor studies suggest that postischemic extramitochondrial accumulation of these intermediates can be disassociated from mechanical dysfunction. Finally, it should be noted that substantial postischemic mechanical dysfunction occurs in isolated hearts supplied with nonlipid substrates as well (Zimmer et al., 1989).

2. Postischemic Glucose and Glycolytic Intermediate Metabolism

While there exists general agreement regarding the preference of the postischemic myocardium for NEFA, there are differing results regarding the activity of the glycolysis and delivery of acetyl CoA into the TCA cycle from the glycolytic pathway. Studies using positron emission tomography have identified increased glucose uptake (via the uptake of fluorodeoxy-glucose, which is transported, phosphorylated via hexokinase, but not metabolized further) in postischemic, reversibly injured myocardium (Schwaiger et al., 1985a). This increased uptake may persist for days after a severe insult (Schwaiger et al., 1985b). In another open-chested canine model, the glycolytic contribution to acetyl CoA formation in reperfused myocardium was approximately twice as much as in normal myocardium (Myears et al., 1987). However, palmitate oxidation still accounted for the preponderance of substrate utilized. In contrast, acetyl CoA contributed from glycolysis (measured by the production of labeled CO_2 for one hour after reperfusion in the presence of adequate arterial concentrations of fatty acids) revealed no increased contribution of glycolytic activity to aerobic ATP production in an open-chest porcine model (Renstrom et al., 1989).

These observations are not necessarily at variance, since increased glucose uptake does not necessarily imply increased production of acetyl CoA from glucose. Restoration of intracellular glycogen stores, increased production of glycerol for triglyceride synthesis, increased hexose monophosphate shunt activity for generation of adenine nucleotides, and restoration of reduced glutathione levels could also increase glucose utilization. The extent of activity in each of these pathways in postischemic myocardium is unknown. The nutritional state of the animal (fed vs. fasting) significantly influences postischemic glucose uptake, with fasted animals showing unchanged rates of glucose uptake from the preischemic state and fed animals showing significant decreases in glucose uptake (Schneider et al., 1991). Finally, several studies have noted an increased contribution of glycolysis early after reperfusion (up to 30 min) (Lopaschuk et al., 1990; Görge et al., 1991). Within an hour, however, glucose oxidation rates become significantly less and are similar to preischemic values.

As mentioned previously, increased postischemic arterial lactate concentrations do not shift metabolism from fatty acid to lactate utilization in the intact heart. Similarily, de novo lactate and pyruvate utilization is reduced and parallels the reduction in the glycolytic contribution to acetyl CoA production (Renstrom et al., 1990a). When fatty acid utilization is blocked with oxyfenicin, pyruvate oxidation increases to levels similar to nonblocked palmitate perfused hearts. This indicates that metabolic flux through pyruvate dehydrogenase is dynamic and does not limit glycolytic flux due to alterations in enzyme function in the postischemic myocardium (Renstrom et al., 1990b). In isolated crystalloid perfused rat hearts, glucose, lactate, and pyruvate can be metabolized in the postischemic myocardium in the absence of exogenous fatty acid. Substrates such as pyruvate or lactate introduced at the time of reperfusion are not associated with improvement in mechanical function (S. Zimmer and K. Sipprell, unpublished). However, isolated rat hearts perfused with pyruvate-glucose or lactate prior to no-flow ischemia or during low-flow ischemia exhibit less mechanical impairment after reperfusion than hearts perfused with palmitate or glucose (Machizuki and Neely, 1980; Bünger et al., 1986; Zimmer et al., 1988a, 1989). In addition, hearts perfused with these substrates exhibit less impairment in oxidative function after an ischemic insult sufficient to induce contracture in glucose-insulin or palmitate-perfused hearts (Zimmer et al., 1989). Both of these glycolytic intermediates may act by reducing fatty acid accumulation during ischemia (Fritz and Kaplan, 1961; Bielefeld et al., 1985; Liedtke et al., 1987). Pyruvate as an alpha-keto acid may act as a free-radical scavenger, thereby reducing any contribution from oxygen-based injury. In addition, perfusion with pyruvate during low-flow ischemia or prior to ischemia appears to modulate the rate of glycolytic activity so that glycolysis continues for a longer duration (Bünger et al., 1986; Zimmer et al., 1989). This longer duration of glycolysis may reduce subsequent mechanical dysfunction by maintaining Na^+-K^+-ATPase activity, thus decreasing Na^+ uptake and thereby decreasing Ca^{2+} uptake upon reperfusion.

3. Methodological Considerations

Most metabolic studies of the heart are time-averaged and therefore may not detect rapidly changing events. This may be especially important in the beginning stages of reperfusion. In terms of mechanical recovery, there is an initial period of several minutes where contractile function is partially restored, an intermediate period of 20–30 minutes until steady-state conditions are observed, and a chronic period of hours to days until complete recovery is obtained. The above metabolic studies primarily address the intermediate period, with some attention directed toward the initial period. Further work is needed to explore the chronic period of postischemic dysfunction in order to understand substrate metabolism in reperfused myocardium and the events that lead to complete recovery. Part of the apparent discrepancy in results between PET methodology and radioactive tracer studies may result from the relative temporal insensitivity of PET.

An additional consideration is that most metabolic studies of the regionally postischemic myocardium spatially average their observations, particularly in the transmural dimension. Because of inhomogenities of perfusion and metabolic demand, the ischemic-reperfusion injury, particularly for lesser degrees of insult, is likely to be nonuniform across the left ventricular wall (Allison et al., 1977; Fiolet et al., 1985). Methods that depend upon sampling the venous effluent or tracer methods such as PET cannot distinguish transmural gradients of metabolites. In addition, in PET studies regional wall motion abnormalities may prevent accurate assessment of underlying tissue tracer concentrations (Parodi et al., 1984). Myocardial biopsies can sample the entire wall but are inherently destructive. For rapidly metabolized metabolites such as creatine phosphate, biopsy methods underestimate the actual tissue content.

NMR spectroscopy has the ability to sample the myocardium transmurally. Figure 8 shows ^{31}P spectra obtained in an open-chest canine preparation be-

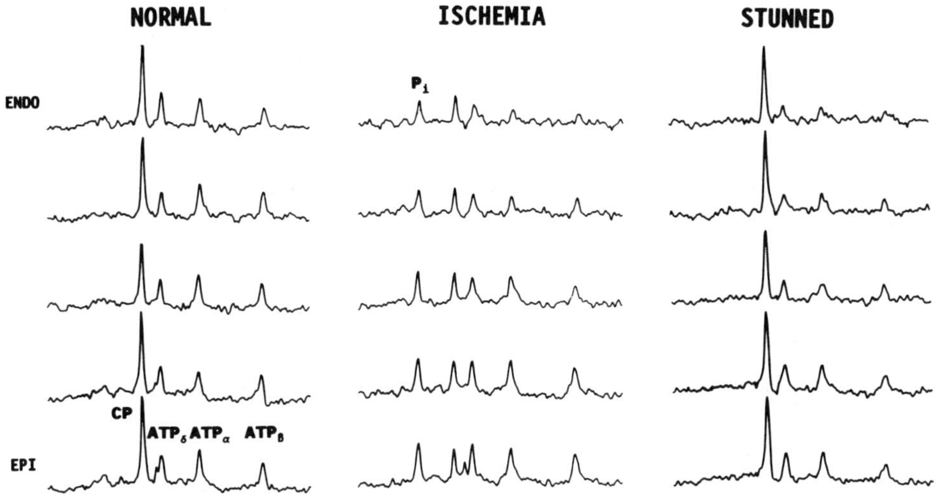

Figure 8 ^{31}P NMR spectra from five transmural left ventricular layers from epicardium (EPI) to endocardium (ENDO) of an open-chest anesthesized dog. Data were obtained during normal control conditions (NORMAL), during a severe coronary artery stenosis (ISCHEMIA), and during reperfusion following three 26-minute periods of coronary artery stenosis, which resulted in persistent systolic dysfunction (STUNNED). During normal conditions phosphocreatine (CP) and the three resonances of ATP were essentially uniform across the left ventricular wall, and inorganic phosphate (Pi) was not detected. Coronary occlusion was associated with depletion of phosphocreatine and, to a lesser degree, ATP, with appearance of a prominent resonance of inorganic phosphate. Following reperfusion, there was rapid repletion of phosphocreatine and disappearance of inorganic phosphate. However, ATP depletion persisted and was most marked in the deeper myocardial layers.

fore, during a severe coronary artery stenosis, and following reflow of the left anterior descending artery. The spectra demonstrate a transmural gradient for CP and ATP during ischemia and a gradient for ATP after ischemia. Figure 9 shows transmural 2-deoxyglucose uptake (as the phosphorylated metabolite) before, during, and after a coronary occlusion in an open-chest canine model. In normal hearts, glucose uptake is nonuniform with the greatest activity seen in the subendocardium. After reperfusion, uptake is enchanced across the entire wall but most elevated in the area of greatest metabolic injury in the subendocardium. Both NMR studies illustrate the heterogenous nature of the insult in the postischemic myocardium. The nonuniformity of metabolites and activity has major implications for the interpretation of metabolic studies in the postischemic myocardium. The ability of NMR spec-

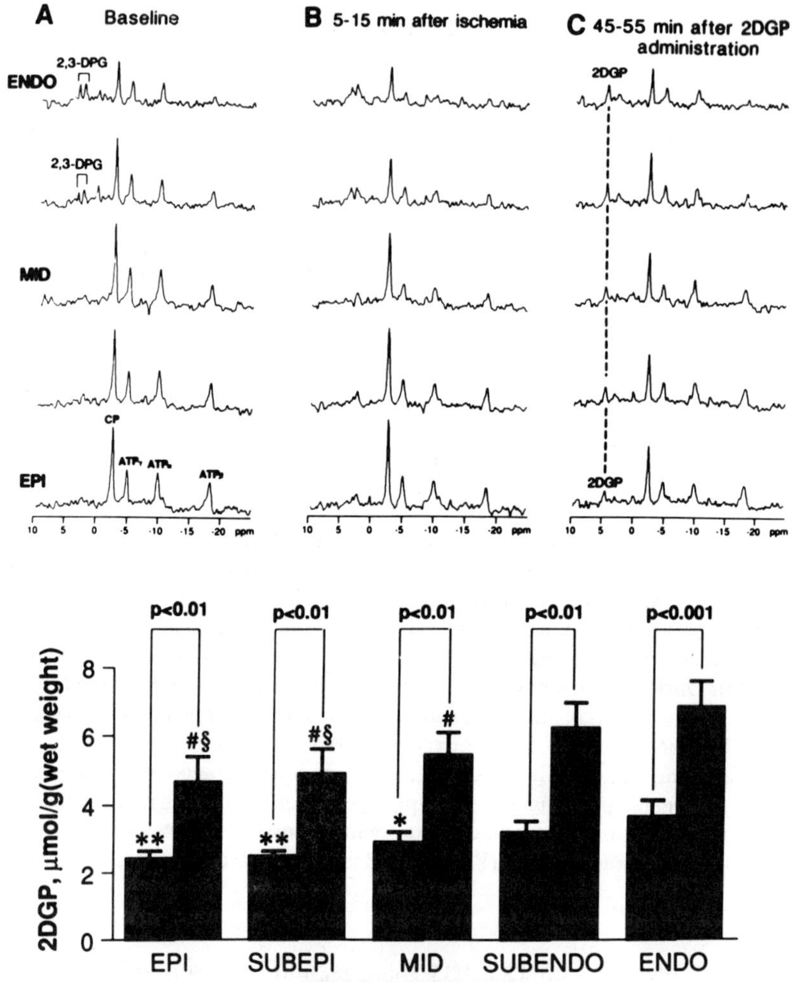

Figure 9 Upper panel: ^{31}P NMR spectra from five transmural left ventricular layers from epicardium (EPI) to endocardium (ENDO) of an open chest anesthesized dog. Data were obtained during normal conditions (A), 5–15 minutes after stenosis (B), and after reperfusion (C). 2-Deoxyglucose was infused after reperfusion (C) and its metabolite, 2-deoxyglucose 6-phosphate, is evident in all layers with the greatest accumulation in the innermost layers. 2, 3-DPG refers to 2, 3-diphosphoglycerate from erythrocytes at the endocardial surface. Lower panel: 2-Deoxyglucose 6-phosphate content (2-DGP) for normal (left bar of each pair) and postischemic hearts (right bar of each pair) from five transmural layers. In normal hearts, significantly greater uptake is evident in the innermost layer (ENDO;* $p < 0.05$, ** $p < 0.01$). In

troscopy to localize metabolic information transmurally and nondestructively with a high degree of sensitivity will be of value in determining the extent of injury and the course of recovery.

C. Summary

Despite profound ischemic-reperfusion injury to the myocardium, carbon substrate preference remains directed toward NEFA utilization. Although the accumulation of NEFA during ischemia is detrimental to function and appears to contribute to the injury, the presence of intracellular accumulations of fatty acid intermediates in the postischemic myocardium is not the cause of mechanical dysfunction. In contrast to the deleterious effects of fatty acids, the preischemic perfusion of pyruvate or lactate can reduce postischemic mechanical dysfunction. Similar to fatty acids, this effect is not seen if these substrates are given during reperfusion alone.

Apparent differences in postischemic glucose utilization can be attributed to limitations in the methodology involved (PET vs. labeled CO_2 production). The glycolytic contribution to oxidative ATP synthesis is minimal after restoration of steady-state postischemic mechanical function. However, in the initial period immediately after reperfusion, glycolysis may be an important source of ATP synthesis. Since PET studies have identified increased glucose uptake several days after an ischemic-reperfusion insult, additional studies are needed to better characterize the temporal course of glycolytic activity. In addition, since increased regional glycolytic activity by PET may reflect an area of limited oxygen availability as well as a recently reperfused area, it is important to characterize the metabolic fate of glucose in the postischemic myocardium. Specifically, it would be important to distinguish glycolytic activity leading to ATP synthesis from glucose utilization via increased hexose monophosphate shunt activity or glycogen synthesis.

The application of this information to human myocardial ischemic syndromes is just beginning. The major question to be addressed the the identification of viable from nonviable myocardium. PET methodology has provided the first link by demonstrating that viable but mechanically depressed myocardium can be identified by continuing uptake of glucose after a variety of ischemic conditions (Camici et al., 1986a,b; Schwaiger et al., 1986;

---

postischemic hearts, uptake of 2-DGP is significantly increased in each transmural layer ($p < 0.01$). 2-DGP uptake in postischemic hearts is also greatest in the two innermost layers (# $p < 0.01$ vs. ENDO of postischemic hearts; § $p < 0.01$ vs. SUBENDO of postischemic hearts). Thus, in normal hearts, transmural inhomogeneities exist in uptake of 2-DGP, and after ischemia and reperfusion these inhomogeneities are increased. (From Yoshiyama et al., 1990.)

Brunken et al., 1987; Hashimoto et al., 1988). Further advances in methodology, particularly NMR spectroscopy, hold promise for transmural identification of detailed metabolic information for clinical decision making.

ACKNOWLEDGMENT

This work was supported by NIH grants HL02014 (SDZ), HL20598 (RJB), and HL32427 (RJB).

REFERENCES

Acad, B. A., and Weiss, H. R. (1969). Regional O_2 consumption and coronary flow during beta-adrenoceptor stimulation in reperfused canine myocardium. *J. pharm. Exp. Ther. 250*: 611.

Adams, R. J., Cohen, D. W., Gupte, S., Johnson, J. D., Wallick, E. T., Wang T., and Schwartz, A. (1979a). "In vitro" effects of palmitoyl-carnitine on cardiac plasma membrane Na, K-ATPase and sarcoplasmic reticulum Ca^{2+}-ATPase and Ca^{2+} transport. *J. Biol. Chem. 254*: 12404.

Adams, R. J., Pitts, B. J. R., Wood, J. M., Gende, O. A., Wallick, E. T., and Schwartz, A. (1979b). Effects of palmitoyl-carnitine on ouabain binding to Na^+, K^+-ATPase. *J. Mol. Cell. Cardiol. 11*: 941.

Allison, T. B., Ramey, C. A., and Holsinger, J. W., Jr. (1977). Transmural gradients of left ventricular tissue metabolites after circumflex artery ligation in dogs. *J. Mol. Cell. Cardiol. 9*: 837.

Asimakis, G. K., and Conti, V. R. (1984). Myocardial ischemia: Correlation of mitrochondrial adenine nucleotide and respiratory function. *J. Mol. Cell. Cardiol. 16*: 439.

Bielefeld, D. R., Vary, T. C., and Neely, J. R. (1985). Inhibition of carnitine palmitoyl-CoA transferase activity and fatty acid oxidation by lactate and oxy fenicine in cardiac muscle. *J. Mol. Cell. Cardiol. 17*: 619.

Blanchard, E. M., and Alpert, N. R. (1987). The effects of isoproterenol, UDCG115, and caffeine on the heart related to excitation-contraction coupling in heart muscle. *Can. J. Physiol. Pharm. 65*: 659.

Blanchard, E. M., Smith, G. L., Allen, D. G., and Alpert, N. R. (1990). The effects of 2,3-butanedione monoxime on initial load tension and aequorin light output of ferret papillary muscles. *Pflugers Arch, 416*: 219.

Bolli, R., Patel, B. S., Hartley, C. J., Thornby, J. I., Jeroudi, M. O., and Roberts, R. (1989). Nonuniform transmural recovery of contractile function in stunned myocardium. *Am. J. Physiol. 257*: H375.

Brunken, B., Schwaiger, M., Grove, V., McKay, M., Phelps, N. E., Tillish, J., and Schelbert, H. R. (1987). Position emission tomography detects tissue metabolic activity in myocardial segments with persistent thallium perfusion defects. *J. Am. Coll. Cardiol. 10*: 557.

Bünger, R., Swindall, B., Brodie, D., Zdunek, D., Stieglen, H., and Walter, G. (1986). Pyruvate attenuation of hypoxia damage in isolated working guinea-pig heart. *J. Mol. Cell. Cardiol. 18*: 423.

Burkhoff, D., Kalil-Filho, R., and Gerstenblith, G. (1990). Oxygen consumption is less in rat hearts arrested by low calcium than by high potassium at fixed flow. *Am. J. Physiol. 259*: H1142.

Camici, P., Aranjo, L., Spinks, T., Lammertsma, A. A., Jones, T., and Maseri, A. (1986a). Myocardial glucose utilization in ischaemic heart disease: Preliminary results with F18-fluorodeoxyglucose and position emission tomography. *Eur. Heart J. 7*(Suppl C): 19.

Camici, P., Aranjo, L. I., Spinks, T., Lammertsma, A. A., Keoki, J. C., Shea, M. J., Selwyn, A. P., Jones, T. and Maseri, A. (1986b). Increased uptake of ^{18}F-fluoro deoxyglucose in postischemic myocardium of patients with exercise-induced angina. *Circulation 74*: 81.

Camici, P., Aranjo, L., Spinks, T., Lammertsma, A. A., Suhanpan, S. K., Jones, T., and Maseri, A. (1988). Prolonged metabolic recovery allows late identification of ischaemia in the absence of electrocardiographic and perfusion changes in patients with exertional angina. *Am. J. Cardiol. 61*(Suppl A): 131.

Corr, P. B., Gross, R. W., and Sobel, B. E. (1982). Arrhythmogenic amphiphilic lipids and the myocardial cell membrane. *J. Mol. Cell. Cardiol. 14*: 619.

Corr, P. B., Gross, R. W., and Sobel, B. E. (1984). Amphipathic metabolites and membrane dysfunction in ischemic myocardium. *Circ. Res. 54*: 135.

Devaux, P. S., Bienvenue, A., Lauquin, G., Brisson, A. D., Vignais, M., and Vignais, P. V. (1975). Interaction between spin-labeled acytl-coenzyme A and the mitochondrial adenosine diphosphate carrier. *Biochemistry 14*: 1272.

Drake-Holland, A. J. (1983). Substrate utilization. In *Cardiac Metabolism* (A. J. Drake-Holland and M. I. M. Noble, eds.), John Wiley, Chichester, England, pp. 201-204.

Edoute, Y., vanderMerwe E., Sanan, D., Kotze, J. C. N., Steinmann, C., and Lochner A. (1983). Normothermic ischemic cardiac arrest of the isolated working rat heart. Effects of time and reperfusion on myocardial ultrastructure, mitochondrial oxidative function, and mechanical recovery. *Circ. Res. 53*: 663.

Finney, R. S., DiNatale, J. M., and Gardner, T. J. (1990). Myocardial oxygen consumption (MVO_2) in regionally stunned myocardium. *Curr. Surg. 47*: 350.

Fiolet, J. W. T., Baartscheer, A., Schumaker, C. A., terWelle, H. F., and Kriegor, W. J. G. (1985). Transmural inhomogeneity of energy metabolism during acute global ischemia in the isolated rat heart: Dependence on environmental conditions. *J. Mol. Cell. Cardiol. 17*: 87.

Fritz, I. B., and Kaplan, F. (1961). Effects of glucose on palmitate esterification by isolated rat diaphragm. *Am. J. Physiol. 200*: 1047.

Fox, K. A. A., Abendschein, D. R., Ambos, H. D., Sobel, B. E., and Bergmann, S. R. (1985). Efflux of metabolized and nonmetabolized fatty acid from canine myocardium. Implications for quantifying myocardial metabolism tomographically. *Circ. Res. 57*: 232.

Görge, G., Chatelain, P., Schaper, J., and Lerch, R. (1991). Effect of increasing degrees of ischemic injury on myocardial oxidative metabolism early after reperfusion in isolated rat hearts. *Circ. Res. 68*: 1681.

Grisham, M. B., and McCord, J. (1986). Chemistry and cytotoxicity of reactive oxygen metabolities. In *Physiology of Oxygen Radicals* (A. E. Taylor, S. Matalon, and P. Ward, eds.), American Physiological Society, Bethesda, MD, p. 4.

Gwathmey, J. K., and Solaro, R. J. (1990). Effects of 2,3-butanedione monoxime on [Ca^{2+}] and myofilament responsiveness. *Biophys. J. 57*: 528a.

Hashimoto, T. Kambara, H., Fudo, T., Hayashi, M., Tamaki, S., Tokunaga, S., Tamaki, N., Yonekwa, Y., Konishi, J., and Kawai, C. (1988). Non-q wave versus q wave myocardial infarction: Regional myocardial metabolism and blood flow assessed by positron emission tomography. *J. Am. Coll. Cardiol. 12*: 88.

Jeremy, R. W., Stahl, L., Gillinor, M., Litt, M., Aversano, T. R., and Becker, L. C. (1989). Preservation of coronary flow reserve in stunned myocardium. *Am. J. Physiol. 256*: H1303.

Kingsley-Hickman, P. B., Sako, E. Y., Ugurbil, K., From, A. H. L., and Foker, J. E. (1990). ^{31}P NMR measurements of mitochondrial uncoupling in isolated rat hearts. *J. Biol. Chem. 265*: 1545.

Kissling, G., and Rupp, H. (1986). The influence of myosin isoenzyme pattern on increase in myocardial oxygen consumption induced by catecholamines. *Basic Res. Cardiol. 81*(Suppl 1): 103.

Koomen, J. M., Schevers, J. A. M., and Noordhock, J. (1983). Myocardial recovery from global ischemia and reperfusion: Effects of pre- and/or post-ischemic perfusion with low- Ca^{2+}. *J. Mol. Cell. Cardiol. 15*: 383.

Krukenkamp, I., Silverman, N., Sorlie, D., Pridjian, A., Feinberg, H., and Levitsky, S. (1986). Oxygen utilization during isovolumic pressure-volume loading: Effects of prolonged extracorporal circulation and cardioplegic arrest. *Ann. Thorac. Surg. 41*: 407.

Kusuoka, H., Porterfield, J. K., Weisman, H. F., Weisfeldt, M. L., and Marban, E. (1987). Pathophysiology and pathogenesis of stunned myocardium. Depressed Ca^{2+} activation of contraction as a consequence of reperfusion-induced cellular calcium overload in ferret hearts. *J. Clin. Invest. 79*: 950.

Kusuoka, H., Koretsune, Y., Chacko, V. P., Weisfeldt, M. L., and Marban, E. (1990). Excitation-contraction coupling in post-ischemic myocardium. Does failure of activation Ca^{2+} transients underlie stunning? *Circ. Res. 66*: 1268.

Laster, S. B., Becker, L. C., Ambrosio, G., and Jacobus, W. E. (1989). Reduced aerobic metabolic efficiency in globally "stunned" myocardium. *J. Mol. Cell. Cardiol. 21*: 419.

Laxson, D. D., Homans, D. C., Dai, X-Z., Sublett, E., and Bache, R. J. (1989). Oxygen consumption and coronary reactivity in postischemic myocardium. *Circ. Res. 64*: 9.

Lee, H-C., Smith, N., Mohabir, R., and Clusin, W. T. (1987). Cytosolic calcium transients from the beating mammalian heart. *Proc. Natl. Acad. SCI. USA 84*: 7793.

Lekven, J., Brusting, L. A., Jessen, M. E., Abd-Elfattah, A. S., Doherty, N. E. III., and Wechslev, A. S. (1988). Myocardial oxygen use during epinephrine administration to ischemically injured canine hearts. *Circulation* Suppl. III *78*: 125.

Li T., Sperelakis, N., Teneick, R. E., Solaro, R. J. (1985). Effect of diacetyl monoxime on cardiac excitation-contraction coupling. *J. Pharm. Exp. Ther. 232*: 688.

Liedtke, A. J., Miller, W. P., and Field, J. M. (1987). Modifying excess-fatty and metabolism in ischemic myocardium. In *Myocardial Metabolism* Vol 2: *Proceedings of the Sixth Joint USA-USSR Symposium*, (V. N. Smirnov and A. M. Katz eds.), Harwood Academic Publishers GmbH, Switzerland, p. 63.

Liedtke, A. J., DeMaison, L., Eggleston, A. M., Cohen, L. M., and Nellis, S. H. (1988). Changes in substrate metabolism and effects of excess fatty acids in reperfused myocardium. *Circ. Res. 62*: 535.

Lopaschuk, G. D., Wall, S. R., Olley, P. M., and Davies, N. J. (1988). Etomoxir, a carnitine palmitoyltransferase I inhibitor, protects hearts from fatty acid-induced ischemic injury independent of changes in long chain acylcarnitine. *Circ. Res. 63*: 1036.

Lopaschuk, G. D., Spafford, M. A., Davies, N. J., and Wall, S. R. (1990). Glucose and palmitate oxidation in isolated working rat hearts reperfused after a period of transient global ischemia. *Circ. Res. 66*: 546.

Marijic, J., Buljubasc, N., Stowe, D. F., Turner, L. A., Kampine, J. P., and Bosnjak, Z. J. (1991). Opposing effects of diacetyl monoxime on contractility and calcium transients in isolated myocardium. *Am. J. Physiol. 260*: H1153.

Mickle, D. A. G., del Nido, P. J., Wilson, G. J., Harding, R. D., and Bomaschin, A. D. (1986). Exogenous substrate preference of the post-ischaemic myocardium. *Cardiovasc. Res. 20*: 256.

Mochizuki, S., and Neely, J. R. (1980) Energy metabolism during reperfusion following ischemia. *J. Physiol., Paris, 76*: 805.

Molaparast-Saless, F., Liedtke, A. J., and Nellis, S. H. (1987). Effects of the fatty acid blocking agents, oxyfenicine and 4-bromocrotonic acid, on performance in aerobic and ischemic myocardium. *J. Mol. Cell. Cardiol. 19*: 509.

Mukherjee, A. L., Buja, M., Kulkayni, P., Nicav, M., Chien, K. R., and Willerson, J. T. (1982). Relationship of mitochondrial alterations and 99m Tc Pyrophosphate uptake during myocardial ischemia *Am. J. Physiol. 243*: H268.

Murphy, M. L., Peng, C. F., Kane, J. J. and Stranb, K. D. (1982). Ventricular performance and biochemical alteration of regional ischemic myocardium after reperfusion in the pig. *Am. J. Cardiol. 50*: 821.

Myears, D. W., Sobel, B. E., and Bergman, S. R. (1987). Substrate use in ischemic and reperfused canine myocardium: quantitative considerations. *Am. J. Physiol. 253*: H107.

Nakahara, T, and Takeo, S. (1986). Irreversible changes in oxidative phosphorylation activity of the mitochondrial membrane from hearts subjected to hypoxia and reoxygenation. *Can. J. Cardiol. 2*: 24.

Neely, J. R., and Morgan, H. E. (1974). Relationship between carbohydrate and lipid metabolism and the energy balance of heart muscle. *Ann. Rev. Physiol.* (J. H. Comroe, R. R. Sonnenschein, and K. L. Zierler, eds), Annual Reviews Inc., Palo Alto, CA, pp. 413-459.

Ohgoshi, Y., Goto Y., Futaki, S., Yaku, H., Kawaguchi, O., and Suga, H. (1991). Increased oxygen cost of contractility in stunned myocardium of dogs. *Circ. Res. 69*: 975.

Ohkusa, T., and Gwathmey, J. K. (1989). The effects of 2,3-butanedione monoxime on twitch force and steady-state force relationships in ferret papillary muscles. *Biophys. J. 55*: 100a.

Owen, P., Dennis, S., and Opie, L. H. (1990). Glucose flux rate regulates onset of ischemic contracture in globally underperfused rat hearts. *Circ. Res. 66*: 344.

Pantely, G. A., Malone, S. A., Rhen, W. S., Angelone, C. G., Arai, A., Bristow, J., and Bristow, J. D. (1990). Regeneration of myocardial phosphocreatine in pigs despite continued moderate ischemia. *Circ. Res. 67*: 1481.

Parodi, O., Schelbert, H. R., Schwaiger, M., Hansen, H., Selin, C., and Hoffman, E. J. (1984). Cardiac emission computed tomography underestimation of regional tracer concentrations due to wall motion abnormalities. *J. Comp. Asst. Tomog. 8*: 1083.

Paulson, D. J., Noonan, J. J., Ward, K. M., Stanley, H., Shevratt, A., and Shug, A. L. (1986). Effects of POCA on metabolism and function in the ischemic rat heart. *Bas. Res. Cardiol. 81*: 180.

Peng, C. F., Murphy, M. L., and Straub, K. D. (1986). Effects of early reperfusion on the mechanism and biochemical characteristics of ischemic myocardium. *J. Surg. Res. 41*: 493.

Renlund, D. G., Gerstenblith, G., Lakatta, E. G., Jacobus, W. E., Kallman, C. H., and Weisfeldt, M. L. (1984). Perfusate sodium during ischemia modifies postischemic functional and metabolic recovery in the rabbit heart. *J. Mol. Cell. Cardiol. 16*: 795.

Renlund, D. G., Lakatta, E. G., Mellits, E. D., and Gerstenblith, G. (1985). Calcium-dependent enhancement of myocardial diastolic tone and energy utilization dissociates systolic work and oxygen consumption during low sodium perfusion. *Circ. Res. 57*: 876.

Renstrom, B., Nellis, S. H., and Liedtke, A. J. (1989). Metabolic oxidation of glucose during early myocardial reperfusion. *Circ. Res. 65*: 1094.

Renstrom, B., Liedtke, A. J., and Nellis, S. H. (1990a). Mechanisms of substrate preference for oxidative metabolism during early myocardial reperfusion. *Am. J. Physiol. 259*: H317.

Renstrom, B., Nellis, S. H., and Liedtke, A. J. (1990b). Metabolic oxidation of pyruvate and lactate during early myocardial reperfusion. *Circ. Res. 66*: 282.

Rosamond, T. L., Abendschein, D. R., Sobel, B. E., Bergmann, S. R., and Fox, K. A. A. (1987). Metabolic fate of radiolabeled palmitate in ischemic canine myocardium: Implications for positron emission tomography. *J. Nucl. Med. 28*: 1322.

Rosamond, T. L., Abendschein, D. R., Sobel, B. E., Bergmann, S. R., and Fox, K. A. A. (1987). Metabolic fate of radiolabeled palmitate in ischemic canine myocardium: Implications for positron emission tomography. *J. Nucl. Med.* 28: 1322.

Sako, E. Y., Kingsley-Hickman, P. B., From, A. H. L., Foker, J. E., and Ugurbil K. (1988). ATP synthesis kinetics and mitochondrial function in the post ischemic myocardium as studied by ^{31}P NMR. *J. Biol. Chem. 263*: 10600.

Schneider, C. A., Nguyen, V. T. B., and Taegtmeyer, H. (1991). Feeding and fasting determine postischemic glucose utilization in isolated working rat hearts. *Am. J. Physiol. 260*: H542.

Schwaiger, M., Schelbert, H. R., Keen, R., Vinten-Johanson, J., Hansen, H., Selin, C., Barrio, J., Huang, S. C., and Phelps, M. E. (1985a). Retention and clearance of C-11 palmitic acid in ischemic and reperfused canine myocardium. *J. Am. Coll. Cardiol. 6*: 311.

Schwaiger, M., Schelbert, H. R., Ellison, D., Hansen, H., Yeatman, L., Vinten-Johnsen, J., Selin, C., Barrio, J., and Phelps, M. E. (1985b). Sustained regional abnormalities in cardiac metabolism after transient ischemia in the chronic dog model. *J. Am. Coll. Cardiol. 6*: 336.

Schwaiger, M., Brunken, R., Grover-McKay, M., Krivokapich, J., Child, J., Tillisch, J. H., Phelps, M., and Shelbert, H. R. (1986). Regional myocardial metabolism in patients with acute myocardial infarction assessed by position emission tomography. *J. Am. Coll. Cardiol. 8*: 800.

Schwaiger, M., Neese, R. A., Aranjo, L., Wyns, W., Wisnest, J. A., Sochov, H., Swank, S., Kulber, D., Selin, C., Phelps, M., Schelbert, H. R., Fishbein, M. C., and Gertz, E. W. (1989). Sustained nonoxidative glucose utilization and depletion of glycogen in reperfused canine myocardium. *J. Am. Coll. Cardiol. 13*: 745.

Shlafer, M., Kirsh, M., Lucchesi, B. R., Slater, A. P., and Warren, S. (1981). Mitochondrial function after global cardiac ischemia and reperfusion: Influences of organelle isolation protocols. *Basic Res. Cardiol. 76*: 250.

Stahl, L. D., Weiss, H. R., and Becker, L. C. (1988). Myocardial oxygen consumption, oxygen supply/demand heterogeneity, and microvascular patency in regionally stunned myocardium. *Circulation 77*: 865.

Steenbergen, C., Murphy, E., Levy, L., and London, R. E. (1987). Elevation in cytosolic free calcium concentration early in myocardial ischemia in perfused rat heart. *Circ. Res. 60*: 700.

Stern, M. D., Weisman, H. F., Renlund, D. G., Gerstenblith, G., Hano, O., Blank, P. S., and Lakatta, E. G. (1989). Laser backscatter studies of intracellular Ca^{2+} oscillations in isolated hearts. *Am. J. Physiol. 257*: H665.

Takayasu, T., Toyo-oka, T., and Hosocka, S. (1990). Waste of ATP for tension development in myocardial acidosis: Chemomechanical uncoupling at myofibrillar level. *J. Mol. Cell. Cardiol. 22*: 127.

Trach, V., Buschmans-Denkel, E., and Schaper, W. (1986). Relation between lipolysis and glycolysis during ischemia in the isolated rat heart. *Bas. Res. Cardiol. 81*: 454.

Upsher, M. E., Joselevitz, Goldman, J., and Weiss, H. R. (1988). Effect of reperfusion on O_2 supply/consumption balance in ischemic canine left ventricle. *Res. Exp. Med 188*: 377.

Wang, J-X., and Lee, N. K. (1990). Primary and secondary effects of 2,3-butanedione monoxime on Ca^{++}. *Biophys. J. 57*: 548a.

Weinstein, E. S., Spector, M. L., Adams, E. M., Yokum, M. D., Humphrey, R. W., and Fry, D. E. (1986). Mitochondrial and myocardial performance: Response to ischemia and reperfusion. *Arch. Surg. 121*: 324.

Weiss, J., and Hiltbrand, B. (1985). Functional compartmentation of glycolytic versus oxidative metabolism in isolated rabbit heart. *J. Clin. Invest. 75*: 436.

Weiss, R. G., Gerstenblith, G., and Lakatta, E. G. (1990). Calcium oscillations index the extent of calcium loading and predict functional recovery during reperfusion in rat myocardium. *J. Clin. Invest. 85*: 757.

Whitmen, J. T., Idell-Wenger, J. A., Poretto, M. J., and Neely, J. R. (1978). Control of fatty acid metabolism in ischemic and hypoxic hearts. *J. Biol. Chem. 253*: 4305.

Wikman-Coffelt, J., Sievers, R., and Parmely, W. W. (1985). Influence of myocardial isomyosins on cardiac performance and oxygen consumption. *Biochem. Biophys. Res. Comm. 130*: 1314.

Yoshiyama, M., Zhang, J., Path, G., Sipprell, K., Merkle, H., Garwood, M., From, A. H. L., Bache, R. J., and Ugurbil, K. (1990). Transmural high-energy phosphate distribution and glucose uptake in stunned myocardium. *Circulation 82* (Suppl III): 684.

Zimmer, S. D., Micharshi, S., Lew, B., Ugurbil, K., and From, A. H. L. (1988a). The protective effects of lactate on mechanical and oxidative function after global myocardial ischemia. Abstract from The Society for Magnetic Resonance in Medicine Meeting, 1988, San Francisco.

Zimmer, S. D., Mohanakrishnon, P., Sipprell, K., Ugurbil, K., and From, A. H. L. (1988b). The post-ischemic efficiency of myocardial oxygen utilization—mechanistic studies with diacetyl monoxime (DAM). Abstract from The Society for Magnetic Resonance in Medicine Meeting, 1988, San Francisco.

Zimmer, S. D., Ugurbil, K., Michurski, S. P., Mohanakrishnan, P., Ulstad, V. K., Foker, J. E., and From, A. H. L. (1989). Alterations in oxidative function and respiratory regulation in the post-ischemic myocardium. *J. Biol. Chem. 264*: 12402.

4

Stunned Myocardium in Models of Repeated Coronary Occlusion

Mengjia Zhao, Stephen M. Factor, and Calvin Eng

Albert Einstein College of Medicine, Bronx, New York

I. INTRODUCTION

The phenomenon of stunned myocardium was originally described in experimental canine studies of a single brief coronary occlusion. Prolonged depression of contractile function was observed despite restoration of coronary blood flow and absence of tissue necrosis (Heyndrickx et al., 1975; Braunwald and Kloner, 1982). Subsequently, repeated brief coronary occlusion models, among others, were utilized to study myocardial stunning (Nicklas et al., 1985; Becker et al., 1986; Zhao et al., 1987; Stahl et al., 1988). Although the total ischemic load is quite different, a similar degree of contractile dysfunction was found in all these models. In light of recent experimental evidence on the preconditioning effect of a brief coronary occlusion (Cohen and Downey, 1990, Murry et al., 1986, 1990), differences in myocardial metabolism and functional characteristics might be expected between a single occlusion model and a repeated occlusion model. In addition, several studies have demonstrated a dichotomy of systolic and diastolic dysfunction and heterogeneous, model-dependent structural changes in the stunned myocardium (Przyklenk et al., 1987, 1990; Zhao et al., 1987; Whittaker et al., 1991). Presently, the concept of myocardial stunning encompasses a wide variety of experimental and clinical settings with major pathophysiological and structural implications. Thus, our evolving understanding of the stunned myocardium, along with an increasing body of clinical and experimental data, necessitates a reevaluation of the standard definition and classification of this phenomenon (Bolli, 1990). In this chapter, our discussion will be focused on the dynamic changes in systolic function and passive properties of myocardium using the canine model of repeated coronary occlusion. Salient features distinctive from the single occlusion model will be evaluated with emphasis on structure-function implications.

II. SYSTOLIC DYSFUNCTION IN REPEATED CORONARY OCCLUSION MODEL

Regional contractile activity disappears completely within 10-15 seconds after coronary occlusion and is replaced by passive bulging of the ischemic segment (Tennant and Wiggers, 1935). If repeated episodes of coronary occlusion are followed by reperfusion, contractile behavior remains depressed despite complete restoration of myocardial flow and absence of tissue necrosis (Nicklas et al., 1985, Zhao et al., 1987). Changes in systolic function are characterized by an initial large decrement in systolic shortening of the ischemic segment after the first postocclusive reperfusion, with progressively smaller decrements in systolic shortening after subsequent occlusions (Fig. 1). The decrease in segmental shortening usually reaches a nadir during the third reperfusion period and remains essentially unchanged thereafter (Nicklas et al., 1985; Zhao et al., 1987; Cohen and Downey, 1990). Although the stunned myocardium can be recruited to contract almost normally by several interventions such as inotropic stimulation, postextrasystolic potentiation (Becker et al., 1986), or enhanced coronary blood flow (Stahl et al., 1986), the systolic dysfunction persists for at least 90 minutes after the final occlusion (Nicklas et al., 1985; Becker et al., 1986; Zhao et al., 1987). There have been no studies performed to define the long-term time course of systolic dysfunction in the repeated occlusion model. Systolic dysfunction lasting as long as 6 hours to 2 days after the restoration of blood flow has been characterized for the single 15-minute coronary occlusion model (Heyndrickx et al., 1975; Bolli et al., 1988; Charlat et al., 1989).

Several factors affect the degree of systolic dysfunction and the rate of functional recovery following repeated ischemic insults. The magnitude of depression is related to the length of the coronary occlusion period. A longer period of ischemia is associated with more severe depression of contractile behavior. Lange et al. (1984) noted that systolic shortening recovered to 60% of control baseline following three 5-minute coronary occlusions as compared to 37% recovery after three 15-minute occlusions. Coronary collateral flow has also been suggested as an important determinant of the degree of systolic dysfunction. In conscious dogs, residual systolic wall thickening 5 minutes following release of a 15-minute coronary occlusion is significantly correlated with collateral flow (Bolli et al., 1988). In the repeated coronary occlusion model, a significant correlation was also noted between collateral flow

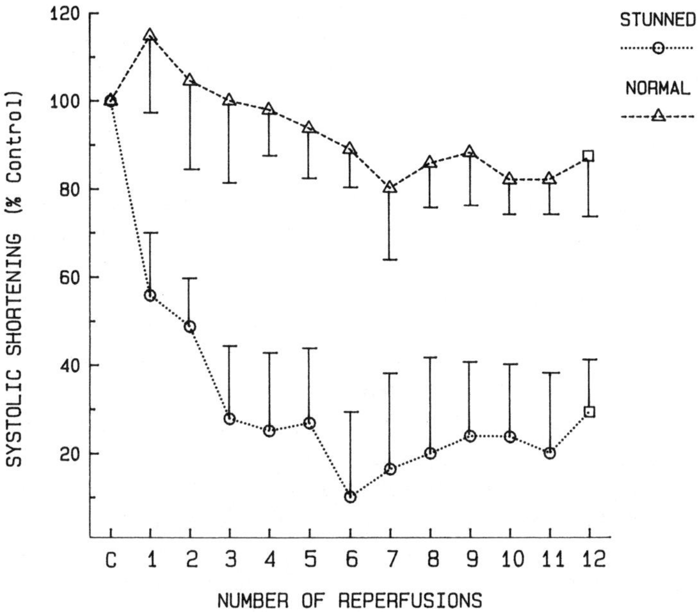

Figure 1 Percent systolic shortening for both normal and stunned regions. Results of contractile function during each reperfusion period is expressed as percent of the baseline. The percent systolic shortening of the stunned region is progressively decreased during the first three reperfusion periods and persists throughout the experiment. The normal zone shortening during the experimental protocol is not significantly different from the baseline. The 12th reperfusion (square) represents the data at the end of the final 90-minute reperfusion period. C, control measurement obtained at baseline. (Reproduced from Zhao et al., 1987, with permission of the American College of Cardiology.)

and the degree of systolic dysfunction following the initial 5-minute occlusion (Cohen and Downey, 1990). However, this correlation deteriorated during subsequent reperfusion periods, implying that other yet unidentified factors also influence the extent of myocardial stunning after the initial one or two reperfusion cycles.

The rate of functional recovery depends on the duration of the reperfusion periods separating the repeated brief occlusions (Wynsen et al., 1991). It is clear that sufficient time is needed for a complete functional recovery after a brief coronary occlusion. When the duration of reperfusion is 5–10 minutes, contractile function recovers incompletely, resulting in a cumulative deterioration of contractile function (Nicklas et al., 1985; Zhao et al., 1987; Cohen and Downey, 1990; Wynsen et al., 1991). If a longer reperfusion period is allowed, systolic shortening returns to near normal level in the ischemic region, and no cumulative effect can be demonstrated (Lange et al., 1984; Wynsen et al., 1991). With 15-minute reperfusion periods, the systolic function was essentially unchanged during the first through fourth reperfusion periods (Wynsen et al., 1991). Therefore, functional recovery correlates positively with the duration of the reperfusion interval.

The relationship between functional recovery and duration of the reperfusion interval could have a biochemical basis. For example, Swain et al. (1984) found that three 12-minute occlusions separated by 10-minute reperfusion did not produce a cumulative depletion of high energy phosphate compounds in the ischemic myocardium. This finding was supported by the study of Reimer et al. (1986), in which four 10-minute coronary occlusions, separated by 20-minute reperfusion, caused no cumulative ATP loss or tissue necrosis. In contrast, Geft et al. (1982) demonstrated a cumulative effect of repeated coronary occlusions in dog heart. Animals were subjected to as many as 18 5, 10, or 15-minute coronary occlusions. More severe tissue injury was associated with longer coronary occlusion time and greater number of occlusions. Patchy subendocardial necrosis was noted in a greater percentage of animals with 15-minute (29%) and 10-minute occlusions (24%) as compared to 9% of animals with 5-minute occlusions. Later studies using 10–16 5-minute coronary occlusions to produce myocardial stunning have not found evidence of tissue necrosis (Nicklas et al., 1985; Zhao et al., 1987; Stahl et al., 1988).

The degree of dyskinesia during occlusion may have an influence on subsequent systolic dysfunction. In a retrospective analysis of the various factors that may potentially affect systolic dysfunction, Przyklenk and Kloner (1989) found that the degree of dyskinesia correlated significantly with functional recovery. In contrast, several hemodynamic factors, including heart rate, aortic pressure, and myocardial blood flow during occlusion, and tissue ATP content did not correlate with the rate of recovery in the stunned myocardium (Przyklenk and Kloner, 1989). Since this analysis was performed on the single 15-minute coronary occlusion model, it is unclear to what degree this finding applies to the repeated coronary occlusion model.

III. DIASTOLIC PROPERTIES IN MYOCARDIUM STUNNED BY REPEATED ISCHEMIA

A dynamic course of changes in the material properties of ischemic muscle can be demonstrated in the stunned myocardium following repeated coronary occlusions. During coronary occlusion, the myocardium is subjected to mechanical shearing and stretching by phasic ventricular pressure. The combined metabolic and mechanical effects of the ischemic insult on muscle cells and their supporting structures may alter the passive or inherent material properties of the ischemic myocardium (Zhao et al., 1987). Regional systolic bulging during ischemia may produce diastolic fiber elongation at cellular and muscle levels and thus result in longer unstressed segment lengths and ventricular chamber dilatation (Edwards et al., 1981). The acute change in unstressed muscle length may have significant implications in ventricular wall remodeling during the recovery phase of the myocardial stunning. Changes in the contractile behavior would also contribute to a positive feedback mechanism via the Laplace law. Despite their importance, diastolic abnormalities and changes in material properties of the ischemic/reperfused tissue remain poorly understood.

A. Changes in End-Diastolic Length

As diastolic length increases in response to higher ventricular pressure and/or mechanical stretching, several processes occur. Myocytes elongate with or without changes in diameter. Myocytes can also be displaced relative to one another (myocellular slippage), resulting in a reduced number of cells across the ventricular wall (Weisman et al., 1988; Olivetti et al., 1990). From a cellular point of view, sarcomere length increases in the ischemic tissue (Crozatier et al., 1977; Zhao et al., 1989a). Furthermore, sarcomeres become misaligned in the stunned tissue (Zhao et al., 1989b), indicating intracellular slippage.

Both inter- and intracellular slippage in the stunned myocardium may contribute to the increase in unstressed muscle length. Nicklas et al. (1985) noted a progressive increase in end-diastolic segment length using a multiple occlusion stunning protocol. Ischemic segment length increased 4% after the first occlusion/reperfusion cycle, 10% after the third occlusion/reperfusion cycle, 19% after the sixteenth occlusion/reperfusion cycle, and 16% after the final 1 hour of reperfusion. However, the influence of diastolic pressure was not controlled since the normal segment length also increased slightly. A similar increase in end-diastolic length was noted by Cohen and Downey (1990). Stahl et al. (1988) also found a 20% increase in ischemic end-diastolic length using the repeated coronary occlusion protocol. In contrast to the results of Nicklas et al. (1985) and Cohen and Downey (1990), the end-diastolic length in the normal region did not change in this study (Stahl et al., 1988). Zhao et al. (1987) found that during coronary occlusion, the ischemic region bulged progressively from the first to twelfth occlusion. The time course for this progressive change was similar to that of end-diastolic length expansion observed by Nicklas et al. (1985). Charney et al. (1989) also noted increased end diastolic length in the stunned region. There was a 5–8% expansion in the stunned region relative to the normal region, which was highly significant.

The end-diastolic segment length measurement is sensitive to the end-diastolic pressure, which is experienced by both the normal and stunned regions at any given time. Figure 2 illustrates a relative expansion index that grossly

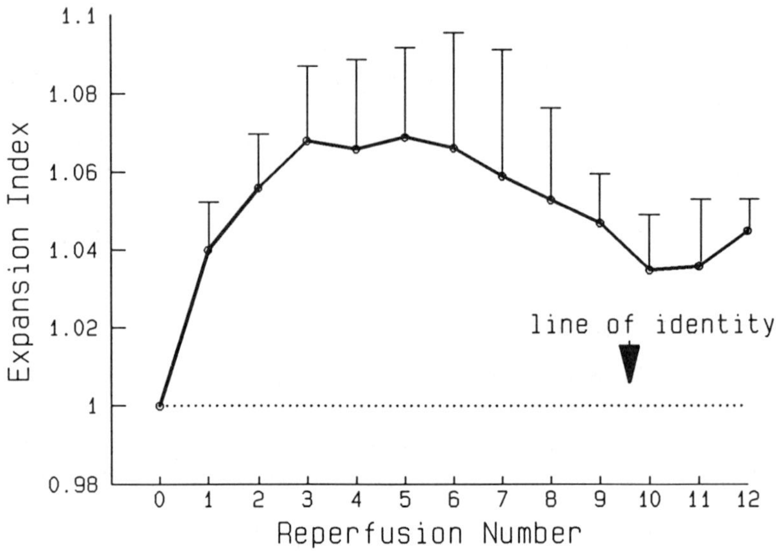

Figure 2 Relative expansion in stunned region. The values represent ratio of the simultaneous % control end-diastolic length for the stunned and normal regions at a given reperfusion period. This expansion index illustrates the relative increase in stunned end diastolic length over and above any changes in normal zone end diastolic length. There is a progressive relative expansion of the stunned region up to 7% at the third reperfusion period. There was a slight but not significant decline in relative explosion during the latter periods of the protocol. (These data are based on the results of 24 experiments from Zhao et al., 1987, and Charney et al., 1989.)

accounts for variability in end-diastolic pressure during the course of the stunning protocol. The data points represent ratios of simultaneous percent control end-diastolic lengths for the stunned and normal regions from 24 experiments in two separate studies from this laboratory (Zhao et al., 1987; Charney et al., 1989). This expansion index illustrates a mild increase in the stunned end diastolic length over and above changes in normal zone end diastolic length. Unlike systolic dysfunction, which demonstrates a rapid onset, diastolic expansion appears more gradual, with a progressive increase in expansion until the fourth to sixth reperfusion period, where it plateaus. The different response patterns may suggest different pathogenetic mechanisms for systolic and diastolic dysfunction in stunned myocardium.

B. Changes in Muscle Compliance

Several studies have demonstrated that ischemia shifts the pressure-dimension relationship to the right, indicating a greater myocardial compliance

(Forrester et al., 1971; Pirzada et al., 1976; Hess et al., 1983). Passive properties of the stunned myocardium were recently studied by Zhao et al. (1989a) using the repeated coronary occlusion model. Regional segment lengths were measured along both circumferential and longitudinal axes of the left ventricle. Passive pressure-length relationships were constructed for both the stunned and normal regions by varying the ventricular distending pressure at the end of the 12th occlusion-reperfusion sequence. The hearts were then perfusion-fixed in glutaraldehyde at a predetermined cavity pressure for ultrastructural analysis of cellular changes in both the stunned and normal tissue. In stunned myocardium, the muscle strain (segment length) was significantly increased in the circumferential direction (Zhao et al., 1989a). In contrast, strain in the longitudinal direction was unchanged compared to the normal region. This directional difference in muscle strain agrees well with the study of Edwards et al. (1981) in which the increase in unstressed segment length due to ischemia was twice as great in the circumferential direction as in the longitudinal direction. The differential changes in muscle compliance along the major and the minor axes could result in ventricular deformation of the heart into a globular configuration following myocardial ischemia.

IV. CELLULAR CHANGES IN REPEATED OCCLUSION MODELS

A. Changes in Sarcomere Length

Sarcomere lengths are markedly increased in the ischemic myocardium despite zero or minimal cavity-distending pressure during fixation (Crozatier et al., 1977). We have quantitated sarcomere length changes in stunned myocardium in hearts fixed at cavity-distending pressures ranging from 0 to 40 mmHg (Zhao et al., 1989a). Sarcomere lengths were significantly longer in all transmural layers of the stunned tissue as compared to the normal tissue at all distending pressures. Most notably, the unstressed (0 mmHg cavity pressure) sarcomere length in the stunned region was about 6–8% greater, resulting in a rightward shift of the pressure-sarcomere length relationship.

The mechanism of sarcomere length increase in ischemic myocardium is not well understood. The stability of sarcomere length depends on the presence of intact cytoskeletal supporting structures (Horowits and Podolsky, 1987). An extensive network of intermediate filaments associated with sarcomeres has been described in adult vertebrate skeletal muscle (Lazarides, 1980; Wang and Ramirez-Mitchell, 1983). The repeated passive stretching during systolic bulging in the repeated occlusion protocol could alter these structures. In addition, ischemia per se may also result in intracellular processes that degrade or depolymerize these cytoskeletal proteins. Other factors, including reperfusion injury mediated by oxygen-derived free radicals, may also contribute to cytoskeletal damage during stunning. Such ischemic damage to the cytoskeleton may affect cell volume in both longitudinal (longer sarcomere length) and transverse (increased myofilament separation) dimensions.

Segment length and sarcomere length represent two simultaneous measurements of linear dimension. The relationship between segment (macroscopic) strain and sarcomere (microscopic) strain reveals information regarding the structural integrity of the intercellular connections (Zhao et al., 1989a). As would be expected, segment strain and sarcomere strain change proportionately in the normal myocardium. Similarly, longitudinal muscle strain was also superimpossible with the sarcomere strain in the stunned myocardium. In contrast, there was a disproportionately greater change in circumferential segment length strain as compared to sarcomere length in stunned myocardium. Thus, a partial uncoupling of the cell and muscle occurred, leading to a greater muscle compliance in stunned myocardium. The changes in segment length cannot be accounted for by changes in sarcomere length, indicating strains or slippage of nonmyofibrillar structures. Damage to the extracellular collagen matrix could account for this decrease in coupling function.

B. Sarcomere Misregistration and Cytoskeletal Damage

Cytoskeletal structures may be damaged in the stunned myocardium, causing sarcomere misregistration. In normal myocardium, sarcomeres are co-aligned in a well-ordered array (Fig. 3A). The cytoskeletal proteins desmin and vimentin surround each myofibril Z disc and form honeycomblike networks within each Z plane of the muscle fiber (Granger and Lazarides, 1979). Based on their structural characteristics, desmin and vimentin may be involved in maintaining the lateral registration of sarcomeres by transversely linking adjacent myofibrils at their Z discs. This linkage would support and integrate the cell as a whole and provide a coupling mechanism for coordinated contraction and relaxation. Structural damage to these proteins would result in sarcomere misalignment. Vinculin forms riblike structures near the Z bands called costameres (Pardo et al., 1983). Costameres are thought to anchor the Z discs to the sarcolemma. Extracellular collagen struts at the lateral surface of the cells anchor at the Z band outside the sarcolemma (Caulfield and Borg, 1979; Robinson et al., 1983). Thus, vinculin may play an important role in transmitting and integrating forces across the cell membrane. Damage to vinculin structures may adversely affect coordinated multicellular contraction. Similarly, disruption of the extracellular collagen matrix during ischemia (Zhao et al., 1987) could also interrupt mechanical coupling across the cell membrane. Mechanical stretching and/or biochemical processes during reversible myocardial ischemia may result in myocyte deformation with increased sarcomere length and sarcomere misregistration.

Whereas sarcomere length could be normal in response to mechanical stretching, sarcomere misregistration must indicate intracellular shearing forces and/or changes in cytoskeletal structures. Significant sarcomere misregistration was found in all layers of the stunned myocardium using morphometric methods (Fig. 3B) (Zhao et al., 1989b). In a preliminary study, we observed a marked and rather uniform decrease in immunolabeling of desmin and vimentin in the stunned tissue, indicating structural damage to the cytoskeleton (Zhao et al., 1992b). Partial loss of vinculin staining was also noted. This latter finding has been observed in irreversible myocardial injury (Steenbergen et al., 1987). The disruption of lateral tethering proteins could explain sarcomere misregistration. It is conceivable that marked sarcomere misregistration may contribute to the macroscopic changes in unstressed muscle length.

C. Increased Myofilament Separation

During myocardial ischemia and subsequent reperfusion, the myocytes lose their normal ability to regulate cell volume, resulting in cell swelling (DiBona and Powell, 1980; Reimer et al., 1981; Jennings et al., 1985; Basuk et al., 1986; Jennings and Reimer, 1986). Myocardial and cellular edema is particularly notable in hearts subjected to repeated episodes of ischemic insults as compared to a single coronary occlusion (Basuk et al., 1986). Tissue water content is significantly increased following multiple coronary occlusion (Charney et al., 1989). At the ultrastructural level, the intracellular space is markedly enlarged with bundles of myofilbrils separated from each other, giving an electron-lucent appearance (Schaper et al., 1979). This increase in diffusional distance between the mitochondria and energy-utilizing contractile proteins could potentially affect cellular function. Abnormalities in energy utilization have been observed in the stunned myocardium following a 15-minute coronary occlusion (Schaper et al., 1985). Increased heterogeneity of oxygen extraction was found in dog hearts subjected to multiple 5-minute coronary occlusions, suggesting inefficient transfer of energy for myocyte contraction (Stahl et al., 1988).

Ischemic reperfusion injury also affects the radial separation distance between thick and thin myofilaments. In stunned myocardium following repeated coronary occlusions, quantitative analysis of interfilament distance revealed that center-to-center thick filament distance was 8% and 12% greater in the stunned region compared with normal control tissue in the subendo-

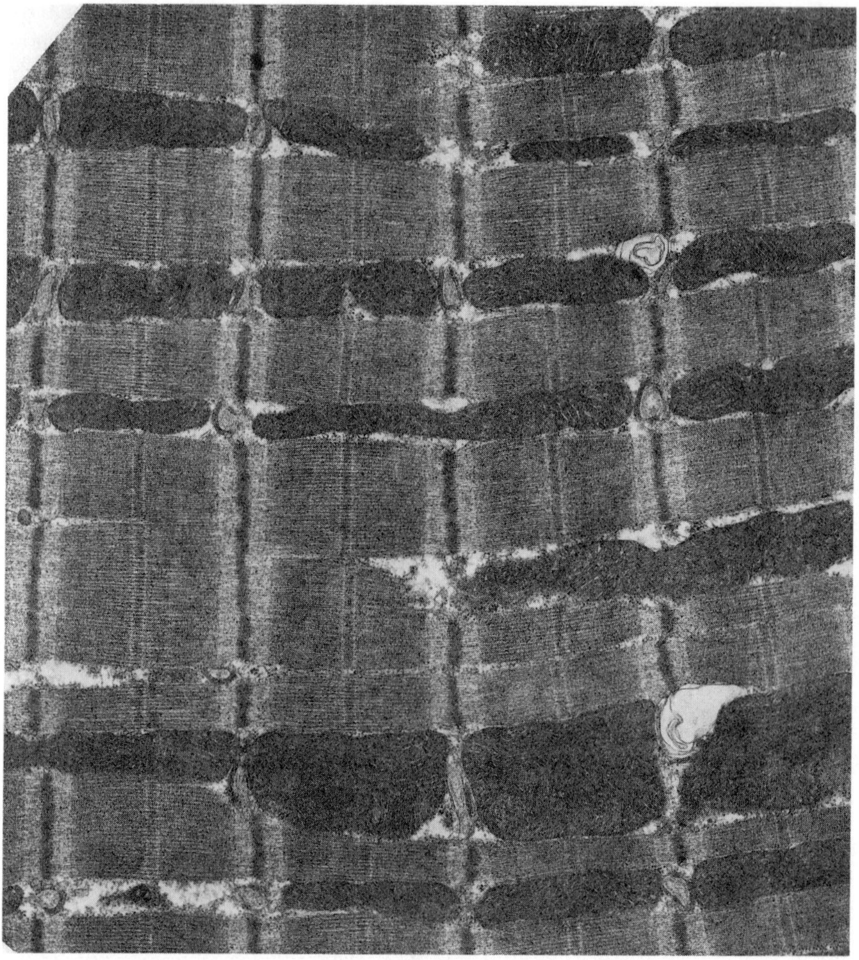

(A)

Figure 3 (A) An electron micrograph from normal myocardium. Sarcomeres are co-aligned in a well-ordered array. The heart was arrested in diastole and perfusion-fixed at 0 mmHg cavity pressure. Sarcomeres are fully relaxed, showing clearly delineated I bands. The sarcomere length in this micrograph is approximately 2.0 μm. (Original magnification: $\times$5000.)

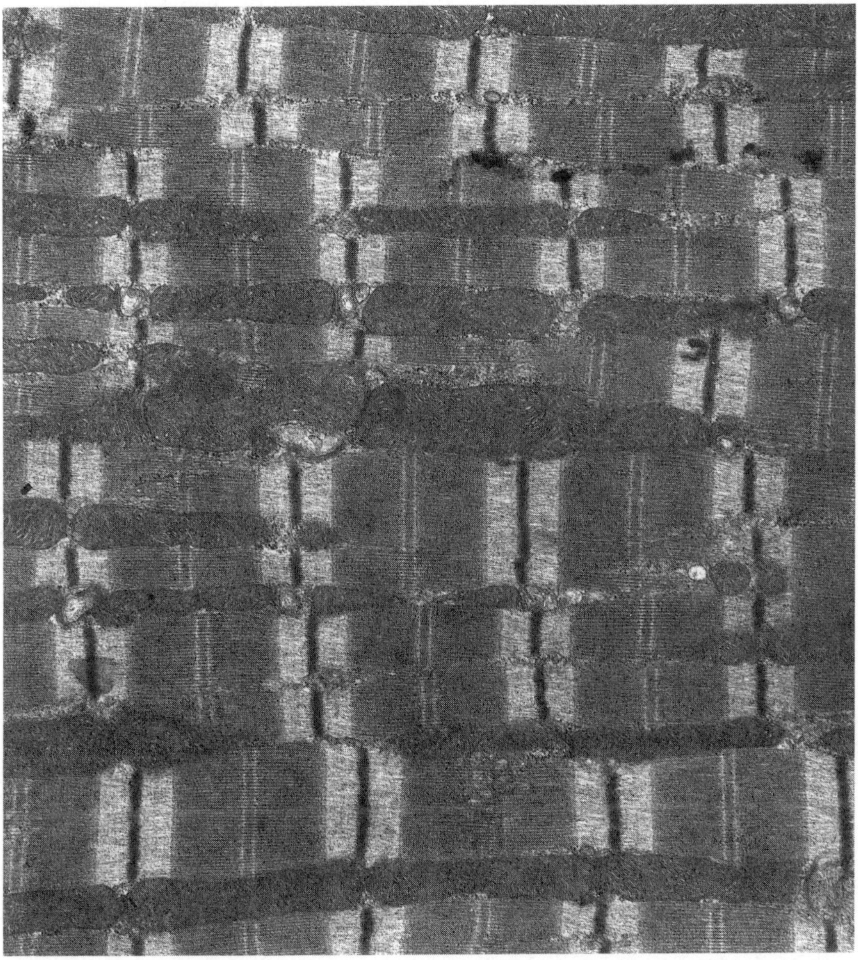

(B)

(B) Electron micrograph of stunned tissue from the same heart as in (A). Sarcomeres are markedly misregistered, probably due to the damage to cytoskeletal structures that normally keep sarcomeres in register. The sarcomere length is increased to approximately 2.2 μm, representing a 10% increase in unstressed sarcomere length as compared to normal tissue from the same heart (A). Wide I bands are apparent. (Original magnification: $\times 5000$.) Similar findings were found by Zhao et al. (1989a).

cardium and subepicardium, respectively (Zhao et al., 1992a). Such an increase in interfilament distance may affect optimal cross-bridge force generation at the molecular level. Myocardial performance in stunned myocardium could be easily affected by these geometric alterations. Experimental studies have demonstrated that alteration in filament separation distance compromises maximal tension development in isolated skeletal muscle preparations (Godt and Maughan, 1981; Krasner and Maughan, 1984; Harrison et al., 1988). Increases in the interfilament distance may result in a decreased calcium sensitivity of the contractile filaments and thereby contribute to myocardial stunning. Kusuoka et al. (1987) found that in isolated ferret hearts subjected to 15 minutes of ischemia, the myocardium exhibited decreased responsiveness to calcium, as manifested by a decrease in the maximal calcium-activated force and a decrease in the myocardial sensitivity to extracellular calcium. It is likely that such a change in calcium sensitivity also occurs in the stunned myocardium following repeated coronary occlusions. In addition to the osmotic stresses during reperfusion injury, cytoskeletal damage may also be a contributing factor to the increased interfilament distance. The Z-band structural proteins, such as desmin, vimentin, alpha-actinin, and possibly M-line proteins, may play a role in the structural stability of the myofilament lattice (Lazarides, 1980; Pardo et al., 1983; Wang and Ramirez-Mitchell, 1983). It remains unclear, however, whether increased myofilament separation is unique to the repeated occlusion model.

V. EXTRACELLULAR COLLAGEN DAMAGE IN STUNNED MYOCARDIUM

In mammalian heart, a complex network of extracellular collagen fibers interconnects myocyte to myocyte, myocyte to capillaries, and myocyte to connective tissue (Fig. 4A) (Caulfield and Borg, 1979; Robinson et al., 1983). It also invests groups of myocytes and binds myocardial mural layers. An increasing body of experimental evidence suggests that the collagen matrix may be a significant source of myocardial stiffness in normal and diseased hearts (Bing et al., 1978; Borg et al., 1981; Weber et al., 1987). A role of collagen in the active properties of muscle has also been suggested (Winegrad and Robinson, 1987). Recently, a knotlike umbilical mass of large coiled collagen fibers has been observed in en face sections of the ventriculuar apex (Factor et al., 1988). These fibers course along the major axis of the left ventricle and anchor at the fibrous annulus at the LV base, providing a mechanical tethering to prevent overstretch along the longitudinal direction of the left ventricle. Thus, it would appear that the structural integrity of the myocardial collagen matrix is needed to maintain an optimal configuration of the heart.

Profound morphological alterations of the extracellular collagen matrix were noted in the stunned myocardium following repeated coronary occlusions (Zhao et al., 1987). Large collagen cables were roughened, uncoiled, and discontinuous. The usual dense collagen weave investing myocytes became patchy or absent. Lateral struts between myocytes were sparse and frequently absent (Fig. 4B). The changes were rapid in onset and occurred prior to irreversible cellular damage. A progressive increase in systolic bulging was found during the 12 coronary occlusion protocol. Although a direct causal effect between collagen loss and progressive systolic bulging has not been firmly established, it is conceivable that some kind of link between the two findings may be present. Similar changes in collagen structures were also found in hearts subjected to repeated coronary occlusion using a different morphological method (Whittaker et al., 1991). In contrast, structural changes in collagen matrix were not apparent in the single occlusion model (Whittaker et al., 1991). In addition, greater systolic bulging was noted following a repeated coronary occlusion protocol (Whittaker et al., 1991), supporting a linkage between structural changes of collagen and the degree of systolic bulging.

Myocardial collagen metabolism is also altered in stunned myocardium following repeated coronary occlusions (Charney et al., 1989). Tissue hydroxyproline content was 10–15% lower in the stunned region as compared to the normal region. In addition, all transmural layers in the stunned myocardium had significant increases in collagenase activity. Furthermore, complete activation of procollagenase forms revealed no differences in fully activated collagenase between the stunned and normal regions. The lysosomal enzymes elastase and cathepsin G were not different between stunned and normal zone tissue, suggesting no exogenous sources of protease in the stunned tissue. These findings are consistent with the histological observation that no inflammatory process is involved in the stunned tissue (Zhao et al., 1987).

VI. MODEL-DEPENDENT FEATURES OF STUNNED MYOCARDIUM

Although systolic dysfunction is a common characteristic in all models of stunned myocardium, there are major biochemical, structural, and perhaps functional differences between the single occlusion and repeated occlusion models. One of the unique features of the repeated coronary occlusion model is the potential influence of the preconditioning effect rendered by the initial brief coronary occlusions. Murry et al. (1990) noted that a brief coronary occlusion slows the rate of ATP depletion in the following episodes of ischemia. Cohen and Downey (1990) suggested that the initial coronary oc-

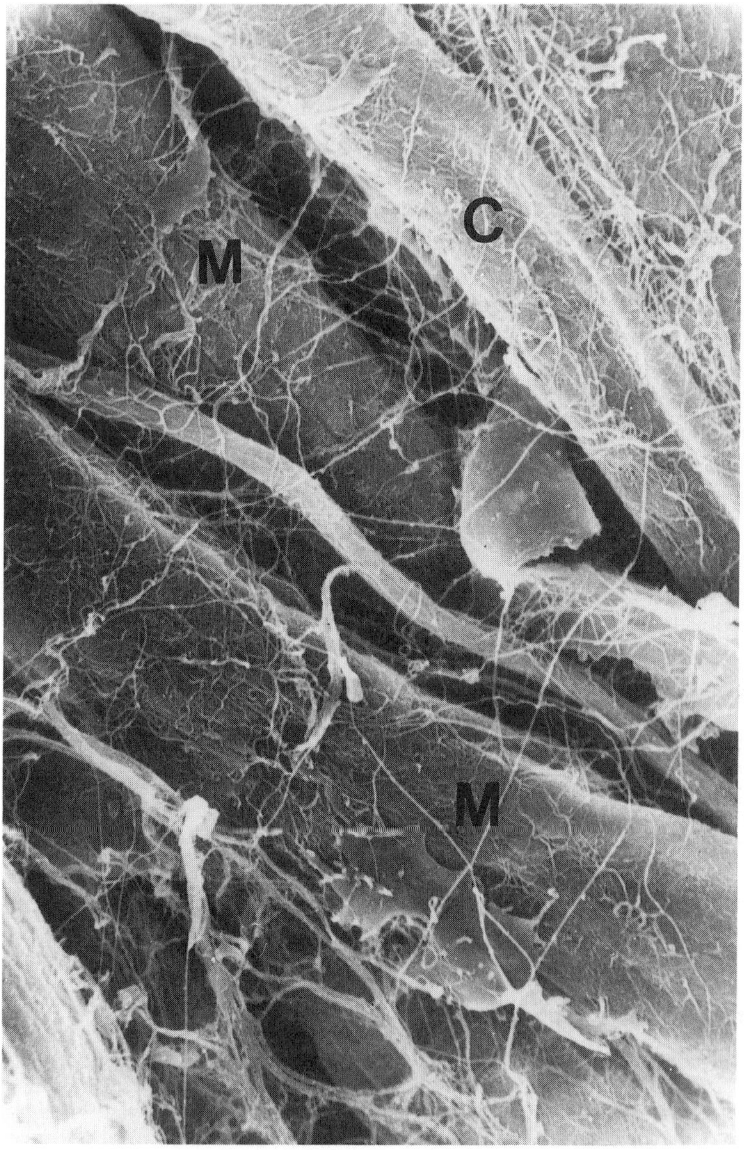

(A)

Figure 4 (A) A scanning electron micrograph from normal tissue showing the usual dense and florid collagen weave investing the individual myocytes (M). Abundant collagen struts interconnect myocyte to myocyte, and myocyte to capillary (C). (Original magnification: ×1500.)

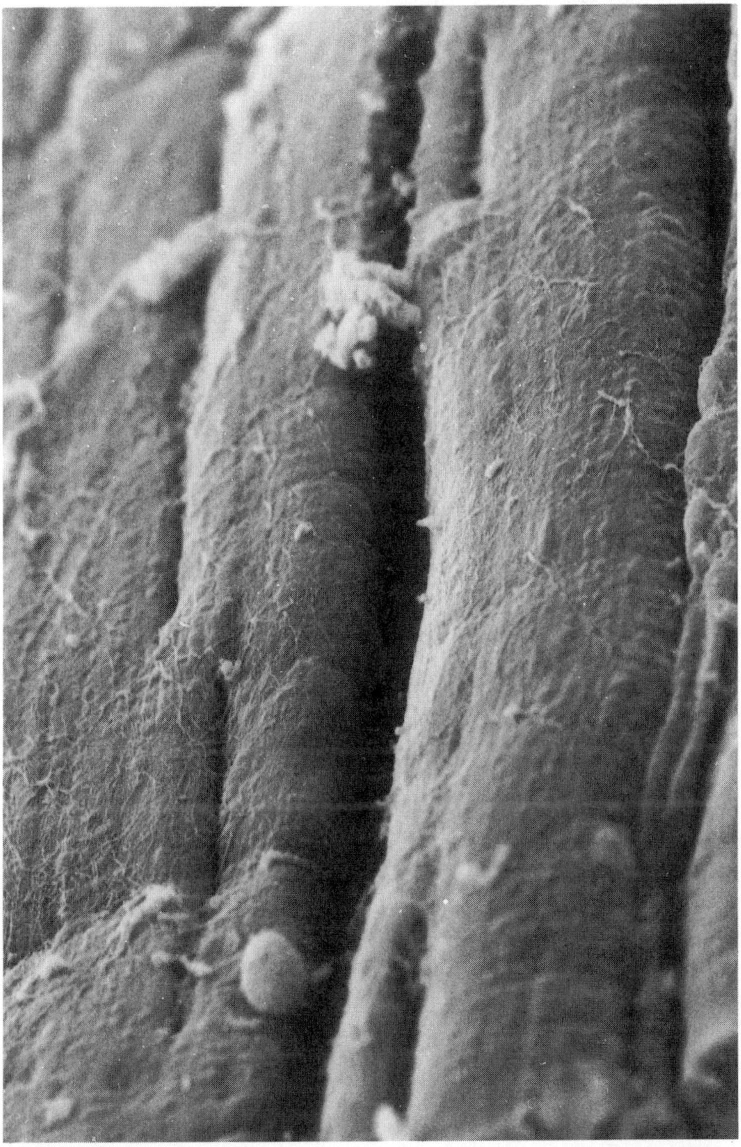

(B)

(B) A scanning electron micrograph of stunned myocardium demonstrating almost complete absence of the perimysial weave. Note the absence of myocyte-to-myocyte struts as compared to their abundance in normal tissue. (Original magnification: ×2100.) Similar findings have been published by Zhao et al. (1987).

clusion offered a preconditioning effect that markedly attenuated the rate of deterioration of systolic shortening in the stunned region. These studies indicate different biochemical and functional considerations that are characteristic of the repeated coronary occlusion model as compared to the single occlusion model of stunned myocardium. The preconditioning effect may prolong the time course of reversible ischemic injury, thereby allowing the collagen and, probably, cytoskeletal damage to take place without tissue necrosis. Thus, the structural changes in the extracellular collagen matrix appears to be a model-dependent phenomenon (Zhao et al., 1987; Whittaker et al., 1991). The degree of myocardial edema may be more severe following multiple coronary occlusion-reperfusion cycles. It is not clear, however, whether cytoskeletal damage and sarcomere misregistration also occur after a single coronary occlusion. Nor is it clear if passive myocardial properties such as unstressed dimension and muscle compliance are altered in the single occlusion model. Further studies are obviously needed to confirm these findings in the repeated occlusion model and define the nature of the differences between myocardium stunned by single vs. repeated occlusions.

VII. IMPLICATIONS FOR VENTRICULAR REMODELING POSTISCHEMIA

Results obtained from the repeated occlusion model suggest that myocardial ischemia affects the extracellular compartment of the heart prior to irreversible structural changes in the cellular compartment. This differential sensitivity to ischemia may have important implications for cardiac enlargement and pathogenetic mechanisms in cardiomyopathy. Ischemic damage to the collagen network could be followed by remodeling of the ventricular geometry into a larger heart size, which is less favorable for contractile function. Remodeling could entrap cells into a new matrix, which could be less efficient in relengthening, compromise intercellular force transmission, and alter restoring forces. This scenario may further load the normal region via the Laplace law, thus creating a positive feedback mechanism that would lead to a larger heart. Interventions that interrupt this feedback loop, such as preserving structural integrity of the collagen matrix and/or reducing pre- and afterloads during the remodeling phase, may provide a rationale for new approaches in the clinical management of ischemic cardiomyopathies and chronic heart failure.

VIII. SUMMARY

Despite extensive investigation of stunned myocardium in recent years, the precise mechanism for this phenomenon has not been firmly established. Part of the difficulty may stem from the use of different experimental models with varying length of coronary occlusion and reperfusion periods. Two experimental approaches with either a single coronary occlusion or repeated coronary occlusions have been commonly used to study myocardial stunning. Although the ischemic load is quite different between the two models, the degree of systolic dysfunction is similar. However, insofar as diastolic abnormalities are concerned, major differences appear to exist between the two models. Apart from a potential protective effect of the initial coronary occlusions on the myocytes, repeated interruptions of the coronary circulation appear to be detrimental to the structural integrity of the myocardial collagen matrix. The destruction of myocardial supporting structures with preservation of viable myocytes sets into motion a positive feedback mechanism that could eventually lead to an enlarged heart via the Laplace law. The natural course of this recovery process remains to be characterized and various influencing factors to be determined. A better understanding of ventricular wall remodeling following myocardial stunning will provide important insights into the mechanism of postischemic recovery and eventually may provide a rationale for new approaches in clinical management of ischemic heart disease.

ACKNOWLEDGMENTS

This work was supported in part by NIH grants HL27219 and HL37412 and a Grant in Aid from the New York Heart Association.

REFERENCES

Basuk, W. L., Reimer, K. A., and Jennings, R. B. (1986). Effect of repetitive brief episodes of ischemia on cell volume, electrolytes and ultrastructure. *J. Am. Coll. Cardiol. 8*: 33A.

Becker, L. C., Levine, J. H., DiPaula, A. F., Guarnieri, T., and Aversano, T. (1986). Reversal of dysfunction in postischemic stunned myocardium by epinephrine and postextrasystolic potentiation. *J. Am. Coll. Cardiol. 7*: 580.

Bing, O. H. L., Fanburg, B. L., Brooks, W. W., and Matsushita, S. (1978). The effect of the lathyrogen B-amino proprionitrile (BAPN) on the mechanical properties of experimentally hypertrophied rat cardiac muscle. *Circ. Res. 43*: 632.

Bolli, R. (1990). Mechanism of myocardial "stunning." *Circulation 82*: 723.

Bolli, R., Zhu, W. X., Thornby, J. I., O'Neill, P. G., and Roberts, R. (1988). Time course and determinants of recovery of function after reversible ischemia in conscious dogs. *Am. J. Physiol. 254*: H102.

Borg, T. K., Ranson, W. F., Moslehy, F. A., and Caulfield, J. B. (1981). Structural basis of ventricular stiffness. *Lab. Invest. 44*: 49.

Braunwald, E. and Kloner, R. A. (1982). The stunned myocardium: prolonged, postischemic dysfunction. *Circulation, 66*: 1146.

Caulfield, J. B., and Borg, T. K. (1979). The collagen network of the heart, *Lab Invest., 40*: 364.

Charlat, M. L., O'Neill, P. G., Hartley, C. J., Roberts, R., and Bolli, R. (1989). Prolonged abnormalities of left ventricular diastolic wall thinning in the "stunned" myocardium in conscious dogs: Time course and relation to systolic function. *J. Am. Col. Cardiol. 13*: 185.

Charney, R. H., Takahashi, S., Zhao, M. J., Sonnenblick, E. H., Factor, S. M., and Eng, C. (1989). Collagen loss in the stunned myocardium, *Circulation. 80* (Supp II):99 (abstract).

Cohen, M. V., and Downey, J. M. (1990). Myocardial stunning in dogs: preconditioning effect and influence of coronary collateral flow. *Am. Heart J.* 120: 282.

Crozatier, E., Ashraf, M., Franklin, D., and Ross, J. (1977). Sarcomere length in experimental myocardial infarction: Evidence for sarcomere overstretch in dyskinetic ventricular regions. *J. Mol. Cell. Cardiol. 9*: 785.

DiBona, D. R., and Powell, W. J. (1980). Quantitative correlation between cell swelling and necrosis in myocardial ischemia in dogs. *Circ. Res. 47*: 653.

Edwards, II, C. H., Rankin, J. S., McHall, P. A., Ling, D., and Anderson, R. W. (1981). Effects of ischemia on left ventricular regional function in the conscious dog. *Am. J. Physiol. 240*: H413.

Factor, S. M., Flomenbaum, M., Zhao, M. J., Eng, C., and Robinson, T. F. (1988). The effects of acutely increased ventricular cavity pressure on intrinsic myocardial connective tissue. *J. Am. Coll. Cardiol. 12*: 1582.

Forrester, J. S., Diamond, G., Parmley, W. W., and Swan, H. J. C. (1972). Early increase in left ventricular compliance after myocardial infarction. *J. Clin. Lab. Invest. 51*: 589.

Geft, I. L., Fishbein, M. C., Ninomiya, K., Hashida, J., Chaux, E., Yano, J., Y-Rit, J., Genov, T., Shell, W., and Ganz, W. (1982). Intermittent brief periods of ischemia have a cumulative effect and may cause myocardial necrosis. *Circulation. 66*: 1150.

Godt, R. E., and Maughan, D. W. (1981). Influence of osmotic compression on calcium activation and tension in skinned muscle fibers of the rabbit. *Pflügers Arch. 391*: 334.

Granger, B. L., and Lazarides, E. (1979). Desmin and vimentin coexist at the periphery of the myofibril Z disc. *Cell 18*: 1053.

Harrison, S. M., Lamont, C., and Miller, D. J. (1988). Hysteresis and the length dependence of calcium sensitivity in chemically skinned rat cardiac muscle. *J. Physiol. 401*: 115.

Hess, O. M., Osakada, G., Lavelle, J. F., Gallagher, K. P., Kemper, W. S., and Ross, J., Jr. (1983). Diastolic myocardial wall stiffness and ventricular relaxation during partial and complete coronary occlusion in the conscious dog. *Circ. Res. 52*: 387.

Heyndrickx, G. R., Millard, R. W., McRitchie, R. J., Maroko, P. R., and Vatner, S. F. (1975). Regional myocardial functional and electrophysiological alterations after brief coronary artery occlusion in conscious dogs. *J. Clin. Invest. 56*: 978.

Horowits, R., and Podolsky, R. J. (1987). The positional stability of thick filaments in activated skeletal muscle depends on sarcomere length: Evidence for the role of thin filaments. *J. Cell Biol. 105*: 2217.

Jennings, R. B., and Reimer, K. A. (1986). Myocardial ischemia revisited. The osmolar load, membrane damage, and reperfusion. *J. Mol. Cell. Cardiol. 18*: 769.

Jennings, R. B., Schaper, J., Hill, M. L., Steenbergen, Jr., C., and Reimer, K. A. (1985). Effect of reperfusion late in the phase of reversible ischemic injury. Changes in cell volume, electrolytes, metabolites, and ultrastructure. *Circ. Res. 56*: 262.

Krasner, B., and Maughan, D. (1984). The relationship between ATP hydrolysis and active force in compressed and swollen skinned muscle fibers of the rabbit. *Pflügers Arch., 400*: 160.

Kusuoka, H., Porterfield, J. K., Weisman, H. F., Weifeldt, M. L., and Marban, E. (1987). Pathophysiology and pathogenesis of stunned myocardium: Depressed Ca^{2+} activation of contraction as a consequence of reperfusion-induced cellular calcium overload in ferret hearts. *J. Clin. Invest. 79*: 950.

Lange, R., Ware, J., and Kloner, R. A. (1984). Absence of a cumulative deterioration of regional function during three repeated 5 or 15 minute coronary occlusions. *Circulation 69*: 400.

Lazarides, E. (1980). Intermediate filaments as mechanical integrators of cell space. *Nature 283*: 249.

Murry, C. E., Jennings, R. B., and Reimer, K. A. (1986). Preconditioning with ischemia: A delay of lethal cell injury in ischemic myocardium. *Circulation 74*: 1124.

Murry, C. E., Richard, V. J., Reimer, K. A., and Jennings, R. B. (1990). Ischemic preconditioning slows energy metabolism and delays untrastructural damage during a sustained ischemic episode. *Circ. Res. 66*: 913.

Nicklas, J. M., Becker, L. C., and Healy-Bulkley, B. (1985). Effects of repeated brief coronary occlusion on regional left ventricular function and dimension in dogs. *Am. J. Cardiol. 56*: 473.

Olivetti, G., Capasso, J. M., Sonnenblick, E. H., and Anversa, P. (1990). Side to side slippage of myocytes participates in ventricular wall remodeling acutely after myocardial infarction in rats. *Circ. Res. 67*: 23.

Pardo, J. V., Silisiano, J. D., and Craig, S. W. (1983). A vinculin-containing cortical lattice in skeletal muscle: Transverse lattice elements ("costameres") mark sites of attachment between myofibrils and sarcolemma. *Proc. Natl. Sci. USA 80*: 1008.

Pirzada, F. A., Ekong, E. A., Vokonas, P. S., Apstein, C. S., and Hood, W. B. (1976). Experimental myocardial infarction. XIII. Sequential changes in left ventricular pressure-length relationships in the acute phase. *Circulation 53*: 970.

Przyklenk, K. and Kloner, R. A. (1989). What factors predict recovery of contractile function in the canine model of the stunned myocardium. *Am. J. Cardiol. 64*: 18F.

Przyklenk, K., Patel, B., and Kloner, R. A. (1987). Diastolic abnormalities of postischemic 'stunned' myocardium. *Am. J. Cardiol. 60*: 1211.

Przyklenk, K., Whittaker, P., and Kloner, R. A. (1990). In vivo infusion of oxygen free radical substrates causes myocardial systolic, but not diastolic dysfunction. *Am. Heart J. 119*: 807.

Reimer, K. A., Jennings, R. B., and Hill, M. L. (1981). Total myocardial ischemia, in vitro, 2. High energy phosphate depletion and associate defects in energy metabolism, cell volume regulation, and sarcolemmal integrity. *Circ. Res. 49*: 901.

Reimer, K. A., Murry, C. E., Yamasawa, I., Hill, M. L., and Jennings, R. B . (1986). Four brief periods of myocardial ischemia cause no cumulative ATP loss or necrosis. *Am. J. Physiol. 251*: H1306.

Robinson, T. F., Cohen-Gould, L., and Factor, S. M. (1983). Skeletal framework of mammalian heart muscle. *Lab. Invest. 49*: 482.

Schaper, J., Mulch, J., Winkler, B., and Schaper, W. (1979). Ultrastructural, functional, and biochemical criteria for estimation of reversibility of ischemic injury: A study on the effects of global ischemia on the isolated dog heart. *J. Mol. Cell. Cardiol. 11*: 521.

Schaper, W., Buchwald, A., Hoffmeister, H. M., and Ito, B. R. (1985). "Stunned" myocardium is a problem of energy utilization and not of energy supply. *Circulation 72*(Supp III): 119. (abstract).

Stahl, L. D., Aversano, T. R., and Becker, L. C. (1986). Selective enhancement of function of stunned myocardium by increased flow. *Circulation 74*: 843.

Stahl, L. D., Weiss, H. R., and Becker, L. C. (1988). Myocardial oxygen consumption, oxygen supply/demand heterogeneity, and microvascular patency in regionally stunned myocardium. *Circulation 77*: 865.

Steenbergen, C., Hill, M. L., and Jennings, R. B. (1987). Cytoskeletal damage during myocardial ischemia: changes in vinculin. Immunofluorescence staining during total in vitro ischemia in canine heart. *Circ. Res. 60*: 478.

Swain, J. L., Sabina, R. L., Hines, J. J., Greenfield, J. C., Jr., and Holmes, E. W. (1984). Repetitive episodes of brief ischaemia (12 min) do not produce a cumulative depletion of high energy phosphate compounds. *Cardiovas. Res. 18*: 264.

Tennant, R., and Wiggers, C. J. (1935). The effect of coronary occlusion on myocardial contraction. *Am. J. Physiol. 112*: 351.

Wang, K., and Ramirez-Mitchell, R. (1983). A network of transverse and longitudinal intermediate filaments is associated with sarcomeres of adult vertebrate skeletal muscle. *J. Cell Biol. 96*: 562.

Weber, K. T., Janicki, J. S., Pick, R., Abrahams, C., Shroff, S. G., Bashey, R. I., and Chen, R. M. (1987). Collagen in the hypertrophied, pressure-overloaded myocardium. *Circulation 75*(Supp 1): 40.

Weisman, H. F., Bush, D. E., Mannisi, J. A., Weisfeldt, M. L., and Healy, B. (1988). Cellular mechanisms of myocardial infarct expansion. *Circulation 78*: 186.

Whittaker, P., Boughner, D. R., Kloner, R. A., and Przyklenk, K. (1991). Stunned myocardium and myocardial collagen damage: Differential effects of single and repeated occlusions. *Am. Heart J. 121*: 434.

Winegrad, S., and Robinson, T. F. (1978). Force generation among cells in the relaxing heart. *Eur. J. Cardiol. 7*(Supp): 63.

Wynsen, J. C., Kenny, D., Brooks, H. L., and Warltier, D. C. (1991). Regional myocardial function after repetitive brief episodes of ischemia: effect of altering the duration of the reperfusion period. *Am. Heart J. 121*: 1331.

Zhao, M. J., Zhang, H., Robinson, T. F., Factor, S. M., Sonnenblick, E. H., and Eng, C. (1987). Profound structural alterations in the extracellular collagen matrix in postischemic dysfunctional ("stunned") but viable myocardium. *J. Am. Coll. Cardiol. 6*: 1322.

Zhao, M. J., Forman, R., Sonnenblick, E. H., Zhang, H., Charney, R. H., Factor, S. M., and Eng, C. (1989a). Pressure-sarcomere length relationship in the stunned myocardium. *Circulation 80*(Supp II): 97 (abstract).

Zhao, M. J., Forman, R., Sonnenblick, E. H., Zhang, H., Charney, R. H., Factor, S. M., and Eng, C. (1989b). Sarcomere misregistration in the stunned myocardium: evidence for intracellular slippage. *Circulation 80*(Supp II): 513 (abstract).

Zhao, M. J., Zhang, H., Sonnenblick, E. H., and Eng, C. (1992a). Increase in myofilament separation in the "stunned" myocardium. *J. Mol. Cell. Cardiol. 24*: (in press).

Zhao, M. J., Sonnenblick, E. H., Zhang, H., Factor, S. M., and Eng, C. (1992b). Cytoskeletal alterations in the stunned myocardium. *FASEB J. 6*: A1245 (abstract).

5

Stunned Myocardium Following Exercise-Induced Ischemia

David C. Homans

University of Minnesota, Minneapolis, Minnesota

I. INTRODUCTION

Myocardial stunning was first described and has been best characterized in models of transient complete coronary artery occlusions in resting animals. Transient, reversible decreases in regional function may also occur following episodes of exercise-induced ischemia (Robertson et al., 1983; Homans et al., 1986). These studies of exercise-induced myocardial stunning may be particularly clinically relevant, since exercise-induced ischemia occurs very frequently in the clinical setting. There are important differences between "high-flow" and "low-flow" ischemia, however, relevent to the stunning that follows these different types of ischemia. These include differences in the oxygen consumption of ischemic myocardium, blood flow to the ischemic zone, duration of ischemic insult, and the mechanical response to ischemia.

II. DIFFERENCES BETWEEN HIGH-FLOW ISCHEMIA AND LOW-FLOW ISCHEMIA

A. Myocardial Oxygen Consumption

During exercise-induced ischemia, myocardial oxygen consumption is increased relative to coronary occlusion at rest. Myocardial oxygen consumption rises during exercise as a result of chronotropic and inotropic stimuli and increases in wall stress resulting from elevated systolic pressure. Although myocardial oxygen consumption during exercise-induced ischemia is less than during exercise without ischemia, it still exceeds that of resting myocardium with a total coronary artery occlusion.

B. Myocardial Blood Flow

Blood flow to the ischemic myocardium is also higher during exercise-induced ischemia. This perfusion to the ischemic zone results from both antegrade flow across the stenotic coronary artery and collateral flow from intercoronary collateral vessels. This residual flow permits continued delivery of oxygen, glucose, and fatty acids to the ischemic tissue, which allows continued myocardial contraction during ischemia and also permits removal of products of anaerobic metabolism and products of ATP catabolism. This is also likely to be associated with less severe alterations in osmolality and tissue pH. In the presence of marked distal coronary vasodilation, severely reduced distal intracoronary pressure, and high heart rates, a steep transmural gradient in perfusion occurs with markedly reduced subendocardial perfusion but residual flow to the subepicardial layers, which may be close to that occurring under basal conditions. This further raises the possibility that significant transmural variations in metabolic or functional derangements may occur.

In the clinical setting, flow during exercise is limited by a relatively fixed coronary artery stenosis, and therefore persistent obstruction to flow occurs in the postexercise period. This continued restriction to flow in the postischemic period differs greatly from the reactive hyperemia that occurs following release of total coronary occlusions in resting animals. In the presence of a severe stenosis, the intense distal coronary vasodilation produced by the episode of ischemia results in continued maldistribution of myocardial blood flow away from the subendocardium in the postexercise period. Therefore, abnormalities of subendocardial perfusion may persist following exercise, which may functionally prolong the period of ischemia (Homans et al., 1986). Differences in the reactive hyperemia that follows an ischemic insult may also have relevance to the mechanisms of myocardial stunning, since the superabundance of oxygen associated with an unimpeded reactive hyperemia would not occur in a setting of a persistent stenosis following exercise. If a rich oxygen supply were to facilitate the generation of oxygen-free radicals in the postischemic period, differences in the reactive hyperemia following ischemia could affect the stunning that follows the ischemic insult.

C. Mechanical Properties

The mechanical response to exercise-induced ischemia may also differ significantly from coronary artery occlusions at rest. Hypoxia, even at constant coronary flow, results in a decrease in distensibility and an increase in wall thickness, whereas ischemia resulting from decreased perfusion results in a decrease in wall thickness and an increase in chamber distensibility (Wyman et al., 1988). In studies of exercising animals, exercise-induced ischemia is generally associated with less regional dilatation and wall thinning than complete coronary artery occlusion. Thus, recovery of mechanical function following exercise-induced ischemia does not require changes in left ventricular geometry, regional wall stress, or fiber length. Second, prolonged episodes of myocardial ischemia in resting animals may result in myocardial necrosis. In the clinical setting, stunned myocardium may occur in regions physically adjacent to areas of myocardial necrosis. These regions of myocardial necrosis may alter regional geometry and regional wall stress even in the postischemic period, which may have implications for the function of noninfarcted adjacent myocardium (Guth et al., 1984; Homans et al., 1985; Gallagher et al., 1986, 1987). These considerations do not apply to exercise-induced ischemia where the intensity and duration of the ischemia insult is too short to produce myocardial necrosis.

D. Conscious vs. Anesthetized Preparations

Finally, studies of exercise-induced ischemia are of necessity conducted in conscious animals free from the acute effects of surgical trauma and anesthesia. These differences in experimental preparations may contribute to differences observed in studies of coronary artery occlusion in anesthetized open-chest animals and studies of exercise-induced ischemia. In our laboratory, it has actually been more difficult to produce stable myocardial stunning by transient total coronary occlusions in unanesthetized, conscious animals than it has been to produce stunning in pentobarbital anesthetized animals with heart rates of 140–160 beats/minute. This may be due to the decreased metabolic demands of the myocardium at the low heart rates present in resting conscious animals. Infusions of catecholamines or rapid atrial pacing have sometimes been required to produce consistent prolonged stunning (Laxson et al., 1988) in these conscious animals with total occlusions. It is even possible that studies performed in acutely anesthetized open-chest animals with high heart rates may actually reflect a state between exercise and the true resting conscious state.

III. MODELS OF EXERCISE-INDUCED ISCHEMIA

Several different models have been utilized to study myocardial ischemia during conditions of high demand and limited myocardial perfusion. Muscular exercise has frequently been utilized as a stimulus that increases myocardial inotropic state, arterial pressure, and heart rate. Differences in exercise intensity and duration may have important effects on the magnitude and duration of postischemic dysfunction (Homans et al., 1991). Therefore, some differences between studies may reflect in part different exercise protocols. The mechanism by which myocardial perfusion is restricted during exercise is also important, and may include ameroid constrictors that gradually occlude a coronary artery over 14–21 days (Tomoike et al., 1983), hydraulic occluders, or models of left ventricular hypertrophy. In ameroid models of coronary artery occlusion, there is little or no antegrade flow through the native coronary artery, and all perfusion reaching the ischemic myocardium is conducted through the intercoronary collateral vessels. The myocardial perfusion during exercise, therefore, will reflect the abundance of intercoronary collateral vessels as well as the vasomotor properties of these vessels (Tomoike et al., 1983). Since coronary collaterals are capable of vasodilation and constriction, and the vasomotor properties of coronary collateral vessels may vary depending on the maturity of these vessels (Hautamaa et al., 1989), the duration of placement of the ameroid constrictor prior to the time of study may influence perfusion and functional abnormalities observed during and following exercise-induced ischemia. Furthermore, chronically hypoperfused vessels may have different vasomotor properties from acutely hypoperfused vessels (Bache et al., 1990), which may contribute to differences between studies performed using ameroid and hydraulic occluders to restrict coronary flow. In studies of exercise in which flow is limited by a hydraulic occluder, residual perfusion into the ischemic myocardium may occur either antegrade through the stenosed, but not occluded, coronary artery or retrograde via intercoronary collateral vessels. Under these circumstances, changes in coronary artery vasomotor tone and pressure gradients across the region of stenosis may influence the severity of coronary artery stenosis during exercise. Thus, even in studies in which the total volume of antegrade coronary flow is held constant, the actual severity of stenosis may change. In models of left ventricular hypertrophy, subendocardial perfusion is limited by coronary vascular resistance and extravascular compressive forces resulting from myocardial hypertrophy, increased systolic wall tension, increased left ventricular end-diastolic pressure, and increased length of coronary vessels traversing the thickened left ventricular wall. These abnormalities of perfusion may also, therefore, be influenced by the vasomotor properties of the coronary circulation and the mechanical properties of the left ventricle, which may differ between resting conditions, exercise, and the early postexercise period. Mechanical differences between the hypertrophied heart and models of regional myocardial ischemia may result from the global nature of the ischemia and mechanical abnormalities in hypertrophy and the increased wall thickness of the hypertrophied ventricle. Finally, other inotropic and/or chronotropic stimuli such as pacing or catecholamine infusions have been used to increase myocardial oxygen consumption in resting animals and to some extent mimic the effects of exercise. The exact clinical relevance of these alternatives to exercise, however, is unknown, since the degree to which these interventions mimic the metabolic, mechanical, and vascular responses to exercise is not yet clear.

IV. CHARACTERISTICS OF EXERCISE-INDUCED STUNNING

A. Postischemic Dysfunction Following Exercise

Studies of regional function during and following high-flow ischemia have noted markedly different degrees of postexercise dysfunction. As noted above, these models have also used different stimuli for increasing myocardial oxygen demand, exercise protocols utilizing different intensities and durations of exercise, different means of reducing perfusion during exercise, and different degrees of restriction of perfusion in the postexercise period. It is probable that these differences contribute importantly to the variability of the results. Tomoike first demonstrated evidence of very brief reductions in regional function following rapid atrial pacing at heart rates of approximately 190 beats/min (Tomoike et al., 1978). A severe coronary artery stenosis was imposed using a hydraulic occluder, which was not released following termination of the pacing. In that study segment shortening was decreased at 1 minute but not 5 minutes, following termination of atrial pacing.

Subsequent studies of dogs with chronically occluded coronary arteries performing exercise 3 to 5 minutes in duration have demonstrated variable periods of postischemic dysfunction ranging from 5 to 30 minutes (Kumada et al., 1980a, Matsuzaki et al., 1984a, b, 1985; Guth et al., 1986, 1987). These studies have further demonstrated that interventions which reduce the severity of ischemia during exercise (beta-blockers, calcium blockers, and nitrates) are, in general, also associated with a more rapid return of function to normal following exercise. Since these antianginal agents were all administered prior to exercise and affected function during as well as following exercise, it seems probable that any beneficial effects on postexercise stunning were due to decreases in the severity of exercised-induced ischemia, and not due to a selective improvement in the myocardial stunning that followed exercise. For example, beta blockade administered prior to exercise resulted in a more rapid return of function following exercise, but is also associated with lower heart rates and improved regional function and blood flow during exercise (Matsuzaki et al., 1984a).

In other studies of myocardial function in the postexercise period, hydraulic occluders have been used to acutely restrict coronary flow during exercise (Homans et al., 1986, 1989, 1991). This model has the advantage of permitting release of the coronary occlusion at the end of exercise so that the precise duration of the ischemic stimulus can be controlled, and any contribution of continuing ischemia in the postexercise period can be eliminated. Using this technique, experimental protocols similar to that depicted in Figure 1 have been utilized. Exercise is begun in the absence of a coronary artery stenosis, during which time both coronary blood flow and regional systolic wall thickening increase moderately. Coronary blood flow is then reduced to control levels by inflation of the hydraulic occluder while exercise is continued. Almost immediately following the decrease in coronary flow, systolic wall thickening falls significantly, but rarely to the extent observed during complete acute coronary artery occlusions at rest. The severity of dysfunction remains constant during the remainder of the exercise, as long as the stenosis remains in place. At the end of exercise, the coronary artery occluder is promptly released, resulting in a brisk reactive hyperemia, which lasts approximately 5–10 minutes following a 10-minute period of exercise. Coronary perfusion then returns to control levels, where it remains constant thereafter. Regional function follows a triphasic course in the postexercise period. There is an early transient recovery of function to near control values, followed by a decline in function with a nadir occurring at 10–15 minutes following exercise. Thereafter, there is a slow return of function towards the preexercise control value, which may take from 30 minutes to 3–4 hours, depending on the exact nature of the ischemic stimulus.

B. Effects of Persistent Ischemia Following Exercise

This experimental model was used to determine whether postischemic dysfunction was due to persistent abnormalities of subendocardial perfusion in the postexercise period (Homans et al., 1986). Animals performed two identical 10-minute periods of exercise in the presence of a coronary artery stenosis. Following one run, the coronary artery occluder was completely released at the end of exercise; following the alternate run, the stenosis remained in place for 20 minutes following exercise. It was found that when the stenosis remained in place after exercise, there were persistent abnormali-

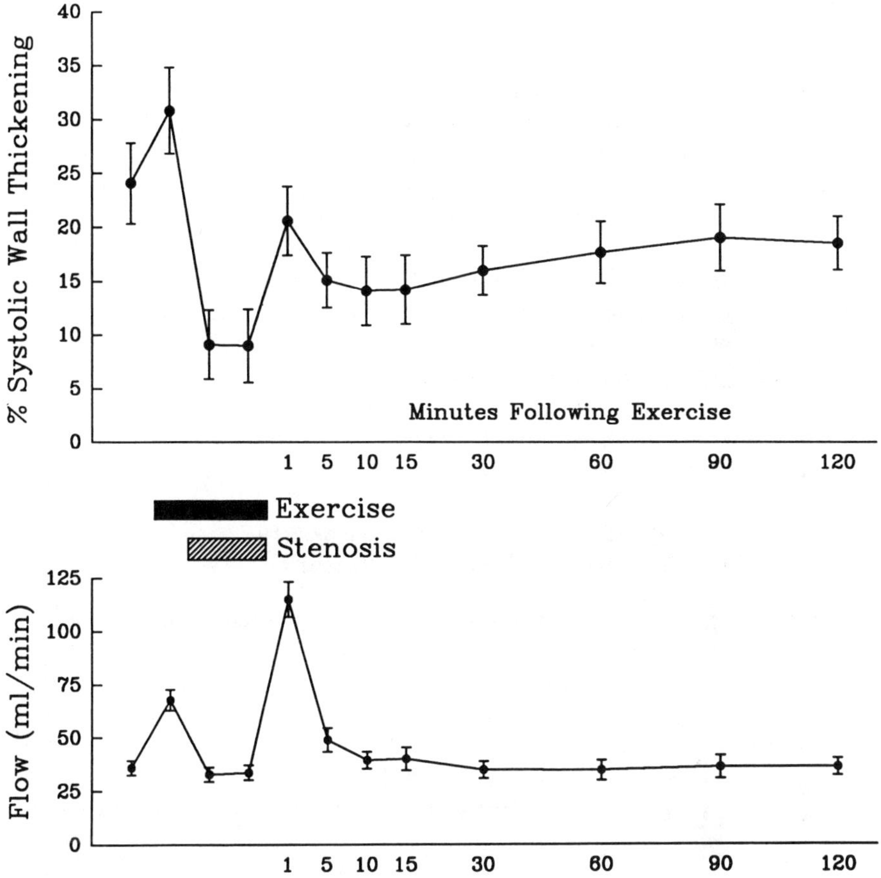

Figure 1 Systolic wall thickening (upper panel) and coronary blood flow (lower panel) during and after exercise. Exercise is begun in the absence of a coronary artery stenosis (solid bar), and subsequently the coronary artery stenosis is applied (diagonal hatched bar). During exercise in the absence of a coronary artery stenosis, there is an increase in both coronary blood flow and systolic wall thickening. When coronary blood flow is returned to control levels by partial inflation of a coronary artery hydraulic occluder, there is a decrease in systolic wall thickening to values well below resting control. Exercise is continued for 10 minutes in the presence of a coronary artery stenosis. At the termination of exercise, the coronary artery stenosis is abruptly released. One minute following exercise there is a marked reactive hyperemia with coronary blood flows rising to approximately four times the control value. This is associated with a transient "rebound" in systolic wall thickening to levels approaching the preexercise control value. Subsequently there is a return of coronary blood flow in the control value where it remains for the rest of the 2-hour observation period. This is associated with an initial decrease in systolic wall thickening followed by a progressive gradual increase in control values. $N = 8$; values are represented as ± 1 standard error of the mean.

ties in the transmural distribution of perfusion with severe reductions in subendocardial blood flow. These were associated with significantly poorer systolic function. This effect on regional function persisted for only approximately 5 minutes, however, after which time regional myocardial function recovered at the same rate whether or not a stenosis remained in place. Thus, functional abnormalities occurring in the first 5 minutes following exercise-induced ischemia are likely to be related to persistent abnormalities of myocardial perfusion, whereas functional abnormalities occurring later than 5 minutes after exercise are unrelated to abnormalities of myocardial perfusion, and therefore represent true myocardial stunning. In the clinical setting, postexercise abnormalities of regional function are therefore probably multifactorial and result from variable degrees of persistent subendocardial ischemia and postexercise stunning.

C. Effects of Exercise Frequency, Intensity, and Duration on Recovery of Function

Several studies have investigated the effects of different characteristics of exercise on the magnitude and duration of postexercise stunning. Repetitive episodes of exercise result in cumulative effects on postexercise stunning. Figures 2 and 3 illustrate the effects of a series of three exercise periods, each 10 minutes in duration and separated by 60-minute rest periods. With repeated episodes of exercise there is a progressive decrease in function at rest following exercise, indicating a cumulative effect on postischemic stunning (Ho-

Figure 2 Strip chart recordings depicting hemodynamic measurements and regional wall thickness measurements recorded during a series of three consecutive exercise periods. The first panel (control) is obtained in the resting animal prior to exercise. The animal performed two 10-minute periods of exercise separated by a 60-minute rest period. Recordings in the second panel were obtained one hour following the second exercise period. Systolic wall thickening in the distribution of the circumflex coronary artery is markedly reduced relative to the control value, despite stable hemodynamics and coronary artery blood flow. Panel 3 was recorded during a third exercise period and was obtained during exercise prior to the application of a coronary artery stenosis. There is a marked increase in systolic wall thickening in the circumflex distribution to levels exceeding the preexercise control. The fourth panel was recorded 2 hours following three periods of exercise-induced ischemia each 10 minutes in duration and separated by 60-minute rest periods. There is persistent severe systolic dysfunction in the distribution of the circumflex coronary artery. Ao = aortic pressure in mmHG; LV dP/dt = first derivative of left ventricular pressure; LV = left ventricular pressure. Dark vertical lines denote the beginning and end of systole. (Adapted from Homans et al., 1989.)

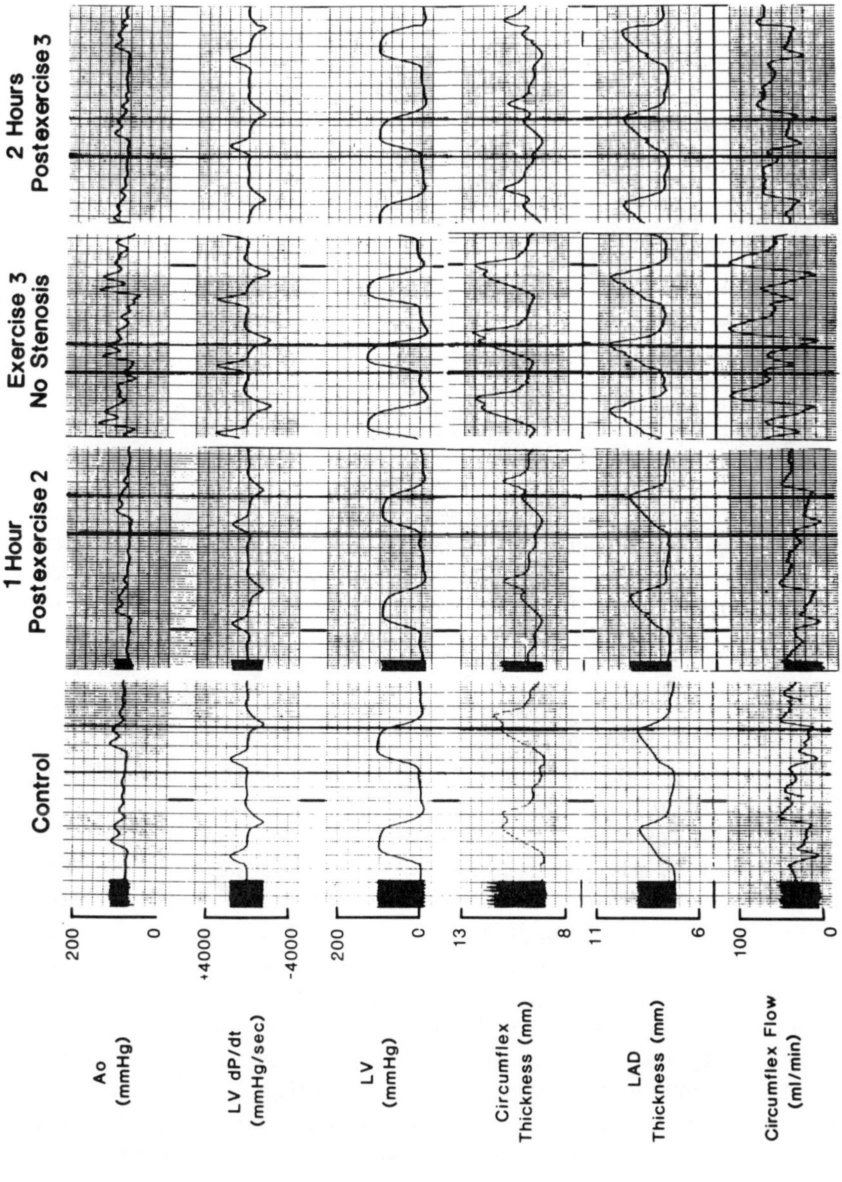
Control
1 Hour
Postexercise 2
Exercise 3
No Stenosis
2 Hours
Postexercise 3
Ao
(mmHg)
200
0
LV dP/dt
(mmHg/sec)
+4000
-4000
LV
(mmHg)
200
C
Circumflex
Thickness (mm)
13
8
LAD
Thickness (mm)
11
6
Circumflex Flow
(ml/min)
100
0

Figure 2

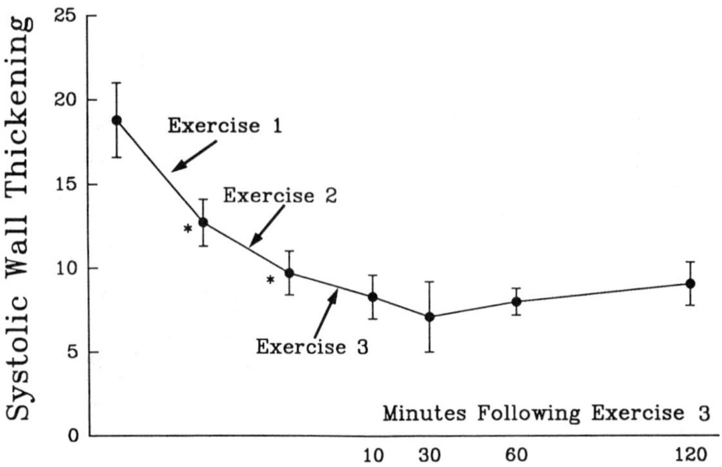

Figure 3 Group data obtained at rest before and after three episodes of exercise-induced ischemia each 10 minutes in duration and separated by 60-minute rest periods. There is a progressive decline in systolic wall thickening after each exercise period with a prolonged stable period of dysfunction after the third exercise period. (Adapted from Homans et al., 1989.)

mans et al., 1989). This postischemic stunning remained quite stable after the end of the last period of exercise.

Exercise intensity and duration both affect the severity of postischemic dysfunction; high-*intensity* exercise is associated with higher heart rates and more severe abnormalities of subendocardial perfusion and regional function during exercise (Homans et al., 1991). This greater degree of exercise-induced ischemia is also associated with more severe and more prolonged periods of postexercise dysfunction. The mechanisms responsible for these different intensities of exercise-induced ischemia may include differences in heart rate, arterial pressure, inotropic stimulation, and coronary vasomotor tone. The most powerful predictor of postexercise stunning was found to be the severity of dysfunction *during* exercise, consistent with earlier observations that interventions which reduce exercise-induced ischemia also decrease postexercise stunning. The degree of postischemic dysfunction also varies with the *duration* of exercise. Although measures of regional function and perfusion were similar at the end of 5 minutes of exercise and 10 minutes of exercise in the presence of a stenosis, myocardial stunning was more severe following a 10-minute period of exercise-induced ischemia than a 5-minute period of exercise-induced ischemia of similar severity (Homans et al., 1991). Although there was no evidence of progressive myocardial dysfunction during the more prolonged period of exercise, it is probable that progressive metabolic abnormalities occurred, resulting in more severe stunning following the longer duration of exercise.

V. TRANSMURAL VARIATIONS IN POSTEXERCISE STUNNING

Exercise-induced ischemia is associated with a steep transmural gradient in myocardial perfusion with severe decreases in perfusion to the subendocardial layers but only modestly impaired subepicardial perfusion (Ball and Bache, 1976). It is possible that these transmural variations in myocardial perfusion might be associated with transmural differences in myocardial function during or following exercise-induced ischemia. Bolli et al. (1989) have demonstrated selective depression of subendocardial thickening following release of coronary artery occlusions in resting animals using an epicardial doppler crystal technique to measure transmural variations in systolic wall thickening. Using separate pairs of pulse transit ultrasonic microcrystals to estimate outer wall and transmural thickening during exercise, however, it was found that exercise-induced ischemia was not associated with transmural variations in systolic wall thickening. There was also no evidence of selective subendocardial stunning in this model. It was further noted that although subendocardial and transmural wall thickening were closely correlated with myocardial blood flow, thickening in the outer layer of the left ventricular wall correlated poorly with perfusion (Homans et al., 1988a). Thus, significant transmural variations in myocardial stunning may not occur following exercise-induced ischemia in a regional ischemia model. This is perhaps due to mechanical "tethering" of subepicardial layers to the dysfunctional subendocardial layers (Weintraub et al., 1981; Gallagher et al., 1982).

Steep transmural gradients in myocardial perfusion may also occur during exercise in the presence of severe left ventricular hypertrophy. Left ventricular hypertrophy has been experimentally induced by aortic banding, and wall thickening was measured using three separate paris of pulse transit ultrasonic microcrystals to measure subendocardial, subepicardial, and transmural wall thickening. Using this model, Hittinger et al. (1990) demonstrated severe subendocardial hypoperfusion during exercise and selective subendocardial dysfunction lasting 30–60 minutes following intense exercise (Hittinger et al., 1990). These data suggest that in the *hypertrophied* ventricle, transmural variations in stunning do occur following exercise-induced ischemia; the greater thickness of the left ventricular wall may result in less "tethering" between the subendocardial and subepicardial layers, or subendocardial wall stresses may be higher in pressure-overloaded hearts.

VI. MECHANISMS OF EXERCISE-INDUCED STUNNING

These demonstrate that the severity of postexercise stunning is related to the intensity, duration, and frequency of the ischemic stimulus. The mechanisms responsible for exercise-induced stunning have not, however, been established. In the setting of total coronary artery occlusions in resting animals, a large body of evidence suggests that free radical mediated damage may be an important cause of postischemic stunning (Bolli, 1990). Preliminary results, however, suggest that the free radical scavengers SOD and catalase are ineffective in attenuating myocardial stunning following exercise-induced ischemia (Homans et al., 1988b). This highlights the model dependency of studies of myocardial stunning and supports the concept that multiple mechanisms contribute to myocardial stunning. The relative importance of each mechanism may vary depending on the precise experimental or clinical characteristics of the ischemic stimulus.

VII. CLINICAL STUDIES OF EXERCISE-INDUCED STUNNING

In addition to the abundant experimental demonstrations of transient reversible myocardial dysfunction following episodes of exercise-induced ischemia, clinical studies have also demonstrated the presence of persistent regional wall motion abnormalities following exercise. Robertson et al. (1983), using exercise echocardiography to assess regional function, noted that 7 of a group of 20 patients had regional wall motion abnormalities which persisted 30 minutes after the end of exercise. There was a trend towards more severe coronary artery disease in this latter group of patients. Delayed recovery of global left ventricular function has also been noted in selected patients using radionuclide ventriculography (Schneider, 1986). The group of patients demonstrating delayed recovery of function had more severe coronary artery disease as indicated by a greater number of diseased vessels. Since left ventricular ejection fraction is an insensitive measure of regional left ventricular dysfunction, and the magnitude of dysfunction resulting from exercise-induced stunning is rather modest (function reduced by 30–40% of the control value), radionuclide studies of left ventricular ejection fraction postexercise are unlikely to demonstrate abnormalities unless severe multivessel disease is present. In the study of Schneider (1986), the group with delayed recovery of function postexercise did not demonstrate lower *ejection fractions* during exercise, but did have more prominent abnormalities of *regional* wall motion during exercise (see also Chapter 20).

The clinical importance of exercise-induced stunning in patients with coronary artery disease probably varies depending on the frequency, severity, and duration of exercise, the severity of coronary artery disease, the degree of collateral growth, and the severity of impairment of left ventricular function. Postexercise-induced stunning may be particularly important in patients with "silent" ischemia who continue exercising, unaware of the presence of myocardial ischemia. It may also assume greater importance in the presence of severe multivessel disease or in the presence of impaired resting left ventricular performance, where it could result in clinically significant left ventricular dysfunction. In caring for patients with ischemic heart disease, it may be useful to appreciate that left ventricular dysfunction may persist long after exercise-induced angina has resolved. Therefore, permitting patients to resume exercising shortly after pain has improved may result in progressive deterioration in regional function.

As noted above, interventions which decrease the severity of exercise-induced ischemia also appear to reduce the duration of postexercise stunning. Thus, therapeutic approaches to postexercise stunning are directed primarily at ameliorating the ischemic insult. Since exercise-induced ischemia can be relatively easily anticipated (unlike sudden coronary artery occlusions), standard interventions that favorably affect the oxygen supply-demand balance during exercise, such as nitrates, beta blockers, and Ca^{2+} blockers, are likely to be effective.

ACKNOWLEDGMENT

The secretarial assistance of Andrea Dahl is greatly appreciated.

REFERENCES

Bache, R. J., Foreman, B. W., Pavek, T., Lindstrom, P., Laxson, D. D., and Homans, D. C. (1990). Acute but not chronic, reduction of myocardial blood flow results in marked subendocardial underperfusion during exercise. *Circulation 82* (Suppl III): III-381 (abstract).

Ball, R. M., and Bache, R. J. (1976). Distribution of myocardial blood flow in the exercising dog with restricted coronary artery inflow. *Circ. Res.* 38: 60.

Bolli, R., Patel, B. S., Hartley, C. J., Thronby, J. I., Jeroudi, M. O., and Roberts, R. (1989). Nonuniform transmural recovery of contractile function in stunned myocardium. *Am. Physiol. Soc. 89*: H375.

Bolli, R. (1990). Mechanism of myocardial "stunning." *Circulation 82*: 723.

Gallagher, K. P., Osakada, G., Hess, O. M., Koziol, J. A., Kemper, W. S., and Ross, J. (1982). Subepicardial segmental function during coronary stenosis and the role of myocardial fiber orientation. *Circ. Res. 50*: 352.

Gallagher, K. P., Gerren, R. A., Stirling, M. C., Choy, M., Dysko, R. C., McManimon, S. P., and Dunham, W. R. (1986). The distribution of functional impairment across the lateral border of acutely ischemic myocardium. Circ. Res. 58: 570.

Gallagher, K. P., Gerren, R. A., Ning, X-H, McManimon, S. P., Stirling, M. C., Shlafer, M., and Buda, A. J. (1987). The functional border zone in conscious dogs. *Circulation 76*: 929.

Guth, B. D., White, F. C., Gallagher, K. P., and Bloor, C. M. (1984). Decreased systolic wall thickening in myocardium adjacent to ischemic zones in conscious swine during brief coronary artery occlusion. *Am. Heart J. 107*: 458.

Guth, B. D., Tajimi, T., Seitelberger, R., Lee, J-D., Matsuzaki, M., and Ross, J. (1986). Experimental exercise-induced ischemia: Drug therapy can eliminate regional dysfunction and oxygen supply-demand imbalance. *J. Am. Coll. Cardiol. 7*: 1036.

Guth, B. D., Heusch, G., Seitelberger, R., and Ross, J. (1987). Mechanism of beneficial effect of β-adrenergic blockade on exercise-induced myocardial ischemia in conscious dogs. *Circ. Res. 60*: 738.

Hautamaa, P. V., Dai, X-Z., Homans, D. C., and Bache, R. J. (1989). Vasomotor activity of moderately well-developed canine coronary collateral circulation. *Am. Physiol. Soc. 89*: H890.

Hittinger, L., Shannon, R. P., Kohin, S., Manders, W. T., Kelly, P., and Vatner, S. F. (1990). Exercise-induced subendocardial dysfunction in dogs with left ventricular hypertrophy. *Circ. Res. 66*: 329.

Homans, D. C., Asinger, R., Elsperger, J., Erlien D., Sublett, E., Mikell, F., and Bache, R. J. (1985). Regional function and perfusion at the lateral border of ischemic myocardium. *Circulation 71*: 1038.

Homans, D. C., Sublett, E., Dai, X-Z., and Bache, R. J. (1986). Persistence of regional left ventricular dysfunction after exercise-induced myocardial ischemia. *J. Clin. Invest. 77*: 66.

Homans, D. C., Sublett, E., Lindstrom, P., Nesbitt, T., and Bache, R. J. (1988). Subendocardial and subepicardial wall thickening during ischemia in exercising dogs, *Circulation 78*: 1267.

Homans, D. C., Sublett, E., Asinger, R., Peterson, D. and Bache, R. J. (1988b). SOD + catalase does not attenuate regional left ventricular dysfunction following exercise induced ischemia. *Circulation 78*(Suppl II): II-76(abstract).

Homans, D. C., Laxson, D. D., Sublett, E., Lindstrom, P., and Bache, R. J. (1989). Cumulative deterioration of myocardial function after repeated episodes of exercise-induced ischemia. *Am. Physiol. Soc. 89*: H1462.

Homans, D. C., Laxson, D. D., Sublett, E., Pavek, T., and Crampton, M. (1991). The effect of exercise intensity and duration on regional function during and following exercise induced ischemia. *Circulation 83*: 2029.

Kumada, T., Gallagher, K. P., Miller, M., McKown, M., White, F., McKown, D., Kemper, W. S., and Ross, R. (1980a). Improvement by isosorbide dinitrate of exercise-induced regional myocardial dysfunction. *Am. Physiol. Soc. 239*: H399.

Kumada, T., Gallagher, K. P., Shirato, K., McKown, D., Miller, M., Kemper, W. S., White, F., and Ross, J. (1980b). Reduction of exercise-induced regional myocardial dysfunction by propranolol. Studies in a canine model of chronic coronary artery stenosis. *Circ. Res. 46*: 190.

Kumada, T., Gallagher, K. P., Battler, A., White, F., Kemper, W. S., and Ross, J. (1982). Comparison of postpacing and exercise-induced myocardial dysfunction during collateral development in conscious dogs. *Circulation 65*: 1178.

Laxson, D. D., Homans, D. C., Dai, X-Z., Sublett, E., and Bache, R. J. (1989). Oxygen consumption and coronary reactivity in postischemic myocardium. *Circ. Res. 64*: 9.

Matsuzaki, M., Patritti, J., Tajimi, T., Miller, M., Kemper, W. S., and Ross, J. (1984a). Effects of β-blockade on regional myocardial flow and function during exercise. *Am. Physiol. Soc. 84*: H52.

Matsuzaki, M., Gallagher, K. P., Patritti, J., Tajimi, T., Kemper, W. S., White, F. C., and Ross, J. (1984b). Effects of a calcium-entry blocker (diltiazem) on regional myocardial flow and function during exercise in conscious dogs. *Circulation 69*: 801.

Robertson, W. S., Feigenbaum, H., Armstrong, W. F., Dillon, J. C., O'Donnell, J., and McHenry, P. W. (1983). Exercise echocardiography: A clinically practical addition in the evaluation of coronary artery disease. *J. Am. Coll. Cardiol. 6*: 1085.

Schneider, R. M. (1986). Rate of left ventricular functional recovery by radionuclide angiography after exercise in coronary artery disease. *Am. J. Cardiol. 57*: 927.

Tomoike, H., Franklin, D., McKown, D., Kemper, W. S., Guberek, M., and Ross, J. (1977). Regional myocardial dysfunction and hemodynamic abnormalities during strenuous exercise in dogs with limited coronary flow. *Circ. Res. 42*: 487.

Tomoike, H., Franklin, D., and Ross, J. (1978). Detection of myocardial ischemia by regional dysfunction during and after rapid pacing in conscious dogs. *Circulation 58*: 48.

Tomoike, H., Inou, T., Watanabe, K., Mizukami, M., Kikuchi, Y., and Nakamura, M. (1983). Functional significance of collaterals during ameroid-induced coronary stenosis in conscious dogs. Interrelationships among regional shortening, regional flow and grade of coronary stenosis. *Circulation 67*: 1001.

Weintraub, W. S., Hattori, S., Agarwal, J. B., Bodenheimer, M. M., Banka, V. S., and Helfant, R. H. (1981). The relationship between myocardial blood flow and contraction by myocardial layer in the canine left ventricle during ischemia. *Circ. Res. 48*: 430.

Wyman, R. M., Farhi, E. R., Bing, O. H. L., Johnson, R. G., Weintraub, R. M., and Grossman W. (1989). Comparative effects of hypoxia and ischemia in the isolated, blood-perfused dog heart: Evaluation of left ventricular diastolic chamber distensibility and wall thickness. *Circ. Res. 64*: 121.

6

Stunned Myocardium in the Isolated Perfused Heart Preparation

Karin Przyklenk

Hospital of the Good Samaritan and University of Southern California, Los Angeles, California

Carl S. Apstein

Boston University School of Medicine and Boston City Hospital, Boston, Massachusetts

I. INTRODUCTION

The term stunned myocardium was initially used to describe postischemic contractile dysfunction in the in vivo canine model of brief coronary artery occlusion followed by reperfusion (Heyndrickx et al., 1975, 1978). In fact, the initial five chapters of this book focus largely on the properties of canine myocardium stunned by one or more episodes of either supply ischemia (i.e., coronary occlusion) or demand ischemia (i.e., ischemia due to increased oxygen demand).

Reports of postischemic dysfunction are not, however, limited to the in vivo setting: numerous investigators have used the isolated perfused heart preparation as a model of the stunned myocardium. Our objectives in this chapter are to describe the consequences of transient ischemia on contractile function and energy metabolism in the various isolated heart models that have been developed and, perhaps most importantly, discuss whether these models truly represent stunned myocardium.

II. STUNNED MYOCARDIUM FOLLOWING BRIEF ISCHEMIA/REPERFUSION

A. The Crucial Caveat

Stunned myocardium is defined as the prolonged but transient contractile dysfunction of viable myocardium that has been salvaged by reperfusion. The crucial caveat in this definition is that *the function of the stunned myocardium, although initially depressed following reflow, will eventually recover to normal values*. Such recovery, however, may take hours to days to weeks, depending upon the severity and duration of the ischemic insult and the conditions during reperfusion. In contrast, myocardium that has been irreversibly injured during a period of ischemia will obviously not show a progressive recovery of function.

Definitive confirmation of viable but stunned myocardium in the isolated perfused heart preparation is limited by the relatively brief period of stability of this model (3–4 hours at most). As stunned myocardium may require days to weeks to recover completely from a severe or prolonged ischemic insult, this crucial component of the definition can often not be met: progressive improvements in function are often not seen, and full recovery can seldom be confirmed in a typical isolated perfused heart study. To determine whether these preparations represent true models of stunned myocardium, additional hallmarks of this phenomenon—including morphological evidence of reversible tissue injury (or an absence of irreversible injury), response to inotropic stimulation, partial preservation of adenosine triphosphate stores, and/or rebound in creatine phosphate concentrations—should be provided as confirmatory evidence in cases where progressive improvement in function cannot be documented.

B. Effects of Global Ischemia in the Isolated Buffer-Perfused Rat Heart

Isolated buffer-perfused hearts subjected to a brief episode of global ischemia followed by reperfusion exhibit transient abnormalities in systolic function and diastolic relaxation analogous to those observed in the in situ canine heart subjected to brief regional ischemia. For example, Apstein and colleagues (1978) assessed mechanical performance in isolated rat hearts subjected to 3 minutes of global ischemia followed by 20 minutes of reperfusion (Fig. 1). Not surprisingly, left ventricular (LV) developed pressure and the rate of change of LV pressure (positive and negative dP/dt) decayed to $<20\%$ of normal preocclusion values during the 3-minute period of ischemia. Following reperfusion, LV developed pressure and positive dP/dt were rapidly (within 30 seconds) restored to 65% of baseline, and then progressively re-

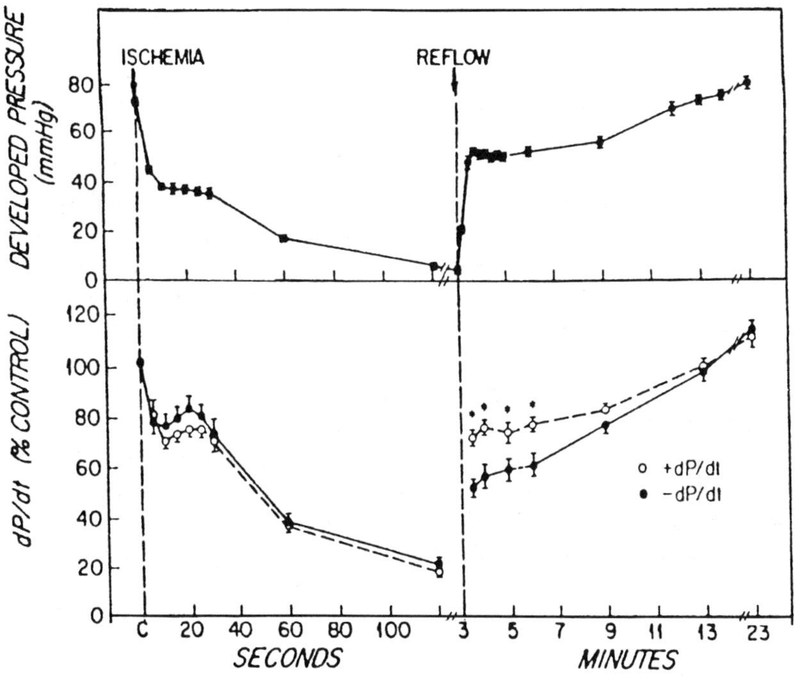

Figure 1 Temporal changes in left ventricular contractility and relaxation in isolated rat hearts ($n = 17$) subjected to 3 minutes of global ischemia and 20 minutes of reperfusion. dP/dt = first derivative of left ventricular pressure. $^{*}p < 0.05$ for +dP/dt vs. -dP/dt. (Reprinted with permission of the American Physiological Society from Apstein et al., 1978.)

covered to baseline values during the subsequent 10 minutes. Interestingly, the maximum rate of LV relaxation (negative dP/dt) exhibited greater postischemic dysfunction than did systolic contraction assessed by LV developed pressure and positive dP/dt. However, both systolic contraction and diastolic relaxation had recovered completely within 20 minutes of reperfusion (Fig. 1) (Apstein et al., 1978). The fact that function was initially depressed upon reflow but then progressively recovered to normal baseline values in this study definitively confirms that the isolated perfused rat heart had been stunned by the 3-minute episode of ischemia.

When the duration of global ischemia is increased to 10 minutes, LV developed tension remains depressed at 60–85% of its preischemia value, with no net improvement during the initial 30 minutes following reperfusion (Nayler et al., 1988, 1990) (see also Chapter 12). Confirmation of stunned myocardium in this protocol is, in principle, confounded by the plateau, or lack of a progressive increase in function, during the 30-minute observation period. However, electron microscopic analysis revealed *no ultrastructural defect that could explain the depressed mechanical performance observed in these hearts following reperfusion*. That is, the myocytes were only mildly and reversibly injured, providing the necessary confirmatory evidence that the tissue was in fact stunned by the brief, 10-minute episode of global ischemia (Nayler et al., 1988). Nayler and colleagues further noted that mechanical performance following reflow could be enhanced by inotropic stimulation (Nayler et al., 1988). Thus, as in the in vivo canine model of regional ischemia, rat hearts stunned by brief global ischemia maintained the latent capacity for normal, active contraction.

Isolated perfused hearts subjected to brief global ischemia/reperfusion also exhibit abnormalities in high energy phosphate metabolism similar to those observed in the in vivo canine model of the stunned myocardium. As expected, both adenosine triphosphate (ATP) and creatine phosphate (CP) stores were markedly depleted during 10 minutes of global ischemia (Fig. 2) (Nayler et al., 1988). Following reflow, ATP content remained mildly depressed at approximately 75% of preischemia values, but, as in the in vivo canine model, CP content rebounded to normal (or even supranormal) values (Fig. 2) (Nayler et al., 1988).

C. Variations of the Model

There is no question that the isolated heart preparation lends itself to virtually endless variation in terms of the species that is used, the route of coronary perfusion (retrograde vs. antegrade), the use of an isovolumic (i.e., balloon in LV) vs. nonisovolumic Langendorff preparation, the nature and composition of the perfusate, and the nature of the insult (ischemia vs. hypoxia). In fact, all of these manipulations have been used singly or in combination by one or more investigators in their efforts to elucidate the mechanisms of the stunned myocardium and/or evaluate the effects of numerous interventions on the recovery of mechanical performance following reflow. The following section provides a brief overview of the various models that have been employed in the study of brief transient ischemia and the effects of manipulating these various parameters on postischemic recovery of function.

1. Route of Perfusion

The route of coronary perfusion does not appear to mediate the consequences of brief global ischemia in the isolated buffer-perfused rat heart. Rat hearts perfused antegrade via the left atrium and subjected to 10–15 minutes of global ischemia followed by antegrade reflow exhibit significant postischemic

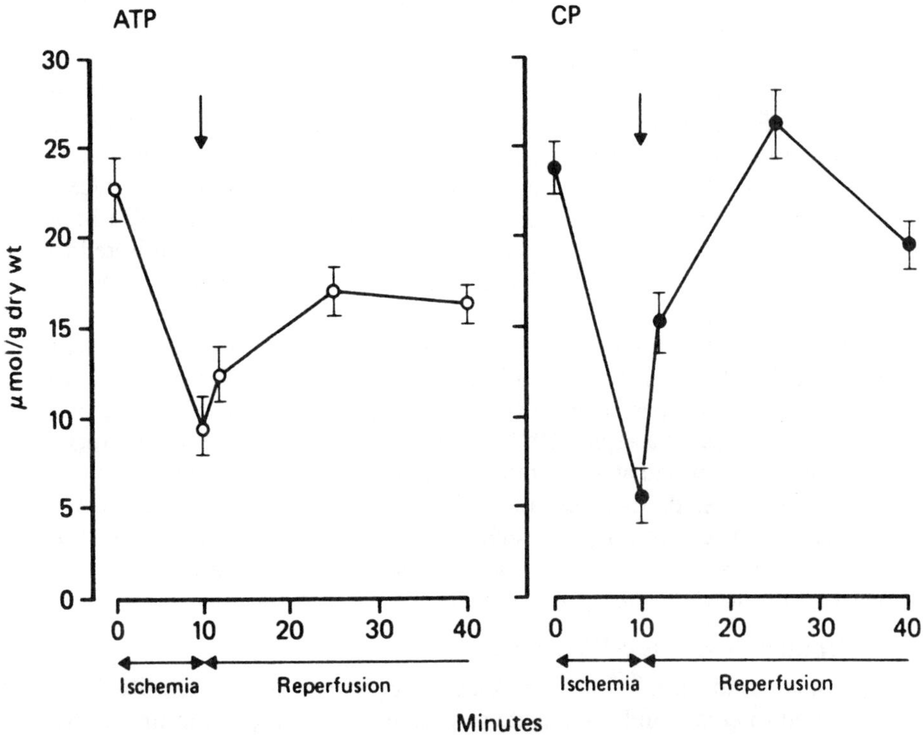

Figure 2 Effect of reperfusion after 10 minutes of global ischemia on adenosine triphosphate (ATP) and creatine phosphate (CP) content in isolated rat hearts. Each point represents the mean ± SEM of 6 experiments. Arrow indicates reperfusion. (Reprinted with permission of the American Physiological Society from Nayler et al., 1988.)

reduction in indices of mechanical performance (including LV developed pressure; developed pressure × heart rate; systolic pressure × cardiac output, etc.) to approximately 80% of preischemia values (Humphrey et al., 1985; Zucchi et al., 1990), depletion of ATP stores to approximately 70% of control values, and rapid restoration of CP content to normal or greater than normal levels (Taegtmeyer et al., 1985; Zucchi et al., 1990). These data are similar to the results obtained following 10 minutes of global ischemia in rat hearts perfused via the aorta in the Langendorff mode.

2. Species

Postischemic dysfunction following brief global ischemia is not limited to the isolated rat heart: postischemic dysfunction has also been described in other species, including the rabbit (Borgers et al., 1987; Ambrosio et al., 1989; Krause, 1990) and ferret (Kusuoka et al., 1987, 1990; Kitakaze et al., 1988). For example, 15–20 minutes of global ischemia followed by reperfusion in isolated, isovolumic Langendorff-perfused rabbit hearts results in postischemic values of LV developed pressure averaging 50–80% of baseline (Ambrosio et al., 1989; Krause, 1990), persistent postischemic depletion of ATP stores at 70% of control values, and recovery of CP content to at least preischemia values (Ambrosio et al., 1989). Similar results have also been obtained using isovolumic Langendorff-perfused ferret hearts subjected to 15 minutes of global ischemia (Kusuoka et al., 1987, 1990; Kitakaze et al., 1988).

In addition, 15–20 minutes of global ischemia in the isovolumic rabbit and ferret heart results in a modest increase in LV end diastolic pressure (7–10 mmHg) following reperfusion (Ambrosio et al., 1989; Krause, 1990; Kitakaze et al., 1988; Kusuoka et al., 1987, 1990). Importantly, these latter experiments were performed at a constant LV volume (achieved by placement of a noncompressible, fluid-filled balloon in the LV): thus, the increase in LV end-diastolic pressure reflects a small but significant reduction in distensibility (or increase in diastolic stiffness) (Apstein et al., 1977a,b; Isoyama et al., 1987) following brief global ischemia.

3. Repeated Brief Global Ischemia

Both single and repeated brief episodes of coronary artery occlusion have been used to create and investigate postischemic dysfunction in the in vivo canine model. For example, data obtained in our laboratory indicate that segment shortening measured 1 hour following 12 repeated 5-minute episodes of coronary occlusion recovers to a mean of 37% of baseline values, with no evidence of significant cumulative deterioration in contractile function between the first and the final ischemia/reperfusion cycles (Whittaker et al., 1991). Furthermore, segment shortening at 1 hour following reflow in the repeated occlusion model was similar to the value of 32% of baseline observed in canine myocardium stunned by a single 15-minute ischemic insult (Whittaker et al., 1991). It is important to note that, although the repeated occlusion protocols in many cases subject the myocardium to a total of ⩾60 minutes of ischemia, these repeated brief episodes of coronary artery occlusion interrupted by reperfusion do not result in myocyte necrosis (Nicklas et al., 1985). Details concerning the properties of canine myocardium stunned by repeated brief occlusions are reviewed in Chapter 4.

Similar results have been observed in isolated buffer-perfused rat hearts subjected to three repeated 10-minute episodes of normothermic global ischemia separated by 15–20 minutes of reflow (Nayler et al., 1988, 1990). Specifically, peak developed tension following the first ischemia/reperfusion sequence recovered to 60% of preischemia values and showed little additional deterioration at 55% and 51% of baseline following the second and third brief ischemic insult (Nayler et al., 1988). Repeated brief ischemia did not, however, result in an increase in resting tension (Nayler et al., 1988).

The effects of repeated brief ischemia have also been evaluated using isovolumic, blood-perfused rabbit hearts (Fig. 3) (Owen et al., 1989). Use of a blood perfusate avoids the potential confounding effects of buffer perfusion: for example, the high coronary flow rates required to adequately oxygenate the tissue during buffer perfusion (on the order of 8 ml/min, or 16 ml/min/g tissue) results in tissue edema (Vogel and Apstein, 1988). Although this edema does not appear to alter systolic function either before or after ischemia, it may influence the diastolic stiffness of the tissue (Vogel et al., 1986; Vogel and Apstein, 1988). In contrast, perfusion of the isolated heart with blood or erythrocyte suspensions permits the use of coronary flow rates on the order of 2 ml/min/g, which fall within the physiological range of 1.8 to 3.4 ml/min/g for the rabbit heart (Vogel et al., 1982). In any case, LV developed pressure following four repeated 5-minute episodes of brief ischemia in this blood-perfused model was depressed at 53% of baseline preischemia values (Fig. 3A) (Owen et al., 1989), in good agreement with the data obtained by Nayler and colleagues in the isolated rat heart. Brief repeated ischemia in this model also resulted in a modest but significant increase in LV end-diastolic pressure (Fig. 3B), similar in magnitude to that observed in isolated rabbit hearts stunned by a single 15- to 20-minute period of sustained global ischemia.

4. Regional Ischemia in the Isolated Heart

It is interesting to note that global ischemia is not a prerequisite for postischemic dysfunction in the isolated heart. Evidence obtained in isolated Langendorff-perfused rat hearts indicates that 15 minutes of regional ischemia (achieved by transient ligation of the left coronary artery) followed by 30 minutes of reflow results in persistent depression of LV pressure generation, rate-pressure product and apex displacement to 30–35% of baseline preischemia values (de Graeff et al., 1986). In fact, recovery of mechanical performance following brief regional ischemia in the isolated heart is similar in magnitude to that observed following a comparable episode of brief global ischemia, probably due to the large proportion (30–50%) of the LV that is rendered ischemic by proximal coronary occlusion in the rat model (Li et al., 1992).

5. "Demand" Ischemia

As described in Chapter 5, stunned myocardium has also been documented in the in vivo canine model of "demand" ischemia: that is, in the setting of

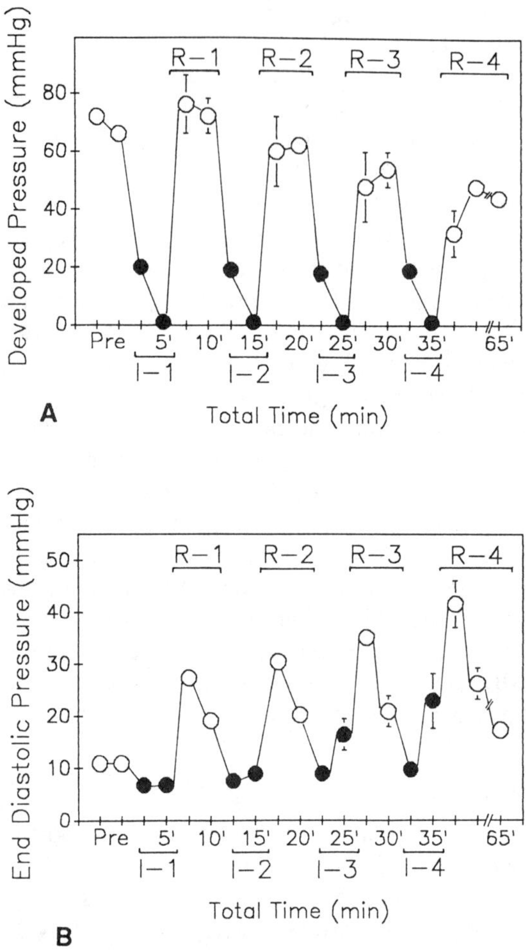

Figure 3 Effect of four repeated 5-minute episodes of global ischemia on: (A) left ventricular developed pressure; and (B) left ventricular end-diastolic pressure in the isovolumic blood-perfused rabbit heart. Measurements obtained during ischemia are indicated by the filled circles. I = ischemia; R = reperfusion. (Adapted with permission from Owen et al., 1989.)

increased myocardial oxygen demand induced by treadmill exercise in dogs instrumented with a coronary artery stenosis. Although placement of the stenosis per se (resulting in a reduction in resting blood flow of <20%) did not alter wall motion as compared with baseline, 10 minutes of treadmill exercise (such that heart rate was increased to 200–240 beats/min) depressed contractile function during ischemia to 40% of baseline values. Furthermore, contractile function remained significantly depressed or stunned at 50–70% of baseline values for the initial 30 minutes following exercise (Homans et al., 1986).

An ex vivo analog of this in vivo canine model has been reported by Isoyama et al. (1987) in the isovolumic blood-perfused rabbit heart. Specifically, Isoyama and colleagues superimposed pacing tachycardia at a frequency of 6.4 Hz on a 6-minute episode of global low-flow ischemia, achieved by reducing coronary perfusion pressure from 100 to 20 mmHg. Following a 6-minute reduction in perfusion pressure at a physiological pacing rate of 4 Hz (the ex vivo equivalent of the "stenosis" alone), LV developed pressure remained mildly stunned at 80–90% of preischemia values. LV end-diastolic pressure gradually recovered to baseline during the first 20 minutes after relief of ischemia (Isoyama et al., 1987; Lorell et al., 1988), and, as in the in vivo canine model of regional ischemia (Przyklenk et al., 1987), diastolic relaxation time T remained persistently evaluated at 120% of baseline values following reperfusion (Isoyama et al., 1987). That is, these data demonstrate postischemic dysfunction both during systole and during diastole in this model. Pacing tachycardia exacerbated the deterioration in developed pressure, increase in end-diastolic pressure, and prolongation of diastolic relaxation time measured during low-flow ischemia, but did not exacerbate the magnitude of postischemic dysfunction observed following reflow (Isoyama et al., 1987). Thus, although the relative contribution of the "stenosis" per se vs. superimposed "demand" ischemia to postischemic dysfunction clearly differs in the isolated rabbit heart vs. the in vivo canine model, there is no doubt that pacing tachycardia superimposed upon global low-flow ischemia represents a model of the stunned myocardium.

6. Hypoxia/Reoxygenation in the Isolated Papillary Muscle

Isolated myocardium exhibits the phenomenon of stunning following hypoxia as well as following ischemia. For example, Figure 4 illustrates posthypoxic dysfunction during both systole and diastole in isolated rat trabecular and papillary muscle subjected to 60 minutes to hypoxia and 30 minutes of reoxygenation (Apstein et al., 1976). Figure 4A shows temporal changes in developed tension throughout the protocol for tissue bathed with substrate containing a normal concentration of glucose, a high concentration of glucose, or a normal concentration of glucose + mannitol. The high glucose group exhibited a progressive improvement in developed tension following reoxygenation, with full recovery to preocclusion values observed within 15 minutes. Thus, there is no question that this group was truly stunned by hypoxia/reoxygenation. In contrast, the groups suffused with normal glucose (with or without mannitol) exhibited a slower rate of recovery of function: developed tension continued to increase throughout the 30 minutes following hypoxia. Whether these groups would have ultimately recovered to base-

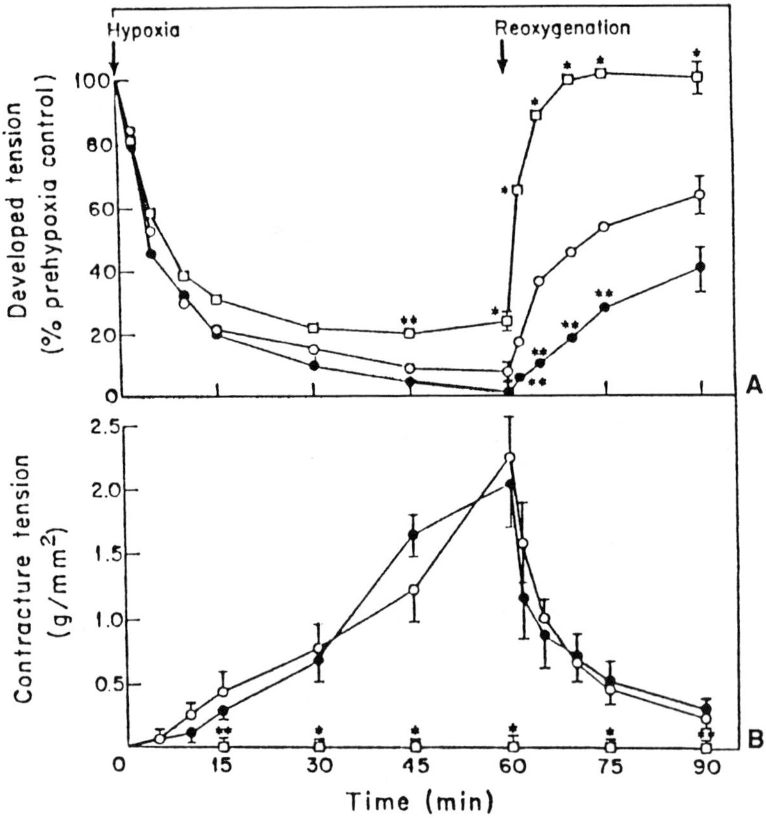

Figure 4 (A and B) Mechanical performance of isolated rat papillary and trabecular muscle subjected to 60 minutes of hypoxia and 30 minutes of reoxygenation. Tissue was hypothermic (28–30 °C) and stimulated to contract at 12 times per minute. Effects of high glucose concentration (open boxes) ($n = 6$), low glucose concentration with mannitol (closed circles) ($n = 5$), and low glucose concentration without mannitol (open circles) ($n = 10$) were evaluated. Note that the high glucose group is stunned following reperfusion. $^{**}p < 0.05$ and $^{*}p < 0.01$ vs. low glucose-no mannitol group. (Reprinted with permission from Apstein et al., 1976.)

line values (that is, whether this tissue was truly stunned) cannot be confirmed from this brief 30-minute observation period.

Figure 4B reports the effects of hypoxia/reoxygenation on diastolic dysfunction as assessed by the increase in resting tension or contracture (Apstein et al., 1976). Tissue bathed with high glucose exhibited no increase in resting tension during the protocol. However, papillary muscles suffused with normal glucose concentrations demonstrated stunning during diastole, in that the intial posthypoxic contracture progressively dissipated to near-normal values during the 30 minutes following reoxygenation.

Despite the apparently prolonged (60-minute) duration of hypoxia in this study, the severity of the hypoxic insult was relatively mild because the tissue was hypothermic (28–30 °C) and because the tissue was stimulated to contract at the relatively low rate of 12 per minute (Apstein et al., 1976). (The ability of hypothermia to attenuate ischemic injury is addressed in further detail in Section III.) Nonetheless, there is no question that the hypoxic/reoxygenated papillary muscles in this study demonstrate the essential features of post-hypoxic stunning.

III. CONSEQUENCES OF PROLONGED GLOBAL ISCHEMIA/REPERFUSION

In the in vivo canine model, increasing the duration of coronary artery occlusion to >30 minutes results in irreversible myocyte injury within the subendocardium: as the duration of occlusion is further increased, cell death progresses as a transmural time-dependent wavefront across the LV wall (Reimer et al., 1977; Reimer and Jennings, 1979). Thus, although 30 minutes to 3 hours of transient coronary occlusion in the canine model results in subendocardial necrosis, the overlying subepicardium remains viable but stunned, exhibiting gradual improvement in contractile function and high energy phosphate metabolism during the initial weeks following reflow (Ellis et al., 1983).

A. Consequences of Prolonged Total Normothermic Global Ischemia

Does prolonged normothermic global ischemia followed by reflow in the isolated perfused heart represent a model of stunned myocardium analogous to that seen in canine myocardium subjected to prolonged but transient coronary artery occlusion (as detailed in Chapter 2) or in patients successfully reperfused for the treatment of acute myocardial infarction (see Chapter 18)? Reperfusion following 30 minutes of total global ischemia at 37 °C in the isolated heart preparation results in some restoration of contractility (Figs. 5,6A): indices of postischemic mechanical performance (e.g., LV developed pressure; developed tension; cardiac output) have ranged from 15 to 40% of baseline in the rabbit (Ambrosio et al., 1987) and rat models (Elz and Nayler, 1988; Nayler et al., 1990; Higgins and Blackburn, 1984; Watts et al., 1985; Kirkels et al., 1988). However, recovery of function is clearly less than that observed after ≤20 minutes of ischemia. In addition, 30 minutes of ischemia

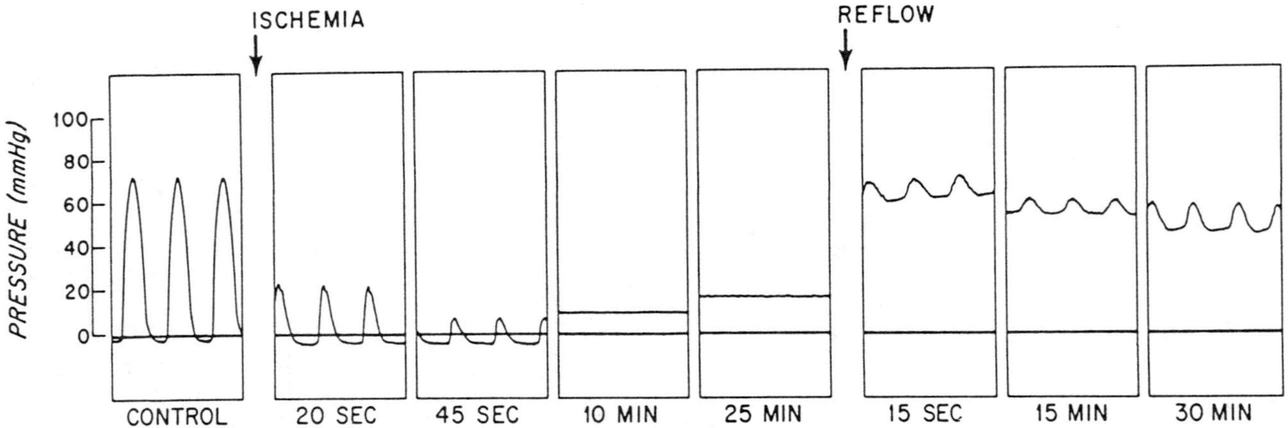

Figure 5 Left ventricular pressure tracing during ischemia and reflow in an isolated rat heart paced at 300 beats/min. Ischemia causes a rapid fall in developed pressure. After 10 minutes, contraction had ceased and mild diastolic contracture or rigor had developed (as reflected by the sustained increase in intraventricular pressure), which increased with subsequent ischemia. Reflow after 30 minutes of ischemia caused a marked increase in contracture and return of contractile activity as a reduced level. (Reprinted from Apstein et al., 1977a, with permission of the American Heart Association.)

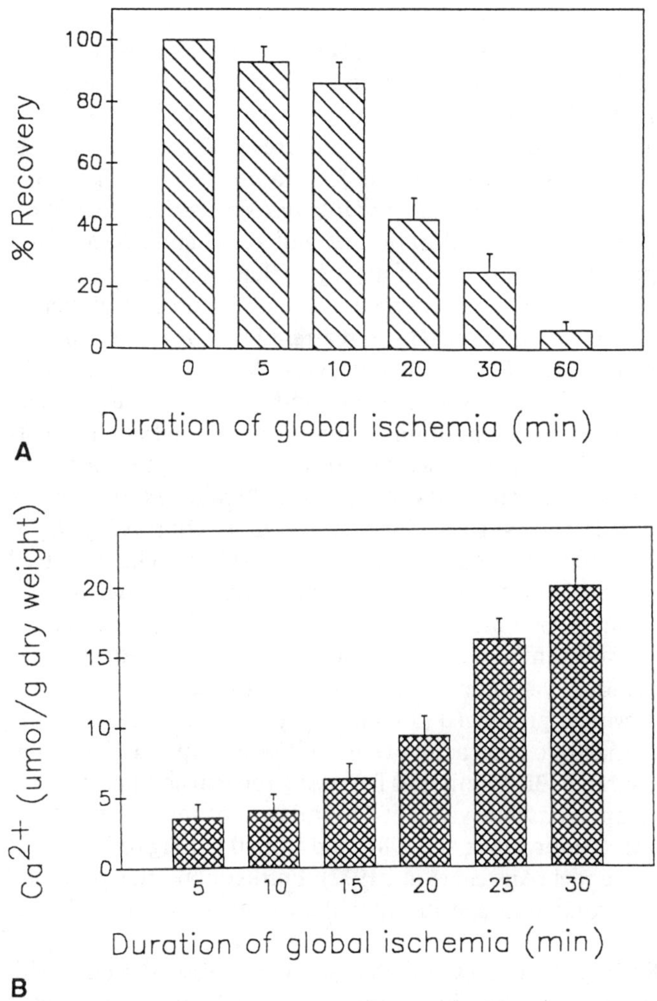

Figure 6 Effect of duration of global ischemia on: (A) % recovery of mechanical function; and (B) reperfusion-induced calcium gain in isolated Langendorff-perfused rat hearts after ischemia/reperfusion. Each point represents the mean ± SEM of six experiments. (Adapted with permission from Nayler et al., 1990.)

followed by reflow results in a more marked depletion of ATP stores to 20-50% of normal (Kirkels et al., 1988; Elz and Nayler, 1988; Ambrosio et al., 1987). However, as illustrated in Figures 5 and 6, 30 minutes of unmodified normothermic global ischemia also results in massive calcium influx upon reperfusion, profound diastolic contracture, and irreversible tissue injury—factors that clearly demonstrate that this slightly more prolonged ischemic insult *does not represent a true model of viable but stunned myocardium.*

Not surprisingly, increasing the duration of global ischemia results in a progressive increase in the proportion of myocytes that become irreversibly injured by the ischemic insult. For example, even 15 minutes of global ischemia in the isolated rabbit heart results in scattered foci of irreversible injury involving approximately 8% of the myocytes. After 30 minutes of ischemia, 80% and 60% of cells in the subendo- and subepicardium, respectively, exhibited cytolysis, pyknosis of nuclei, and contraction band necrosis (Borgers et al., 1987). Similar evidence of irreversible myocyte injury has been documented in isolated rat hearts subjected to 30 minutes of ischemia followed by reflow (Elz and Nayler, 1988). However, in contrast to the in vivo canine model, global ischemia in the isolated heart is not characterized by a time-dependent transmural gradient in cell vulnerability and death (Borgers et al., 1987). That is, 30 minutes of normothermic ischemia in the isolated heart results in substantial cell death: the proportion of myocytes that are viable (and presumably stunned) following reperfusion is small.

Reperfusion following a prolonged (30-minute) episode of global ischemia results in profound diastolic contracture (Fig. 5). For example, LV end-diastolic pressure measured at 30-45 minutes following reperfusion has been reported to increase from a baseline value of 11 mmHg to 65 mmHg in the isovolumic rabbit model (Ambrosio et al., 1987) and from 0 mmHg to 34 mmHg in the isovolumic rat model (Apstein et al., 1977). Furthermore, this profound contracture persists throughout reperfusion in these studies, with no evidence of recovery.

Reperfusion following 30 minutes of global ischemia is also associated with massive and uncontrolled calcium influx into the previously ischemic cells. For example, total tissue calcium content averages approximately 4-6 μmol/g dry weight in normoxic buffer-perfused rat hearts (Fig. 6B) (Elz and Nayler, 1988; Nayler et al., 1988, 1990). Brief global ischemia (15 minutes) is characterized by subtle but significant increases in peak systolic *intracellular* calcium concentration in the reversibly injured tissue, resulting in an increase in the amplitude of the intracellular calcium transient between systole and diastole (Kusuoka et al., 1990). In fact, as discussed in Chapter 9, this subtle temporal abnormality in intracellular calcium homeostasis has been hailed as an important mechanism in the pathophysiology of the stunned myocardium. However, *total tissue calcium concentration* remains essentially unchanged at approximately 4-6 μmol/g after 10–15 minutes of global ischemia and 15 minutes of reflow (Elz and Nayler, 1988; Nayler et al., 1988, 1990).

In contrast, total tissue calcium content increases markedly to 20–27 μmol/g after 30 minutes of ischemia and 15 minutes of reperfusion (Fig. 6B) (Elz and Nayler, 1988; Nayler et al., 1988, 1990). This massive calcium influx is attributed both to membrane damage per se and inadequate supplies of high energy phosphate stores needed to maintain calcium (and other ion) gradients across the sarcolemma, sarcoplasmic reticulum, and mitochondrial membranes (Opie, 1991; Barry, 1991). There is no question that calcium overload has dire consequences, including loss of mitochondrial function, wasting of energy due to activation of Ca^{2+}-sensitive ATPases and persistent tension development during diastole, and tissue injury due to activation of Ca^{2+}-sensitive phospholipases (Nayler, 1982). In fact, an uncontrolled increase in total tissue calcium content in the isolated perfused heart had been associated with electron microscopic evidence of irreversible myocyte injury (Borgers et al., 1987).

Injury due to ischemia is a continuum: the number of cells that progress from reversible to irreversible injury increases as a function of the duration and severity of the ischemic insult. Thus, any sharp distinction between "brief" ischemia and "prolonged" ischemia is somewhat arbitrary. However, the data clearly indicate that a 30-minute episode of normothermic global ischemia in the isolated perfused heart model results in a heterogenous population of both irreversibly injured and viable but stunned myocytes. Furthermore, the apparent absence of a transmural wavefront of cell death, combined with the global indices of contractile performance and metabolic status typically used in these models, confounds any efforts to focus on the properties of the stunned myocytes per se in the setting of prolonged total global ischemia followed by reperfusion.

B. Variations of the Model

Although 30 minutes of sustained normothermic global ischemia does not represent a homogeneous (or readily measurable) model of the stunned myocardium, prolonged ischemia in the isolated heart can be manipulated such that the tolerance of the myocytes to ischemia is increased and irreversible injury is thereby minimized. Numerous investigators have employed countless interventions in an effort to minimize ischemic injury in the isolated heart model, and a comprehensive review of these studies is beyond the scope of this chapter. Rather, we focus on three specific and important variations of the model—reduction in temperature, the use of prolonged low-flow (rather than total) ischemia, and manipulation of metabolic substrates—that have all been shown to attenuate injury due to prolonged ischemia in the isolated perfused heart. This reduction in ischemic injury increases the proportion of viable (and presumably stunned) cells present at the time of reperfusion, and thereby modifies the preparation such that it reverts to a model of the stunned myocardium.

1. Hypothermia and Cardioplegia

There is no question that cooling of the heart (with and without potassium-induced cardiac arrest) enhances the tolerance of the myocardium to prolonged global ischemia: this is best illustrated by the overwhelming evidence that hypothermic cardioplegia protects the myocardium, at least in part, from prolonged ischemia during cardiac surgery. For example, Nayler (1982) used isolated Langendorff-perfused rabbit hearts to assess recovery of function and energy metabolism following 60 minutes of total global ischemia at temperatures ranging from 37 °C to 5 °C (Fig. 7). As expected, reperfusion following 60 minutes of normothermic ischemia was associated with poor recovery of active tension generation to only 5% of preischemia values and persistent severe depletion of ATP stores at 20% of baseline values. Furthermore, the mitochondria developed massive (>300%) calcium overload and were essentially unable to generate ATP (Fig. 7) (Nayler, 1982). This tissue

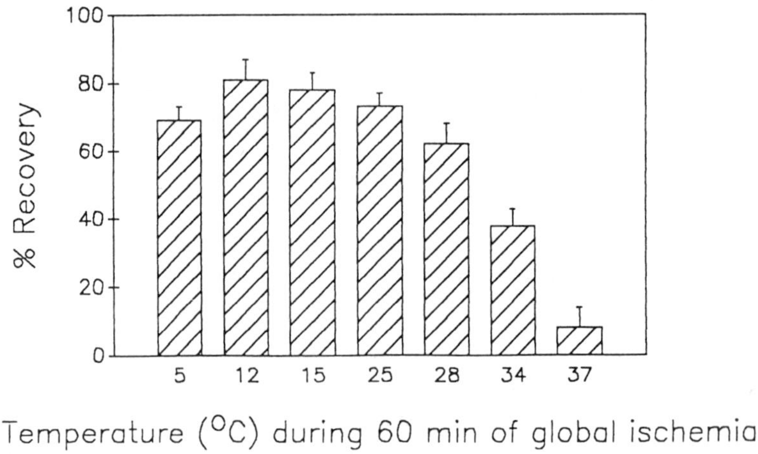

A

Figure 7 Effect of temperature during ischemia on: (A) % recovery of mechanical function; (B) % retention of mitochondrial ATP producing activity; and (C) % increase in mitochondrial calcium content in isolated Langendorff-perfused rabbit hearts subjected to 60 minutes of global ischemia followed by normothermic reperfusion. (Adapted with permission from Nayler, 1982.)

subjected to prolonged normothermic ischemia was, for the most part, necrotic.

Hypothermia during the ischemic insult was cardioprotective, with the greatest protection achieved at temperatures of 12–15 °C (Fig. 7): active tension following reflow recovered to 80% of preischemia values, tissue ATP content averaged 65% of normal, mitochondrial calcium overload was limited to approximately 10%, and the mitochondria maintained approximately 60% of their ability to synthesize ATP (Nayler, 1982). These data imply that the

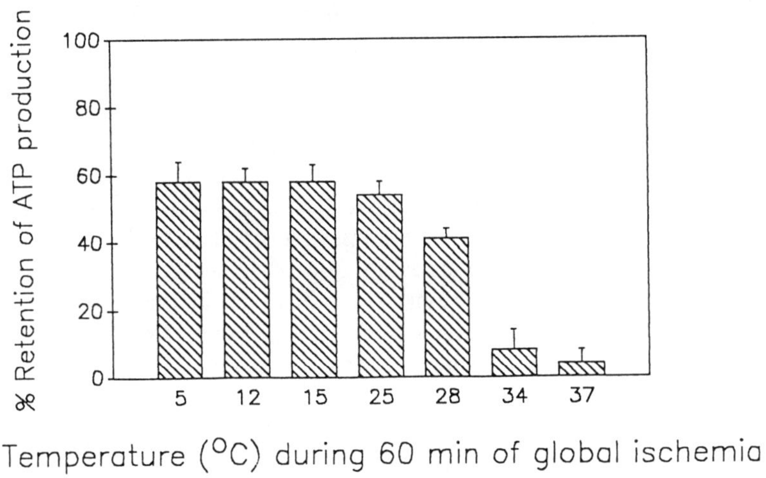

B

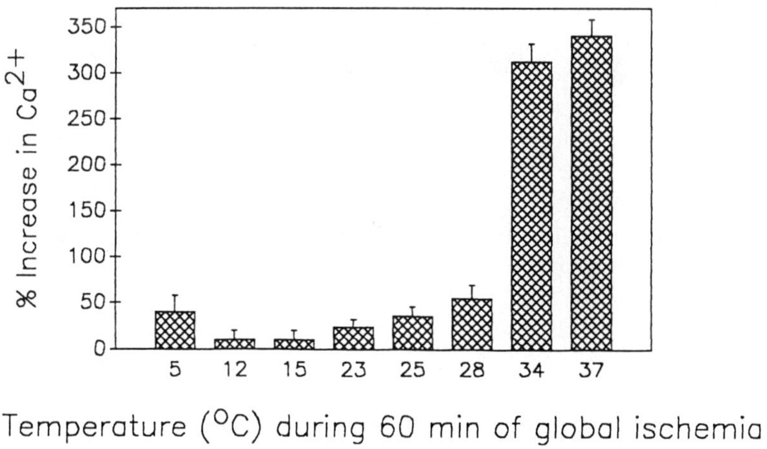

C

isolated hearts subjected to hypothermic global ischemia were viable but stunned following reflow. However, as described in Section II, complete recovery of this tissue (as per the definition of stunned myocardium) could not be documented or confirmed during the time course of the experiment.

Potassium-induced cardioplegia has similarly been shown to enhance recovery of contractile and metabolic performance following prolonged global ischemia. Furthermore, the protective effects of hypothermia and potassium-induced cardioplegia have been shown to be additive (Rosenfeldt et al., 1980). Not surprisingly, the protective effects of both hypothermia and cardioplegia have been attributed to an energy-sparing mechanism: cooling the heart slows the rate of cardiac metabolism, and the rapid arrest of the heart achieved by addition of potassium to the perfusate further attenuates the metabolic requirements of the tissue (Nayler, 1982).

A comprehensive review of the cardioprotective effects of hypothermia, cardioplegia (and a host of pharmacological interventions) in isolated perfused hearts subjected to global ischemia, in experimental models of cardiopulmonary bypass, and patients undergoing cardiac surgery has been provided by McGoon (1985). These data leave little doubt that myocardium subjected to prolonged hypothermic global ischemia (or prolonged hypothermic arrest) followed by reperfusion is viable but stunned.

2. Prolonged Low-Flow Ischemia

While 30 minutes of total normothermic global ischemia in the isolated heart results in irreversible tissue injury, partial or low-flow ischemia results in reversible injury to the myocytes. Recovery of function following transient low-flow ischemia has been assessed by Apstein et al. (1977) in isovolumic buffer-perfused rat hearts perfused for 30 minutes at 0, 0.04, 0.4, and 0.8 ml/min (or 0, 0.5, 5, and 10% of baseline coronary flow rates) (Fig. 8). Following severe ischemia (flow rates of 0 and 0.04 ml/min), developed pressure at 30 minutes following reflow recovered to only 16–25% of preischemia values. In addition, these hearts showed enzymatic evidence of irreversible tissue injury. In contrast, developed pressure following more moderate ischemia (flow rates of 0.4 and 0.8 ml/min) progressively recovered to 85–94% of baseline values within the initial 20 minutes of reflow (Fig. 8A) (Apstein et al., 1977).

All four groups exhibited significant increases in LV end-diastolic pressure during the ischemic episode (Fig. 8B). Diastolic contracture persisted following reflow in hearts perfused at 0 and 0.04 ml/min, with end-diastolic pressure remaining markedly elevated at 34–48 mmHg. In contrast, diastolic pressure recovered to near-normal values of 4–5 mmHg following reperfusion in hearts perfused at 0.4 and 0.8 ml/min during ischemia (Fig. 8B) (Apstein et al., 1977). That is, myocardium subjected to prolonged, 30-minute perfu-

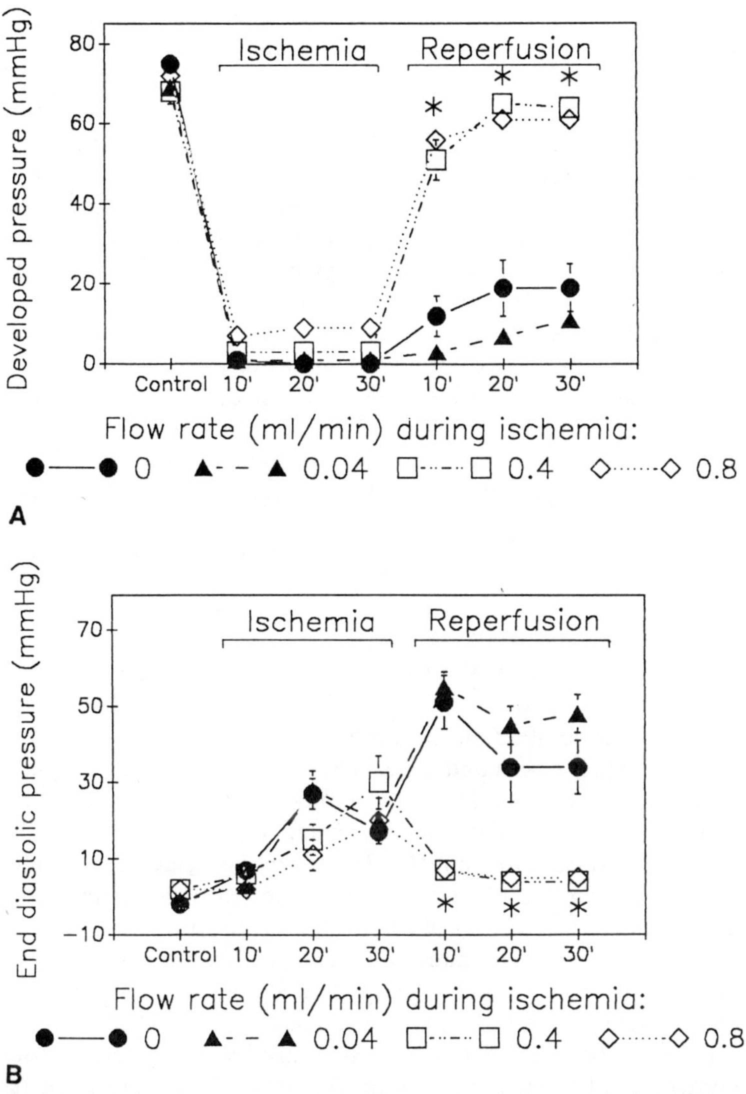

Figure 8 (A) Left ventricular developed pressure and (B) left ventricular end-diastolic pressure in isolated buffer-perfused rat hearts subjected to 30 minutes of low-flow ischemia at flow rates of 0, 0.04, 0.4, and 0.8 ml/min (or 0, 0.5, 5, and 10% of baseline values) followed by 30 minutes of reperfusion. $^*p < 0.001$ for either the 0 or 0.04 ml/min groups vs. either the 0.4 and 0.08 ml/min groups. (Adapted from Apstein et al., 1977.)

sion at 5–10% of baseline coronary flow rates was able to tolerate the moderate ischemic result and remained viable but stunned.

Similar results have been reported by Ferrari et al. (1988) using isolated rabbit hearts perfused for 30 minutes at 4% of baseline coronary flow rates. Peak systolic pressure was restored to 92% of baseline following reflow, with no evidence of diastolic contracture or calcium overload. In addition, ATP and CP content were only mildly depressed, and normal mitochondrial function was resumed following reperfusion (Ferrari et al., 1988). Not surprisingly, however, the preparation cannot be maintained indefinitely under these conditions: when the duration of low-flow ischemia was extended to 90 minutes, there was essentially no recovery of function following reflow, the hearts developed contracture with LV end-diastolic pressure averaging 55 mmHg, ATP and CP stores were severely depleted, and the tissue was overloaded with calcium (Ferrari et al., 1988). Prolonged perfusion at even slightly higher flow rates (90 minutes at 11% of baseline coronary flow rates) were better tolerated, with maximal developed pressure returning to 41% of baseline after reperfusion, partial depletion of ATP stores at 50% of normal, and only mild depression of CP stores at 85% of normal (Vogel and Apstein, 1988).

3. Increased Glycolytic Substrate

High concentrations of glucose + insulin added to the perfusate have been shown to protect the isolated rabbit heart from prolonged periods of moderate (but not total) normothermic ischemia (Apstein et al., 1983; Eberli et al., 1991). For example, Eberli and colleagues recently reported the effects of hyperglycemia + insulin on recovery of function in isovolumic rabbit hearts following 2.5 hours of moderate ischemia, achieved by lowering the coronary perfusion pressure to 8 mmHg. Treatment with glucose + insulin protected the hearts against injury during ischemia and thus, not surprisingly, resulted in superior recovery of systolic and diastolic function following reperfusion. Specifically, at 30 minutes after reflow, LV developed pressure averaged 68% vs. 17% of baseline values, while LV end-diastolic pressure averaged 68 vs. 23 mmHg in control vs. treated hearts (Fig. 9) (Eberli et al., 1991). Similar improved recovery with high concentrations of glucose + insulin as also observed following 3 hours of moderate ischemia achieved by reducing the coronary perfusion rate to 1 ml/min (Apstein et al., 1983). Apstein and colleagues further noted a progressive increase (rather than plateau) in function following reflow and provided electron microscopic evidence of reversible (rather than irreversible) injury in hearts treated with glucose + insulin.

Possible mechanisms for this cardioprotection with glucose + insulin are complex and may involve such diverse concepts as increased blood osmolarity, increased glycolytic flux, replenishment of potassium ions, esterifi-

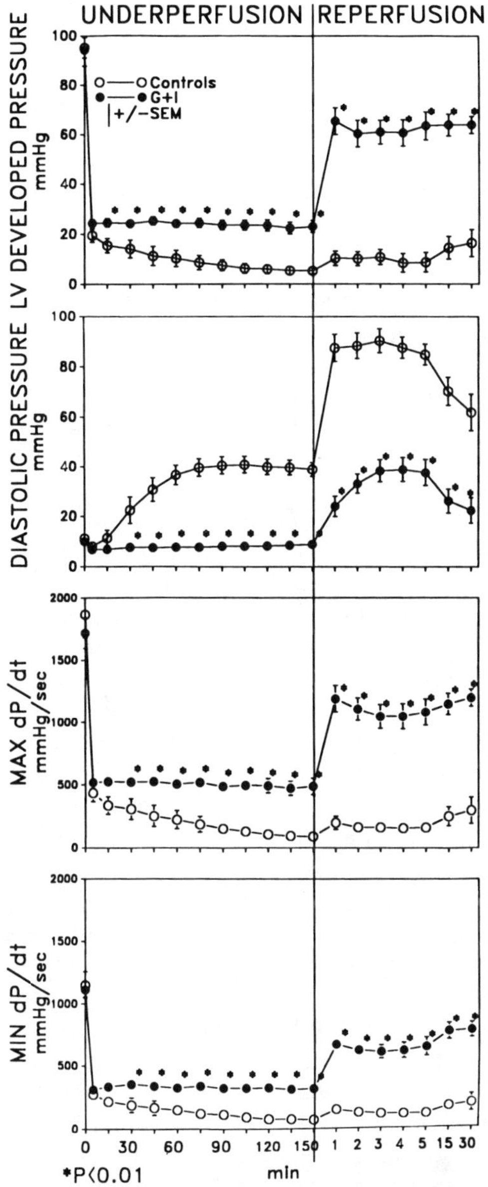

Figure 9 Effect of 2.5 hours of moderate global ischemia (perfusion pressure of 8 mmHg) followed by 30 minutes of reperfusion in isovolumic rabbit hearts perfused with erythrocyte suspensions. Data were obtained for control hearts (n = 8) and hearts perfused with high levels of glucose + insulin (G + I) (n = 8). LV = left ventricle; dP/dt = first derivative of LV pressure. *$p < 0.01$ vs. control. (Reprinted with permission of the American Heart Association from Eberli et al., 1991.)

cation of intracellular free fatty acids, and even scavenging of free radicals (Eberli et al., 1991). In any case, glucose + insulin clearly protected against ischemic injury in this model and, as a result, these hearts appeared to be reversibly injured and stunned following prolonged moderate ischemia/reperfusion.

IV. ROLE OF THE ISOLATED HEART MODEL IN THE STUDY OF STUNNED MYOCARDIUM

Isolated perfused hearts subjected to brief global ischemia, repeated episodes of brief global ischemia, regional ischemia, demand ischemia, prolonged hypothermic global ischemia, or prolonged low-flow ischemia exhibit the characteristic hallmarks of the stunned myocardium: persistent systolic and diastolic dysfunction, partial depletion of ATP content, and rapid resumption of oxidative phosphorylation (as indicated by the rebound in CP stores) in viable, previously ischemic tissue salvaged by reperfusion.

Contractile and metabolic function of stunned myocardium will, as defined from the in vivo models, recover to normal values during the days to weeks following reflow. Eventual long-term recovery following transient ischemia—the caveat in the definition of the stunned myocardium—clearly cannot be confirmed in most studies involving the isolated perfused heart model: this represents an important consideration in determining whether postischemic dysfunction in these models truly represents stunned myocardium. Perhaps even more importantly, acute dysfunction observed during the initial 30-60 minutes following reflow in the isolated heart may be a consequence of both stunned myocardium and *instability of the preparation*. For example, although most investigators are careful to document and confirm the stability of a well-oxygenated preparation over the time course of their experiments, Duan and Karmazyn (1989) reported that developed force in control hearts deteriorated to 65% of baseline values—in the absence of ischemia/reperfusion—during 80 minutes of normoxic buffer perfusion.

Despite these important limitations, the isolated heart model provides numerous advantages over the in vivo model in the study of the stunned myocardium. Specifically, measurement of postischemic dysfunction following global ischemia/reperfusion is not confounded by hemodynamic or neurohumoral effects or by hypercontractility of adjacent, nonischemic tissue. Furthermore, the importance of a specific component of the perfusate, or the effects of subtle variations in the severity of ischemia, can be assessed in a highly controlled and accurate manner. Perhaps the most obvious and direct application of results obtained from the isolated heart model involves the recovery of function following cardiac surgery. However, the isolated heart preparation has also provided our first insights into the role of both oxygen-derived free radicals and intracellular calcium homeostasis in the pathophysiology of postischemic dysfunction (see Chapters 8 and 9). There is no doubt that data derived from the isolated perfused heart model will continue to make important contributions to our understanding of the stunned myocardium.

REFERENCES

Ambrosio, G., Jacobus, W. E., Bergman, C. A., Weisman, H. F., and Becker, L. C. (1987). Preserved high energy phosphate metabolic reserve in globally "stunned" hearts despite reduction of basal ATP content and contractility. *J. Mol. Cell. Cardiol. 19*: 953.

Ambrosio, G., Jacobus, W. E., Mitchell, M. C., Litt, M. R., and Becker, L. C. (1989). Effects of ATP precursors on ATP and free ADP content and functional recovery of postischemic hearts. *Am. J. Physiol. 256*: H560.

Apstein, C. S., Bing, O. H. L., and Levine, H. J. (1976). Cardiac muscle function during and after hypoxia: effects of glucose concentration, mannitol and isoproterenol. *J. Mol. Cell Cardiol. 8*: 627.

Apstein, C. S., Mueller, M., and Hood, W. B. (1977a). Ventricular contracture and compliance changes with global ischemia and reperfusion, and their effects on coronary resistance in the rat. *Circ. Res. 41*: 206.

Apstein, C. S., Deckelbaum, L., Mueller, M., Hagopian, L., and Hood, W. B. (1977b). Graded global ischemia and reperfusion: cardiac function and lactate metabolism. *Circulation 55*: 864.

Apstein, C. S., Deckelbaum L., Hagopian, L., and Hood, W. B. (1978). Acute cardiac ischemia and reperfusion: contractility, relaxation, and glycolysis. *Am. J. Physiol. 235*: H637.

Apstein, C. S., Gravino, F. N., and Haudenschild, C. C. (1983). Determinants of a protective effect of glucose and insulin on the ischemic myocardium: effects on contractile function, diastolic compliance, metabolism and ultrastructure during ischemia and reperfusion. *Circ. Res. 52*: 515.

Barry, W. H. (1991). Calcium and ischemic injury. *Trends Cardiovasc. Med. 1*: 162.

Borgers, M., Shu, L. G., Xhonneux, R., Thone, F., and van Overloop, P. (1987). Changes in ultrastructure and Ca^{2+} distribution in the isolated working rabbit heart after ischemia: a time-related study. *Am. J. Pathol. 126*: 92.

de Graeff, P. A., van Gilst, W. H., de Langen, C. D. J., Kingma, J. H., and Wesseling, H. (1986). Concentration-dependent protection by captopril against ischemia-reperfusion injury in the isolated rat heart. *Arch. Int. Pharmacodyn. Ther. 280*: 181.

Duan, J., and Karmazyn, M. (1989). Relationship between oxidative phosphorylation and adenine nucleotide translocase activity of two populations of cardiac mitochondria and mechanical recovery of ischemic hearts following reperfusion. *Can. J. Physiol. Pharmacol. 67*: 704.

Eberli, F. R., Weinberg, E. O., Grice, W. N., Horowitz, G. L., and Apstein, C. S. (1991). Protective effect of increased glycolytic substrate against systolic and diastolic dysfunction and increased coronary resistance from prolonged global underperfusion and reperfusion in isolated rabbit hearts perfused with erythrocyte suspensions. *Circ. Res. 68*: 466.

Ellis, S. G., Henschke, C. I., Sandor, T., Wynne, J., and Braunwald, E. (1983). Time course of functional and biochemical recovery of myocardium salvaged by reperfusion. *J. Am. Coll. Cardiol. 1*: 1047.

Elz, J. S., and Nayler, W. G. (1988). Contractile activity and reperfusion-induced calcium gain after ischemia in the isolated rat heart. *Lab. Invest. 58*: 653.

Ferrari, R., Ceconi, C., Currelo, S., Cargnoni, A., Condorelli, E., Belloli, S., Albertini, A., and Visioli, O. (1988). Metabolic changes during post-ischemic reperfusion. *J. Mol. Cell. Cardiol. 20*(Suppl. II): 119.

Heyndrickx, G. R., Millard, R. W., McRitchie, R. J., Maroko, P. R., and Vatner, S. F. (1975). Regional myocardial function and electrophysiological alterations after brief coronary artery occlusion in conscious dogs. *J. Clin. Invest. 56*: 978.

Heyndrickx, G. R., Baig, H., Nellens, P., Leusen, I., Fishbein, M. C., and Vatner, S. F. (1978). Depression of regional blood flow and wall thickening after brief coronary occlusions. *Am. J. Physiol. 234*: H635.

Higgins, A. J., and Blackburn, K. J. (1984). Prevention of reperfusion damage in working rat hearts by calcium antagonists and calmodulin antagonists. *J. Mol. Cell. Cardiol. 16*: 427.

Homans, D. C., Sublett, E., Dai, X. Z., and Bache, R. J. (1986). Persistence of regional left ventricular dysfunction after exercise-induced myocardial ischemia. *J. Clin. Invest 77*: 66.

Humphrey, S. M., Hollis, D. G., and Seelye, R. N. (1985). Myocardial adenine pool depletion and recovery of mechanical function following ischemia. *Am. J. Physiol. 248*: H644.

Isoyama, S., Apstein, C. S., Wexler, L. F., Grice, W. N., and Lorell, B. H. (1987). Acute decrease in left ventricular diastolic chamber distensibility during simulated angina in isolated hearts. *Circ. Res. 61*: 925.

Kirkels, J. H., Ruigrok, T. J. C., van Echteld, C. J. A., and Meijler, F. L. (1988). Protective effect of pretreatment with the calcium antagonist anipamil on the ischemic-reperfused rat myocardium: a phosphorous-31 nuclear magnetic resonance study. *J. Am. Coll. Cardiol. 5*: 1087.

Kitakaze, M., Weisfeldt, M. L., and Marban, E., (1988). Acidosis during early reperfusion prevents myocardial stunning in perfused ferret hearts. *J. Clin. Invest. 82*: 920.

Krause, S. M. (1990). Effect of global myocardial stunning on Ca^{2+}-sensitive myofibrillar ATPase activity and creatine kinase kinetics. *Am. J. Physiol. 259*: H813.

Kusuoka, H., Porterfield, J. K., Weisman, H. F., Weisfeldt, M. L., and Marban, E. (1987). Pathophysiology and pathogenesis of stunned myocardium: depressed Ca^{2+} activation of contraction as a consequence of reperfusion-induced cellular calcium overload in ferret hearts. *J. Clin. Invest. 79*: 950.

Kusuoka, H., Koretsune, Y., Chacko, V. P., Weisfeldt, M. L., and Marban, E. (1990). Excitation-contraction coupling in postischemic myocardium: does failure of activator Ca^{2+} transients underlie stunning? *Circ. Res. 66*: 1268.

Li, Y., Whittaker, P., and Kloner, R. A. (1991). The transient nature of the effect of ischemic preconditioning on myocardial infarct size and ventricular arrhythmias. *Am. Heart J. 123*: 346.

Lorell, B. H., Isoyama, S., Grice, W. N., Weinberg, E. O., and Apstein, C. S. (1988). Effects of ouabain and isoproterenol on left ventricular diastolic function during low-flow ischemia in the isolated, blood-perfused rabbit heart. *Circ. Res. 63*: 457.

McGoon, D. C. (1985). The ongoing quest for ideal myocardial protection: a catalogue of the recent English literature. *J. Thorac. Cardiovasc. Surg. 89*: 639.

Nayler, W. G. (1982). Protection of the myocardium against postischemic reperfusion damage: combined effect of hypothermia and nifedipine. *J. Thorac. Cardiovasc. Surg. 84*: 897.

Nayler, W. G., Elz, J. S., and Buckley, D. J. (1988). The stunned myocardium: effects of electrical and mechanical arrest and osmolarity. *Am. J. Physiol. 254*: H60.

Nayler, G. W., Liu, J., and Panagiotopoulos, S. (1990). Nifedipine and experimental cardioprotection. *Cardiovasc. Drugs Ther. 4*: 879.

Nicklas, J. M., Becker, L. C., and Healy-Bulkley, B. (1985). Effects of repeated brief coronary occlusion on regional left ventricular function and dimension in dogs. *Am. J. Cardiol. 56*: 473.

Opie, L. H. (1991). Role of calcium and other ions in reperfusion injury. *Cardiovasc. Drugs Ther. 5*: 237.

Owen, A. N., Grice, W. N., Vogel, W. M., and Apstein, C. S. (1989). Improved diastolic function during repetitive ischemia and reperfusion by beta adrenergic stimulation. *J. Mol. Cell. Cardiol. 21* (Suppl. III): S21 (abstract).

Przyklenk, K., Patel, B., and Kloner, R. A. (1987). Diastolic abnormalities of postischemic stunned myocardium. *Am. J. Cardiol. 60*: 1211.

Reimer, K. A., Lowe, J. E., Rasmussen, M. M., and Jennings, R. B. (1977). The "wavefront" phenomenon of ischemic cell death. I. Myocardial infarct size vs. duration of coronary occlusion in dogs. *Circulation 56*: 786.

Reimer, K. A., and Jennings, R. B. (1979). The "wavefront" phenomenon of myocardial ischemic cell death. II. Transmural progression of necrosis within the framework of ischemic bed size (myocardium at risk) and collateral flow. *Lab. Invest. 40*: 633.

Rosenfeldt, F. L., Hearse, D. J., Cankovic-Darracott, C., and Baimbridge, M. V. (1980). The additive protective effects of hypothermia and chemical cardioplegia during ischemic cardiac arrest in the dog. *J. Thorac. Cardiovasc. Surg. 79*: 29.

Taegtmeyer, H., Roberts, A. F. C., and Raine, A. E. G. (1985). Energy metabolism in reperfused heart muscle: metabolic correlates to return of function. *J. Am. Coll. Cardiol. 6*: 864.

Vogel, W. M., Apstein, C. S., Briggs, L. L., Gaasch, W. H., and Ahn, J. (1982). Acute alterations in left ventricular diastolic chamber stiffness: role of the "erectile" effect of coronary arterial pressure and flow in normal and damaged hearts. *Circ. Res. 51*: 465.

Vogel, W. M., Cerel, A. W., and Apstein, C. S. (1986). Postischemic cardiac chamber stiffness and coronary vasomotion: the role of edema and affects of dextran. *J. Mol. Cell. Cardiol. 18*: 1207.

Vogel, W. M., and Apstein, C. S. (1988). Effects of alloxan-induced diabetes on ischemia-reperfusion injury in rabbit hearts. *Circ. Res. 62*: 975.

Watts, J. A., Maiorano, L. J., and Maiorano, P. C. (1985). Comparison of the protective effects of verapamil, diltiazem, nifedipine, and buffer containing low calcium upon global myocardial ischemic injury. *J. Mol. Cell Cardiol. 18*: 255.

Whittaker, P., Boughner, D. R., Kloner, R. A., and Przyklenk, K. (1991). Stunned myocardium and myocardial collagen damage: differential effects of single and repeated occlusions. *Am. Heart J. 121*: 434.

Zucchi, R., Limbruno, U., di Vincenzo, A., Mariani, M., and Ronca, G. (1990). Adenine nucleotide depletion and contractile dysfunction in the stunned myocardium. *Cardiovasc. Res. 24*: 440.

7

Is Stunned Myocardium a Protective Mechanism?

Keith A. Reimer and Robert B. Jennings

Duke University Medical Center, Durham, North Carolina

I. INTRODUCTION

A brief episode of myocardial ischemia causes reversible myocyte injury, defined by the fact that early restoration of arterial flow prevents infarction (Jennings et al., 1960) and permits eventual restoration of normal myocardial structure, function, and metabolism. This reversible injury phase exists for at least 15 minutes of coronary occlusion in dogs. Moreover, although myocyte death begins to occur shortly after this time in the severely ischemic subendocardial zone, moderately ischemic myocytes in the subepicardial zone of an ischemic region may remain reversibly injured for as long as 3–6 hours (Reimer and Jennings, 1979).

The postischemic recovery of reversibly injured myocardium is not immediate; in a variety of experimental models, profound metabolic and functional abnormalities have been observed for hours or days after only 5–15 minutes of coronary occlusion. A substantial loss of adenine nucleotides occurs during ischemia (Jennings et al., 1985) and repletion may not be completed for as long as 4 days following reflow (Reimer et al., 1981; Swain et al., 1982). Also, postischemic contractile dysfunction occurs and may persist for 2–4 days postreperfusion. The latter phenomenon, first reported by

Heyndrickx et al. (1975) and later termed "myocardial stunning" by Braunwald and Kloner (1982) is, of course, the subject of this book.

The phenomenon of stunning occurs after a single brief episode of regional ischemia, but also occurs in a variety of other experimental and clinical settings. For example, postischemic contractile dysfunction gradually improves following longer periods of regional ischemia associated with subendocardial necrosis. The likely explanation for functional improvement in this setting is that, although the subendocardial zone undergoes infarction, the subepicardial zone, which still is salvaged by reperfusion, is stunned. In the clinical setting of interventional reperfusion, this combination of subendocardial necrosis and subepicardial stunning is undoubtedly far more common than pure stunning without necrosis.

Temporary cardiac dysfunction also is a common sequella of cardiac surgery when global ischemia is used during cardioplegic arrest. This too probably is a manifestation of stunning.

Exercise in animals or patients with a flow-limiting coronary stenosis also has been associated with persistent postexercise contractile abnormalities (Homans et al., 1986). Thus, stunning may be caused by high-flow ischemia resulting from increased oxygen requirements rather than reduced coronary blood flow.

In each of these circumstances, the existence of stunned myocardium is potentially detrimental by virtue of its negative impact on overall cardiac function. On the contrary, in the setting of brief periods of ischemia followed by reperfusion, the phenomenon of myocardial stunning is paralleled by adaptive changes in the myocardium which have been termed *ischemic preconditioning* (Murry et al., 1986). This term recently has been used to include several phenomena which may or may not be related. In the present chapter, the term will be defined narrowly as the phenomenon in which sublethal episode(s) of ischemia result in increased tolerance to a later, potentially lethal episode of ischemia. This increased tolerance is manifest by a slower rate of ischemic metabolism: adenosine triphosphate (ATP) utilization is slowed markedly so that depletion of ATP stores is delayed, even though the major source of ATP synthesis, namely anaerobic glycolysis, also is markedly slowed (Murry et al., 1990). This is accompanied by a delayed onset of irreversible cell injury, which translates into limitation of infarct size if the subsequent episode of ischemia is terminated by timely reperfusion (Murry et al., 1986).

Thus, the titular question of whether stunning is a protective mechanism can be rephrased as, Is ischemic preconditioning a consequence or manifestation of myocardial stunning? In order to address this question, we shall first provide a brief general review of the phenomenon of ischemic preconditioning and then discuss several hypotheses regarding its pathogenesis.

II. ISCHEMIC PRECONDITIONING: DEFINITION AND CHARACTERISTICS

A. Background

The recognition that a single brief episode of ischemia may cause prolonged depletion of adenine nucleotides initially raised the concern that recurrent brief episodes of ischemia (e.g., in patients with angina pectoris) might have cumulative effects, producing progressively worsening metabolic and functional deficits, and perhaps even lethal myocyte injury. However, this concern was not substantiated by experimental results. For example, we observed that four 10-minute episodes of ischemia caused virtually no myocyte necrosis (Reimer et al., 1986). This is in marked contrast to an uninterrupted 40-minute episode of ischemia, which typically results in a confluent subendocardial infarct. Other studies of repeated brief ischemic episodes also revealed minimal structural damage or necrosis (Geft et al., 1982; Henrichs et al., 1987; Basuk et al., 1986), and little cumulative effect on tissue adenine nucleotide content (Swain et al., 1984; Lange et al., 1984; Reimer et al., 1986; Hoffmeister, Mauser and Schaper, 1986; Henrichs et al., 1987). Also, postischemic contractile function deteriorates only slightly from one occlusion to another, with a cumulative effect detected in some studies only with multiple occlusions (Lange et al., 1984a; Schroder et al., 1987; Nicklas et al., 1985).

The metabolic consequences of repeated ischemic episodes (Reimer et al., 1986) were particularly intriguing: in our studies, a single 10-minute episode of ischemia caused loss of 60% of ATP. In addition, only half of the lost ATP was resynthesized by rephosphorylation of AMP and ADP during a 20-minute period of reperfusion. Nevertheless, a second, third, and fourth 10-minute episode of ischemia caused no cumulative ATP depletion. ATP and adenine nucleotide content were similar after four, vs. only one 10-minute ischemic episode(s). Moreover, although substantial quantities of adenine nucleosides and bases (products of adenine nucleotide degradation) were produced in the first ischemic episode, much less were produced in later episodes. These results were the first indication that the rate of energy metabolism of ischemic myocardium was different if the myocardium already had been recently exposed to ischemia.

The most striking observation, however, was that myocardial infarct size produced by a 40-minute test period of coronary occlusion was reduced by 75% (from 29% to 7% of the ischemic vascular bed at risk) when the myocardium first had been subjected to four 5-minute episodes of coronary occlusion, each separated by 5 minutes of reperfusion (Fig. 1) (Murry et al., 1986). It was this phenomenon that initially was termed *ischemic preconditioning*.

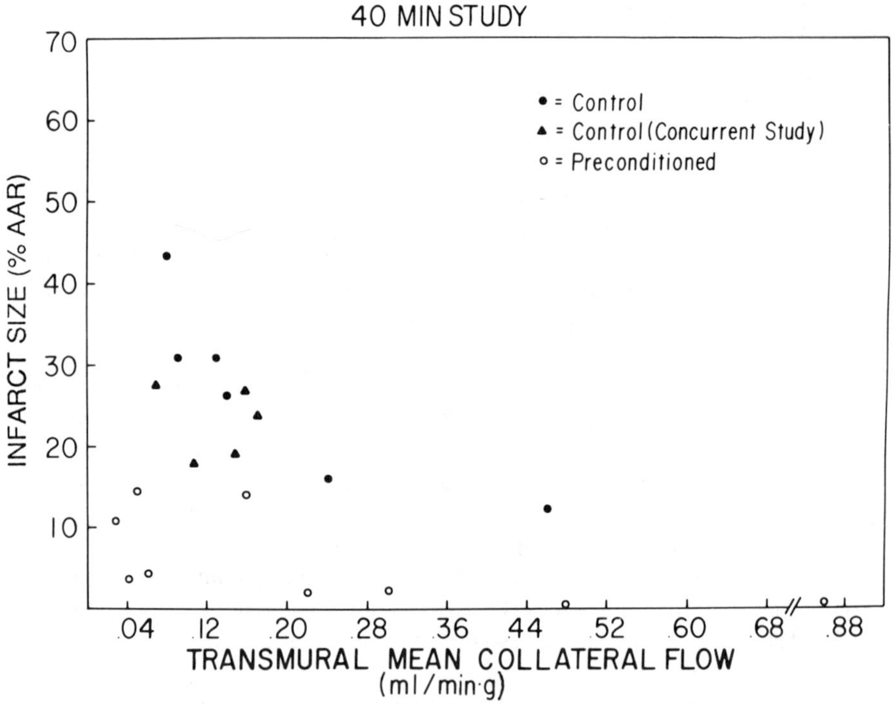

Figure 1 Myocardial infarct size, measured in dogs after 40 minutes of coronary occlusion and 4 days of reperfusion, is plotted with respect to collateral blood flow, a major predictor of infarct size in nonpreconditioned (control) animals. Infarct size is inversely related to the amount of collateral blood flow during the period of ischemia, but averages between 20 and 30% of the ischemic vascular bed at risk of infarction. When the 40-minute episode of ischemia was preceded by four 5-minute episodes of ischemia, infarct size was markedly limited at any level of collateral blood flow. Thus, the brief episodes of ischemia and/or reperfusion induced an adaptive response so that myocardium now could tolerate 40 minutes of ischemia without being lethally injured. (Reprinted from Murry et al., 1986, with permission of the American Heart Association.)

This phenomenon now has been observed by several investigators and is known to occur in dogs (Li et al., 1990), pigs (Schott et al., 1990), and rabbits (Downey and Jordan, 1989; Iwamoto et al., 1991). Moreover, recent clinical studies have provided indirect evidence that ischemic preconditioning occurs in humans, in the setting of ischemia induced by balloon inflation during coronary angioplasty (Deutsch et al., 1990).

B. General Biology

Any mechanism proposed to explain ischemic preconditioning must be consistent with its general biology. Three aspects of the general biology of ischemic preconditioning need to be considered: (1) the number and duration of preconditioning episodes of ischemia required to induce the adaptive response; (2) the duration of reperfusion during which the adaptation persists and (3) the maximum duration of the test episode of ischemia during which myocyte death can be prevented.

In the initial description of ischemic preconditioning in dogs, the preconditioning protocol was comprised of four 5-minute episodes of ischemia interspersed by 5-minute periods of reperfusion (Murry et al., 1986). Subsequent studies have shown that an equivalent degree of protection can be achieved in dogs with a single preconditioning episode ranging from 5 to 15 minutes in duration (Murry et al., 1991; MacDonald et al., 1991; Auchampach and Gross, 1991). Moreover, preliminary experimental results from our laboratory and the aforementioned clinical studies (Deutsch et al., 1990) suggest that the required duration may be as little as a single 90-second episode. Conversely, two 2-minute episodes of ischemia reportedly did not induce preconditioning in rabbits, although either one or two 5-minute episodes did (Van Winkle et al., 1991).

The minimum duration of reperfusion required between the preconditioning episode(s) and test episode of ischemia has not been established. Clearly reperfusion of some duration must be required, or the preconditioning episode(s) would only serve to prolong the test episode. It seems likely that one or more minutes of reperfusion would be required to achieve uniform washout of the ischemic vasculature. We have observed limitation of necrosis when 5-minute periods of reperfusion were used (Murry et al., 1986) and have observed the characteristic metabolic alterations of ischemic preconditioning when the test episode of ischemia followed the preconditioning episode(s) by either 5 or 20 minutes of reperfusion (Reimer et al., 1986; Murry et al., 1990). Most subsequent studies of preconditioning have used reperfusion times in this window.

The adaptive response appears to be relatively short lived. We recently have observed that protection is substantially attenuated if the test episode of ischemia is delayed for two hours after the preconditioning episodes (Fig. 2) (Murry et al., 1991). In rabbits, Van Winkle et al. (1991) have reported loss of protection between 60 and 90 minutes of reperfusion, whereas Miura et al. (1990a) reported that protection began to dissipate by as early as 30 minutes of reperfusion.

Ischemic preconditioning initially was defined from the observation that infarct size resulting from a 40-minute episode of coronary occlusion and

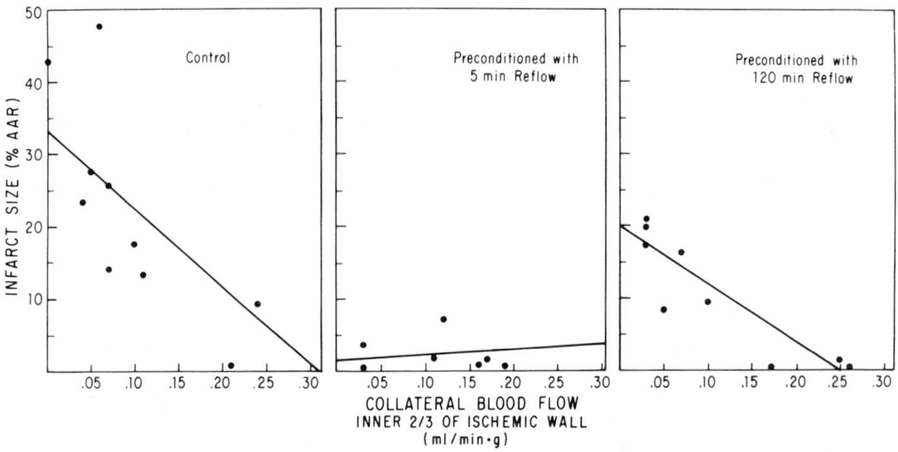

Figure 2 Infarct size vs. collateral blood flow in control and ischemically preconditioned myocardium subjected to 40 minutes of circumflex coronary occlusion. Preconditioning was established with a single 15-minute occlusion. In one preconditioned group the preconditioning and test episodes of ischemia were separated by only 5 minutes of reperfusion, and in the other group the two ischemic episodes were separated by 120 minutes of reperfusion. Marked limitation of infarct size by preconditioning was observed when the two episodes were separated by only 5 minutes of reperfusion. However, this protective effect was partially lost when the reperfusion interval was prolonged to 2 hours. Fifteen minutes of ischemia resulted in severe myocardial stunning, and there was no sign of functional recovery throughout 2 hours of reperfusion. Thus, sustained stunning does not translate into sustained preconditioning; stunning per se is insufficient to explain the preconditioning phenomenon. (Reprinted with permission from Murry et al., 1991.)

subsequent reperfusion could be reduced markedly by a preceeding series of short nonlethal ischemic episodes. From this observation it was clear that lethal cell injury in the subendocardial zone of severe ischemia could be *delayed* for at least 40 minutes (Murry et al., 1986). Conversely, it is now generally accepted that no cardioprotective intervention can delay cell death indefinitely in the absence of restoration of myocardial blood flow. Our initial studies showed a loss of protection if the test episode of ischemia was 3 hours (Murry et al., 1986). More recent studies suggest that the delay of cell death may not last for as long as 90 minutes (Nao et al., 1990). The delay *does* persist through 60 minutes of ischemia in both dogs and pigs, based on observations from several laboratories (Schott et al., 1990; Li et al., 1990; Auchampach and Gross, 1991; Nao et al., 1990). The duration of protection has not been studied in detail in rabbits, but limitation of infarct size has been observed in two laboratories using a 30-minute test episode of ischemia (Iwamoto et al., 1991; Van Winkle et al., 1991).

III. MECHANISM OF ISCHEMIC PRECONDITIONING

The general biology of ischemic preconditioning reviewed above establishes a basic framework within which potential mechanisms can be considered. Specifically, we now know that the adaptive response occurs almost immediately, and certainly within 5 minutes of reperfusion, after being induced by 5 minutes or less of ischemic stress (Murry et al., 1986). We also know that the protective effect dissipates after as little as 2 hours of reperfusion (Murry et al., 1991). Moreover, we know that the prevention of cell death is associated with a marked slowing of ischemic metabolism in the early period of the test episode of ischemia (Murry et al., 1990). Thus, a credible hypothetical mechanism to explain ischemic preconditioning must occur within these time constraints and should also provide a plausible explanation for the concurrent slowing of ischemic metabolism.

A general working hypothesis for ischemic preconditioning is illustrated in Figure 3 (Murry et al., 1990) and is stated as follows: A brief episode of ischemia in some, as yet undetermined way, reduces the demand for high energy phosphates (HEP) when myocardium is subjected to the test episode of ischemia.

To gain further insight into the metabolic slowing in preconditioned myocardium, it is useful to consider the major cellular reactions producing and utilizing ATP in myocardium (Fig. 4). With the inhibition of mitochondrial respiration in ischemia, the major source of HEP is anaerobic glycolysis; the principal substrate is glucose-1-phosphate derived from glycogenolysis (Jennings et al., 1981). Through an as yet undefined mechanism, the rate of anaerobic glycolysis appears to be controlled by the rate of HEP utilization; when ATP utilization is rapid, the rate of anaerobic glycolysis is rapid, and when ATP utilization is slowed, anaerobic glycolysis also is slowed (Murry et al., 1990; Jennings et al., 1981, 1991). However, under no circumstances does the supply of ATP produced by anaerobic glycolysis meet the demand for HEP. Thus, the reduction of demand for HEP can slow, but not prevent, the depletion of HEP stores.

A. Is Ischemic Preconditioning a Consequence of Concurrent Stunning?

In normally perfused myocardium, most of the ATP produced is utilized for contractile function. With the onset of ischemia, contractile function is depressed markedly. Nevertheless, continued calcium cycling occurs as the cell

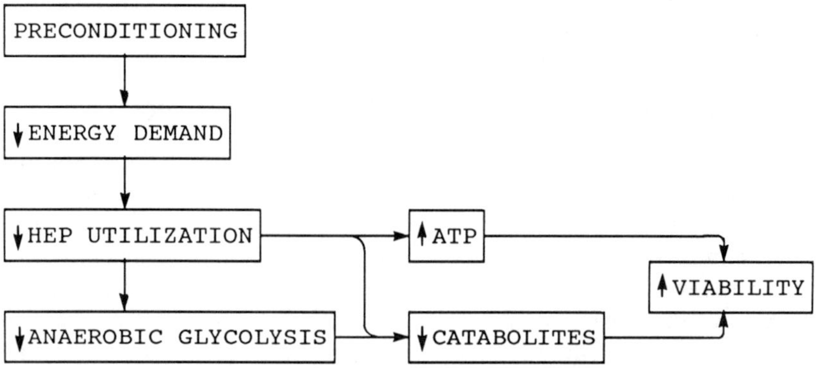

Figure 3 Proposed mechanism for myocardial protection by preconditioning. Ischemic preconditioning reduces myocardial energy demand during the early phase of a subsequent ischemic episode and thereby slows the rate of ATP depletion, slows the rate of anaerobic glycolysis, and thereby slows the accumulation of ischemic catabolites. Either preservation of ATP or limitation of catabolite accumulation (or both) may be responsible for slowing the rate of ischemic cell death. Major unanswered questions are: (1) What is the mechanism leading to reduced energy demand and reduced ischemic metabolism? and (2) Is the benefit of reduced ischemic metabolism a benefit of slower high energy phosphate loss or of slower catabolite accumulation, and how does such benefit prevent cell death? (Reprinted from Murry et al., 1990, with permission of the American Heart Association.)

attempts to contract, and this cycling activity continues to contribute to ATP utilization during ischemia. Thus, one explanation for the metabolic features of ischemically preconditioned myocardium is that it uses less ATP because it is concurrently stunned and therefore uses less ATP in its feeble attempts to contract (Murry et al., 1991). The possibility that stunning could account for the reduced ATP demand of preconditioned myocardium has been addressed directly or indirectly in several studies. For example, indirect evidence favoring the hypothesis (Schroder et al., 1987) is provided by the observation that a brief episode of ischemia followed by reperfusion results in a more rapid onset of contractile failure during a subsequent episode. On the other hand, the observation that four 5-minute episodes of coronary occlusion, which formed the first preconditioning protocol from which dramatic protection was achieved, cause relatively mild stunning (C. E. Murry, R. B. Jennings, and K. A. Reimer, unpublished observations) is indirect evidence against the hypothesis that preconditioning is a manifestation of stunning.

In a direct study of the link between stunning and preconditioning, we observed that a single 15-minute episode of ischemia caused severe stunning,

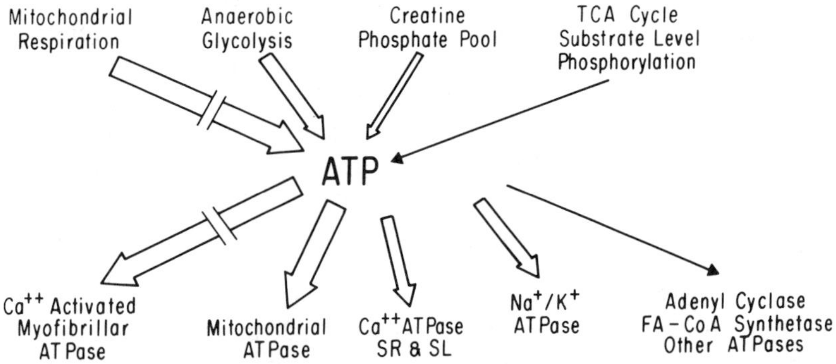

Figure 4 The principal reactions producing and utilizing high energy phosphates in ischemic myocardium. The width of the arrows indicates the estimated quantitative importance of the various reactions. In severe ischemia, aerobic respiration is abolished. The preexisting stores of high energy phosphate, in the form of creatine phosphate (CP) and ATP, are relatively small. Thus, anaerobic glycolysis becomes the principal source of energy, producing about 80% of the high energy phosphate bonds that can be utilized by severely ischemic tissue. Substrate-level phosphorylation of alpha-ketoglutarate in the mitochondria does not require O_2, but the tissue content of substrates that can be shuttled to alpha-ketoglutarate is small. Energy utilization also is reduced markedly during ischemia. Cardiac contraction, mediated by the Ca^{2+} activated myofibrillar ATPase, consumes much of the ATP produced in aerobic myocardium. However, contraction is markedly depressed in areas of severe ischemia. Some ATP still is required to remove Na^+ from the cell, to keep Ca^{2+} sequestered in the sarcoplasmic reticulum, and for a variety of other cellular processes. However, recent studies indicate that a major cause of ATP degradation in ischemia is the squandering of ATP by the mitochondrial ATPase (reverse function of the ATP synthase). (Adapted from Jennings and Reimer, 1981.)

which persisted throughout 2 hours of reperfusion (Murry et al., 1991). When the 40-minute test episode of ischemia was induced 5 minutes after the 15-minute episode, there was marked limitation of infarct size. Thus, both stunning and preconditioning were present. However, when the 40-minute test episode was deferred until 2 hours after the 15-minute episode, the cellular protection was partially lost even though severe stunning still was present (see Fig. 2) (Murry et al., 1991). Similar results have been observed in studies using rabbits (Miura et al., 1990b). Thus, these results indicate that the presence of *stunning alone is insufficient* to achieve the full protective effect of ischemic preconditioning.

Other studies have provided at least preliminary evidence that *stunning is unnecessary* for preconditioning to occur. In a recent study (Jennings et al., 1991), we tested the effects of in vivo preconditioning on myocardial metabolism during a subsequent period of total ischemia in vitro. After preconditioning, hearts were arrested with KCl to abolish all electrical and contractile activity. When this arrested myocardial tissue was subjected to total ischemia, the initial rates of both ATP depletion and anaerobic glycolysis were much slower in preconditioned vs. control myocardium, even though contractile activity was abolished by potassium arrest in both. Thus, the difference in metabolic activity between control and preconditioned tissue persisted during total ischemia, despite abolition of possible differences in contractile effort.

Rohman et al. (1991) have addressed the same question in vivo using pigs. In their study, two 10-minute episodes of ischemia, 30 minutes apart, caused both stunning and preconditioning. The latter was confirmed from measurements of the size of infarcts produced by a 60-minute test occlusion initiated 30 minutes after the preconditioning protocol. In this same protocol, pretreatment with nifedipine prior to the preconditioning episodes prevented myocardial stunning but did not attenuate the protective effect on subsequent infarct size. Thus, these results also suggest that stunning is not a necessary prerequisite for preconditioning.

We also have addressed this issue using a 15-minutes episode of coronary artery occlusion to induce both severe stunning and preconditioning in dogs (M. Matsuda, R. B. Jennings, and K. A. Reimer, unpublished observations). Preconditioning was confirmed by a limitation of infarct size following a 40-minute test occlusion. In another group of dogs, dobutamine was infused after the 15-minute occlusion, titrating the concentration to restore segmental shortening of the stunned region back to baseline (to overcome stunning through inotropic stimulation). This infusion of dobutamine was continued through the subsequent 40-minute test episode of ischemia. Even this inotropic treatment did not abolish the protective effect of preconditioning, despite the observation that a similar infusion of dobutamine in nonpreconditioned dogs resulted in an increased infarct size.

The possibility that ischemic preconditioning might be a favorable consequence of oxygen-derived free radical-mediated injury was suggested as a corollary of the "stunning mediates preconditioning" hypothesis (Murry et al., 1988). Specifically, it was proposed that because substantial evidence implicates oxygen-derived free radicals as contributory causes of stunning (see Chapter 8) and if stunning mediates preconditioning, then free radical injury could indirectly mediate preconditioning. Preliminary studies from our laboratory (C. E. Murry, R. B. Jennings, and K. A. Reimer,, unpublished observations) confirmed that superoxide dismutase (SOD) plus catalase could substantially attenuate the severe stunning resulting from a 15-minute episode of ischemia. However, this anti-free radical treatment did not further attenuate the mild degree of stunning observed following four 5-minute episodes of ischemia (Murry et al., 1989), nor did it abolish the protective effect of preconditioning in three of the six dogs studied. However, protection was abolished in the other three dogs treated with SOD plus catalase, suggesting that free-radical injury might contribute to preconditioning through a nonstunning mechanism (Murry et al., 1988). However, the explanation for this nonuniform effect of treatment with SOD plus catalase remains unexplained. Meanwhile, a study by Iwamoto et al. (1991) has shown no effect of anti-free radical therapy on ischemic preconditioning in rabbits, raising further doubts about the hypothesis. On balance, the evidence available indicates that stunning and preconditioning are phenomena that generally occur concurrently, but that stunning is not the primary cause of preconditioning.

B. Alternative Explanations for Ischemic Preconditioning

1. Increased Collateral Blood Flow

Increased collateral blood flow is not the explanation for preconditioning. Although multiple short episodes of ischemia are known to induce increased collateral blood flow in several species, including dogs (Yamamoto et al., 1984), measurements of collateral flow during the test episode of ischemia showed no differences between control and preconditioned groups. Moreover, infarct size was limited markedly at any given level of collateral blood flow (see Figs. 1 and 2) (Murry et al., 1986; Miyazaki and Zipes, 1989; Li et al., 1900). The fact that ischemic preconditioning also occur in pigs (Schott et al., 1990) and rabbits (Iwamoto et al., 1991), two species largely devoid of native collateral flow, also provides strong evidence against the idea that an acute increase in collateral blood flow is the explanation for preconditioning.

2. Genetic Mechanism

It has been proposed that a brief episode of ischemia might induce the transcription of new messenger RNA and subsequent synthesis of one or more protective proteins, akin to the heat shock response, that somehow might protect the myocardium. Several observations support the plausibility of a stress protein scenario. First, heat shock of rats was reported to have a cardioprotective effect against a myocardial ischemic insult 24 hours later (Currie et al., 1988). Second, a nonlethal episode (10 or 15 minutes) of ischemia was found to induce the synthesis of mRNA for stress proteins, detectable as early as 60 minutes after the initial ischemic insult in dogs (Fleischman et al., 1990).

However, it seems unlikely that such a mechanism could be consistent with the time frame of preconditioning: (1) The protein message would presumably have to be produced within a few minutes after reperfusion; and

(2) the message would have to be lost or countermanded after 90 to 120 minutes, even though the quantities of the known stress proteins have been observed to continue increasing much beyond these times (Dillmann et al., 1986; Currie, 1987). Indeed, recent evidence has cast doubt on the hypothesis. For example, exposure of canine myocardium to regional hyperthermia one hour before a 60-minute coronary occlusion did not limit myocardial infarct size, even though synthesis of stress proteins was detected before the onset of ischemia (Schott et al., 1990). In other studies, neither inhibition of transcription using actinomycin D nor inhibition of translation (protein synthesis) with cycloheximide attenuated the protective effect of ischemic preconditioning in rabbits (Thornton et al., 1990; Iliodromites et al., 1991). In addition, whereas the protective effect of ischemic preconditioning disappears by 2 hours in this rabbit model, the synthesis of the HSP-70 protein itself continues thereafter (Kucukoglu et al., 1991). These studies suggest that preconditioning is not dependent on synthesis of a new class of proteins. Of course, this does not rule out the possibility that translocation of preformed proteins including stress proteins might play a role in the preconditioning response.

3. Inhibition of Mitochondrial ATPase

Recent studies have indicated that ATP hydrolysis by the mitochondrial ATPase (reverse function of the mitochondrial ATP synthetase) is a major cause of ATP utilization in ischemia (Rouslin et al., 1986; Jennings et al., 1990, 1991). In addition, ATP utilization by the mitochondrial ATPase is slower in "slow-heart rate" species, including rabbits and larger mammals, because the cardiac mitochondria in such species contain a natural protein inhibitor of this ATPase, which binds to the enzyme during mitochondrial acidosis induced by ischemia (Rouslin and Pullman, 1987). This inhibitor slows the ATPase activity by 50% or more (Jennings et al., 1990). If this inhibition persisted during the intervening period of reperfusion or recurred more quickly or more completely during a second episode of ischemia, it could explain the preconditioning effect.

Preliminary results from our laboratory (R. S. Vander Heide, K. A. Reimer, and R. B. Jennings, unpublished observations) indicate that the ATPase activity in submitochondrial particles isolated from canine myocardium that had been ischemic for 5 minutes in vivo is reduced substantially compared to ATPase activity in submitochondrial particles from the nonischemic control regions of the same hearts. These data are consistent with the hypothesis that the slower ischemic energy utilization of preconditioned myocardium may be explained by an effect of preconditioning on the mitochondrial ATPase. However, we have not yet established whether such inhibition plays a role in ischemic preconditioning.

4. Activation of Adenosine A_1 Receptor

Another recent proposal is that ischemic preconditioning may be mediated through activation of the A_1 adenosine receptor by adenosine produced in the preconditioning episode (Thornton et al., 1990b). Preliminary evidence supporting this hypothesis has been obtained from rabbits in which myocardial infarcts were produced by 30 minutes of ischemia. The A_1 adenosine receptor agonist, N^6 1-phenyl-2R-propyladenosine (PIA), administered prior to ischemia in nonpreconditioned hearts, was able to mimic the effects of a 5-minute episode of ischemic preconditioning in limiting myocardial infarct size. Conversely, administration of the nonspecific (both A_1 and A_2) adenosine receptor blocker 8(*p*-sulfophenyl) theophylline (SPT) abolished the protective effect of preconditioning.

How activation of adenosine receptors might be translated into cardiac protection remains to be determined. Because preconditioning is not associated with an increase in collateral blood flow, the vasodilatory action of adenosine is unlikely to be involved. Alternatively, adenosine is known to inhibit neutrophil function, and neutrophil content of myocardium has been observed to be reduced following a sublethal (12-minute) episode of ischemia in dogs (Go et al., 1988). However, it is unclear how a reduction in myocardial neutrophil content could mediate the slower rate of ischemic metabolism during the later test episode of ischemia. A third effect of adenosine A_1 receptor activation is stimulation of glycolysis (Wyatt et al., 1989). However, it is clear that stimulation of glycolysis during the test episode of ischemia cannot explain ischemic preconditioning because the rate of anaerobic glycolysis is *decreased* during the test episode of ischemia. A fourth way through which activation of the adenosine A_1 receptor might be protective could be through a G-protein-mediated opening of the ATP-regulated K^+ channel (Kirsch et al., 1990).

5. Opening of ATP-Regulated K^+ Channels

Perhaps related to the aforementioned fourth action of adenosine is a recent proposal that ischemic preconditioning might cause a persisting or more rapidly recurring opening of the ATP-regulated K^+ channel. One way in which the early opening of this channel might be protective is through a shortening of the action potential duration and concomitant shortening of time during which there is an inward flux of Ca^{2+}. Preliminary evidence supporting this hypothesis is that treatment of dogs with glibenclamide, an inhibitor of this K^+ channel, abolished the protective effect of ischemic preconditioning (Auchampach and Gross, 1991). Moreover, K^+ channel openers nicorandil and pinacidil have been reported to have anti-ischemic properties in the absence of ischemic preconditioning (Gross et al., 1989; Glover et al., 1990). However, contradictory results have been observed in rabbits, in which glibenclamide did not attenuate the protection from ischemic preconditioning (J. M. Downey, personal communication).

IV. CONCLUSIONS

Ischemic preconditioning and stunning are two consequences of reversible cell injury, the first being an adaptive response to ischemic stress, the other a manifestation of delayed recovery from reversible ischemic injury and/or nonlethal reperfusion injury. Although both preconditioning and stunning may occur concurrently, the fact that the preconditioning phenomenon is *not* present in all circumstances in which severe stunning exists indicates that stunning is not sufficient to cause the cardioprotection of preconditioning. Moreover, several preliminary lines of evidence suggest that the preconditioning effect may be achieved even though concurrent stunning is either prevented, reversed with inotropic agents, or made irrelevant by complete cardiac arrest. Thus, presently available evidence supports the conclusion that stunning is neither necessary nor sufficient to cause ischemic preconditioning. It follows that there is no evidence that stunning per se is a protective mechanism.

REFERENCES

Auchampach, J. A., and Gross, G. J. (1991). Myocardial preconditioning is mediated by activation of the ATP-regulated potassium channel. *FASEB J. 5*: A1103 (Abstract).

Basuk, W. L., Reimer, K. A., and Jennings, R. B. (1986). Effect of repetitive brief episodes of ischemia on cell volume, electrolytes, and ultrastructure. *J. Am. Coll. Cardiol. 8*(Suppl. A): A33.

Braunwald, E., and Kloner, R. A. (1982). The stunned myocardium: Prolonged, postischemic ventricular dysfunction. *Circulation 66*: 1146.

Currie, R. W. (1987). Effects of ischemia and perfusion temperature on the synthesis of stress-induced rat (heat shock) proteins in isolated and perfused rat hearts. *J. Mol. Cell. Cardiol. 19*: 795.

Currie, R. W., Karmazyn, M., Kloc, M., and Mailer, K. (1988). Heat-shock response is associated with enhanced postischemic ventricular recovery. *Circ. Res. 63*: 543.

Deutsch, E., Berger, M., Kussmaul, W. G., Hirshfeld, J. W., Jr., Hermann, H. C., and Laskey, W. K. (1990). Adaptation to ischemia during PTCA: Clinical, hemodynamic and metabolic features, *Circulation 82*: 2044.

Dillmann, W. H., Mehta, H. B., Barrieux, A., Guth, B. D., Neeley, W. E., and Ross, J., Jr. (1986). Ischemia of the dog heart induces the appearance of a cardiac mRNA coding for a protein with migration characteristics similar to heat-shock/stress protein 71. *Circ. Res. 59*: 110.

Downey, J. M., and Jordan, M. (1989). Preconditioning limits infarct size in rabbits. *Circulation 80* (Suppl. II): II-238 (Abstract).

Fleischman, K. E., Brand, T., Sharma, H. S., Duncker, D. J., Sassen, L. M. A., McFalls, E. O., Verdouw, P. D., and Schaper, W. (1990). Gene expression in a preconditioning model. *Circulation 82*(Suppl. III): III-464 (Abstract).

Geft, I. L., Fishbein, M. C., Ninomiya, K., Hashida, J., Chaux, E., Yano, J., Y-Rit, J., Genov, T., Shell, W., and Ganz, W. (1982). Intermittent brief periods of ischemia have a cumulative effect and may cause myocardial necrosis. *Circulation 66*: 1150.

Glover, G. J., McCullough, J. R., Henry, D. E., Conder, M. L., and Sleph, P. G. (1990). Anti-ischemic effects of the potassium channel activators pinacidil and cromakalim and the reversal of these effects with the potassium channel blocker glyburide. *J. Pharm. Exp. Ther. 251*: 98.

Go, L. O., Murry, C. E., Richard, V. J., Weischedel, G. R., Jennings, R. B., and Reimer, K. A. (1988). Myocardial neutrophil accumulation during reperfusion after reversible and irreversible ischemic injury. *Am. J. Physiol. 255*: H1188.

Gross, G., Pieper, G., Faber, N. E., Warltier, D., and Hardman, H. (1989). Effects of nicorandil on coronary circulation and myocardial ischemia. *Am. J. Cardiol. 63*: 11J.

Henrichs, K. J., Matsuoka, H., and Schaper, J. (1987). Influence of repetitive coronary occlusions on myocardial adenine nucleosides, high energy phosphates and ultrastructure. *Bas. Res. Cardiol. 82*: 557.

Heyndrickx, G. R., Millard, R. W., McRitchie, R. J., Maroko, P. R., and Vatner, S. F. (1975). Regional myocardial functional and electrophysiological alterations after brief coronary artery occlusion in conscious dogs. *J. Clin. Invest 56*: 978.

Hoffmeister, H. M., Mauser, M., and Schaper, W. (1986). Repeated short periods of regional myocardial ischemia: effect on local function and high energy phosphate levels. *Bas. Res. Cardiol. 81*: 361.

Homans, D. C., Sublett, E., Dai, X. Z., and Bache, R. J. (1986). Persistence of regional left ventricular dysfunction after exercise-induced myocardial ischemia. *J. Clin. Invest. 77*: 66.

Iliodromites, E., Kucukoglu, S., Marber, M. S., Walker, J. M., Latchman, D. S., and Yellon, D. M. (1991). Preconditioning protects the rabbit myocardium independent of de novo protein synthesis. *Eur. Heart J.* in press: (Abstract).

Iwamoto, T., Miura, T., Adachi, T., Noto, T., Ogawa, T., Tsuchida, A., and Iimura, O. (1991). Myocardial infarct size-limiting effect of ischemic preconditioning was not attenuated by oxygen free-radical scavengers in the rabbit. *Circulation 83*: 1015.

Jennings, R. B., Sommers, H. M., Smyth, G. A., Flack, H. H., and Linn, H. (1960). Myocardial necrosis induced by temporary occlusion of a coronary artery in the dog. *Arch. Pathol. 70*: 68.

Jennings, R. B., and Reimer, K. A. (1981). Lethal myocardial ischemic injury. *Am. J. Pathol. 102*: 241.

Jennings, R. B., Reimer, K. A., Hill, M. L., and Mayer, S. E. (1981). Total ischemia in dog hearts in vitro. 1. Comparison of high energy phosphate production, utilization and depletion and of adenine nucleotide catabolism in total ischemia in vitro vs. severe ischemia in vivo. *Circ. Res. 49*: 892.

Jennings, R. B., Schaper, J., Hill, M. L., Steenbergen, C., Jr., and Reimer, K. A. (1985). Effect of reperfusion late in the phase of reversible ischemic injury. Changes in cell volume, electrolytes, metabolites and ultrastructure. *Circ. Res. 56*: 262.

Jennings, R. B., Reimer, K. A., and Steenbergen, C. (1990). Effect of inhibition of the mitochondrial ATPase on net myocardial ATP in total ischemia. *J. Mol. Cell. Cardiol.*

Jennings, R. B., Murry, C. E., and Reimer, K. A. (1991a). Heart surgery. In *Energy Metabolism in Regional and Total Ischemia: Role of the Mitochondrial ATPase* (L. C. D'Alessandro, ed.), Casa Editrice Internazionale, Rome, p. 395.

Jennings, R. B., Murry, C. E., and Reimer, K. A. (1991b). Preconditioning myocardium with ischemia. *Cardiovasc. Drugs Ther.* in press.

Kirsch, G. E., Codina, J., Birnbaumer, L., and Brown, A. M. (1990). Coupling of ATP-sensitive K+ channels to A1 receptors by G proteins in rat ventricular myocytes. *Am. J. Physiol. 259*: H820.

Kucukoglu, S., Iliodromites, E., Van Winkle, D. M., Downey, J. M., Marber, M. S., Heads, R. J., and Yellon, D. M. (1991). Protection by ischemic preconditioning appears independent of stress protein synthesis. *J. Mol. Cell. CArdiol. 23* (Suppl. V.): S.71 (Abstract).

Lange, R., Ingwall, J. S., Hale, S. L., Alker, K. J., and Kloner, R. A. (1984). Effects of recurrent ischemia on myocardial high energy phosphate content in canine heart. *Bas. Res. Cardiol. 79*: 469.

Lange, R., Ware, J., and Kloner, R. A. (1984). Absence of a cumulative deterioration of regional function during three repeated 5 or 15 minute coronary occlusions. *Circulation 69*: 400.

Li, G. C., Vasquez, J. A., Gallagher, K. P., and Lucchesi, B. R. (1990). Myocardial protection with preconditioning. *Circulation 82*: 609.

MacDonald, B. R., Chastain, M., Simpson, P. J., and Hahn, R. A. (1991). Protection of canine ischemic myocardium by single event preconditioning without attenuation of neutrophil recruitment or superoxide production. *Faseb J. 5* (5): A1047 (Abstract).

Miura, T., Ogawa, T., Iwamoto, T., Tsuchida, A., and Iimura, O. (1990a). Infarct size limiting effect of preconditioning: Its duration and "dose-response" relationship. *Circulation 82* (Suppl. III): III-271 (Abstract).

Miura, T., Noto, T., Adachi, T., Enoh, A., Goto, M., Urabe, K., and Iimura, O. (1990b). Does myocardial stunning contribute to infarct size limitation by preconditioning? *Circulation 82* (Suppl. III): III-40 (Abstract).

Miyazaki, T., and Zipes, D. P. (1989). Protection against automatic denervation following acute myocardial infarction by preconditioning ischemia. *Circ. Res. 64*: 437.

Murry, C. E., Jennings, R. B., and Reimer, K. A. (1986). Preconditioning with ischemia: a delay of lethal cell injury in ischemic myocardium. *Circulation 74*: 1124.

Murry, C. E., Richard, V. J., Jennings, R. B., and Reimer, K. A. (1988). Preconditioning with ischemia: is the protective effect mediated by free radical-induced myocardial stunning? *Circulation 78* (Suppl II): 77 (Abstract).

Murry, C. E., Richard, V. J., Jennings, R. B., and Reimer, K. A. (1989). Free radicals do not cause myocardial stunning after four 5 minute coronary occlusions. *Circulation 80* (Suppl. II): 296 (Abstract).

Murry, C. E., Richard, V. J., Reimer, K. A., and Jennings, R. B. (1990). Ischemic preconditioning slows energy metabolism and delays ultrastructural damage during a sustained ischemic episode. *Circ. Res. 66*: 913.

Murry, C. E., Richard, V. J., Jennings, R. B., and Reimer, K. A. (1991). Myocardial protection is lost before contractile function recovers from ischemic preconditioning. *Am. J. Physiol. (Heart Circ. Physiol.) 260* (29): H796.

Nao, B. S., McClanahan, T. B., Groh, M. A., Schott, R. J., and Gallagher, K. P. (1990). The time limit of effective ischemic preconditioning in dogs. *Circulation 88* (Suppl. III): III-271 (Abstract).

Nicklas, J. M., Becker, L. C., and Bulkley, B. H. (1985). Effects of repeated brief coronary occlusion on regional left ventricular function and dimension in dogs. *Am. J. Cardiol. 56*: 473.

Reimer, K. A., and Jennings, R. B. (1979). The "wavefront phenomenon" of myocardial ischemic cell death. II. Transmural progression of necrosis within the framework of ischemic bed size (myocardium at risk) and collateral flow. *Lab. Invest. 40*: 633.

Reimer, K. A., Hill, M. L., and Jennings, R. B. (1981). Prolonged depletion of ATP and of the adenine nucleotide pool due to delayed resynthesis of adenine nucleotides following reversible myocardial ischemic injury in dogs. *J. Mol. Cell. Cardiol. 13*: 229.

Reimer, K. A., Murry, C. E., Yamasawa, I., Hill, M. L., and Jennings, R. B. (1986). Four brief periods of myocardial ischemia cause no cumulative ATP loss or necrosis. *Am. J. Physiol. 251*: H1306.

Rohmann, S., Scott, R. J., Harting, J., and Schaper, W. (1991). Ischemic preconditioning is not a function of stunned myocardium, *J. Mol. Cell. Cardiol. 23* (Suppl. V): S.71 (Abstract).

Rouslin, W., Erickson, J. L., and Solaro, R. J. (1986). Effects of oligomycin and acidosis on rates of ATP depletion in ischemic heart muscle. *Am. J. Physiol. 250*: H503.

Rouslin, W., and Pullman, M. E. (1987). Protonic inhibition of the mitochondrial adenosine 5′-triphosphatase in ischemic cardiac muscle. Reversible binding of the ATPase inhibitor protein to the mitochondrial ATPase during ischemia. *J. Mol. Cell. Cardiol. 19*: 661.

Schott, R., Nao, B., Strieter, R., Groh, M., Kunkel, S., McClanahan, T., Schaper, W., and Gallagher, K. (1990a). Heat shock does not "precondition" canine myocardium. *Circulation 82* (Suppl. III): III-464 (Abstract).

Schott, R. J., Rohmann, S., Braun, E. R., and Schaper, W. (1990b). Ischemic preconditioning reduces infarct size in swine myocardium. *Circ. Res. 66*: 1133.

Schroder, E., Kieso, R. A., Laughlin, D., Schroder, M., Meng, R., and Kerber, R. E. (1987). Altered response of reperfused myocardium to repeated coronary occlusion in dogs. *J. Am. Coll. Cardiol. 10*: 898.

Swain, J. L., Sabina, R. L., McHale, P. A., Greenfield, J. C., Jr., and Holmes, E. W. (1982). Prolonged myocardial adenine nucleotide depletion after brief ischemia in the open-chest dog. *Am. J. Physiol. 242*: H818.

Swain, J. L., Sabina, R. L., Hines, J. J., Greenfield, J. C., Jr., and Holmes, E. W. (1984). Repetitive episodes of brief ischaemia (12 min) do not produce a cumulative depletion of high energy phosphate compounds. *Cardiovasc. Res. 18*: 264.

Thornton, J., Striplin, S., Liu, G. S., Swafford, A., Stanley, A. W. H., Van Winkle, D. M., and Downey, J. M. (1990a). Inhibition of protein synthesis does not block myocardial protection afforded by preconditioning. *Am. J. Physiol. (Heart Circ. Physiol.), 259* (28): H1822.

Thornton, J. D., Van Winkle, D. M., and Downey, J. M. (1990b). Preconditioning protection is mediated through adenosine receptors. *Circulation 82* (Suppl. III): III-464 (Abstract).

Van Winkle, D. M., Thornton, J. D., Downey, D. M., and Downey, J. M. (1991). The natural history of preconditioning: Cardioprotection depends on duration of transient ischemia and time to subsequent ischemia. *Coronary Artery Disease 2*: 613.

Wyatt, D. A., Edmunds, M. C., Rubio, R., Berne, R. M., Lasley, R. D., and Mentzer, R. M., Jr. (1989). Adenosine stimulates glycolytic flux in isolated perfused rat hearts by A1-adenosine receptors. *Am. J. Physiol. 257* (6): H1952.

Yamamoto, H., Tomoike, H., Shimokawa, H., Nabeyama, S., and Nakamura, M. (1984). Development of collateral function with repetitive coronary occlusion in a canine model reduces myocardial reactive hyperemia in the absence of significant coronary stenosis. *Circ. Res. 55*: 623.

Part II

Mechanisms of Postischemic Dysfunction

From the very first reports that apparently viable myocardium salvaged by timely reflow exhibits profound abnormalities in contractile function, the search has been on for the cause(s) or mechanism(s) of the stunned myocardium. In fact, Heyndrickx and colleagues in their seminal report (1978) postulated that the postischemic contractile dysfunction they observed may be due in part to "certain damage to the contractile proteins that occurs during ischemia"—a general concept that has not been entirely ruled out. During the subsequent decade, investigators have offered no fewer than eight seemingly diverse theories to explain this enigma.

Our objective in this section is to provide a comprehensive overview of the major hypotheses for the stunned myocardium. The roles of oxygen-derived free radicals, abnormal calcium homeostasis, and alterations in the cyclooxygenase pathway—the current frontrunners in terms of scientific evidence and popular opinion—are critically reviewed by Drs. Bolli, Kusuoka, Marban, Farber, and Gross, the investigators who were instrumental in developing these concepts. Additional theories that fleetingly captured the imagination of investigators—including perturbations in myocardial perfusion, conduction, energy metabolism, sympathetic neural responsiveness, and collagen integrity—are summarized and placed into perspective. It would be naive to expect, however, that the stunned myocardium is a simple, unifactorial process: in the final chapter of this section, Dr. Nayler attempts to provide a unified and integrated approach to this complex phenomenon. Although the precise cellular basis for postischemic contractile dysfunction has, to date, eluded explanation, this section aims to separate myth from fact concerning our current knowledge of the pathogenesis of the stunned myocardium.

REFERENCE

Heyndrickx, G. R., Baig, H., Nellens, P., Leusen, I., Fishbein, M. C., and Vatner, S. F. (1978). Depression of regional blood flow and wall thickening after brief coronary occlusions. *Am. J. Physiol. 2234*: H653.

8

Role of Oxygen Radicals in Myocardial Stunning

Roberto Bolli

Baylor College of Medicine, Houston, Texas

In recent years, several experiments have been reported that suggest that myocardial stunning is mediated in part by the generation of cytotoxic oxygen-derived free radicals. As a result of these investigations, the "oxyradical hypothesis" has emerged as one of the leading theories regarding the pathogenesis of postischemic contractile dysfunction. The purpose of this chapter is to critically review the evidence supporting this hypothesis and to discuss its pathophysiological and clinical implications. The major unresolved issues and areas for future research will be identified, and an attempt will be made to integrate the oxyradical hypothesis and other leading theories into a unifying pathogenetic paradigm. Many of the concepts discussed in this chapter have been presented in a recent review (Bolli, 1990).

I. HISTORICAL PERSPECTIVE

Since its introduction in the mid-1980s (Myers et al., 1985; Przyklenk and Kloner, 1986; Gross et al., 1986), the oxyradical hypothesis of stunning has undergone a remarkably rapid development: from 1985 to 1991, at least 51 full-length articles have been published on the relation between oxidative stress and postischemic dysfunction, and the issue continues to be vigorously pursued. The development of this hypothesis can be divided into three sequential phases, which reflect a logical, progressive effort to gain more cogent evidence and to obtain a more complete understanding. In the first phase, the approach to the problem was indirect, much as in other areas of biology in which a free radical involvement was postulated. Evidence for a role of free radicals was sought by administering a putative antioxidant and by measuring protection in terms of enhanced recovery of contractile function. This indirect approach has been useful because it has permitted formulation of the oxyradical hypothesis; however, it is inherently limited because it relies on the unproven assumptions that free radicals are indeed generated and that the drugs under examination do indeed act by scavenging these species. Therefore, in the second phase of investigation, a more direct approach to the problem was sought. Free radical generation in the stunned myocardium was measured directly, and the ability of antioxidants to inhibit this process was correlated with their ability to enhance recovery of function. This direct approach has been useful because it has dissipated the ambiguities raised by the potential nonspecific effects of many antioxidants and thus has provided convincing evidence for a pathogenetic role of oxyradicals in stunning. However, the question of how free radicals produce contractile dysfunction remains unanswered. Consequently, in the third phase of investigation (which is just beginning), the focus will be the identification of the molecular mechanisms by which a brief oxidative stress leaves behind a prolonged depression of contractility.

II. HETEROGENEITY OF EXPERIMENTAL MODELS OF MYOCARDIAL STUNNING

One of the major problems in elucidating the pathogenesis of myocardial stunning is that this term has been applied to a wide variety of experimental settings that have major pathophysiological differences, and that may or may not share a common pathogenesis (Bolli, 1990). In order to avoid misleading generalizations, it is important to recognize that concepts derived from one experimental setting cannot be automatically extrapolated to another one. Detailed discussions of the various models of stunning have been published elsewhere (Bolli, 1990) (see Section I) and are beyond the scope of this chapter. Briefly, the available observations can be grouped into the following categories (Table 1): (1) stunning after a single, completely reversible episode of regional ischemia (e.g., a coronary occlusion < 20 minutes in the dog); (2) stunning after multiple, completely reversible episodes of regional ischemia (e.g., repeated 5- or 10-minute coronary occlusions in the dog); (3) stunning after a single, partly irreversible episode of regional ischemia (subendocar-

Table 1 Classification of Myocardial Stunning and Evidence for the Various Mechanisms Proposed in Experimental Animals

	Evidence for a pathogenetic role of			
Experimental setting	Oxygen radicals	Sarcoplasmic reticulum dysfunction	Calcium overload	Reduced calcium sensitivity
Stunning due to decreased blood flow				
Regional ischemia				
Single, completely reversible ischemic episode	+ +	?	?	−
Multiple, completely reversible ischemic episodes	+	+	?	−
Single, partly irreversible ischemic episode (subendocardial infarction)	±	?	?	?
Global ischemia				
Isolated heart in vitro	+	?	+	+
Cardioplegic arrest in vivo	+	?	?	?
Stunning due to increased O_2 demand				
Exercise-induced ischemia	−	?	?	?

+, Published studies support this mechanism.
+ +, Published studies from multiple laboratories consistently support this mechanism; evidence is also available in conscious animal preparations.
−, Published studies do not support this mechanism.
±, Published studies are conflicting.
?, No data available.
Source: Adapted with permission of the American Heart Association from *Circulation 82*: 723-738, 1990.

dial infarction) (e.g., a coronary occlusion > 20 minutes but < 3 hours in the dog); (4) stunning after global ischemia in isolated hearts; (5) stunning after global ischemia in vivo (cardioplegic arrest); and (6) stunning after exercise-induced ischemia (high flow ischemia). Because of the obvious heterogeneity of these experimental preparations, the role of oxygen radicals will be examined separately for each of the settings listed above.

III. ROLE OF OXYGEN RADICALS IN MYOCARDIAL STUNNING AFTER A SINGLE, REVERSIBLE EPISODE OF REGIONAL ISCHEMIA

Most of the evidence supporting the oxyradical hypothesis has been obtained in models of myocardial stunning produced by a single, completely reversible episode of regional ischemia (i.e., a 15-minute coronary occlusion in the dog). It is, therefore, appropriate to devote the larger part of this chapter to a discussion of the role of oxygen radicals in this model.

A. Effect of Antioxidants in Anesthetized Animals

In the mid-1980s a number of investigators, including ourselves, postulated that myocardial stunning is caused in part by the generation of reactive oxygen metabolites, such as superoxide anion ($\cdot O_2^-$), hydrogen peroxide (H_2O_2), and hydroxyl radical ($\cdot OH$), and began a series of experiments designed to test this hypothesis. We used an open-chest dog preparation in which the left anterior descending coronary artery was occluded for 15 min and then reperfused (Zhu et al., 1986). In the first study (Myers et al., 1985), we found that administration of superoxide dismutase (SOD) (an enzyme that catalyzes the dismutation of $\cdot O_2^-$ to O_2 and H_2O_2) and catalase (an enzyme that reduces H_2O_2 to O_2 and H_2O) significantly enhanced recovery of function after reperfusion. Attenuation of myocardial stunning by SOD and catalase has also been observed by other investigators using similar experimental preparations (15-minute occlusion) in dogs (Gross et al., 1986; Przyklenk and Kloner, 1986; Murry et al., 1989) and rabbits (Koerner et al., 1991). In a subsequent study (Jeroudi et al., 1990), we found that neither SOD alone nor catalase alone significantly improved recovery of function in the stunned myocardium; however, when the two enzymes were combined, contractile recovery was significantly greater than that observed in controls or in dogs receiving either enzyme alone. These results suggest that both $\cdot O_2^-$ and H_2O_2 contribute to the cellular damage responsible for myocardial stunning, and that combined administration of SOD and catalase is more likely to be effective against stunning than separate administration. Similar results have been recently reported in rabbits (Koerner et al., 1991). The inability of SOD alone to mitigate postischemic dysfunction has also been observed in a pig model (Buchwald et al., 1989a).

Although both $\cdot O_2^-$ and H_2O_2 appear to contribute to stunning, it remains uncertain whether they do so by direct cytotoxicity or via formation of other species. $\cdot O_2^-$ and H_2O_2 can interact through the metal-catalyzed Haber-Weiss reaction to generate the highly reactive $\cdot OH$ radical (Halliwell and Gutteridge, 1984). Consequently, accumulation of $\cdot O_2^-$ and H_2O_2 could produce postischemic dysfunction, at least in part, indirectly through generation of $\cdot OH$. To elucidate this problem, we evaluated dimethylthiourea, an $\cdot OH$ scavenger that is more effective than traditional $\cdot OH$ scavengers and does not react with $\cdot O_2^-$ or H_2O_2 in vitro (Bolli et al., 1987a). We observed that dimethylthiourea produced a significant and sustained improvement in the function of the stunned myocardium (Bolli et al., 1987a). These results were further corroborated in studies using *N*-2-mercaptopropionyl glycine (MPG), a free radical scavenger that readily enters the intracellular space and is active orally. MPG was found to be a powerful scavenger of ·OH with no effect on $\cdot O_2^-$ or H_2O_2 in vitro (Bolli et al., 1989c) and to effectively attenuate myocardial stunning in vivo (Myers et al., 1986a; Bolli et al., 1989c). The protective effects of MPG against stunning have been recently confirmed in rabbits (Koerner et al., 1991). Taken together, these results suggest that the ·OH radical (or one of its reactive products) is a mediator of postischemic dysfunction and that the beneficial effects of SOD and catalase previously demonstrated (Myers et al., 1985; Gross et al., 1986; Przyklenk and Kloner, 1986; Murry et al., 1989; Jeroudi et al., 1990, Koerner et al., 1991) are due in part to prevention of ·OH generation. This conclusion is also consistent with the finding that the iron chelator, desferrioxamine, attenuates postischemic dysfunction (Bolli et al., 1987b; Farber et al., 1988). Because iron catalyzes the formation of ·OH (through the Haber-Weiss or Fenton mechanisms) as well as the propagation of ·OH-initiated lipid peroxidation (Halliwell and Gutteridge, 1984), the protective effects of desferrioxamine are compatible with the view that ·OH is a mediator of myocardial stunning.

The effectiveness of antioxidants that scavenge ·OH or prevent its generation should not be construed as evidence that *all* of the damage initiated by oxygen is mediated via ·OH. It is generally agreed that H_2O_2 is a relatively nonreactive species and its toxicity may be largely due to its reduction to ·OH (Halliwell and Gutteridge, 1984). However, there is evidence that $\cdot O_2^-$ in itself can directly cause cellular toxicity in vitro (Schrier and Hess, 1988; reviewed in DiGuiseppi and Fridovich, 1982). Furthermore, since catalase alone prevents formation of ·OH by removing H_2O_2, the fact that SOD has to be added to catalase to produce significant attenuation of stunning in vivo (Jeroudi et al., 1990; Koerner et al., 1991) implies the existence of a component of damage specifically due to $\cdot O_2^-$. It appears, therefore, that all three species ($\cdot O_2^-$, H_2O_2, and ·OH) are important in postischemic dysfunction ($\cdot O_2^-$ and ·OH as mediators of injury and H_2O_2 as a precursor of ·OH) (Jeroudi et al., 1990).

Other antioxidant therapies, such as probucol, have been recently shown to attenuate myocardial stunning after a 15-minute coronary occlusion in the rabbit (Dage et al., 1991). In contrast, a 1-week pretreatment with α-tocopherol failed to enhance recovery of function after an 8-minute coronary occlusion in pigs (Buchwald et al., 1989b).

In summary, numerous investigations from several independent laboratories (Myers et al., 1985, 1986a; Gross et al., 1986; Przyklenk and Kloner, 1986; Bolli et al., 1987a,b, 1989c; Farber et al., 1988, Murry et al., 1989; Jeroudi et al., 1990; Koerner et al., 1991; Dage et al., 1991) uniformly suggest that oxygen metabolites play a significant role in the genesis of myocardial stunning after a 15-minute period of ischemia. The relative contributions of the various metabolites have not been definitively established. It seems clear that a portion of the damage is mediated by ·OH. However, the available evidence suggests that myocardial stunning cannot be simplistically ascribed to a single oxygen species, and that all of the three initial metabolites of oxygen ($\cdot O_2^-$, H_2O_2, and ·OH) contribute to the cellular injury responsible for postischemic dysfunction. Iron also appears to play a role in stunning, presumably by catalyzing the formation of ·OH.

B. Effect of Antioxidants in Conscious Animals

Although the studies discussed above (Myers et al., 1985, 1986a; Gross et al., 1986; Przyklenk and Kloner, 1986; Bolli et al., 1987a,b, 1989c; Farber et al., 1988, Murry et al., 1989; Jeroudi et al., 1990; Koerner et al., 1991; Dage et al., 1991) consistently support the oxyradical hypothesis, their significance is limited by the fact that they were all performed in anesthetized, open-chest animal preparations, which are subject to the confounding influence of many unphysiologic conditions. Thus, artifacts due to the combined effects of anesthesia, hypothermia, surgical trauma, lack of integrity of the chest wall, abnormal hemodynamic conditions, excessive release of catecholamines, volume and ionic imbalances, and other metabolic abnormalities cannot be excluded. Certain conclusions derived from open-chest preparations have subsequently been found not to be applicable to conscious animals (see Triana et al., 1991). Indeed, observations in our laboratory (Triana et al., 1991) demonstrate that both the severity and the duration of myocardial stunning are greatly exaggerated in the barbiturate-anesthetized, open-chest dog as compared with the conscious dog, even when differences in collateral perfusion and hemodynamic variables are taken into account and arterial blood gases, hematocrit, and body temperature are carefully kept within the normal range: after an identical period of ischemia (a 15-minute coronary occlusion), approximately half of the postischemic depression of contractility noted in open-chest dogs was not observed in conscious dogs, and thus appears to be an artifact of the acute preparation (Triana et al., 1991). This striking disparity raises the question of whether the oxyradical hypothesis (predicated exclusively on open-chest preparations) is applicable to conscious animals. Clearly, the lack of supporting evidence in more physiological animal models represents a significant limitation of the oxyradical hypothesis of stunning (and, for that matter, of any other hypothesis): in my opinion, before results obtained in open-chest models can be extrapolated to humans, it is essential that they be tested in awake animals. In a recent experiment (Triana et al., 1991), we observed that the combined administration of SOD and catalase significantly enhanced the recovery of function after a 15-minute coronary occlusion in conscious, unsedated dogs, and that this effect was sustained for at least 6 hours after reflow (Fig. 1). The magnitude of this beneficial effect was a function of the severity of ischemia: the lower the collateral perfusion, the greater the improvement effected by the enzymes (Fig. 2). The accelerated recovery produced by SOD and catalase was not followed by any subsequent deterioration of contractility (Figs. 1, 2), suggesting that postischemic dysfunction is not a teleologically "protective" response to injury (Triana et al., 1991).

In summary, studies in conscious dogs suggest that oxygen radicals play a pathogenetic role in myocardial stunning that is independent of the abnormal conditions associated with the open-chest preparation. Therefore, despite the large differences between anesthetized and awake models, it appears that the oxyradical hypothesis derived from acute studies (Myers et al., 1985,

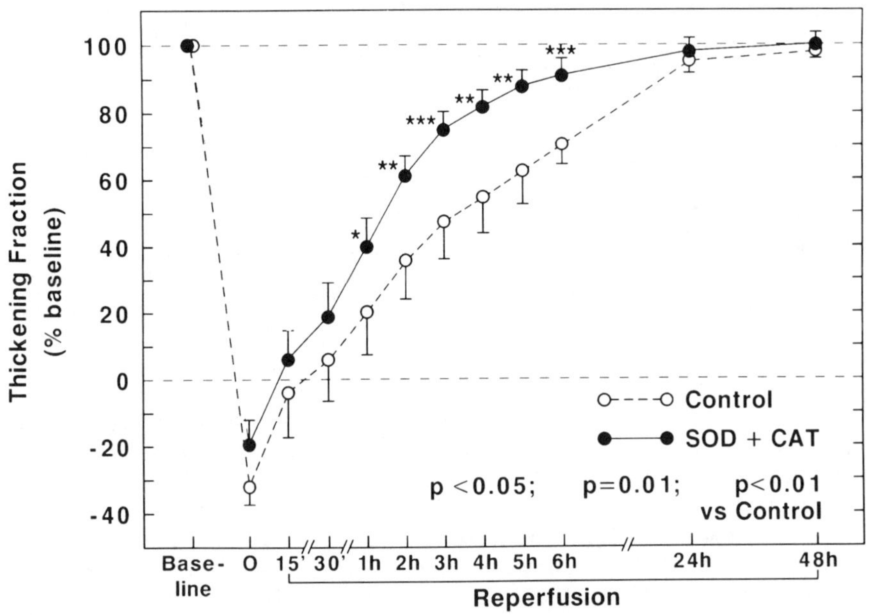

Figure 1 Systolic thickening fraction in the ischemic/reperfused region 5 minutes after coronary occlusion (○) and at selected times after reperfusion in control (dashed line with open circles) and SOD and catalase-treated (continuous line with solid circles) conscious dogs. Thickening fraction is expressed as percent of baseline values. The data pertain to all of the conscious dogs studied (controls, $n = 19$; treated, $n = 21$). Data are mean ± SEM. (Reproduced from Triana et al., 1991, with permission of The American Heart Association.)

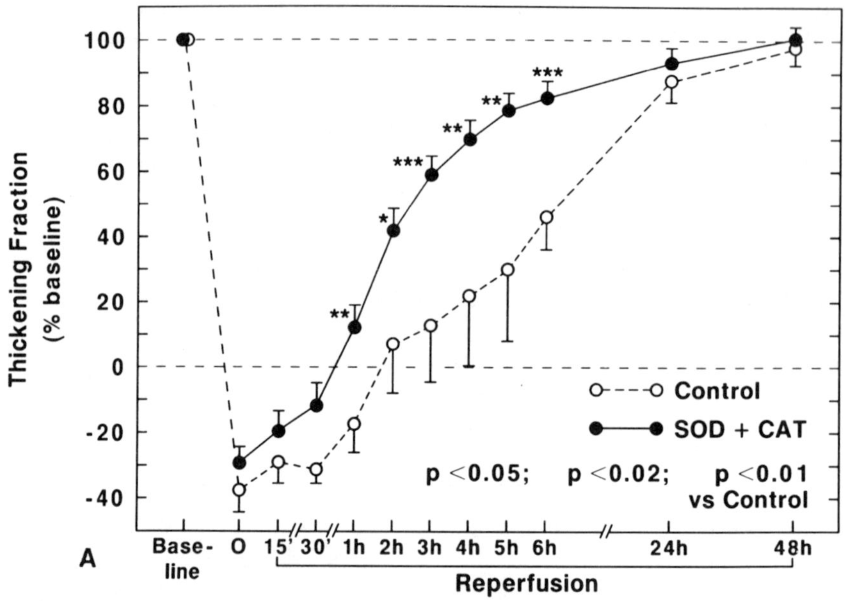

Figure 2 Systolic thickening fraction in the ischemic/reperfused region 5 minutes after coronary occlusion (○) and at selected times after reperfusion in subset (A), subset II (B), and subset III (C) of the conscious dogs. Control dogs are represented by the dashed line with open circles; SOD and catalase-treated dogs are represented by the continuous line with solid circles. Thickening fraction is expressed as percent of baseline values. Data are mean ± SEM. Subset I was formed by dogs with collateral flow < 10% of nonischemic zone flow (NZF); subset II included animals with collateral flow between 10 and 30% of NZF; subset III consisted of dogs with collateral flow > 30% of NZF. In subset I, transmural ischemic zone flow averaged 0.07 ± 0.02 ml/min/g in controls (n = 7) and 0.09 ± 0.01 ml/min/g in treated animals (n = 11) (4.1 ± 1.1% and 5.9 ± 0.9% of NZF, respectively). In subset II, ischemic zone flow was 0.25 ± 0.04 ml/min/g in controls (n = 7) and 0.31 ± 0.03 ml/min/g in treated dogs (n = 5) (15.7 ± 2.0% and 23.0 ± 2.6% of NZF, respectively). In subset III, ischemic zone flow averaged 0.52 ± 0.06 ml/min/g in controls (n = 5) and 0.63 ± 0.04 ml/min/g in treated dogs (n = 5) (43.2 ± 4.2% and 41.6 ± 4.9% of NZF, respectively). (Reproduced from Triana et al., 1991, with permission of The American Heart Association.)

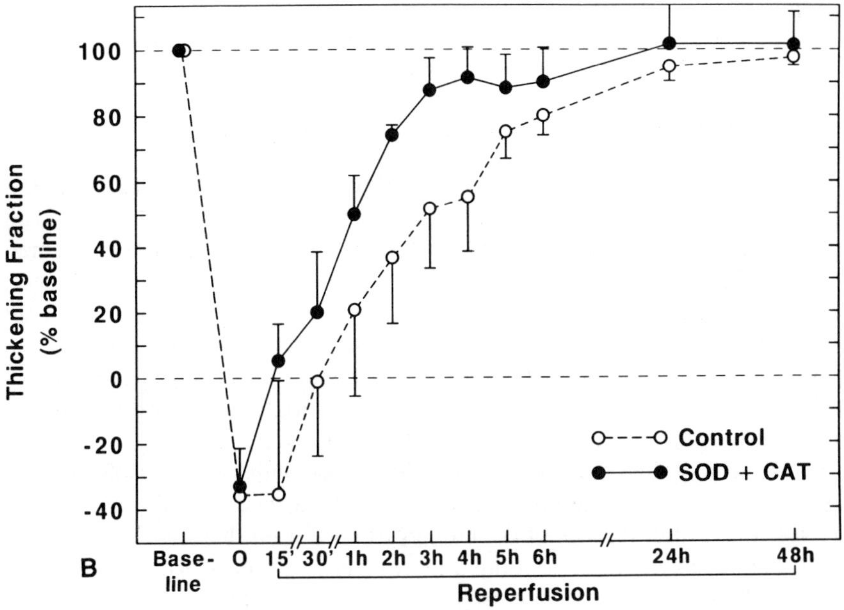

Thickening Fraction (% baseline)
100
80
60
40
20
0
-20
-40
Control
SOD + CAT
Base-line
O
15'
30'
1h
2h
3h
4h
5h
6h
24h
48h
Reperfusion

B

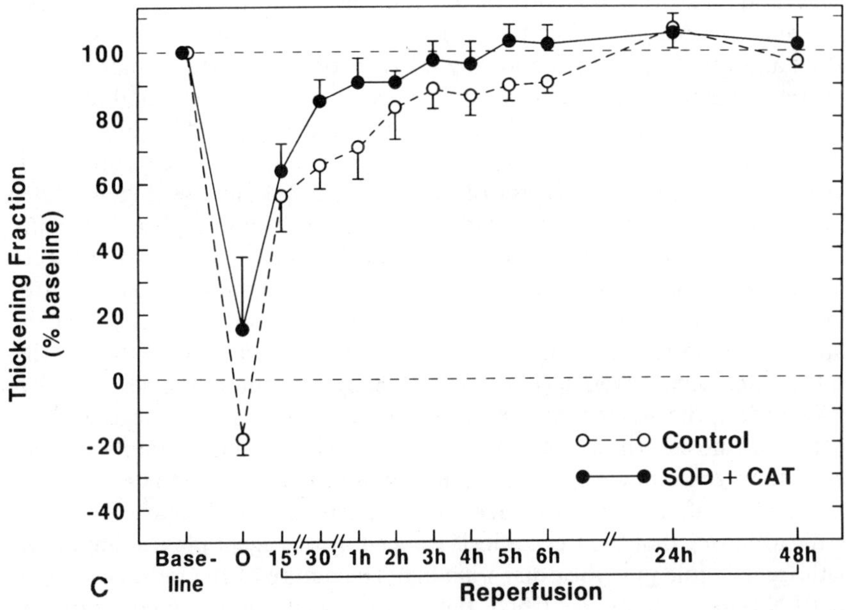

Thickening Fraction (% baseline)
100
80
60
40
20
0
-20
-40
Control
SOD + CAT
Base-line
O
15'
30'
1h
2h
3h
4h
5h
6h
24h
48h
Reperfusion

C

1986a; Gross et al., 1986; Przyklenk and Kloner, 1986; Bolli et al., 1987a, b, 1989c; Farber et al., 1988; Murry et al., 1989; Jeroudi et al., 1990; Koerner et al., 1991; Dage et al., 1991) is applicable to the conscious animal.

C. Direct Evidence for the Oxyradical Hypothesis

A major limitation of the studies reviewed to this point (Myers et al., 1985, 1986a; Gross et al., 1986; Przyklenk and Kloner, 1986; Bolli et al., 1987a, b, 1989c; Farber et al., 1988; Murry et al., 1989; Jeroudi et al., 1990; Koerner et al., 1991; Dage et al., 1991; Triana et al., 1991) is that all of the evidence provided by these investigations is indirect and, therefore, inconclusive. In my opinion, in order to definitively confirm a causative role of oxygen metabolites in postischemic dysfunction, it is necessary to directly demonstrate and quantitate free radical generation in the stunned myocardium in the presence and absence of antioxidant interventions.

Production of free radicals has been directly demonstrated in isolated rabbit or rat hearts, undergoing global ischemia and reperfusion (reviewed in Davies, 1989), but because of the numerous important differences in experimental conditions, results obtained in vitro cannot necessarily be extrapolated to the intact animal. We used the spin trap, α-phenyl *N-tert*-butyl nitrone (PBN), and electron paramagnetic resonance (EPR) spectroscopy to detect and measure production of free radicals in our in vivo model of postischemic dysfunction (15-minute coronary occlusion in open-chest dogs) (Bolli and McCay, 1990). Following infusion of PBN, EPR signals characteristic of PBN radical adducts were detected in the venous blood draining from the ischemic-reperfused vascular bed (Bolli et al., 1988b) (Fig. 3). The myocardial production of radicals began during coronary occlusion but increased dramatically after reperfusion, peaking at 2–4 minutes (Fig. 4). After this initial burst, production of radicals abated but did not cease, persisting up to 3 hours after reflow (Bolli et al., 1988b) (Fig. 4). As shown in Figure 5, there was a linear, positive relation between the magnitude of adduct production and the magnitude of ischemic flow reduction, indicating that the intensity of free radical generation after reflow is determined by the severity of the antecedent ischemia (Bolli et al., 1988b): the greater the degree of hypoperfusion, the greater the subsequent production of free radicals and, by inference, the severity of reperfusion injury. These findings imply that interventions that improve perfusion during ischemia will attenuate free radical reactions after reflow. Further, PBN in itself enhanced recovery of function, suggesting that the free radicals trapped by this agent play an important pathogenetic role in myocardial stunning. The nature of the radicals trapped by PBN remains to be identified, but they are likely to be a mixture of carbon-centered and oxygen-centered species, such as alkyl and alkoxyl radi-

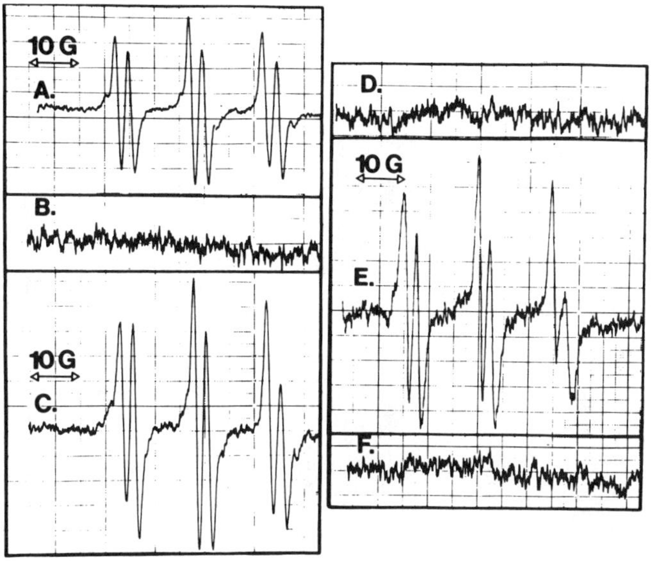

Figure 3 Representative electron paramagnetic resonance (EPR) spectra of PBN radical adducts detected in the coronary venous effluent blood in open-chest dogs. Dogs underwent a 15-minute coronary occlusion followed by reperfusion. The spin trap, α-phenyl *N-tert*-butyl nitrone (PBN), was infused intracoronarily beginning 5 minutes before occlusion and continuing until 10 minutes after reperfusion (group I), beginning 20 seconds before reperfusion and continuing until 10 minutes after reperfusion (group II), or beginning 30 minutes after reperfusion and continuing until 40 minutes after reperfusion (group III). The average rate of infusion was 4.4 mg/min. Blood samples were obtained from a vein draining the ischemic/reperfused region and the plasma lipids were extracted by the Folch procedure and analyzed by EPR spectroscopy. Shown in this figure are signals from plasma samples obtained: (A) 3 minutes after reperfusion in a dog from group I (PBN infusion started 5 minutes before ischemia) ($a_N = 14.75$, $a^H_\beta = 2.69$ G; gain, 5×10^5); (B) at corresponding time after start of PBN infusion in a control dog (gain, 1×10^6); (C) 5 minutes after reperfusion in a dog in group II (PBN infusion started 20 seconds before reperfusion) $a_N = 14.77$, $a^H_\beta = 2.69$ G; gain, 5×10^5); (D) at corresponding time after start of PBN in a second control dog (gain, 1×10^6); (E) 35 minutes after reperfusion in a dog in group III (PBN infusion started 30 minutes after reperfusion) ($a_N = 15.00$, $a^H_\beta = 2.78$ G; gain, 2×10^6); (F) at corresponding time after start of PBN in a third control dog (gain, 1×10^6). The signals observed are characteristic of radical adducts of PBN. These results demonstrate that free radicals are generated in the stunned myocardium in the intact dog. The spectrometer settings were as follows: microwave power, 19.7 mW; modulation amplitude, 1 G; time constant, 1.25 seconds; scan range, 100 G; and scan time, 8 minutes. All spectra were recorded at room temperature (25 °C). (Reproduced with permission from Bolli et al., 1988b.)

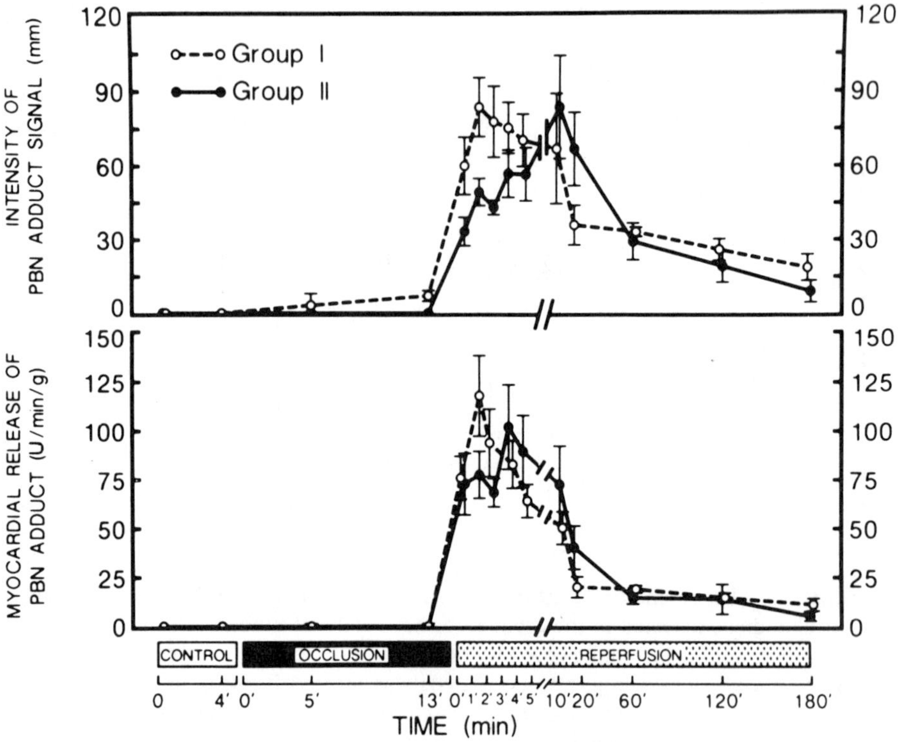

Figure 4 (Upper panel) Intensity of the electron paramagnetic resonance spectroscopy signals detected in the coronary venous effluent blood in groups I and II. (Lower panel) Time course of myocardial release of PBN adducts in groups I and II. Data are mean ± SEM. Open-chest dogs underwent a 15-minute coronary occlusion followed by reperfusion. Group I received intracoronary PBN starting 5 minutes before occlusion and continuing until 10 minutes after reperfusion ($n = 5$); group II received intracoronary PBN starting at reperfusion and ending 10 minutes thereafter ($n = 5$). Reperfusion after 15 minutes of ischemia was associated with a burst of free radical generation, which abated by 10 minutes but continued up to 3 hours after reflow. PBN, α-phenyl *N-tert*-butyl nitrone. (Reproduced with permission from Bolli et al., 1988b.)

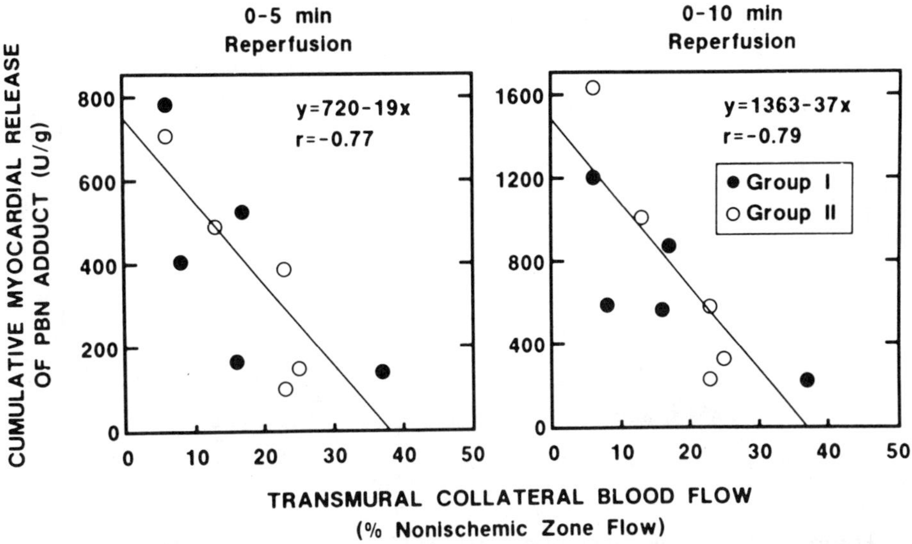

Figure 5 Relationship between mean transmural collateral blood flow to the ischemic region during coronary occlusion (horizontal axis) and total cumulative myocardial release of PBN adducts during the first 5 minutes (left) and 10 minutes (right) of reperfusion. Collateral flow is expressed as percentage of simultaneous nonischemic zone flow; adduct release is expressed in arbitrary units per gram of myocardium. Solid circles represent dogs in group I (PBN given before ischemia); open circles represent dogs in group II (PBN given at reperfusion). In both groups, the myocardial production of PBN adducts after coronary reperfusion was linearly and inversely related to collateral flow during the antecedent occlusion. These data suggest that the severity of the ischemic injury is the major determinant of the severity of the subsequent reperfusion injury. PBN, α-phenyl *N-tert*-butyl nitrone. (Reproduced with permission from Bolli et al., 1988b.)

cals, both of which are known to be byproducts of oxyradical-initiated lipid peroxidation (Thompson and Hess, 1986) and both of which can be trapped by PBN (Bolli and McCay, 1990). Generation of free radicals in in vivo models of regional myocardial stunning has also been reported by Weglicki's group (Leiboff et al., 1988).

In a subsequent study (Bolli et al., 1989b), we found that SOD plus catalase suppressed the production of free radicals in the stunned myocardium (Fig. 6), indicating that these radicals are derived from univalent reduction of oxygen; furthermore, the inhibition of free radical production was associated with inhibition of myocardial stunning (Bolli et al., 1989b). More re-

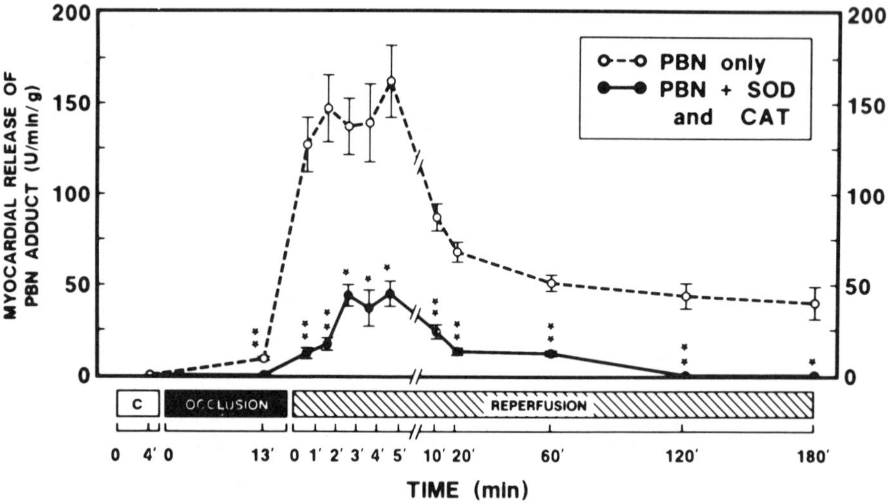

Figure 6 Time course of myocardial release of PBN adducts in group I (PBN only, $n = 6$) and group II (PBN plus superoxide dismutase and catalase, $n = 6$). Data are mean ± SEM. Administration of superoxide dismutase and catalase markedly inhibited production of free radicals in the stunned myocardium after 15 min of regional ischemia. $^{*}p < 0.05$; $^{**}p < 0.01$ vs. group I. PBN, α-phenyl *N-tert*-butyl nitrone. (Reproduced from Bolli et al., 1989b.)

cently, we observed that MPG (Bolli et al., 1989c) or desferrioxamine (Bolli et al., 1990), administered just before reperfusion, markedly attenuated myocardial stunning and the associated production of PBN adducts; however, the same agents given 1 minute after reperfusion did not attenuate myocardial stunning or initial PBN adduct production (Figs. 7–10). Thus, three different antioxidant interventions (SOD plus catalase, MPG, and desferrioxamine) reduced postischemic dysfunction at the same doses and under the same experimental conditions in which they reduced formation of PBN adducts. This consistent association between the two effects suggest that the production of free radicals in the stunned myocardium plays a causal role in the depression of contractility.

More recently, we have demonstrated, using PBN, that free radicals are also produced in the stunned myocardium in the conscious dog after a 15-minute occlusion (Zughayb et al., 1991), with a time course similar to that observed in the open-chest dog. These results (Zughayb et al., 1991) suggest that the generation of free radicals observed in anesthetized animals (Bolli et al., 1988b, 1989b,c, 1990; Leiboff et al., 1988; Bolli and McCay, 1990) is not an artifact due to the unphysiological conditions associated with this

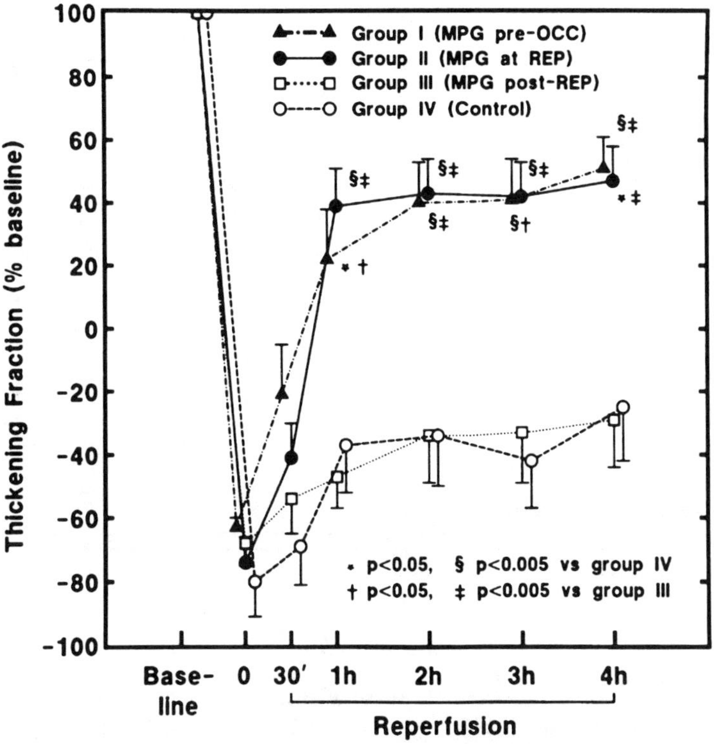

Figure 7 Systolic thickening fraction in the ischemic/reperfused region 5 minutes after coronary occlusion (○) and at selected times after reperfusion in the following groups: Group I (MPG infusion started 15 min before ischemia, $n = 8$), group II (MPG started 1 minute before reperfusion, $n = 9$), group III (MPG infusion started 1 minute after reperfusion, $n = 10$), and group IV (controls, $n = 10$). Thickening fraction is expressed as percent of baseline values. Data are mean ± SEM. MPG attenuated postischemic dysfunction in a similar extent irrespective of whether the infusion was started before ischemia or just before reperfusion; however, infusion started 1 minute after reperfusion was ineffective, suggesting that the critical radical-mediated injury occurs in the first few minutes after reperfusion. MPG, *N*-2-mercaptopropionyl glycine. (Reproduced from Bolli et al., 1989c, with permission of The American Heart Association.)

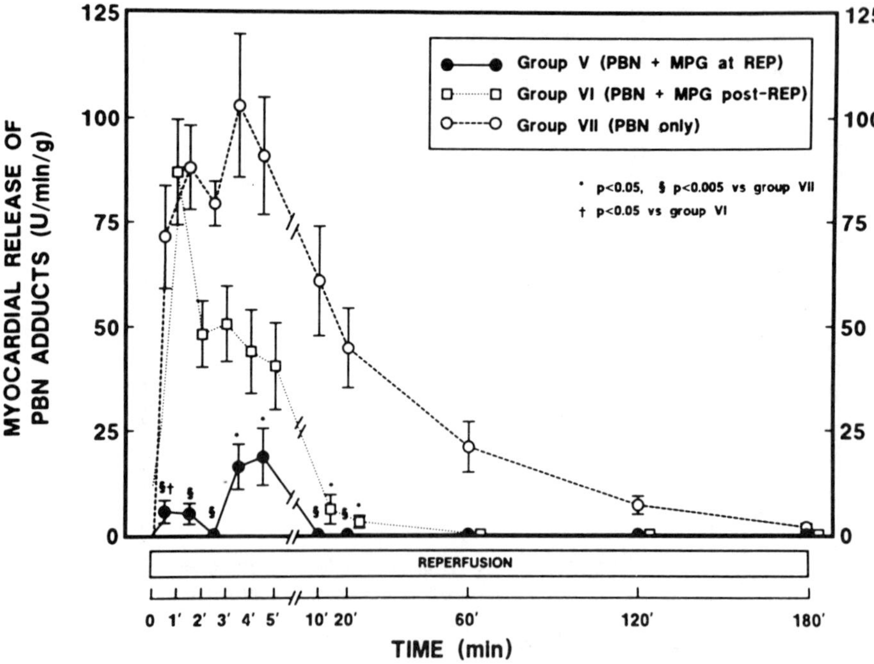

Figure 8 Time course of myocardial release of PBN adducts in group V (MPG infusion started 1 minute after reperfusion, $n = 5$), group VI (MPG infusion started 1 min after reperfusion, $n = 5$), and group VII (controls, $n = 6$). Data are mean ± SEM. All groups received PBN by the intracoronary route. Infusion of MPG started 1 minute before reperfusion markedly suppressed production of free radicals in the stunned myocardium. Infusion of MPG started 1 minute after reperfusion did not affect the initial production of free radicals and produced a delayed suppression, which became evident by 10 minutes of reflow. Since only MPG given as in group V attenuated postischemic dysfunction (whereas MPG given as in group VI did not) (see Fig. 1), these data suggest that the free radicals important in myocardial stunning are those generated immediately after reperfusion. MPG, *N*-2-mercaptopropionyl glycine; PBN, α-phenyl *N-tert*-butyl nitrone. (Reproduced from Bolli et al., 1989c, with permission of The American Heart Association.)

preparation. In another recently reported study (Bolli et al., 1991), we have used aromatic hydroyxylation of phenylalanine to investigate whether the hydroxyl radical is generated in the stunned myocardium. We have found that hydroxylated derivatives of phenylalanine (*ortho-*, *meta-*, and *para*-tyrosine) are released in the local coronary venous blood during the first few minutes of reperfusion after a 15-minute occlusion, both in open-chest and in conscious dogs (Bolli et al., 1991a), indicating that ·OH is produced in

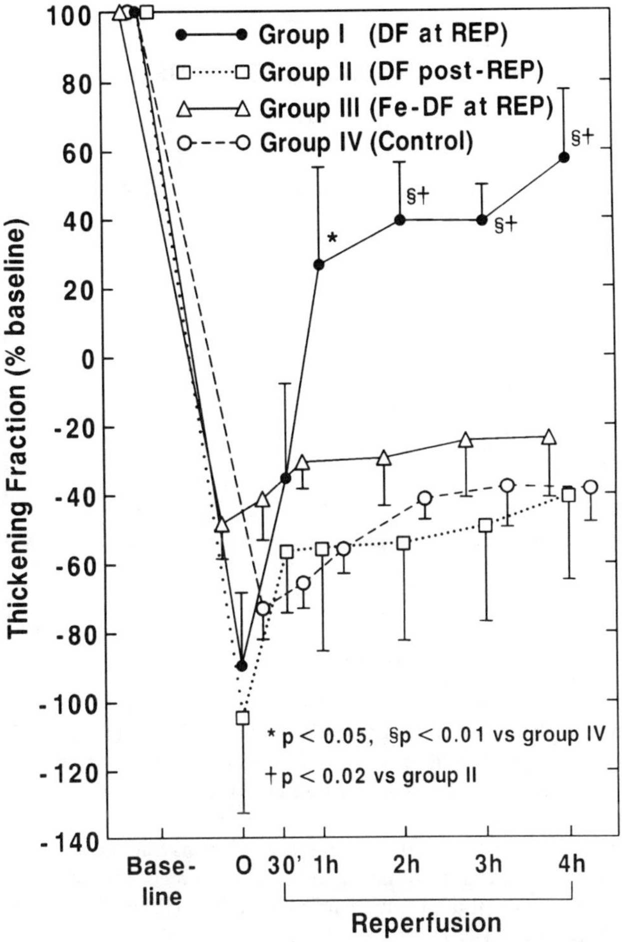

Figure 9 Systolic thickening fraction in the ischemic/reperfused region 5 minutes after coronary occlusion (○) and at selected times after reperfusion in the following groups: Group I [desferrioxamine (DF) administration started 2 minutes before reperfusion (REP), $n = 8$], group II (DF administration started 1 minute after reperfusion, $n = 6$), group III [iron-loaded desferrioxamine (Fe-DF) administration started 2 minutes before reperfusion, $n = 7$], and group IV (controls, $n = 8$). Thickening fraction is expressed as percent of baseline values. Data are mean ± SEM. Desferrioxamine attenuated postischemic dysfunction when started just before reperfusion; however, administration started 1 minute after reperfusion was ineffective, suggesting that the critical iron-mediated injury occurs in the first few moments after reperfusion. (Reproduced with permission from Bolli et al., 1990.)

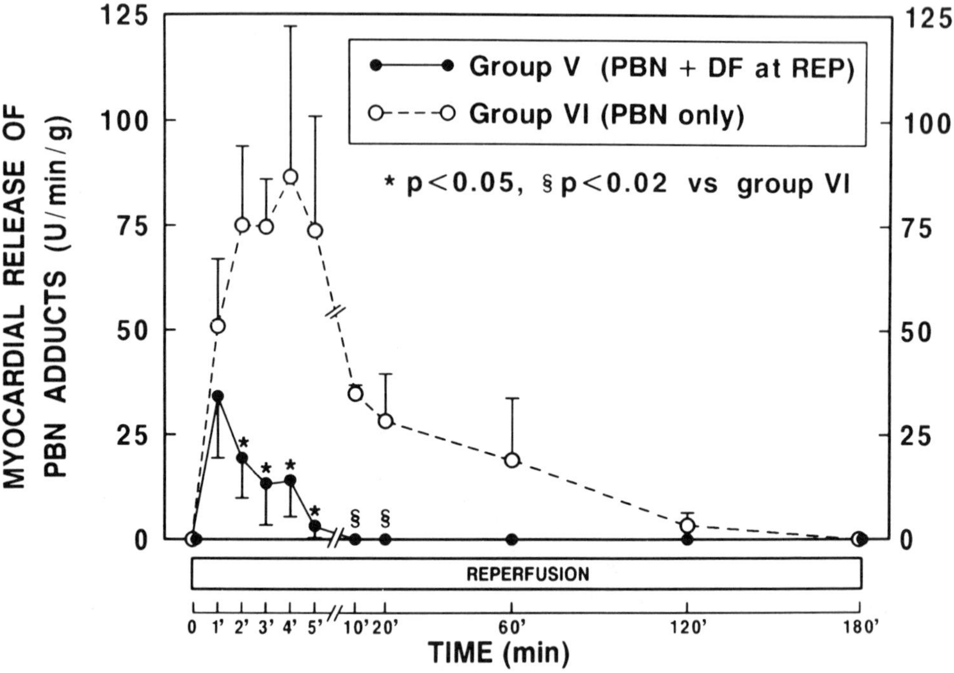

Figure 10 Time course of myocardial release of PBN adducts in group V [desferrioxamine (DF) administration started 2 minutes before reperfusion (REP), $n = 4$] and group VI (controls, $n = 5$). Data are mean ± SEM. Both groups received PBN by the intracoronary route. Infusion of desferrioxamine started 2 minutes before reperfusion markedly suppressed production of free radicals in the stunned myocardium. Since desferrioxamine given as in Group V attenuated postischemic dysfunction (see Fig. 8), these data suggest that iron-mediated free radical reactions occurring immediately after reperfusion contribute to myocardial stunning. (Reproduced with permission from Bolli et al., 1990.)

the stunned myocardium upon reperfusion. The similarity of the results obtained in our canine model of stunning with two completely different techniques—spin trapping (Bolli et al., 1988b, 1989b,c, 1990; Leiboff et al., 1988; Bolli and McCay, 1990; Zughayb et al., 1991) and aromatic hydroxylation (Bolli et al., 1991)—further corroborates the concept that reactive oxygen species play a significant role in the pathogenesis of postischemic ventricular dysfunction.

In summary, the results of the studies that have measured free radicals in the stunned myocardium (Bolli et al., 1988b, 1989b,c, 1990, 1991; Leiboff et al., 1988b; Bolli and McCay, 1990; Zughayb et al., 1991) provide direct evidence supporting a pathogenetic role of oxygen metabolites. Specifically, these studies indicate that (1) free radicals are produced in the stunned myocardium in both open-chest and conscious dogs after reversible regional ischemia; (2) the univalent pathway of reduction of oxygen is the source of the radicals; and (3) inhibition of free radical reactions results in enhanced recovery of contractility (i.e., the radical reactions are necessary for postischemic dysfunction to occur).

D. Time Course of Free Radical-Induced Damage in the Stunned Myocardium

When exactly in the ischemia/reperfusion sequence that leads to stunning does the crucial free radical-induced damage take place? We have observed that infusion of the antioxidant, MPG, attenuated postischemic dysfunction to a similar extent whether the infusion was started before ischemia or 1 minute before reperfusion; however, infusion started 1 minute after reflow was ineffective (Bolli et al., 1989c), suggesting that the critical radical-mediated injury occurs in the first few moments of reperfusion (Fig. 7). We have subsequently obtained similar results with desferrioxamine (Bolli et al., 1990) (Fig. 9). Furthermore, the spin trap, PBN, enhances contractile recovery even when the infusion is commenced 20 seconds before reflow; the magnitude of the protective effect is similar to that observed when the infusion is commenced before ischemia (Bolli et al., 1988b). Captopril, an angiotensin-converting enzyme inhibitor with free radical scavenging properties, has been reported to produce similar attenuation of postischemic dysfunction when the administration is started before ischemia and when it is started 2 minutes before reperfusion (Westlin and Mullane, 1988). Antioxidant therapy started just before reperfusion has also been shown to reduce myocardial stunning in the rabbit (Koerner et al., 1991). The conclusion that a substantial portion of the cellular damage responsible for stunning occurs immediately after reflow is further corroborated by direct measurements of free radicals (Bolli et al., 1988b, 1989b,c) and lipid peroxidation products (Romaschin et al., 1987) in the stunned myocardium, both of which have shown a burst in the initial moments after restoration of flow. If free radical production is inhibited during this initial burst, postischemic dysfunction is mitigated; however, if free radical production is inhibited after the first 5 minutes of reperfusion (i.e., after the initial burst), no functional improvement is observed (Bolli et al., 1989c) (Fig. 8). These observations suggest that the free radicals important in causing myocardial stunning are those produced immediately after reflow.

In summary, myocardial stunning appears to be, in part, a form of oxyradical-mediated "reperfusion injury." This concept may have significant therapeutic implications, because it suggests that antioxidant therapies begun *after* the onset of ischemia could still be effective in preventing postischemic dysfunction; however, a delay in the implementation of such therapies until *after reperfusion* would result in loss of efficacy. It is important to keep in mind, however, that not all of the postischemic loss of contractility can be attributed to injurious events associated with reperfusion; part of the postischemic dysfunction undoubtedly represents a slow process of recovery from the damage incurred during ischemia (Hearse, 1991).

E. Sources of Oxygen Radicals in the Stunned Myocardium

Three potential mechanisms of oxyradical generation in the stunned myocardium have been explored thus far, namely, the enzyme xanthine oxidase, the activated neutrophil, and the arachidonate cascade. We found that the xanthine oxidase inhibitor allopurinol produced a marked improvement in the functional recovery of the stunned myocardium (Charlat et al., 1987). Furthermore, allopurinol inhibited the increased cardiac production of urate observed in control dogs during ischemia and early reperfusion, indicating effective inhibition of xanthine oxidoreductase (Charlat et al., 1987). Attenuation of stunning has also been demonstrated with oxypurinol after 15 minutes (Holzgrefe and Gibson, 1988) and 90 minutes (Puett et al., 1987) of ischemia and reperfusion. These data suggest that xanthine oxidase is one of the sources of the oxygen radicals that contribute to postischemic dysfunction in the dog. Whether this concept applies to humans remains uncertain because the myocardial content of xanthine oxidase is species dependent. Reports regarding the myocardial content of the enzyme in the human heart are conflicting (Jarasch et al., 1986; Eddy et al., 1987; Muxfeldt and Schaper, 1987; Huizer et al., 1989; Grum et al., 1989).

In contrast to these earlier reports (Charlat et al., 1987; Puett et al., 1987; Holzgrefe and Gibson, 1988), in a recent study (Werns et al., 1989) oxypurinol and amflutizole, two xanthine oxidase inhibitors, failed to mitigate stunning after 15 minutes of ischemia in dogs. Whether the discrepancy is due to different degrees of inhibition of xanthine oxidoreductase or to other reasons is presently unclear. In any case, the role of this enzyme in postischemic myocardial dysfunction does not seem to be critical because antioxidant therapy has been found to attenuate stunning in the rabbit (Koerner et al., 1991; Dage et al., 1991), a species that apparently lacks myocardial xanthine oxidase activity; this indicates that there are other important sources of free radicals in the stunned myocardium besides xanthine oxidase.

Leukocytes are another potential source of oxygen metabolites. However, several investigators have found that myocardial stunning is not attenuated by depletion of neutrophils with antiserum (Shea et al., 1987; O'Neill et al., 1989) or with filtration (Jeremy and Becker, 1989), by administration of nafazatrom, which inhibits production of leukotrienes (O'Neill et al., 1987) by administration of antibodies to the adhesion-promoting Mo1 glycoprotein (Schott et al., 1989), and by administration of dextran, which inhibits leukocyte adherence to the endothelium (Kerber et al., 1989). Recent studies have shown that the neutrophil content of the stunned myocardium after a 12-minute period of ischemia is decreased (Go et al., 1988) and that myeloperoxidase activity (a marker of neutrophils) in myocardium stunned by a 15-minute occlusion is not different from nonischemic myocardium (Schott et al., 1989). Furthermore, myocardial stunning occurs in isolated heart preparations that are devoid of circulating neutrophils. Taken together, these results (Shea et al., 1987; O'Neill et al., 1987, 1989; Go et al., 1988; Jeremy and Becker, 1989; Schott et al., 1989; Kerber et al., 1989) suggest that granulocytes do not play a major role in the genesis of postischemic dysfunction after brief, reversible ischemia, although they appear to be major mediators of irreversible tissue injury and vascular obstruction following prolonged periods of ischemia (Lucchesi and Mullane, 1986; Engler et al., 1986; Engler, 1987).

In contrast to the aforementioned findings, however, others have reported that depletion of granulocytes by Leukopak filtration prevents (Engler and Covell, 1987) or alleviates (Westlin and Mullane, 1989) postischemic dysfunction after a 15-minute coronary occlusion. The reasons for the differences between these studies (Engler and Covell, 1987; Westlin and Mullane, 1989) and the aforementioned investigations (Shea et al., 1987; O'Neill et al., 1987, 1989; Jeremy and Becker, 1989; Schott et al., 1989; Kerber et al., 1989) are presently unclear and warrant further research.

Metabolism of arachidonic acid via the cyclooxygenase pathway is another potential source of oxygen radicals. However, administration of indomethacin in doses that effectively inhibit cardiac production of TxB_2 and 6-keto-$PGF_{2\alpha}$ has no appreciable effect on myocardial stunning (Farber and Gross, 1990), suggesting that oxygen radicals generated by the arachidonate cascade do not contribute significantly to postischemic dysfunction.

In summary, in the canine model of myocardial stunning produced by a single, reversible ischemic episode, xanthine oxidase may be a source of free radicals (although the data are not entirely consistent), whereas the weight of the evidence suggests that neutrophils are relatively unimportant. Arachidonate metabolism also does not appear to be a significant source of oxyradicals. Of course, many other processes could lead to formation of O_2^- and H_2O_2 during myocardial ischemia and reperfusion, including autooxidation of catecholamines and other compounds, ischemia-induced damage of the electron transport chain in the mitochondria, and accumulation of reducing equivalents. It will be difficult to selectively assess the role of these potentially important mechanisms in a complex system such as the intact animal. Identification of the sources of oxyradicals in the stunned myocardium represents a major unresolved issue.

IV. ROLE OF OXYGEN RADICALS IN OTHER FORMS OF MYOCARDIAL STUNNING

The investigations reviewed thus far employed a single brief (≤15 minutes) coronary occlusion. The 15-minute coronary occlusion model of myocardial stunning has been investigated more extensively than any other model with respect to the potential pathogenetic role of oxygen radicals. As shown in Table 2, a large number of investigations from different laboratories have consistently shown improved contractile recovery with antioxidant therapy.

Table 2 Effect of Antioxidants on Myocardial Stunning After a Coronary Occlusion ≤15 min

Antioxidant	Preparation	Protection	Ref.
SOD + CAT	Open-chest dog	Yes	Myers et al., 1985
SOD + CAT	Open-chest dog	Yes	Przyklenk and Kloner, 1986
SOD + CAT	Open-chest dog	Yes	Gross et al., 1986
SOD + CAT	Open-chest dog	Yes	Murry et al., 1989
SOD + CAT	Open-chest dog	Yes	Bolli et al., 1989b
SOD + CAT	Open-chest dog	Yes	Jeroudi et al., 1990
SOD alone		No	
CAT alone		No	
SOD + CAT	Conscious dog	Yes	Triana et al., 1991
SOD + CAT	Open-chest rabbit	Yes	Koerner et al., 1991
MPG		Yes	
SOD alone	Open-chest pig[a]	No	Buchwald et al., 1989a
MPG	Open-chest dog	Yes	Myers et al., 1986a
MPG	Open-chest dog	Yes	Bolli et al., 1989c
DMTU	Open-chest dog	Yes	Bolli et al., 1987a
Desferrioxamine	Open-chest dog	Yes	Bolli et al., 1987b
Desferrioxamine	Open-chest dog	Yes	Farber et al., 1988
Allopurinol	Open-chest dog	Yes	Charlat et al., 1987
PBN	Open-chest dog	Yes	Bolli et al., 1988b
PBN	Open-chest dog	Yes	Bolli et al., 1989b
Probucol	Open-chest rabbit	Yes	Dage et al., 1991
α-Tocopherol	Open-chest pig[a]	No	Buchwald et al., 1989b

SOD, superoxide dismutase; CAT, catalase; MPG, *N*-2-mercaptopropionyl glycine; DMTU, dimethylthiourea; PBN, α-phenyl *N*-*tert*-butyl nitrone.
[a]The duration of occlusion was 8 minutes, not 15 minutes.
Source: Adapted with permission from *Cardiovasc. Drugs Ther.* 5: 249–268, 1991.

The evidence for a pathogenetic contribution of oxygen radicals in this model is overwhelming and represents one of the few areas in which a general consensus has been achieved regarding the importance of reactive oxygen species. The 15-minute occlusion model has the advantage that it is not associated with any infarction, so that the mechanical dysfunction observed can be entirely ascribed to stunning. But what is the role of oxygen metabolites in other forms of postischemic dysfunction?

In recent studies in our laboratory (Triana et al., 1990) we found that the ·OH scavenger, MPG, markedly improves contractile recovery after 10 repeated 5-minute coronary occlusions separated by 10-minute reflow periods in open-chest dogs. Furthermore, each occlusion-reperfusion cycle was associated with a burst of free radical production (measured by spin trapping techniques), which was markedly blunted by MPG (unpublished observations). Thus, oxyradicals also appear to contribute to the genesis of myocardial stunning after multiple brief ischemic episodes. Further, numerous studies from the surgical literature suggest that oxygen radicals contribute to postischemic dysfunction after global ischemia in in vivo models of cardioplegic arrest (Stewart et al., 1983; Johnson et al., 1987; Gardner, 1988; Illes et al., 1989), and there is evidence that oxidative stress contributes to postoperative dysfunction in patients undergoing cardiac surgery (Ferrari et al., 1990). Finally, antioxidants consistently alleviate mechanical dysfunction after global ischemia in isolated hearts (Shlafer et al., 1982a,b; Casale et al., 1983; Menasche et al., 1986; Myers et al., 1986b; Ambrosio et al., 1987a,b; Ytrehus et al., 1987) but the relevance of these in vitro preparations to myocardial stunning is uncertain because it is unclear whether the postischemic depression of contractility in these models is fully reversible (i.e., whether it is due to stunning or to cell death) (Bolli, 1990).

Data regarding the role of oxygen radicals in myocardial stunning after a prolonged coronary occlusion associated with subendocardial infarction are conflicting (Table 3). Three studies failed to detect improvement in functional recovery with SOD and catalase after coronary occlusions lasting 1 hour (Asinger et al., 1988), 90 minutes (Nejima et al., 1989), and 2 hours (Przyklenk and Kloner, 1989) in open-chest (Przyklenk and Kloner, 1989) or conscious dogs (Asinger et al., 1988; Nejima et al., 1989). We (Patel et al., 1990) also observed that SOD fails to enhance recovery of contractility after a 2-hour coronary occlusion in anesthetized dogs. These results suggest that short-term administration of antioxidant enzymes is not effective in mitigating myocardial stunning associated with subendocardial infarction. It may be that the postischemic dysfunction that follows a prolonged, partly irreversible ischemic insult (Table 3) differs from the dysfunction that follows a short, completely reversible insult (Table 2). However, other studies (Puett et al., 1987; Forman et al., 1988; Klein et al., 1991) have shown that the cell-per-

Table 3 Effect of Antioxidants on Myocardial Stunning After a Coronary Occlusion >20 min

Antioxidant	Preparation	Duration of ischemia	Protection	Ref.
SOD + CAT	Conscious dog	1 h	No	Asinger et al., 1988
SOD	Closed-chest dog	1 h	No	Vanhaecke et al., 1988
SOD + CAT	Conscious dog	90 min	No	Nejima et al., 1989
SOD + CAT	Open-chest dog	2 h	No	Przyklenk and Kloner, 1989
SOD	Closed-chest dog	2 h	No	Patel et al., 1990
Oxypurinol	Closed-chest dog	90 min	Yes	Puett et al., 1987
N-Acetylcysteine	Closed-chest dog	90 min	Yes	Forman et al., 1988
Trolox	Open-chest pig	45 min	Yes	Klein et al., 1991
α-Tocopherol + ascorbate	Open-chest pig	45 min	No	Klein et al., 1989

SOD, superoxide dismutase; CAT, catalase.
Source: Adapted with permission from *Cardiovasc. Drugs Ther. 5*: 249-268, 1991.

meant antioxidants, oxypurinol, *N*-acetylcysteine, and Trolox, attenuate myocardial stunning independently of infarct size limitation in closed-chest dogs subjected to 90 minutes of coronary occlusion and 24 hours of reflow (Puett et al., 1987; Forman et al., 1988) and in open-chest pigs subjected to 45 minutes of coronary occlusion and 72 hours of reperfusion (Klein et al., in press), although in the latter model pretreatment with α-tocopherol and ascorbate did not seem to enhance functional recovery (Klein et al., 1989) (Table 3). These observations raise the possibility that only small, cell-permeant antioxidants are effective in the setting of subendocardial infarction. Initial observations (Homans et al., 1988) indicate that SOD and catalase do not alleviate exercise-induced stunning.

In summary, there is strong evidence that oxyradicals contribute to postischemic dysfunction after global ischemia in vitro as well as in vivo and after multiple episodes of regional ischemia. They do not appear to contribute to exercise-induced postischemic dysfunction. The role of oxygen radicals in myocardial stunning after a prolonged, partly irreversible ischemic insult remains uncertain and represents a major unresolved problem. Elucidation of this issue will be difficult because the dysfunction is due in part to the presence of infarction and in part to the presence of stunning—a situation that complicates the evaluation of therapy.

V. RELATION BETWEEN SEVERITY OF ISCHEMIA AND INTENSITY OF OXIDATIVE STRESS

Several lines of evidence suggest that the intensity of the oxidative stress responsible for stunning is inversely related to the severity of the antecedent ischemia. First, the magnitude of postischemic loss of contractility is inversely related to the magnitude of the preceding reduction of flow. For example, in conscious dogs undergoing a 15-minute coronary occlusion, there is a sensitive coupling between the degree of myocardial dysfunction after reperfusion and the degree of blood flow reduction during the previous period of ischemia, whereby even small differences in ischemic perfusion are associated with large differences in postischemic recovery (Bolli et al., 1988a). [In open-chest dogs this correlation is weaker (Gross et al., 1986), probably because of the confounding effects of anesthesia and trauma.] Furthermore the severity of stunning is greater in the inner layers of the left ventricular wall, which are the most severely ischemic, than in the outer layers (Bolli et al., 1989a). These observations indicate that, whatever the precise mechanism responsible for stunning may be, the intensity of such mechanism must be modulated by the severity of the antecedent ischemia. Second, direct measurements of free radical production in stunned myocardium have demonstrated a linear, negative relationship between the magnitude of free radical production and the magnitude of collateral perfusion (Fig. 5), indicating that the intensity of free radical generation after reflow is determined by the severity of the previous ischemia (Bolli et al., 1988b): the greater the degree of hypoperfusion, the greater the subsequent production of free radicals. Third, in conscious dogs undergoing a 15-minute coronary occlusion, antioxidant therapy produces the greatest improvement of function in the animals with the lowest collateral flows during coronary occlusion (Fig. 2); as collateral flow increases, the improvement of function decreases (Fig. 2) (Triana et al., 1991). Taken together, these results suggest that the intensity of the oxyradical-mediated damage responsible for stunning is determined primarily by the severity of the antecedent ischemic insult: the more severe the ischemia, the more pronounced the subsequent oxyradical injury and thus the more effective antioxidant therapy. This paradigm has important pathophysiological, methodological, and therapeutical implications.

A. Pathophysiological Implications

It has been proposed (Thompson and Hess, 1986) that the perturbations occurring during ischemia "prime" the myocardium for production of free radicals upon reperfusion. Such perturbations may include the accumulation of reducing equivalents, the disruption of the mitochondrial electron transport chain, the conversion of xanthine dehydrogenase to xanthine oxidase, the activation of the arachidonate cascade, the increased release of catecholamines, and the activation of chemotactic mechanisms for neutrophils. The inverse relationship between collateral flow during coronary occlusion and oxidative stress after reperfusion provides evidence supporting this view. Specifically, it suggests that (1) the mechanisms responsible for the generation of radicals after reperfusion are activated by events taking place during ischemia and (2) the intensity of such activation is determined by the intensity of flow reduction. In a sense, it appears that the amount of oxyradical-mediated injury that will occur after reperfusion is already "predetermined," at least in part, before flow is restored.

B. Methodological Implications

Studies of antioxidants in models of myocardial stunning should probably be restricted to animals with relatively low collateral perfusion, since it is in these animals that both oxyradical-mediated injury and antioxidant-induced protection are maximal. Demonstrating a protective effect of antioxidant therapy in animals with relatively high collateral perfusion would be difficult because the magnitude of the benefit would be relatively small and very large sample sizes would be needed to achieve statistical significance.

C. Therapeutical Implications

Because the severity of oxidative stress is determined to a large extent by the severity of the antecedent ischemia, any intervention that improves perfusion during ischemia would be expected to attenuate stunning after reflow. Reducing the severity of ischemia is probably the most effective way to reduce the severity of postischemic dysfunction. In addition, antioxidant therapy would be expected to be most useful in those patients who are prone to develop the most severe postischemic dysfunction.

It is important to distinguish severity and duration of ischemia. The concepts discussed above suggest that, for a given duration of coronary occlusion (i.e., 15 minutes), the intensity of oxidative stress increases with the severity of flow deprivation. Whether the intensity of oxidative stress also increases with the duration of coronary occlusion is unknown. The available evidence seems to suggest that the importance of free radicals as mediators of stunning actually decreases as the duration of ischemia is extended beyond 15 min (Bolli, 1991): for example, antioxidant treatments that attenuate post-ischemic dysfunction after a 15-minute occlusion fail to do so after a 60-minute or 90-minute occlusion, as discussed above.

VI. EFFECT OF OXYGEN RADICALS ON CARDIAC FUNCTION

The ability of oxygen metabolites to depress myocardial function has been directly demonstrated in vitro and in vivo. Exposure of isolated rabbit interventricular septa (Burton et al., 1984), isolated rat (Blaustein et al., 1986) or rabbit (Schrier and Hess, 1988) papillary muscles, and isolated rat (Schattock et al., 1982; Ytrehus et al., 1986; Miki et al., 1988) or rabbit (Jackson et al., 1986; Goldhaber et al., 1988) hearts to free radical-generating solutions or pure H_2O_2 has uniformly resulted in decreased mechanical function and ATP levels, i.e., in changes similar to those observed in the stunned myocardium. In most of the studies in which an attempt was made to discern the relative roles of different oxygen species (Burton et al., 1984; Blaustein et al., 1986; Jackson et al., 1986; Miki et al., 1988), it was found that the deleterious effects could be prevented by catalase or by ·OH scavengers, but not by SOD, suggesting that H_2O_2 or its byproduct, ·OH, were the oxygen metabolites responsible for the observed depression of contractile function. In one study (Schrier and Hess, 1988), however, SOD was protective, whereas catalase had no effect, implying that the major negative inotropic agent was $\cdot O_2^-$. These in vitro observations have been recently expanded by Przyklenk et al. (1990), who reported that infusion of xanthine oxidase plus purine plus iron-loaded transferrin, administered through a coronary vein in open-chest dogs, resulted in the development of significant wall motion abnormalities.

In summary, it is clear that reactive oxygen species depress myocardial contractility both in vitro and in vivo. The precise role of each species remains to be defined. There is considerable evidence that the detrimental effects of $\cdot O_2^-$ and H_2O_2 on cardiac function are mediated in part by generation of ·OH. This is in accordance with the results of in vivo studies (Myers et al., 1986a; Bolli et al., 1987a,b, 1989c; Farber et al., 1988), which suggest an important role of ·OH as a mediator of stunning. However, there is also evidence for a direct negative inotropic action of $\cdot O_2^-$, which is also congruent with observations in vivo (Jeroudi et al., 1990).

VII. MECHANISM OF OXYRADICAL-MEDIATED CONTRACTILE DYSFUNCTION

The precise mechanism whereby oxygen metabolites depress contractile function remains speculative and represents one of the major unresolved issues pertaining to the pathogenesis of myocardial stunning. Free radicals are reactive species that have no specific target and can attack virtually all cellular components. In theory, every abnormality thus far described in the stunned myocardium could be caused by oxyradicals. At least two key cellular components, proteins and lipids, are likely to be involved in free radical-initiated reactions in the postischemic myocardium. It is well established that activated oxygen species can denaturate proteins and inactivate enzymes, mainly by oxidation of reduced sulfhydryl groups (Davies, 1987). Furthermore, oxygen metabolites can produce peroxidation of the polyunsaturated fatty acids contained in cellular membranes (Thompson and Hess, 1986), which would impair selective membrane permeability and interfere with the function of various cellular organelles.

There is some evidence for the occurrence of lipid peroxidation in settings of myocardial stunning caused by global ischemia in vivo. Romaschin et al. (1987) observed increased myocardial concentration of hydroxy conjugated dienes (products of free fatty acid oxidation) during and after a 45-minute period of global normothermic ischemia in open-chest dogs. The maximal concentration of conjugated dienes was measured at 5 minutes of reflow. Importantly, the tissue examined after reperfusion was dysfunctional but not necrotic, thus representing stunned myocardium. Weisel et al. (1989) subsequently reported that in patients undergoing cardioplegic arrest during coronary artery bypass surgery, there was myocardial release of conjugated dienes in the coronary sinus blood at 3 and 60 minutes of reperfusion, which was associated with a decrease in the myocardial concentration of the antioxidant α-tocopherol. However, it is important to point out that evidence for the occurrence of lipid peroxidation in the 15-minute occlusion model of regionally stunned myocardium is still lacking. One possibility is that in this experimental setting the peroxidative changes may be subtle and thus difficult to detect. A recent study (Lesnefsky et al., 1991) found that 15 minutes of ischemia followed by 30 minutes of reperfusion in dogs did not alter myocardial GSH, GSSG, GSH/GSSG ratio, total SH groups, or protein SH groups, but did significantly reduce the non-GSH, nonprotein SH pool (composed of cysteine, cysteamine, and other low molecular weight SH groups). These results suggest that a 15-minute ischemic period causes a mild oxidative injury, sufficient to produce a selective depletion of the non-GSH, nonprotein SH pool but insufficient to affect GSH or other SH pools (Lesnefsky et al., 1991).

Dysfunction of the sarcoplasmic reticulum may be an important mechanism whereby oxyradicals mediate the contractile abnormalities observed after reversible ischemia. Recent studies have demonstrated that both calcium uptake and Ca^{2+},Mg^{2+}-ATPase activity are significantly depressed in sarcoplasmic reticulum isolated from stunned myocardium (Krause et al., 1989). A similar decrease in calcium uptake and Ca^{2+},Mg^{2+}-ATPase activity is observed in isolated sarcoplasmic reticulum after exposure to oxygen radicals (Rowe et al., 1983; Thompson and Hess, 1986), and oxyradical scavengers (particularly those that remove ·OH or prevent its generation) preserve sarcoplasmic reticulum function (Rowe et al., 1983; Thompson and Hess, 1986).

Other studies suggest that the sarcolemma may be a critical target of free radical-mediated damage. Oxyradicals have been shown to interfere with calcium transport and calcium-stimulated ATPase activity in the sarcolemma (Kaneko et al., 1989a,b). Oxygen radicals have also been shown to interfere with the Na^+-Ca^{2+} exchange (Reeves et al., 1986) and to inhibit the Na^+-K^+-ATPase activity (Kramer et al., 1984). Furthermore, the sarcolemmal Na^+-K^+-ATPase activity is impaired in reperfused myocardium, and this impairment is prevented by antioxidants (Kim and Akera, 1987). Impairment of the Na^+-K^+-ATPase activity would result in Na^+ overload, with consequent activation of the Na^+-Ca^{2+} exchange activity (Grinwald, 1982; Renlund et al., 1984). All of these observations imply that excessive production of oxyradicals could result in increased transarcolemmal calcium influx and cellular calcium overload.

It is important to point out that the foregoing postulated mechanisms involve alterations in calcium homeostasis, and thus would reconcile the oxyradical hypothesis and the calcium overload hypothesis of stunning into one pathogenetic mechanism.

VIII. INTEGRATION OF THE OXYRADICAL HYPOTHESIS AND THE "CALCIUM HYPOTHESES"

Although this chapter has focused on the role of oxygen radicals in stunning, it is important to emphasize that oxidative stress is only one facet of the problem and that other plausible theories have been proposed (for review see Bolli, 1990). In particular, there is considerable evidence suggesting that perturbations of calcium homeostasis contribute importantly to the genesis of myocardial stunning (Bolli, 1990; Kusuoka and Marban, in press). Such perturbations may include a transient calcium overload during the early phase of reperfusion, which could produce a long-lasting damage of the contractile apparatus (Marban et al., 1990), inadequate delivery of calcium to the contractile proteins secondary to sarcoplasmic reticulum dysfunction, which would cause excitation-contraction uncoupling (Krause et al., 1989), and/or decreased sensitivity of myofilaments to calcium, which would result in reduced force generation for any given level of $[Ca]_i$ (Kusuoka et al., 1987). Given the ubiquitous role of calcium as a modulator of myocardial contractile function, it seems probable that one or more of the aforementioned abnormalities does indeed contribute to postischemic dysfunction.

If calcium is involved in stunning, how can one reconcile its role with that of oxygen radicals? Integration of the "oxyradical" and "calcium" hypotheses is complicated by the fact that, for the most part, each of them has been developed in a different experimental preparation (Table 1). Nevertheless, it is important to emphasize that these hypotheses are not mutually exclusive and in fact may represent different parts of the same pathophysiological sequence. There is considerable evidence to suggest a link between generation of oxygen radicals and impaired calcium homeostasis in the setting of reperfusion injury. For example, the damage associated with the "calcium paradox" resembles that associated with the "oxygen paradox" and probably shares a similar pathogenetic mechanism (Hearse et al., 1978). Furthermore, as discussed above, oxyradicals generated upon reperfusion can cause dys-

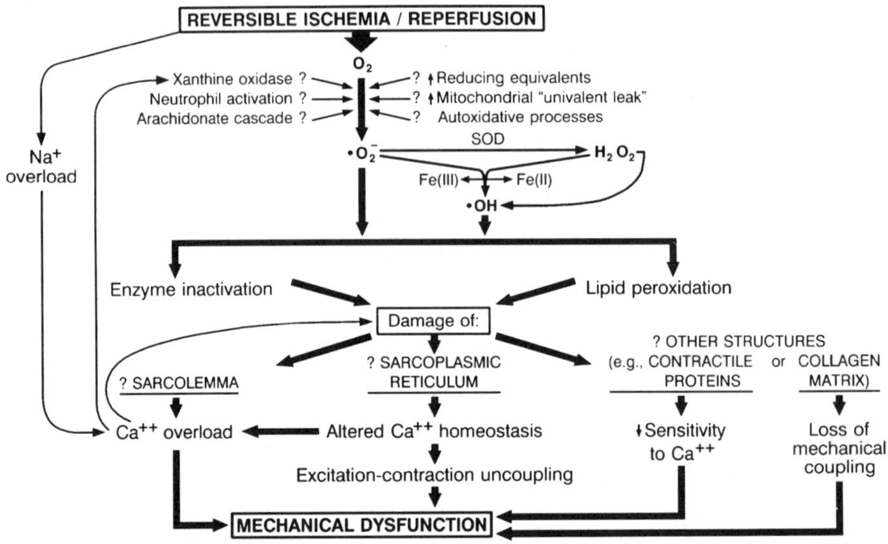

Figure 11 Illustration of the proposed pathogenesis of postischemic myocardial dysfunction. This proposal integrates and reconciles different mechanisms into a unifying pathogenetic hypothesis. Transient reversible ischemia followed by reperfusion could result in increased production of superoxide radicals ($\cdot O_2^-$) through several mechanisms, including (1) increased activity of xanthine oxidase; (2) activation of neutrophils; (3) activation of the arachidonate cascade; (4) accumulation of reducing equivalents during oxygen deprivation; (5) derangements of the intramitochondrial electron transport system resulting in increased univalent reduction of oxygen; and (6) autoxidation of catecholamines and other substances. Superoxide dismutase (SOD) dismutates $\cdot O_2^-$ to hydrogen peroxide (H_2O_2); in the presence of catalytic iron, $\cdot O_2^-$ and H_2O_2 interreact in a Haber-Weiss reaction to generate the hydroxyl radical ($\cdot OH$). H_2O_2 can also generate $\cdot OH$ in the absence of $\cdot O_2^-$ through a Fenton reaction provided that other substances (such as ascorbate) reduce Fe(III) to Fe(II). $\cdot O_2^-$ and $\cdot OH$ attack proteins and polyunsaturated fatty acids, causing enzyme inactivation and lipid peroxidation, respectively.

In the setting of reversible ischemia, the intensity of this damage is not sufficient to cause cell death, but is sufficient to produce dysfunction of key cellular organelles. Postulated targets of free radical damage include: (1) The sarcolemma, with consequent loss of selective permeability, impairment of calcium-stimulated ATPase activity and calcium transport out of the cell, and impairment of the Na^+-K^+-ATPase activity. The net result of these perturbations would be increased transarcolemmal calcium influx and cellular calcium overload. (2) The sarcoplasmic reticulum, with consequent impairment of calcium-stimulated ATPase activity and calcium transport. This would result in impaired calcium homeostasis: specifically, decreased calcium sequestration, which would contribute to increase free cytosolic calcium, and decreased calcium release during systole, which would cause excitation-contraction unfunction of the sarcoplasmic reticulum (Rowe et al., 1983; Thompson and Hess, 1986) and alter calcium flux across the sarcolemma (Kramer et al., 1984; Reeves et al., 1986; Kim and Akera, 1987; Kaneko et al., 1989a,b). The result of these actions would be excitation-contraction uncoupling and cellular calcium overload, respectively (Thompson and Hess, 1986; Kaneko et al., 1989a). The concept that oxidative stress can cause profound disturbances of calcium homeostasis is strongly supported by recent observations. For example, reoxygenation of cultured myocytes results in Ca^{2+} overload, which can be greatly attenuated by antioxidant enzymes (Murphy et al., 1988). Isolated rabbit hearts exposed to 30 minutes of ischemia followed by reperfusion exhibit a rise in intracellular sodium, an increase in the uptake of $^{45}Ca^{2+}$, and a depression of contractile performance, all of which can be reduced by SOD and catalase (Tani, 1990). Exposure of cultured myocytes to a free radical-generating system capable of producing superoxide and hydroxyl radicals results in a marked increase in $[Ca]_i$, which is accompanied by increased levels of conjugated dienes and increased release of [^{3}H] arachidonate, suggesting that the altered ionic homeostasis is associated with peroxidative damage of cellular membranes (Burton et al., 1990a,b). Similarly, a brief (4-minute) perfusion of isolated rabbit hearts with a hydroxyl radical-generating solution causes a rise in $[Ca]_i$ concomitant with a decline in ventricular function (Corretti et al., 1990). In addition to causing calcium overload, oxygen radicals could also damage the proteins of the contractile machinery in a manner that reduces their responsiveness to calcium (Kusuoka and Marban, in press). On the other hand, calcium overload may exaggerate oxyradical production by promoting the conversion of xanthine dehydrogenase to xan-

---

coupling. (3) Possibly other structures, such as the extracellular collagen matrix (with consequent loss of mechanical coupling) or the contractile proteins (with consequent decreased sensitivity to calcium). At the same time, reversible ischemia/reperfusion could cause cellular Na^+ overload due to (1) inhibition of sarcolemmal Na^+-K^+-ATPase, and (2) acidosis and Na^+-H^+ exchange. This could further exaggerate calcium overload via increased Na^+-Ca^{2+} exchange. An increase in free cytosolic calcium would activate phospholipases and other degradative enzymes and further exacerbate the injury to the aforementioned key subcellular structures (sarcolemma, sarcoplasmic reticulum, and contractile proteins). Thus, calcium overload could serve to amplify the damage initiated by oxygen radicals. In addition, calcium overload could in itself impair contractile performance and contribute to mechanical dysfunction. It is also possible that the increase in free cytosolic calcium could increase oxyradical production by promoting the conversion of xanthine dehydrogenase to xanthine oxidase. The ultimate consequence of this complex series of perturbations is a reversible depression of contractility. (Reproduced from Bolli, 1990, with permission of The American Heart Association.)

thine oxidase, which appears to be mediated by a calcium-dependent protease (McCord, 1985).

In view of these considerations, it is my opinion that both oxidative stress and altered calcium homeostasis contribute to myocardial stunning. In this regard, it must be emphasized that neither the oxyradical theory nor the calcium theories (Table 1) explain the entire cascade of events that culminates in postischemic contractile failure: for example, the oxyradical hypothesis does not explain how reactive oxygen species cause mechanical dysfunction, and the calcium theories do not explain why the contractile proteins and/or the sarcoplasmic reticulum are damaged. Clearly, it would be naive to assume that a single abnormality is solely responsible for postischemic dysfunction. Myocardial stunning is probably a *multifactorial* process that involves complex sequences of cellular perturbations and the interaction of multiple pathogenetic mechanisms.

In Figure 11, I propose a unifying hypothesis for the pathogenesis of postischemic dysfunction (detailed description of the postulated mechanisms is provided in the figure legend). This paradigm is largely speculative, but is nevertheless based on the evidence available at this time and discussed in this review. According to this conceptual scheme, oxyradical generation, calcium overload, sarcoplasmic reticulum dysfunction and reduced sensitivity of myofilaments to calcium can be viewed as different aspects of the same pathogenetic mechanism, thereby reconciling the major current hypotheses of myocardial stunning.

In summary, the pathogenesis of myocardial stunning has not been definitively ascertained. Thus far, the attention of experimentalists has focused on the identification of individual mechanisms of injury. Oxyradical generation, calcium overload, excitation-contraction uncoupling, and decreased calcium responsiveness have emerged as likely contributing factors (although in different experimental preparations), and in vitro evidence suggests that they are interrelated. I believe it is now essential to clarify the precise interactions among these factors in vivo and the role that each of them plays in the various experimental settings of myocardial stunning.

IX. CLINICAL IMPLICATIONS OF THE OXYRADICAL HYPOTHESIS

If the results obtained in experimental animals are applicable to humans, prevention of myocardial stunning may soon become a clinical reality. The evidence reviewed in this chapter suggests that postischemic recovery of contractility can be significantly attenuated by the prophylactic administration of antioxidant agents before reflow. Some of these drugs (allopurinol, desferrioxamine, and mercaptopropionyl glycine) are already used clinically for other reasons, whereas other therapies (e.g., human recombinant superoxide dismutase) are being developed rapidly. Indeed, initial clinical trials are being (or will soon be) conducted to examine the effect of antioxidants (in particular, desferrioxamine and human superoxide dismutase) in patients undergoing myocardial reperfusion after open-heart surgery or after myocardial infarction. Compared with inotropic stimulation, antioxidant agents represent a novel approach; by interfering with the mechanisms of cell injury, they can *prevent*, rather than simply temporarily correct, postischemic dysfunction. This approach appears desirable also because it is uncertain whether prolonged inotropic stimulation of stunned myocardium has deleterious effects.

X. SUMMARY

The pathogenesis of myocardial stunning has not been definitively determined. Among the numerous theories proposed, two have emerged as the most plausible: (1) generation of oxygen radicals, and (2) perturbations of calcium homeostasis (i.e., calcium overload, excitation-contraction uncoupling, and/or decreased sensitivity of myofilaments to calcium).

A. Oxyradical Hypothesis

The evidence for a pathogenetic role of oxygen-derived free radicals in myocardial stunning is overwhelming. In the setting of a single 15-minute coronary occlusion, mitigation of stunning by antioxidants has been reproducibly observed by several independent laboratories. Similar protection has been recently demonstrated in the conscious animal, i.e., in the most physiological experimental preparation available. Furthermore, generation of free radicals in the stunned myocardium has been directly demonstrated by spin trapping techniques, and attenuation of free radical generation has been repeatedly shown to result in attenuation of contractile dysfunction. Numerous observations suggest that oxyradicals also contribute to stunning in other settings: after global ischemia in vitro, after global ischemia during cardioplegic arrest in vivo, and after multiple brief episodes of regional ischemia in vivo. Compelling evidence indicates that the critical free radical damage occurs in the initial moments of reflow, so that myocardial stunning can be viewed, in part, as a sublethal form of oxyradical-mediated "reperfusion injury."

B. Calcium Hypothesis

There is also considerable evidence that a transient calcium overload during early reperfusion and/or a persistently reduced sensitivity of contractile proteins to calcium contribute to postischemic dysfunction after global ischemia in vitro; however, the importance of these mechanisms in in vivo models remains to be defined. In addition, inadequate release of calcium by the sarcoplasmic reticulum, with consequent excitation-contraction uncoupling, may occur after multiple brief episodes of regional ischemia, but its role in other forms of postischemic dysfunction has not been explored.

It is probable that multiple mechanisms contribute to the pathogenesis of myocardial stunning. The hypotheses outlined above are not mutually exclusive and in fact may represent different steps of the same pathophysiological cascade. Thus, generation of oxyradicals may cause sarcoplasmic reticulum dysfunction, and both of these processes may lead to calcium overload, which in turn could exacerbate the damage initiated by oxygen species. The concepts discussed in this chapter should provide not only a conceptual framework for further investigation of the pathophysiology of reversible ischemia/reperfusion injury, but also a rationale for developing clinically applicable interventions designed to prevent postischemic ventricular dysfunction.

ACKNOWLEDGMENTS

The thoughtful discussion of Dr. Marcel Zughayb and the excellent secretarial assistance of Valerie R. Price are gratefully acknowledged. The work reported here was supported in part by NIH Grants HL-43151 and by NIH SCOR Grant HL-42267.

REFERENCES

Ambrosio, G., Weisfeldt, M. L., Jacobus, W. E., et al. (1987a). Evidence for a reversible oxygen radical-mediated component of reperfusion injury: Reduction by recombinant human superoxide dismutase administered at the time of reflow. *Circulation 75*: 282.

Ambrosio, G., Zweier, J. L., Jacobus, W. E., Weisfeldt, M. L., and Flaherty, J. T. (1987b). Improvement of postischemic myocardial function and metabolism induced by administration of desferrioxamine at the time of reflow: The role of iron in the pathogenesis of reperfusion injury. *Circulation 76*: 906.

Asinger, R. W., Peterson, D. A., Elsperger, K. J., and Homans, D. (1988). Long-term recovery of LV wall thickening after 1 hour of ischemia is not affected when superoxide dismutase and catalase are administered during the first 45 minutes of reperfusion. *J. Am. Coll. Cardiol. 2*: 163A (Abstract).

Blaustein, A. S., Schine, L., Brooks, W. W., Fanburg, B. L., and Bing, O. H. L. (1986). Influence of exogenously generated oxidant species on myocardial function. *Am. J. Physiol. 250*: H595.

Bolli, R., Zhu, W. X., Hartley, C. J., Michael, L. H., Repine, J., Hess, M. L., Kukreja, R. C., and Roberts, R. (1987a). Attenuation of dysfunction in the postischemic "stunned" myocardium by dimethylthiourea. *Circulation 76*: 458.

Bolli, R., Patel, B. S., Zhu, W. X., O'Neill, P. G., Charlat, M. L., and Roberts, R. (1987b). The iron chelator desferrioxamine attenuates postischemic ventricular dysfunction. *Am. J. Physiol. 253*: H1372.

Bolli, R., Zhu, W. X., Thornby, J. I., O'Neill, P. G., and Roberts, R. (1988a). Time-course and determinants of recovery of function after reversible ischemia in conscious dogs. *Am. J. Physiol. 254*: H102.

Bolli, R., Patel, B. S., Jeroudi, M. O., Lai, E. K., and McCay, P. B. (1988b). Demonstration of free radical generation in "stunned" myocardium of intact dogs with the use of the spin trap α-phenyl *N-tert*-butyl nitrone. *J. Clin. Invest 82*: 476.

Bolli, R., Patel, B. S., Hartley, C. J., Thornby, J. I., Jeroudi, M. O., and Roberts, R. (1989a). Nonuniform transmural recovery of contractile function in the "stunned" myocardium. *Am. J. Physiol. 257*: H375.

Bolli, R., Jeroudi, M. O., Patel, B. S., DuBose, C. M., Lai, E. K., Roberts, R., and McCay, P. B. (1989b). Direct evidence that oxygen-derived free radicals contribute to postischemic myocardial dysfunction in the intact dog. *Proc. Natl. Acad. Sci. U.S.A. 86*: 4695.

Bolli, R., Jeroudi, M. O., Patel, B. S., Aruoma, O. I., Halliwell, B., Lai, E. K., and McCay, P. B. (1989c). Marked reduction of free radical generation and contractile dysfunction by antioxidant therapy began at the time of reperfusion: evidence that myocardial "stunning" is a manifestation of reperfusion injury. *Circ. Res. 65*: 607.

Bolli, R. (1990). Mechanism of myocardial "stunning." *Circulation 82:* 723.

Bolli, R., and McCay, P. B. (1990a). Use of spin traps in intact animals undergoing myocardial ischemia/reperfusion: A new approach to assessing the role of oxygen radicals in myocardial "stunning." *Free Rad. Res. Comms. 9*: 169.

Bolli, R., Patel, B. S., Jeroudi, M. O., Li, X. Y., Triana, J. F., Lai, E. K., and McCay, P. B. (1990). Iron-mediated radical reactions upon reperfusion contribute to myocardial "stunning." *Am. J. Physiol. 259*: H1901.

Bolli, R., Kaur, H., Li, X. Y., Triana, J. F., and Halliwell, B. (1991). Demonstration of hydroxyl radical generation in "stunned" myocardium of intact dogs using aromatic hydroxylation of phenylalanine. *FASEB J. 5*: A704.

Bolli, R. (1991). Superoxide dismutase 10 years later: A drug in search of a use. *J. Am. Coll. Cardiol. 18*: 231.

Buchwald, A., Klein, H. H., Lindert, S., Pich, S., Nebendahl, K., Wiegand, V., and Kreuzer, H. (1989a). Effect of intracoronary superoxide dismutase on regional function in stunned myocardium. *J. Cardiovasc. Pharmacol. 13*: 258.

Buchwald, A., Klein, H. H., Lindert, S., Pich, S., Oberschmidt, R., Nebendahl, K., and Kreuzer, H. (1989b). Effect of α-tocopherol (vitamin E) in a porcine model of stunned myocardium. *J. Cardiovasc. Pharmacol. 14*: 46.

Burton, K. P., McCord, J. M., and Ghai, G. (1984). Myocardial alterations due to free-radical generation. *Am. J. Physiol. 246*: H776.

Burton, K. P., Morris, A. C., Massey, K. D., Buja, L. M., and Hagler, H. K. (1990a). Free radicals alter ionic calcium levels and membrane phospholipids in cultured rat ventricular myocytes. *J. Mol. Cell. Cardiol. 22*: 1035.

Burton, K. P., Nazeran, H., and Hagler, H. K. (1990b). Free radicals alter ionic calcium transients observed in isolated adult rat cardiac myocytes. *Circulation 82* (Suppl. III): 452 (Abstract).

Casale, A. S., Bulkley, G. B., Bulkley, B. H., Flaherty, J. T., Gott, V. L., and Gardner, T. J. (1983). Oxygen free radical scavengers protect the arrested globally ischemic heart upon reperfusion. *Surg. Forum. 34*: 313.

Charlat, M. L., O'Neill, P. G., Egan, J. M., Abernethy, D. R., Michael, L. H., Myers, M. L., Roberts, R., and Bolli, R. (1987). Evidence for a pathogenetic role of xanthine oxidase in the "stunned" myocardium. *Am. J. Physiol. 252*: H566.

Corretti, M. C., Koretsune, Y., Chacko, V. P., Zweier, J. L., and Marban, E. (1990). Intracellular calcium overload and glycolytic inhibition as consequences of exogenously-generated free radicals in rabbit hearts. *Circulation 82*(Suppl III): 700 (Abstract).

Dage, R. C., Anderson, B. A., Mao, S. J. T., and Koerner, J. E. (1991). Probucol reduces myocardial dysfunction during reperfusion after short-term ischemia in rabbit heart. *J. Cardiovasc. Pharmacol. 17*: 158.

Davies, K. J. A. (1987). Protein damage and degradation by oxygen radicals. I. General aspects. *J. Biol. Chem. 262*: 9895.

Davies, M. J. (1989). Direct detection of radical production in the ischaemic and reperfused myocardium: current status. *Free Rad. Res. Comms. 7*: 275.

DiGuiseppi, J., and Fridovich, I. (1982). Oxygen toxicity in *Streptococcus sanguis*: The relative importance of superoxide and hydroxyl radicals. *J. Biol. Chem. 257*: 4046.

Eddy, L. J., Stewart, J. R., Jones, H. P., Engerson, T. D., McCord, J. M., and Downey, J. M. (1987). Free radical-producing enzyme, xanthine oxidase, is undetectable in human hearts. *Am. J. Physiol. 253*: H709.

Engler, R. L., Dahlgren, M. D., Morris, D. D., Peterson, M. A., and Schmid-Schonbein, G. W. (1986). Role of leukocytes in response to acute myocardial ischemia and reflow in dogs. *Am. J. Physiol. 251*: H314.

Engler, R. (1987). Granulocytes and oxidative injury in myocardial ischemia and reperfusion. *Fed. Proc. 46*: 2395.

Engler, R., and Covell, J. W. (1987). Granulocytes cause reperfusion ventricular dysfunction after 15-minute ischemia in the dog. *Circ. Res. 61*: 20.

Farber, N. E., Vercellotti, G. M., Jacob, H. S., Pieper, G. M., and Gross, G. J. (1988). Evidence for a role of iron-catalyzed oxidants in functional and metabolic stunning in the canine heart. *Circ. Res. 63*: 351.

Farber, N. E., and Gross, G. J. (1990). Prostaglandin redirection by thromboxane synthetase inhibition: attenuation of myocardial stunning in canine heart. *Circulation 81*: 369.

Ferrari, R., Alfieri, O., Curello, S., Ceconi, A., Cargnoni, A., Marzollo, P., Pardini, A., Caradonna, E., and Visioli, O. (1990). Occurrence of oxidative stress during reperfusion of the human heart. *Circulation 81*: 201.

Forman, M. B., Puett, D. W., Cates, C. U., McCroskey, D. E., Beckman, J. K., Greene, H. L., and Virmani, R. (1988). Glutathione redox pathway and reperfusion injury. Effect of *N*-acetylcysteine on infarct size and ventricular function. *Circulation 78*: 202.

Gardner, T. J. Oxygen radicals in cardiac surgery. *Free Radical Biol. Med. 4*: 45.

Go, L. O., Murry, C. E., Richard, V. J., Jennings, R. B., Weischedel, G. R., and Reimer, K. A. (1988). Myocardial neutrophil accumulation during reperfusion after reversible or irreversible ischemic injury. *Am. J. Physiol. 255*: H1188.

Goldhaber, J. I., Ji, S., Lamp, S. T., and Weiss, J. N. (1988). Effects of exogenous free radicals on electromechanical function and metabolism in isolated rabbit and guinea pig ventricle: Implications for ischemia and reperfusion injury. *J. Clin. Invest. 83*: 1800.

Grinwald, P. M. (1982). Calcium uptake during postischemic reperfusion in the isolated rat heart: Influence of extracellular sodium. *J. Mol. Cell. Cardiol. 14*: 359.

Gross, G. J., Farber, N. E., Hardman, H. F., and Warltier, D. C. (1986). Beneficial actions of superoxide dismutase and catalase in stunned myocardium of dogs. *Am. J. Physiol. 250*: H372.

Grum, C. M., Gallagher, K. P., Kirsh, M. M., and Shlafer, M. (1989). Absence of detectable xanthine oxidase in human myocardium. *J. Mol. Cell. Cardiol. 21*: 263.

Halliwell, B., and Gutteridge, J. M. C. (1984). Oxygen toxicity, oxygen radicals, transition metals and disease. *Biochem. J. 219*: 1.

Hearse, D. J., Humphrey, S. M., and Bullock, G. R. (1978). The oxygen paradox and the calcium paradox: two facets of the same problem? *J. Mol. Cell. Cardiol. 10*: 641.

Hearse, D. J. (1991). Stunning: A radical re-view. *Cardiovasc. Drugs. Ther. 5*: 853.

Holzgrefe, H. H., and Gibson, J. K. (1988). Enhanced function recovery in the stunned canine myocardium by pretreatment with oxypurinol. *J. Am. Coll. Cardiol. 11*: 208A (Abstract).

Homans, D. C., Sublett, E., Asinger, R., Peterson, D., and Bache, R. J. SOD + catalase does not attenuate regional left ventricular dysfunction following exercise induced ischemia. *J. Am. Coll. Cardiol. 78*: II-76 (Abstract).

Huizer, T., de Jong, J. W., Nelson, J. A., Czarnecki, W., Serruys, P. W., Bonnier, J. J. R. M., and Troquay, R. (1989). Urate production by human heart. *J. Mol. Cell. Cardiol. 21*: 691.

Illes, R. W., Silverman, N. A., Krukenkamp, I. B., del Nido, P. J., and Levitsky, S. (1989). Amelioration of postischemic stunning by deferoxamine-blood cardioplegia. *Circulation 80*(Suppl. III): III-30.

Jackson, C. V., Mickelson, J. K., Pope, T. K., Rao, P. S., and Lucchesi, B. R. (1986). O_2 free radical-mediated myocardial and vascular dysfunction. *Am. J. Physiol. 251*: H1225.

Jarasch, E. D., Bruder, G., and Heid, H. W. (1986). Significance of xanthine oxidase in capillary endothelial cells. *Acta Physiol. Scand. 548*(Suppl.): 39.

Jeremy, R. W., and Becker, L. C. (1989). Neutrophil depletion does not prevent myocardial dysfunction after brief coronary occlusion. *J. Am. Coll. Cardiol. 13*: 1155.

Jeroudi, M. O., Triana, F. J., Patel, B. S., and Bolli, R. (1990). Effect of superoxide dismutase and catalase, given separately, on myocardial "stunning." *Am. J. Physiol. 259*: H889.

Johnson, D. L., Horneffer, P. J., Dinatale, J. M. Jr., Gott, V. L., and Gardner, T. J. (1987). Free radical scavengers improve functional recovery of stunned myocardium in a model of surgical coronary revascularization. *Surgery 102*: 334.

Kaneko, M., Beamish, R. E., and Dhalla, N. S. (1989a). Depression of heart sarcolemmal Ca^{2+}-pump activity by oxygen free radicals. *Am. J. Physiol. 256*: H368.

Kaneko, M., Elimban, V., and Dhalla, N. S. (1989b). Mechanism for depression of heart sarcolemmal Ca^{2+} pump by oxygen free radicals. *Am. J. Physiol. 257*: H804.

Kerber, R. E., Shasby, D. M., Seabold, J., Kieso, R., Fox-Eastham, K. (1989). Does reduction of leukocyte accumulation in reperfused myocardium affect stunning? *Circulation 80*(Suppl. II): II-401 (Abstract).

Kim, M.-S., and Akera, T. (1987). O_2 free radicals: Cause of ischemia-reperfusion injury to cardiac Na^+-K^+-ATPase. *Am. J. Physiol. 252*: H252.

Klein, H. H., Pich, S., Lindert, S., Nebendahl, K., Niedmann, P., and Kreuzer, H. (1989). Combined treatment with vitamins E and C in experimental myocardial infarction in pigs. *Am. Heart J. 118*: 667.

Klein, H. H., Pich, S., Schuff-Werner, P., Niedmann, P., Blattmann, U., and Nebendahl, K. (1991). The effects of Trolox, a water-soluble vitamin E analogue, in regionally ischemic, reperfused porcine hearts. *Int. J. Cardiol. 32*: 291.

Koerner, J. E., Anderson, B. A., and Dage, R. C. (1991). Protection against postischemic myocardial dysfunction in anesthetized rabbits with scavengers of oxygen-derived free radicals: Superoxide dismutase plus catalase, *N*-2-mercaptopropionyl glycine and captopril. *J. Cardiovasc. Pharmacol. 17*: 185.

Kramer, J. H., Mark, I. T., and Weglicki, W. B. (1984). Differential sensitivity of canine cardiac sarcolemmal and microsomal enzymes to inhibition by free radical induced lipid peroxidation. *Circ. Res. 55*: 120.

Krause, S. M., Jacobus, W. E., and Becker, L. C. (1989). Alterations in cardiac sarcoplasmic reticulum calcium transport in the postischemic "stunned" myocardium. *Circ. Res. 65*: 526.

Kusuoka, H., Porterfield, J. K., Weisman, H. F., Weisfeldt, M. L., and Marban, E. (1987). Pathophysiology and pathogenesis of stunned myocardium. Depressed Ca^{2+} activation of contraction as a consequence of reperfusion-induced cellular calcium overload in ferret hearts. *J. Clin. Invest. 79*: 950.

Kusuoka, H., and Marban, E. (1992). Cellular mechanisms of myocardial stunning. *Annul. Rev. Physiol. 54*: 243.

Leiboff, R. L., Arroyo, C. M., Schaer, G. L., Mergner, G. W., Kramer, J. H., Miller, D. L., Visner, M. S., and Weglicki, W. B. (1988). Free radical generation in an in vivo model of regional myocardial stunning. *FASEB J. 2*: A818 (Abstract).

Lesnefsky, E. J., Dauber, I. M., and Horwitz, L. D. (1991). Myocardial sulfhydryl pool alterations occur during reperfusion after brief and prolonged myocardial ischemia in vivo. *Circ. Res. 68*: 605.

Lucchesi, B. R., and Mullane, K. M. (1986). Leukocytes and ischemia-induced myocardial injury. *Ann. Rev. Pharmacol. Toxicol. 26*: 201.

Marban, E., Kitakaze, M., Koretsune, Y., Yue, D. T., Chacko, V. P., and Pike, M. M. (1990). Quantification of $[Ca^{2+}]i$ in perfused hearts: Critical evaluation of the 5F-BAPTA and nuclear magnetic resonance method as applied to the study of ischemia and reperfusion. *Circ. Res. 66*: 1255.

McCord, J. M. (1985). Oxygen-derived free radicals in postischemic tissue injury. *N. Engl. J. Med. 312*: 159.

Menasche, P., Grousset, C., Gauduel, Y., and Piwnica, A. (1986). A comparative study of free radical scavengers in cardioplegic solutions. Improved protection with peroxidase. *J. Thorac. Cardiovasc. Surg. 92*: 264.

Miki, S., Ashraf, M., Salka, S., and Sperelakis, N. (1988). Myocardial dysfunction and ultrastructural alterations mediated by oxygen metabolites. *J. Mol. Cell. Cardiol. 20*: 1009.

Murphy, J. G., Smith, T. W., and Marsh, J. D. (1988). Mechanisms of reoxygenation-induced calcium overload in cultured chick embryo heart cells. *Am. J. Physiol. 254*: H1133.

Murry, C. E., Richard, V. J., Jennings, R. B., and Reimer, K. A. (1989). Free radicals do not cause myocardial stunning after four 5 minute coronary occlusions. *Circulation 80*(Suppl. II): II-296 (Abstract).

Muxfeldt, M., and Schaper, W. (1987). The activity of xanthine oxidase in hearts of pigs, guinea pigs, rats, and humans. *Basic Res. Cardiol. 82*: 486.

Myers, M. L., Bolli, R., Lekich, R. F., Hartley, C. J., and Roberts, R. (1985). Enhancement of recovery of myocardial function by oxygen free-radical scavengers after reversible regional ischemia. *Circulation 72*: 915.

Myers, M. L., Bolli, R., Lekich, R. F., Hartley, C. J., Michael, L. H., and Roberts, R. (1986a). *N*-2-Mercaptopropionylglycine improves recovery of myocardial function following reversible regional ischemia. *J. Am. Coll. Cardiol. 8*: 1161.

Myers, C. L., Weiss, S. J., Kirsh, M. M., Shepard, B. M., and Shlafer, M. (1986b). Effects of supplementing hypothermic crystalloid cardioplegic solution with catalase, superoxide dismutase, allopurinol, or deferoxamine on functional recovery of globally ischemic and reperfused isolated hearts. *J. Thorac. Cardiovasc. Surg. 91*: 281.

Nejima, J., Knight, D. R., Fallon, J. T., Uemura, N., Manders, W. T., Canfield, D. R., Cohen, M. V., and Vatner, S. F. (1989). Superoxide dismutase reduces reperfusion arrhythmias but fails to salvage regional myocardial function or myocardium at risk in conscious dogs. *Circulation 79*: 143.

O'Neill, P. G., Charlat, M. L., Kim, H.-S., Pocius, J., Michael, L. H., Hartley, C. J., Roberts, R., and Bolli, R. (1987). Lipoxygenase inhibitor nafazatrom fails to attenuate postischemic ventricular dysfunction. *Cardiovasc. Res. 21*: 755.

O'Neill, P. G., Charlat, M. L., Michael, L. H., Roberts, R., and Bolli, R. (1989). Influence of neutrophil depletion on myocardial function and flow after reversible ischemia. *Am. J. Physiol. 256*: H341.

Patel, B. S., Jeroudi, M. O., O'Neill, P. G., Roberts, R., and Bolli, R. (1990). Effect of human recombinant superoxide dismutase on canine myocardial infarction. *Am. J. Physiol. 258*: H369.

Przyklenk, K., and Kloner, R. A. (1986). Superoxide dismutase plus catalase improve contractile function in the canine model of the "stunned" myocardium. *Circ. Res. 58*: 148.

Przyklenk, K. and Kloner, R. A. (1989). "Reperfusion injury" by oxygen-derived free radicals? Effect of superoxide dismutase plus catalase, given at the time of reperfusion, on myocardial infarct size, contractile function, coronary microvasculature, and regional myocardial blood flow. *Circ. Res. 64*: 86.

Przyklenk, K., Whittaker, P., and Kloner, R. A. (1990). In vivo infusion of oxygen free radical substrates causes myocardial systolic, but not diastolic dysfunction. *Am. Heart J. 119*: 807.

Puett, D. W., Forman, M. B., Cates, C. U., Wilson, B. H., Hande, K. R., Friesinger, G. C., and Virmani, R. (1987). Oxypurinol limits myocardial stunning but does not reduce infarct size after reperfusion. *Circulation 76*: 678.

Reeves, J. P., Bailey, C. A., and Hale, C. C. (1986). Redox modification of sodium-calcium exchange activity in cardiac sarcolemmal vesicles. *J. Biol. Chem. 261*: 4948.

Renlund, D. G., Gerstenblith, G., Lakatta, E. G., Jacobus, W. E., Kallman, C. H., and Weisfeldt, M. L. (1984). Perfusate sodium during ischemia modifies postischemic functional and metabolic recovery in the rabbit heart. *J. Mol. Cell. Cardiol. 16*: 795.

Romaschin, A. D., Rebeyka, I., Wilson, G. J., and Mickle, D. A. G. (1987). Conjugated dienes in ischemic and reperfused myocardium: An in vivo chemical signature of oxygen free radical mediated injury. *J. Mol. Cell. Cardiol. 19*: 289.

Rowe, G. T., Manson, N. H., Caplan, M., and Hess, M. L. (1983). Hydrogen peroxide and hydroxyl radical mediation of activated leukocyte depression of cardiac sarcoplasmic reticulum: participation of the cyclooxygenase pathway. *Circ. Res. 53*: 584.

Schott, R. J., Nao, B. S., McClanahan, T. B., Simpson, P. J., Stirling, M. C., Todd, R. F., III, and Gallagher, K. P. (1989). $F(ab')_2$ Fragments of anti-mo1 (904) monoclonal antibodies do not prevent myocardial stunning. *Circ. Res. 65*: 1112.

Schrier, G. M., and Hess, M. L. (1988). Quantitative identification of superoxide anion as a negative inotropic species. *Am. J. Physiol. 24*: H138.

Shattock, M. J., Manning, A. S., and Hearse, D. J. (1982). Effects of hydrogen peroxide on cardiac function and postischemic functional recovery in the isolated "working" rat heart. *Pharmacol. 24*: 118.

Shea, M. J., Simpson, P. J., Werns, S. W., Buda, A. J., Alborzy-Khaghany, A. S., Hoff, P. T., and Lucchesi, B. R. (1987). Effect of neutrophil depletion on recovery of "stunned" myocardium. *Clin. Res. 35*: 327A (Abstract).

Shlafer, M., Kane, P. F., and Kirsh, M. M. (1982a). Superoxide dismutase plus catalase enhances the efficacy of hypothermic cardioplegia to protect the globally ischemic, reperfused heart. *J. Thorac. Cardiovasc. Surg. 83*: 830.

Shlafer, M., Kane, P. F., Wiggins, V. Y., and Kirsh, M. M. (1982b). Possible role for cytotoxic oxygen metabolites in the pathogenesis of cardiac ischemic injury. *Circulation 66*(Suppl I): I-85.

Stewart, J. R., Blackwell, W. H., Crute, S. L., Loughlin, V., Greenfield, L. J., and Hess, M. L. (1983). Inhibition of surgically induced ischemia/reperfusion injury by oxygen free radical scavengers. *J. Thorac. Cardiovasc. Surg. 86*: 262.

Tani, M. (1990). Effects of anti-free radical agents on Na^+, Ca^{2+}, and function in reperfused rat hearts. *Am. J. Physiol. 259* (*Heart Circ. Physiol. 28*): H137.

Thompson, J. A., and Hess, M. L. (1986). The oxygen free radical system: A fundamental mechanism in the production of myocardial necrosis. *Prog. Cardiovasc. Dis. 28*: 449.

Triana, J. F., Jamaluddin, U., Li, X. Y., and Bolli, R. (1990). Oxygen free radicals cause myocardial stunning after repetitive ischemia. *Circulation 82*: III-36 (Abstract).

Triana, J. F., Li, X. Y., Jamaluddin, U., Thornby, J. I., and Bolli, R. (1991). Postischemic myocardial "stunning": Identification of major differences between the open-chest and the conscious dog and evaluation of the oxy-radical hypothesis in the latter model. *Circ. Res. 69*: 731.

Weisel, R. D., Mickle, D. A. G., Finkle, C. D., Tumiati, L. C., Madonik, M. M., Ivanov, J., Burton, G. W., and Ingold, K. U. (1989). Myocardial free-radical injury after cardioplegia. *Circulation 80*(Suppl III): III-14.

Werns, S., Ventura, A., Li, G. C., and Lucchesi, B. R. (1989). Amflutizole, a xanthine oxidase inhibitor, does not attenuate myocardial stunning in the canine heart. *Circulation 80*(Suppl. II): II-295 (Abstract).

Westlin, W., and Mullane, K. M. (1988). Does captopril attenuate reperfusion-induced myocardial dysfunction by scavenging free radicals? *Circulation 77*(Suppl. I): I-30.

Westlin, W., and Mullane, K. M. (1989). Alleviation of myocardial stunning by leukocyte and platelet depletion. *Circulation 80*: 1828.

Ytrehus, K., Myklebust, R., and Mjos, O. D. (1986). Influence of oxygen radicals generated by xanthine oxidase in the isolated perfused rat heart. *Cardiovasc. Res. 20*: 597.

Ytrehus, K., Gunnes, S., Myklebust, R., and Mjos, O. D. (1987). Protection by superoxide dismutase and catalase in the isolated rat heart reperfused after prolonged cardioplegia: A combined study of metabolic, functional and morphometric ultrastructural variables. *Cardiovasc. Res. 21*: 492.

Zhu, W. X., Myers, M. L., Hartley, C. J., Roberts, R., and Bolli, R. (1986). Validation of a single crystal for measurement of transmural and epicardial thickening. *Am. J. Physiol. 251*: H1045.

Zughayb, M., Sekili, S., Li, X. Y., Triana, J. F., McCay, P. B., and Bolli, R. (1991). Detection of free radical generation in the "stunned" myocardium in the conscious dog using spin trapping techniques. *FASEB J. 5*: A704.

9

Role of Altered Calcium Homeostasis in Stunned Myocardium

Hideo Kusuoka* and Eduardo Marban

Johns Hopkins University School of Medicine, Baltimore, Maryland

I. INTRODUCTION

"Stunning" describes the impairment of contraction observed in myocardium that has been reperfused after brief periods of ischemia (Braunwald and Kloner, 1982). The paradox of long-lasting dysfunction in completely viable tissue has captured the imagination of clinicians while presenting an interesting challenge to experimental physiologists. Although the investigation of excitation-contraction coupling in isolated cells is highly refined (Wier, 1990), many of the experimental tools used in single cells cannot be brought to bear directly on the problem because stunning, by definition, is an after-effect of ischemia. Unlike metabolic inhibition or hypoxia, ischemia is a vascular phenomenon; therefore, the only unequivocal models are those in which the heart can be made ischemic and reperfused via its native coronary circulation.

The simplest model in which stunning has been investigated is the isolated, crystalloid-perfused heart, in which global contractile parameters can be measured straightforwardly, and several new techniques can be applied to measure intracellular free Ca^{2+} concentration ($[Ca^{2+}]_i$) and other metabolites. Figure 1 shows how stunning is manifested in the isolated ferret heart. The

*Current affiliation: Osaka University, Osaka, Japan

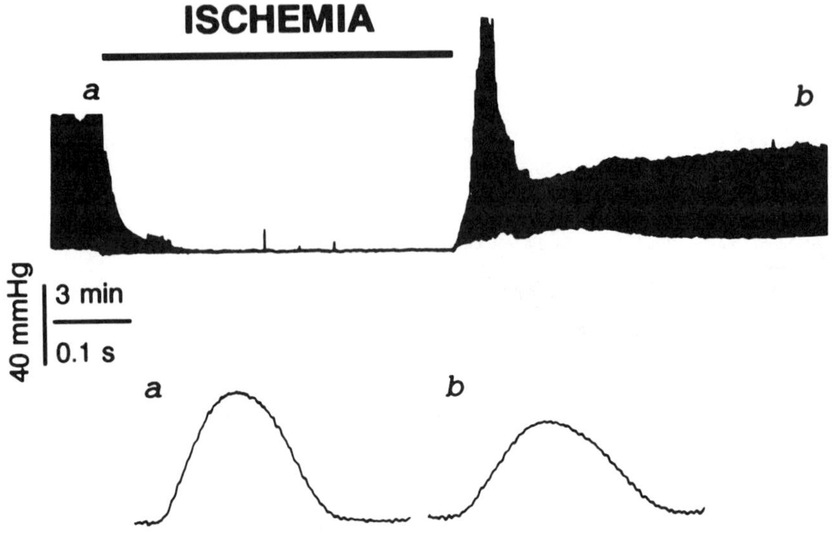

Figure 1 Myocardial stunning in an isolated perfused ferret heart. (Top) Continuous record of isovolumic left ventricular pressure during control, 15-minute global ischemia (37°C), and reperfusion. (Bottom) Rapid time-base records from the points *a* and *b* indicated in the top panel. (Reproduced from Kusuoka and Marban, 1992, by permission of the authors.)

upper panel is a continuous record of isovolumic left ventricular pressure before, during, and after 15 minutes of total global ischemia. Pressure development drops quickly when coronary flow is interrupted (Koretsune et al., 1991). Reperfusion elicits a period of arrhythmia punctuated by some very strong (potentiated) beats, after which contractile pressure settles in to a steady value distinctly lower than the control. The two twitches in the lower panel were sampled before (a) and after (b) ischemia. By extrapolation from intact animal models, the postischemic depression of pressure generation apparent in (b) would be expected to persist for several days before finally resolving completely (Braunwald and Kloner, 1982). Nevertheless, routine histological and metabolic analysis of stunned heart muscle has yielded remarkably benign findings and, as a result, few clues as to the origins of the dysfunction (Braunwald and Kloner, 1985).

Here we review the potential mechanisms of myocardial stunning, with a special emphasis on concepts of how calcium might contribute to this reversible form of cellular injury. A condensed version of this review appeared recently (Kusuoka and Marban, 1992).

II. EXCITATION-CONTRACTION COUPLING IN STUNNED MYOCARDIUM

We first turn our attention to the question of how excitation-contraction coupling might be impaired in stunned myocardium. The contractility lesion in stunned myocardium might affect one of three major links in force generation, as illustrated in Figure 2 (Kusuoka et al., 1987; Marban, 1991). The first of these is the change in intracellular free Ca^{2+} concentration, $[Ca^{2+}]_i$, during each cardiac cycle (the calcium transient), depicted schematically on the left. The second major link is the responsiveness of the contractile machinery to Ca^{2+}. Myofilament Ca^{2+} responsiveness itself consists of two parameters: the myofilament sensitivity to Ca^{2+}, which describes the range of $[Ca^{2+}]_i$ that activates contraction, and maximal Ca^{2+}-activated force, which determines the magnitude of the contractile response. Both of these are subsumed within the apparent Ca^{2+}-tension relation diagrammed above the arrow linking $[Ca^{2+}]_i$ and force. A disturbance in any of these three basic steps could account for the contractile dysfunction of stunned myocadium.

A. Excitability and Transsarcolemmal Ion Transport

The most obvious way that activator Ca^{2+} availability might be restricted would be if excitability were decreased. Despite an isolated report to the contrary (Levine et al., 1987), neither action potentials nor cell-cell coupling appear to be compromised in stunned myocardium (Hanich et al., 1989; Coetzee et al., 1990). The available data are scanty but appear to exclude the gross

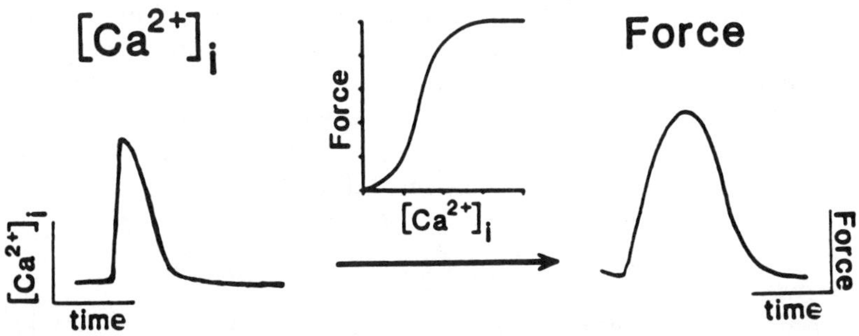

Figure 2 Schematic representation of the components in force generation. This shows a schematic $[Ca^{2+}]$ transient on the left, and a twitch contraction on the right. The $[Ca^{2+}]$ transient and force are linked by an arrow, which represents the $[Ca^{2+}]_i$-force relation. (Adapted from Marban, 1991. Reproduced by permission of the American Heart Association.)

abnormalities in membrane currents or gap junctions that would be required to produce persistent dysfunction.

Few studies have focused on the properties of specific sarcolemmal ion transport pathways in stunned myocardium. Chemnitius et al. (1985) found no change in Na^+,K^+-ATPase activity after repeated cycles of ischemia and reperfusion. The sarcolemmal Ca^{2+}-ATPase activity was reduced in rate and in maximal capacity, which, if anything, would tend to increase rather than decrease activator Ca^{2+} availability. An increase in Ca^{2+} uptake has been detected in reperfused (Tani and Neely, 1989) or reoxygenated (Weiss et al., 1990) rat hearts and attributed to Na^+/Ca^{2+} exchange. Since it is thought to be secondary to changes in $[Na^+]_i$ (Grinwald 1982; Pike et al., 1990), the increase in Ca^{2+} uptake can easily be explained without postulating any inherent modification of the Na^+/Ca^{2+} exchanger.

B. Calcium Release and Calcium Uptake by Sarcoplasmic Reticulum

A fundamentally different way of altering cytoplasmic Ca^{2+} availability would involve changes in calcium transport across the membrane of the sarcoplasmic reticulum (SR). Krause et al. (1989) measured Ca^{2+} uptake and ATPase activity in SR vesicles from regionally stunned canine myocardium. The maximal oxalate-supported Ca^{2+} transport rate was reduced by 17%, paralleled by a similar decrease in maximal Ca^{2+}, Mg^{2+}-ATPase activity. The reduction in SR Ca^{2+} uptake was even greater when the free Mg^{2+} concentration ($[mg^{2+}]_i$) was increased from 0.6 to 1.5 μM (Krause and Rozanski, 1990) to simulate the recently detected elevation of $[Mg^{2+}]_i$ in reperfused myocardium (Borchgrevink et al., 1989; Murphy et al., 1989). Limbruno et al. (1989) have found similar changes in Ca^{2+} uptake by the SR; in addition, their data indirectly support the notion that there is a superimposed decrease in Ca^{2+} release from SR in reperfused myocardium. Krause et al. (1989) reached the opposite conclusion regarding Ca^{2+} release, arguing (also indirectly) that the SR actually becomes somewhat leaky to Ca^{2+} after reperfusion. Regarding Ca^{2+} release from SR, the origin of the discrepant interpretations from the two groups is unclear, but the observations regarding SR Ca^{2+} uptake are mutually consistent.

The physiological implications of the decrease in maximal Ca^{2+} uptake rate and in Ca^{2+},Mg^{2+}-ATPase activity are difficult to predict. Acutely, less Ca^{2+} sequestration would lead to an increase in cytoplasmic Ca^{2+} (if less gets taken up by SR, more remains in the cytosol); in the longer term, reduced Ca^{2+} sequestration by the SR means that less Ca^{2+} will be available to be released from the SR during each beat, so that Ca^{2+} transients might be reduced. On the other hand, if the increase in $[Ca^{2+}]_i$ just offsets the decline of Ca^{2+}-

sensitivity of Ca^{2+} uptake by SR, depletion of SR calcium may not occur and Ca^{2+} release from SR would be maintained. The only parameter of excitation-contraction coupling that directly reflects the rate of Ca^{2+} uptake by the SR is the rate of decline of the Ca^{2+} transient (Wier, 1990), which in turn could influence the rate of mechanical relaxation. Thus, the changes in Ca^{2+} uptake by SR may be manifested most strikingly in the impaired relaxation that is sometimes evident in stunned myocardium (e.g., Fig. 1) (see also Pyzyklenk et al., 1987), rather than in the decline of systolic force generation.

C. Steady-State Intracellular Cation Concentrations

The significance of the various disturbances in ion transport identified in isolated membrane preparations can be gauged by consideration of whether the distribution of the ion of interest is affected. Consistent with the finding that Na^+,K^+-ATPase activity remains intact in sarcolemma from reperfused hearts, steady-state Na^+ concentration is not significantly different from control (Jennings et al., 1985; Pike et al., 1990). Total cellular calcium is not appreciably increased in the stunned heart (Jennings et al., 1985), but since the overwhelming majority of total calcium is tightly bound or resides in noncytosolic compartments (Wier, 1990), changes in $[Ca^{2+}]_i$ cannot be excluded on the basis of these data alone.

D. Calcium Transients

The advent of several new techniques for quantifying $[Ca^{2+}]_i$ in intact perfused hearts has made it possible to determine directly whether or not activator Ca^{2+} is decreased. Two complementary techniques have been brought to bear on the problem, both in ferret hearts: Kusuoka et al. (1990) performed gated nuclear magnetic resonance (NMR) measurements of the Ca^{2+} indicator 5F-BAPTA, while Guarnieri (1989) microinjected the Ca^{2+}-sensitive photoprotein aequorin into ventricular cells.

Gated ^{19}F-NMR spectroscopy revealed paradoxical increases in systolic $[Ca^{2+}]_i$ and in the amplitude of the Ca^{2+} transient after stunning (Fig. 3) (Kusuoka et al., 1990). The slight increase in diastolic $[Ca^{2+}]_i$ was not significant (0.18 ± 0.03 μM in control vs. 0.24 ± 0.03 μM in stunned hearts), but $[Ca^{2+}]_i$ at peak systole did increase (0.61 ± 0.06 μM in control vs. 1.03 ± 0.13 μM in stunned hearts). Concomitantly, the amplitude of Ca^{2+} transients in stunned myocardium was significantly higher than that measured before ischemia. We also ascertained whether the time course of the Ca^{2+} transients was altered. Neither the average time to peak $[Ca^{2+}]_i$ nor the time constant of the declining phase of the Ca^{2+} transient was significantly changed, thus simplifying the interpretation of the results. These findings demonstrate that contractile failure during reflow is not due to a critical failure of any of the mechanisms that regulate cytoplasmic activator Ca^{2+}.

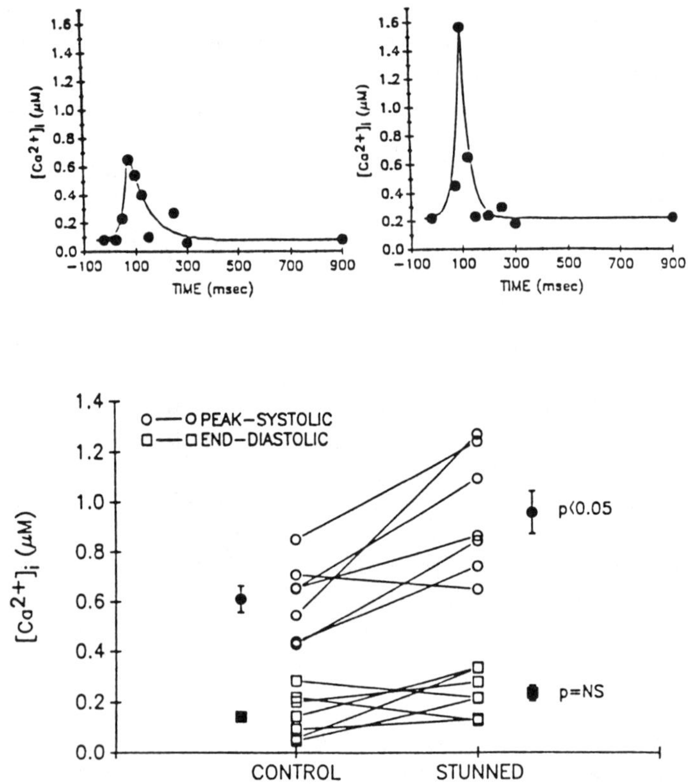

Figure 3 Changes in Ca transients observed before and after stunning. Upper panel shows the Ca transients in the control (left) and stunned (right) conditions in one heart obtained by gated ^{19}F-NMR technique. Lower panel shows pooled data for $[Ca^{2+}]_i$ at end diastole and at peak systole. (From Kusuoka et al., 1990. Reproduced by permission of the American Heart Association.)

The aequorin results concurred in the finding that Ca^{2+} transients are not reduced; although tendencies toward increases in systolic $[Ca^{2+}]_i$ and Ca^{2+} transient amplitude were also observed, these did not reach statistical significance in Guarnieri's work (1989). The main conclusion of both groups was identical: Ca^{2+} availability is not the limiting factor in stunning.

E. Myofilament Ca^{2+} Responsiveness

1. Ca^{2+} Sensitivity and Maximal Ca^{2+}-Activated Force

The observations that Ca^{2+} transients are preserved in stunned myocardium imply that the responsiveness of the myofilaments to Ca^{2+} must be reduced.

This conclusion is further bolstered by deductions regarding myofilament Ca^{2+} responsiveness under conditions in which contractile activation by Ca^{2+} is likely to be maximal. Although complete contractile activation is never reached physiologically, intact hearts can be forced to reach the top of their dynamic range during tetani elicited by rapid electrical stimulation after exposure to ryanodine or other agents that interfere with SR function (Marban et al., 1986). Maximal Ca^{2+}-activated pressure (MCAP), the whole-heart correlate of maximal Ca^{2+}-activated force, is obtained as developed pressure during tetani when such pressure has reached saturation with respect to extracellular [Ca] ($[Ca]_o$) (Marban et al., 1986).

In stunned myocardium, developed pressure during twitches decreased by 35% relative to control values (Kusuoka et al., 1987). Developed pressure during tetani was also depressed after stunning; MCAP in stunned myocardium was significantly smaller than control (Kusuoka et al., 1987). The ratio of developed pressure at different $[Ca]_o$ to MCAP, i.e., Ca_o sensitivity, also decreased in stunned myocardium, indicating that either decreased myofilament Ca^{2+} sensitivity or a decrease in the Ca^{2+} transient additionally occurs in stunned myocardium (Kusuoka et al., 1987).

The new information regarding the amplitude of Ca^{2+} transients now allows us to dissect out the individual components of this decrease in Ca_o sensitivity. As indicated above, maximal Ca^{2+}-activated pressure is decreased in stunned myocardium. Can the decrease in maximal Ca^{2+}-activated pressure account entirely for the decrease in myofilament Ca^{2+} responsiveness in stunned myocardium? When the relation between the amplitude of Ca^{2+} transients and developed pressure was normalized by the corresponding maximal Ca^{2+}-activated pressures, the difference was still significant (Kusuoka et al., 1990). Thus, two distinct forms of decreased myofilament Ca^{2+} responsiveness combine to account for stunning: maximal force is decreased, and the myofilaments are also less sensitive even at submaximal $[Ca^{2+}]_i$.

2. Possible Mechanism of the Change in Ca^{2+} Responsiveness

The evidence favoring a reduction in myofilament Ca^{2+} responsiveness remains largely physiological rather than biochemical. Hess et al. (1980) demonstrated a decrease in maximal Ca^{2+}-activated myofibrillar ATPase activity and a shift in the Ca^{2+} sensitivity of the ATPase after 30 minutes of ischemia, but Krause (1990) found no change in either parameter with reperfusion after only 15 minutes of ischemia (which sufficed to stun). Myofibrillar force was not measured in conjunction with ATPase activity in either study, and Krause (1990) was careful to acknowledge that the ATPase might become relatively uncoupled from cross-bridge cycling. When force and ATPase activity are measured simultaneously in skinned skeletal muscle, the Ca^{2+} activation of isometric force occurs at higher Ca^{2+} concentrations than does the activation of actomyosin ATPase (Kerrick et al., 1991). Interestingly, the discrepancy between force and ATPase activity becomes greater at higher $[Mg^{2+}]$; since $[Mg^{2+}]_i$ is elevated in reperfused hearts (Borchgrevink et al., 1989; Murphy et al., 1989), ATPase activity may well become even more dissociated from changes in force than it would be under control conditions.

Given that there is a reduction of myofilament Ca^{2+} responsiveness, what might be its cause? The usual suspects, pH and inorganic phosphate (Marban and Kusuoka, 1987), return to normal within 30 seconds of reperfusion. As a potential culprit, magnesium merits much closer attention: Murphy et al. (1989), using a fluorinated NMR-detectable Mg^{2+} indicator, found that $[Mg^{2+}]_i$ rises from 0.8 mM to 2.1 mM during ischemia and remains elevated at ≥ 1.5 mM for at least 20 minutes of reflow. Indirect NMR measurements of $[Mg^{2+}]_i$ from the chemical shift of ATP reveal similar qualitative changes (Borchgrevink et al., 1989). Skinned muscle experiments have revealed that, as $[Mg^{2+}]_i$ rises, the $[Ca^{2+}]$-tension relation is shifted to higher $[Ca^{2+}]$ (Fabiato and Fabiato, 1975). Accurate predictions of the likely impact of this change in the intact heart are complicated by the need for numerous assumptions, but the observed change in $[Mg^{2+}]_i$ is certainly of the right magnitude to explain much of the observed fall in force in the stunned heart, even if the Mg^{2+} effect were partially offset by a modest increase in Ca^{2+} transients.

An increase in $[Mg^{2+}]_i$ cannot explain the decrease in maximal force, since the only clear-cut effect of elevated $[Mg^{2+}]_i$ observed in skinned fibers has been a desensitizing shift in the $[Ca^{2+}]$-tension relation. Thus, the origin of the decrease in maximal force remains unclear, although several lines of evidence (reviewed below) suggest that it is an aftereffect of transient calcium overload in the early moments of reperfusion. The available data are consistent with the idea that the Mg^{2+}-independent changes in the myofilaments reflect covalent modification of the contractile proteins due either to Ca^{2+}-mediated phosphorylation or to proteolysis (Kusuoka et al., 1990).

III. PATHOGENESIS OF STUNNED MYOCARDIUM

Beyond the characterization of force generation in stunned myocardium remains the question of the underlying mechanism of cellular injury. Cellular Ca overload is well-recognized as an etiological factor in irreversible reperfusion injury after a long duration of ischemia. Several lines of evidence from our laboratory also give credence to the hypothesis that cellular Ca overload during ischemia and/or reperfusion produces stunning.

A. ATP Depletion

The only consistent metabolic abnormality that has been observed in stunned myocardium examined by conventional methods is a modest reduction of the bulk ATP concentration (DeBoer et al., 1980). Because this resolves with a time course roughly parallel to that of functional recovery (Ellis et al., 1983), considerable emphasis was initially placed on the role of ATP in stunning. Several lines of evidence now make it quite clear that ATP depletion does not play a major pathogenetic role. Treatment with ATP precursors can restore ATP but not ameliorate stunning (Ambrosio et al., 1989); furthermore, functional recovery can be improved by modifications of the reperfusion protocol that do not affect ATP concentration (Kusuoka et al., 1987; Kitakaze et al., 1988a).

B. Calcium Overload

1. Ca Homeostasis During Ischemia and Reperfusion

Cellular Ca overload will occur if Ca^{2+} influx pathways that are inhibited during ischemia are reactivated upon reperfusion. One specific hypothesis involves Na^+-Ca^{2+} exchange (Renlund et al., 1984). This pathway normally extrudes Ca^{2+} from the cell at the expense of the transsarcolemmal Na^+ gradient. Under conditions of high intracellular Na^+ the direction of exchange is reversed, favoring Na^+-induced cellular Ca^{2+} gain. During ischemia, the Na^+,K^+-ATPase is inhibited by metabolic suppression, so that intracellular Na^+ accumulates (Grinwald, 1982; Pike et al., 1990). At the same time Na^+-Ca^{2+} exchange may be inhibited by intracellular acidosis. Upon reperfusion, intracellular pH returns to normal very rapidly, removing the inhibition of Na^+-Ca^{2+} exchange. When Na^+-Ca^{2+} exchange is reactivated under these conditions, intracellular [Na^+] is still elevated, and consequently the Na^+ gradient drives Ca^{2+} into the cells.

In stunned myocardium, the histological changes are not pathognomonic for Ca^{2+}-mediated injury, as they are in reperfusion after longer periods of ischemia. Nevertheless, our study using the ^{19}F-NMR technique recently revealed that $[Ca^{2+}]_i$ increases during ischemia and in the early phase of reperfusion: during 20 minutes of total global ischemia at 30 °C, time-averaged $[Ca^{2+}]_i$ increased significantly, reaching peak values roughly three times control at 15-20 minutes (Marban et al., 1990). Reperfusion resulted in a persistent elevation of $[Ca^{2+}]_i$ during the first 5 minutes, but not afterward. During 15 minutes of global ischemia at 37 °C, a significant increase in $[Ca^{2+}]_i$ was observed at 10–15 minutes (Steenbergen et al., 1987; Marban et al., 1989). Thus, stunning may share the same basic mechanism as reperfusion injury, with the major difference being one of degree of injury. We therefore sought evidence to link the transient Ca overload to the pathogenesis of stunning.

2. Does the Prevention of Ca Overload Diminish Stunning?

To elucidate whether or not blunting Ca overload during reperfusion could prevent stunning, we reperfused hearts with different Ca concentrations

($[Ca]_o$) after the same ischemic duration as in the conventional stunning group (Kusuoka et al., 1987). We reasoned as follows: if Ca^{2+} influx occurs upon reperfusion and is required for stunning, then reduction of $[Ca]_o$ in the reperfusate will decrease stunning by decreasing the driving force for Ca^{2+} influx. Hearts were reperfused with low-$[Ca]_o$ solution (0.1 mM during the initial 7 minutes, 0.2 mM during 7–14 minutes; 0.5 mM during the 14–21 minutes) before returning to the standard perfusate ($[Ca]_o$ = 2 mM). Remarkably, these hearts exhibited developed pressure and maximal Ca^{2+}-activated pressure comparable to nonischemic controls and significantly higher than in the stunned group.

Reperfusion with acidic solution represents a different strategy from the low-$[Ca]_o$ reperfusion, but shares the goal of blunting Ca overload during reperfusion (Kitakaze et al., 1988a). Because acidosis is known to antagonize Ca^{2+} influx and the intracellular binding of Ca^{2+}, acidosis during reperfusion may prevent the effects of Ca^{2+} overload and thereby ameliorate myocardial stunning. Hearts were subjected to the same ischemic protocol as in the conventional stunning group and reperfused with acidic solution (pH 6.6 during 0–3 minutes; pH 7.0 during 4–6 minutes) before returning to the standard perfusate (pH 7.4). Intramyocardial pH was lower in the acidic group than in the stunned group during early reperfusion. Both Ca_o responsiveness and maximal Ca^{2+}-activated pressure were greater in the acidic group than in the stunned group. These results obtained with low-$[Ca]_o$ reperfusion and acidic reperfusion indicate that transient calcium overload during early reperfusion plays a major role in the pathogenesis of myocardial stunning.

3. Does Transient Ca Overload Produce "Stunning"?

The next question is whether or not transient Ca overload without ischemia can produce contractile dysfunction that mimics stunned myocardium. Several lines of experimental evidence have answered the question positively.

Isolated ferret hearts after three 5-minute periods of perfusion with 10 mM $[Ca]_o$ solution without ischemia showed a decrease in both Ca_o responsiveness and maximal Ca^{2+}-activated pressure virtually indistinguishable from that observed in postischemic, reperfused myocardium (Kitakaze et al., 1988b). Developed pressure at 2 mM $[Ca]_o$ decreased by 28.5% after exposure to high-$[Ca]_o$ solution. Mean MCAP in the high-$[Ca]_o$ group was smaller than that in control. Histological examination of the hearts perfused with high-$[Ca]_o$ solution exhibited rare foci of predominantly reversible injury similar to that in stunned myocardium. Phosphorus NMR spectra revealed a decline in intramyocardial ATP content by 30–40% after exposure to high $[Ca]_o$. Inorganic phosphate, phosphocreatine, and pH remained unchanged. These results indicate that transient exposure to high $[Ca]_o$ without ischemia leaves behind distinctive contractile, metabolic, and histological sequelae that mimic those of stunned myocardium.

Recent observations regarding intracellular free calcium in ventricular fibrillation also support the hypothesis of a pathogenetic role of Ca overload in stunned myocardium (Koretsune and Marban, 1989). During ventricular fibrillation induced by burst pacing, $[Ca^{2+}]_i$, measured by F-NMR with 5F-BAPTA, rose rapidly and dramatically, exceeding the control by a factor of four within 5 minutes. $[Ca^{2+}]_i$ remained markedly elevated throughout 20 minutes of fibrillation, but returned to control values shortly after defibrillation. The increase in $[Ca^{2+}]_i$ was independent of myocardial ischemia, because hearts operating at a very low wall stress showed similar increases in $[Ca^{2+}]_i$ despite the absence of ischemic changes. Developed pressure did not recover to control levels after defibrillation (about 50% of control) even in the hearts with low wall stress during ventricular fibrillation. These results also support the notion that a transient increase in $[Ca^{2+}]_i$ leaves behind lingering contractile dysfunction.

Yet another form of support to the "Ca-overload" hypothesis comes from observations of the acute cardiotoxic effect of adriamycin (Kusuoka et al., 1991). Time-averaged $[Ca^{2+}]_i$ measured at 10-minute resolution with 5F-BAPTA increased to more than twice the control during 30-minute perfusion with adriamycin (30 mg/1). Developed pressure decreased during exposure to adriamycin and did not recover after washout. Phosphorus NMR spectra revealed no significant change in myocardial energy metabolism during and after the exposure. These results indicate that transient Ca overload induced by adriamycin is associated with acute contractile failure. Adriamycin has been reported to inhibit Na^{+}-Ca^{2+} exchange (Caroni et al., 1981) and to affect the gating of Ca^{2+} release channels in sarcoplasmic reticulum (Holmberg and Williams, 1990). Whatever the cause of the calcium overload, the fact that dysfunction persists as an aftereffect of adriamycin is consistent with the hypothesis that transient calcium overload, even in the absence of ischemia, can cause long-lasting contractile dysfunction.

4. Role of Ca Overload in Stunning Process

The lines of experimental evidence mentioned above are summarized as follows: $[Ca^{2+}]_i$ rises appropriately; removal of Ca^{2+} attenuates stunning; elevation of Ca^{2+} without ischemia mimics stunning. Thus, these fulfill Koch's postulates to indicate that stunning is a lingering aftereffect of a transient increase in $[Ca^{2+}]_i$ during ischemia and early reflow.

Elevated $[Ca^{2+}]_i$ might bring about its ill consequences by activating protein kinases (Hochachka 1986; Marban et al., 1989) to change Ca^{2+} sensitivity and/or maximal Ca^{2+}-activated force through phosphorylation of one or more of the contractile proteins. Although a decreased Ca^{2+} sensitivity of the contractile proteins represents a plausible, and testable, mechanism for stunning, no evidence for or against such a phenomenon has yet been reported in response to Ca^{2+}-induced phosphorylation. Degradation of contractile proteins by Ca^{2+}-activated proteases also merits future consideration. If such degradation in fact occurs, it would help explain why stunning reverses over several days, a time course consistent with the rate of protein degradation and de novo protein synthesis (McKee et al., 1978).

C. Free Radical Generation

More recently the focus has turned to free radicals as the proximate cause of stunning. In contrast to the controversy that surrounds the question of whether free radicals figure prominently in the irreversible tissue injury following longer periods of ischemia (Downey, 1990), agreement regarding the importance of free radicals in stunning is virtually unanimous (Bolli, 1988, 1990; Kloner et al., 1989). This consensus is based upon two general categories of experimental evidence: first, measurements of free radical generation, which have revealed the transient elaboration of hydroxyl and superoxide radicals just after reperfusion (Zweier et al., 1987); second, improvement of functional recovery by free radical scavengers and related strategies (Bolli, 1988, 1990; Kloner et al., 1989). As far as it goes, the evidence is compelling, but two major gaps remain. First, it has yet to be demonstrated that free radical generation suffices to produce stunning. Numerous strategies have been employed to elaborate free radicals in the absence of ischemia (Blaustein et al., 1986; Goldhaber et al., 1988), and, not surprisingly, such strategies generally result in functional and metabolic damage to myocardial cells. The damage is variously manifested by action potential prolongation and afterpotentials (Goldhaber et al., 1988), calcium overload (Josephson et al., 1991; Matsuura and Shattock, 1991), contracture (Goldhaber et al., 1988), and/or metabolic rundown (Goldhaber et al., 1988; Chatham et al., 1989). The effects of exogenous radicals in isolated tissue preparations are distinctive, with only superficial resemblance to stunning. If anything, the picture is much closer to that of irreversible reperfusion damage in which contracture and severe calcium overload are prominent features (Shen and Jennings, 1972). The failure so far to mimic stunning convincingly with free radicals in isolated tissues may not be fundamental, but rather may be attributable to unrealistic concentrations of exogenous radicals (too high), duration of exposure (too long), or site of radical elaboration (strictly extracellular in most models). Second, the work on free radicals has focused largely on these agents as specific initiators of injury rather than on the mechanism of their deleterious effects, which remains mysterious. More recent in vivo evidence does, however, indicate that infusion of exogenous oxygen radicals in the absence of ischemia can result in myocardial dysfunction without ultrastructural evidence of irreversible tissue injury (Prasad et al., 1989; Przyklenk et al., 1990).

The possibility that radicals stun by perturbing calcium homeostasis is particularly intriguing. As Bolli (1990) has been careful to point out, the "radical hypothesis" and the "calcium hypothesis" are not mutually exclusive. Indeed, recent evidence (Josephson et al., 1991; Corretti et al., 1991) indicates that exogenous radical generation leads to cellular calcium overload. If radicals contribute to calcium overload upon reperfusion, the "radical hypothesis" could turn out to be an explicit elaboration upon the "calcium hypothesis." Although it is not yet apparent how free radicals perturb Ca^{2+} homeostasis, clues may be gleaned from two sets of seemingly disparate observations. First, glycolysis (as opposed to oxidative phosphorylation) appears to play a favored role in maintaining transmembrane ion gradients in general (Weiss and Hiltbrand, 1985; Owen et al., 1990), and perhaps even more so in the stunned heart: Jeremy et al. (1989) have found that reperfusion with the glycolytic inhibitor iodoacetate, in concentrations that do not affect nonischemic hearts, prevents functional recovery and restoration of calcium homeostasis after 20 minutes of ischemia in rabbit hearts. Second, free radicals are known to inactivate the key glycolytic enzyme glyceraldehyde-3-phosphate dehydrogenase (Chatham et al., 1989). It is intriguing to wonder whether the two phenomena, inhibition of glycolysis and disruption of calcium homeostasis, might have a cause-and-effect relationship when free radicals are elaborated. Corretti et al. (1991) have tested this notion with simultaneous NMR measurements of $[Ca^{2+}]_i$ and high-energy phosphates. In response to exogenous hydroxyl radical generation in rabbit hearts, these investigators found that glycolytic inhibition occurs hand-in-hand with the rise in $[Ca^{2+}]_i$. Corretti et al. (1991) hypothesized that radicals inhibit glycolysis, glycolytic inhibition in turn leads to deranged Ca^{2+} homeostasis, and the resultant calcium overload produces dysfunction. Whether this mechanism will stand up to further scrutiny, particularly in stunning, is not yet clear. Regardless, the results give reason to expect that our understanding of the critical links among radicals, calcium and energy metabolism will soon be considerably more refined.

ACKNOWLEDGMENTS

Supported by the National Institutes of Health (RO1 HL 44065 and Research Career Development Award KO4 HL 01872).

REFERENCES

Ambrosio, G., Jacobus, W. E., Mitchell, M. C., Litt, M. R., and Becker, L. C. (1989). Effects of ATP precursors on ATP and free ADP content and functional recovery of postischemic hearts. *Am. J. Physiol. 256*: H560.

Blaustein, A. S., Schine, L., Brooks, W. W., Fanburg, B. L., and Bing, O. H. L. (1986). Influence of exogenously generated oxidant species on myocardial function. *Am. J. Physiol. 250*: H595.

Bolli, R. (1988). Oxygen-derived free radicals and postischemic myocardial dysfunction ("stunned myocardium"). *J. Am. Coll. Cardiol. 12*: 239.
Bolli, R. (1990). Mechanism of myocardial "stunning." *Circulation 82*: 723.
Borchgrevink, P. C., Bergan, A. S., Bakoy, O. E., and Jynge, P. (1989). Magnesium and reperfusion of ischemic rat heart as assessed by ^{31}P-NMR. *Am. J. Physiol. 256*: H195.
Braunwald, E., and Kloner, R. A. (1982). The stunned myocardium: Prolonged, postischemic ventricular dysfunction. *Circulation 66*: 1146.
Braunwald, E., and Kloner, R. A. (1985). Myocardial reperfusion: a double-edged sword? *J. Clin. Invest. 76*: 1713.
Caroni, P., Villiani, F., and Carafoli, E. (1981). The cardiotoxic antibiotic doxorubicin inhibits the Na^+/Ca^{2+} exchange of dog heart sarcolemmal vesicles. *FEBS Lett. 130*: 184.
Chatham, J., Gilbert, H. F., and Radda, G. K. (1989). The metabolic consequences of hydroperoxide perfusion on the isolated rat heart. *Eur. J. Biochem. 184*: 657.
Chemnitius, J. M., Sasaki, Y., Burger, W., and Bing, R. J. (1985). the effect of ischemia and reperfusion on sarcolemmal function in perfused canine hearts. *J. Mol. Cell. Cardiol. 17*: 1139.
Coetzee, W. A., King, L. M., Shattock, M. J., and Matsuura, H. (1990). Electrophysiology of rat hearts and rabbit ventricular myocytes during reperfusion after transient ischemia. In *Ionic Currents and Ischemia* (J. Vereecke, P. P. van Bogaert, F. Verdonck, eds.), Leuven University Press, Leuven, p. 285.
Corretti, M. C., Koretsune, Y., Kusuoka, H., Chacko, V. P., Zweier, J. L., and Marban, E. (1991). Glycolytic inhibition and calcium overload as consequences of exogenously-generated free radicals in rabbit hearts. *J. Clin. Invest.*
DeBoer, F. W. V., Ingwall, J. S., Kloner, R. A., and Braunwald, E. (1980). Prolonged derangements of canine myocardial purine metabolism after a brief coronary artery occlusion not associated with anatomic evidence of necrosis. *Proc. Natl. Acad. Sci. USA 77*: 5471.
Downey, J. M. (1990). Free radicals and their involvement during long-term myocardial ischemia and reperfusion. *Annu. Rev. Physiol. 52*: 487.
Ellis, S. G., Henschke, C. I., Sandor, T., Wynne, J., Braunwald, E., and Kloner, R. A. (1983). Time course of functional and biochemical recovery of myocardium salvaged by reperfusion. *J. Am. Coll. Cardiol. 1*: 1047.
Fabiato, A., and Fabiato, F. (1975). Effects of magnesium on contractile activation of skinned cardiac cells. *J. Physiol. (Lond.) 249*: 497.
Goldhaber, J. I., Ji, S., Lamp, S. T., and Weiss, J. N. (1988). Effect of exogenous free radicals on electromechanical function and metabolism in isolated rabbit and guinea pig ventricle: Implications for ischemia and reperfusion injury. *J. Clin. Invest. 83*: 1800.
Grinwald, P. M. (1982). Calcium uptake during post-ischemic reperfusion in the isolated rat heart: Influence of extracellular sodium. *J. Mol. Cell. Cardiol. 14*: 359.
Guarnieri, T. (1989). Direct measurement of $[Ca^{2+}]_i$ in early and late reperfused myocardium. *Circulation 80*: II-241 (Abstract).
Hanich, R. F., Levine, J. H., Prood, C., Spear, J. F., and Moore, E. N. (1989). Stunned myocardium: A form fruste of electromechanical dissociation? *J. Am. Coll. Cardiol. 13*: 90A (Abstract).

Hess, M. L., Krause, S. M., and Greenfield, L. J. (1980). Assessment of hypothermic, cardioplegic protection to the global ischemic canine myocardium. *J. Thorac. Cardiovasc. Surg. 80*: 293.

Hochachka, P. W. (1986). Defense strategies against hypoxia and hypothermia. *Science 231*: 234.

Holmberg, S. R. M., and Williams, A. J. (1990). Patterns of interaction between anthraquinone drugs and the calcium-release channel from cardiac sarcoplasmic reticulum. *Circ. Res. 67*: 272.

Jennings, R. B., Schaper, J., Hill, M. L., Steenbergen, Jr., C., and Reimer, K. A. (1985). Effect of reperfusion late in the phase of reversible ischemic injury. *Circ. Res. 56*: 262.

Jeremy, R., Lewis, R., and Becker, L. (1989). Relation of glycolysis and calcium during reflow to function of stunned myocardium. *Circulation 80*: II-235 (Abstract).

Josephson, R. A., Silverman, H. S., Lakatta, E. G., Stern, M. D., and Zweier, J. L. (1991). Study of the mechanisms of hydrogen peroxide and hydroxyl free radical induced cellular injury and calcium overload in cardiac myocytes. *J. Biol. Chem. 266*: 2354.

Kerrick, W. G. L., Potter, J. D., and Hoar, P. E. (1991). The apparent rate constant for the dissociation of force generating myosin crossbridges from actin decreases during Ca^{2+} activation of skinned muscle fibres. *J. Musc. Res. Cell Motil. 12*: 53.

Kitakaze, M., Weisfeldt, M. L., and Marban, E. (1988a). Acidosis during early reperfusion prevents myocardial stunning in perfused hearts. *J. Clin. Invest. 82*: 920.

Kitakaze, M., Weisman, H. F., and Marban, E. (1988b). Contractile dysfunction and ATP depletion after transient calcium overload in perfused ferret hearts. *Circulation 77*: 685.

Kloner, R. A., Przyklenk, K., and Whittaker, P. (1989). Deleterious effects of oxygen radicals in ischemia/reperfusion. Resolved and unresolved issues. *Circulation 80*: 1115.

Koretsune, Y., and Marban, E. (1989). Cell calcium in the pathophysiology of ventricular fibrillation and in the pathogenesis of post-arrhythmic contractile dysfunction. *Circulation 80*: 369.

Koretsune, Y., Corretti, M. C., Kusuoka, H., and Marban, E. (1991). Mechanism of early contractile failure. Inexcitability, metabolite accumulation, or vascular collapse? *Circ. Res. 68*: 255.

Krause, S. M. (1989). Myocardial stunning opens the Ca^{2+} release channel in cardiac sarcoplasmic reticulum. *Circulation 80*: II-601 (Abstract).

Krause, S. M., Jacobus, W. E., and Becker, L. C. (1989). Alterations in cardiac sarcoplasmic reticulum calcium transport in the postischemic "stunned" myocardium. *Circ. Res. 65*: 526.

Krause, S. (1990). Effect of global myocardial stunning on Ca^{2+}-sensitive myofibrillar ATPase activity and creatine kinase kinetics. *Am. J. Physiol. 259*: H813.

Krause, S. M., and Rozanski, D. J. (1990). Increased free $[Mg^{2+}]_i$ following myocardial stunning potentiates the depression in sarcoplasmic reticulum (SR) Ca^{2+} transport. *Circulation 82*: III-272 (Abstract).

Kusuoka, H., Porterfield, J. K., Weisman, H. F., Weisfeldt, M. L., and Marban, E. (1987). Pathophysiology and pathogenesis of stunned myocardium: Depressed

Kusuoka, H., Porterfield, J. K., Weisman, H. F., Weisfeldt, M. L., and Marban, E. (1987). Pathophysiology and pathogenesis of stunned myocardium: Depressed Ca^{2+} activation of contraction as a consequence of reperfusion-induced cellular calcium overload in ferret hearts. *J. Clin. Invest.* *79*: 950.

Kusuoka, H., Koretsune, Y., Chacko, V. P., Weisfeldt, M. L., and Marban, E. (1990). Excitation-contraction coupling in postischemic myocardium: Does failure of activator Ca^{2+} transients underlie "stunning"? *Circ. Res.* *66*: 1268.

Kusuoka, H., Futaki, S., Koretsune, Y., Kitabatake, A., Suga, H., Kamada, T., and Inoue, M. (1991). Alterations of intracellular calcium homeostasis and myocardial energetics in acute adriamycin-induced heart failure. *J. Cardiovasc. Pharmacol.* (in press).

Kusuoka, H., and Marban, E. (1992). Cellular mechanisms of myocardial stunning. *Annu. Rev. Physiol.* *54*: (in press).

Levine, J. H., Moore, E. N., Weisman, H. F., Kadish, A. H., Becker, L. C., and Spear, J. F. (1987). Depression of action potential characteristics and a decreased space constant are present in postischemic, reperfused myocardium. *J. Clin. Invest.* *79*: 107.

Limbruno, U., Zucchi, R., Ronca-Testoni, S., Galbani, P., Ronca, G., and Mariani, M. (1989). Sarcoplasmic reticulum function in the "stunned" myocardium. *J. Mol. Cell. Cardiol.* *21*: 1063.

Marban, E., Kusuoka, H., Yue, D. T., Weisfeldt, M. L., and Wier, W. G. (1986). Maximal Ca^{2+}-activated force elicited by tetanization of ferret papillary muscle and whole heart: Mechanism and characteristics of steady contractile activation in intact myocardium. *Circ. Res.* *59*: 262.

Marban, E., and Kusuoka, H. (1987). Maximal Ca^{2+}-activated force and myofilament Ca^{2+} sensitivity in intact mammalian hearts. Differential effects of inorganic phosphate and hydrogen ion. *J. Gen. Physiol.* *90*: 609.

Marban, E., Koretsune, Y., Corretti, M., Chacko, V. P., and Kusuoka, H. (1989). Calcium and its role in myocardial cell injury during ischemia and reperfusion. *Circulation* *80*: IV-17.

Marban, E., Kitakaze, M., Koretsune, Y., Yue, D. T., Chacko, V. P., and Pike, M. M. (1990). Quantification of $[Ca^{2+}]_i$ in perfused hearts: critical evaluation of the 5F-BAPTA/NMR method as applied to the study of ischemia and reperfusion. *Circ. Res.* *66*: 1255.

Marban, E. (1991). Myocardial stunning and hibernation. *Circulation* *83*: 681.

Matsuura, H., and Shattock, M. J. (1991). Membrane potential fluctuations and transient inward currents induced by reactive oxygen intermediates in isolated rabbit ventricular cells. *Circ. Res.* *68*: 319.

McKee, E. E., Cheung, J. Y., Rannels, D. E. and Morgan, H. E. (1978). Measurement of the rate of protein synthesis and compartmentation of heart phenylalanine. *J. Biol. Chem.* *253*: 1030.

Murphy, E., Steenbergen, C., Levy, L. A., Raju, B., and London, R. E. (1989). Cytosolic free magnesium levels in ischemic rat heart. *J. Biol. Chem.* *264*: 5622.

Owen, P., Dennis, S., and Opie, L. H. (1990). Glucose flux rate regulates onset of ischemic contracture in globally underperfused rat hearts. *Circ. Res.* *66*: 344.

Pike, M. M., Kitakaze, M., and Marban, E. (1990). ^{23}Na-NMR measurements of intracellular sodium in intact perfused ferret hearts during ischemia and reperfusion. *Am. J. Physiol.* *259*: H1767.

Prasad, K., Kalra, J., Chan, W. P., and Chaudhary, A. K. (1989). Effect of oxygen free radicals on cardiovascular function at the organ and cellular level. *Am. Heart J. 117*: 1196.

Przyklenk, K., Patel, B., and Kloner, R. A. (1987). Diastolic abnormalities of post-ischemic "stunned" myocardium. *Am. J. Cardiol. 60*: 1211.

Przyklenk, K., Whittaker, P., and Kloner, R. A. (1990). In vivo infusion of oxygen free radical substrates causes myocardial systolic, but not diastolic dysfunction. *Am. Heart J. 119*: 807.

Renlund, D. G., Gerstenblith, G., Lakatta, E. G., Jacobus, W. E., Kallman, C. H., and Weisfeldt, M. L. (1984). Perfusate sodium during ischemia modifies post-ischemic functional and metabolic recovery in the rabbit heart. *J. Mol. Cell. Cardiol. 16*: 795.

Shen, A. C., and Jennings, R. B. (1972). Myocardial calcium and magnesium in acute ischemic injury. *Am. J. Pathol. 67*: 417.

Steenbergen, C., Murphy, E., Levy, L., and London, R. E. (1987). Elevation in cytosolic free calcium concentration early in myocardial ischemia in perfused rat heart. *Circ. Res. 60*: 700.

Tani, M., and Neely, J. R. (1989). Role of intracellular Na^+ and Ca^{2+} overload and depressed recovery of ventricular function of reperfused ischemic rat hearts. Possible involvement of H^+-Na^+ and Na^+-Ca^+ exchange. *Circ. Res. 65*: 1045.

Weiss, J., and Hiltbrand, B. (1985). Functional compartmentation of glycolytic versus oxidative metabolism in isolated rabbit heart. *J. Clin. Invest. 75*: 436.

Weiss, R. G., Lakatta, E. G., and Gerstenblith, G. (1990). Effects of amiloride on metabolism and contractility during reoxygenation in perfused rat hearts. *Circ. Res. 66*: 1012.

Wier, W. G. (1990). Cytoplasmic $[Ca^{2+}]_i$ in mammalian ventricle: Dynamic control by cellular processes. *Annu. Rev. Physiol. 52*: 467.

Zweier, J. L., Flaherty, J. T., and Weisfeldt, M. L. (1987). Direct measurement of free radical generation following reperfusion of ischemic myocardium. *Proc. Natl. Acad. Sci. USA 84*: 1404.

10

Role of the Cyclooxygenase Pathway in Stunned Myocardium

Neil E. Farber and Garrett J. Gross

Medical College of Wisconsin, Milwaukee, Wisconsin

I. INTRODUCTION

During ischemia, the activity of myocardial lipases, such as phospholipase A_2, is significantly enhanced at acidic pH, which results in a significant accumulation of free fatty acids. These fatty acids, as structural components of cellular membranes, are also precursors of many lipid mediators. One such class of mediators, known as the eicosanoids, are peroxidation products of arachidonic acid and include prostaglandins, thromboxane (Tx), endoperoxides, and leukotrienes. Cyclooxygenase, which is inhibited by aspirinlike drugs, converts arachidonic acid first into the cyclic endoperoxide intermediates PGG_2 and PGH_2 and finally to the formation of prostaglandins and Tx. The major cyclooxygenase product released from the intact heart appears to be prostacyclin (PGI_2), mainly from endothelial cells and, to a lesser extent, smooth muscle cells of the vasculature. Thromboxane A_2 (TxA_2) is the major arachidonate metabolite in platelets, yet may also be released in small amounts from the ischemic myocardium. Neutrophils, which have been suggested to be a cause of myocardial stunning, are also a potential source of TxA_2.

Disturbances in the balance of PGI_2 and TxA_2 formation have been associated with many disease states including sudden cardiac death, atherosclerosis, arterial thrombosis, diabetes, hyperlipidemia, reperfusion arrhythmias, spontaneous and effort-induced angina, and other forms of ischemic heart disease (Ogletree, 1987; FitzGerald et al., 1987). Such observations have led to the suggestion that cyclooxygenase inhibitors may prove to be useful in treating or preventing certain types of cardiovascular disease. Several new classes of compounds have been recently synthesized which have the specific effect of inhibiting thromboxane or mimicking prostacyclin, thus increasing the PGI_2/TxA_2 balance. Recent animal and experimental studies indicate that these agents may be beneficial in irreversible ischemia-induced myocardial injury. The role of TxA_2 as a possible mediator of the prolonged abnormalities in myocardial function and metabolism and the importance of the TxA_2/PGI_2 balance in the stunned myocardium will be examined in this chapter.

II. CYCLOOXYGENASE

Inherent in cyclooxygenase blockade for preventing cardiovascular disease is the belief that platelet-mediated thrombosis is an important initiating event in precipitating acute myocardial infarction. Persistent coronary occlusion may result from severe spasm causing a plaque to rupture, and there is growing evidence that in many cases, acute myocardial ischemia results from a combination of fixed and dynamic obstructions. Cyclooxygenase inhibitors such as nonsteroidal anti-inflammatory drugs (NSAIDs; e.g., indomethacin) inhibit both platelet and endothelial enzymes in a dose-dependent fashion. Clinical evidence links platelets to ischemic heart disease since an increase in circulating platelet microthrombi after myocardial infarction (Mehta and Mehta, 1979) as well as an increase in platelet activation and secretion in patients with unstable angina has been observed (Sobel et al., 1981). However, reports concerning the effects of NSAIDs on experimental myocardial ischemic damage are conflicting. NSAIDs, including indomethacin, have been shown to reduce both the release of phosphocreatine and lactate dehydrogenase upon reperfusion of isolated globally ischemic rat hearts, without enhancing recovery of mechanical function (Karmazyn, 1983). Several studies have examined the effects of NSAIDs on experimental infarct size (Lepran et al., 1981; Jugdutt et al., 1979). Jugdutt and coworkers (1979) found no beneficial responses on myocardial infarct size in conscious dogs after indomethacin administration. Lepran and coworkers (1981) observed no decrease in infarct size in rats treated with one of three different cyclooxygeanse inhibitors, including indomethacin. However, these authors noted a protective effect of cyclooxygenase blockade on decreasing the severity and duration or arrhythmias during the acute phase of coronary occlusion. In addition, decreasing the number of circulating platelets with antiplatelet antiserum had no effect on myocardial infarct size in dogs after prolonged coronary occlusion and reperfusion (Mullane and McGiff, 1985). In these studies, neutrophils, which were only slightly reduced in the ischemic myocardium, were a possible source of the TxA_2 being released. In support of a neutrophil-mediated rather than a platelet-mediated progression of long-term ischemic damage, ibuprofen (Kirlin et al., 1982) and BW755C (Jolly and Lucchesi, 1983), which are able to inhibit both cyclooxygenase and lipoxygenase, as well as decrease several aspects of neutrophil function, have both been shown to decrease infarct size. As a cyclooxygenase inhibitor, indomethacin decreases arachidonic acid metabolites and may consequently increase metabolites of the lipoxygenase pathway.

While agents that inhibit both PGI_2 and TxA_2 synthesis appear to be only moderately efficacious in human subjects and animal models, a Veterans Administration Cooperative Study (Lewis et al., 1983) demonstrated that a single daily administration of aspirin begun within 51 hours of admission to the hospital significantly decreased the 12-week incidence of acute myocardial infarction or death by 51% in men with unstable angina. Indeed, the use of aspirin clinically in the treatment of unstable angina has now become routine. Thus, while literature on the effects of NSAIDs in irreversible myocardial ischemia is abundant, only one study has examined the effects of this class of drugs in the stunned myocardium.

Farber and Gross (1990) recently investigated the effect of preocclusion treatment with indomethacin on the recovery of regional systolic shortening in anesthetized dogs subjected to 15 minutes of coronary artery occlusion followed by 3 hours of reperfusion. As expected there was a significant decrease of both TxB_2 and 6-keto-$PGF_{1\alpha}$, the stable hydration products of TxA_2 and PGI_2, respectively, within 10–30 minutes after administration (Figs. 1 and 2). However, indomethacin exhibited no beneficial effect on recovery of regional myocardial function as compared to controls ($5 \pm 6\%$ vs. $12 \pm 11\%$) (Fig. 3). In addition, indomethacin did not preserve adenine nucleotide levels or prevent the rebound increase in phosphocreatine that occurs after a brief episode of ischemia and subsequent reperfusion (unpublished observations). This lack of a beneficial action of indomethacin on functional and metabolic recovery in the presence of markedly depressed levels of coronary venous TxA_2 may not be surprising since PGI_2 was also significantly decreased. While these findings do not definitively exclude a role for platelets in the pathogenesis of myocardial stunning, since platelet aggregation induced by agents other than TxA_2 (e.g., epinephrine, thrombin, or collagen) may still occur, they do indicate that either the TxA_2/PGI_2 balance is important in the stunned myocardium, but that inhibition of PGI_2 concomitant with TxA_2 is not bene-

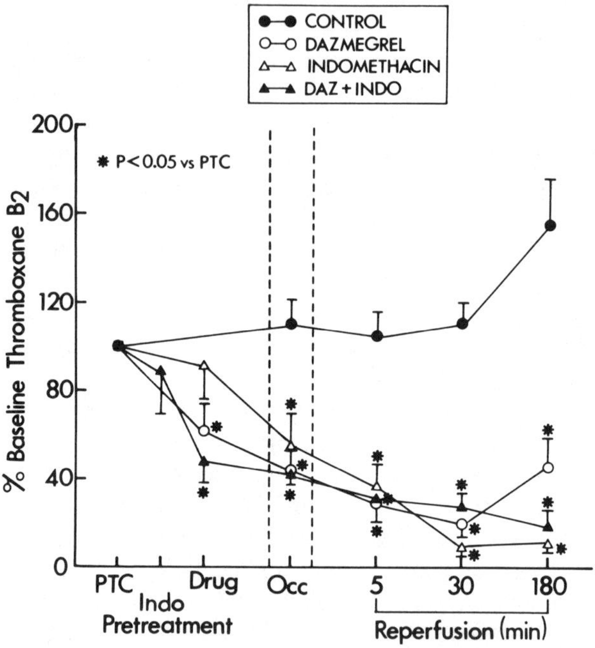

Figure 1 Coronary venous levels of thromboxane as a percent of the pretreatment control (PTC), 10 minutes postindomethacin pretreatment, 10 minutes postdrug (Drug), coronary occlusion (Occ), and during reperfusion in control (saline); dazmegrel 3 mg/kg; indomethacin 5 mg/kg; and dazmegrel + indomethacin-treated dogs. *, Significant difference ($p < 0.05$) from the absolute levels of TxB_2 measured at PTC. (Reprinted by permission from Farber and Gross, 1990.)

ficial, or that other possibly beneficial arachidonic acid metabolites are inhibited by indomethacin. Alternatively, TxA_2 may not be an important mediator of reversible postischemic dysfunction.

III. THROMBOXANE A_2 (TxA_2)

Since the discovery of a strongly vasospastic compound released during anaphylaxis and the subsequent identification of the main component as the arachidonic acid metabolite, TxA_2, there have been many studies using TxA_2 synthesis inhibitors or receptor blockers that suggest a role for TxA_2 as a pathophysiological mediator in thrombosis, vasospasm, arrhythmias, and in the progression of ischemic damage following coronary artery occlusion.

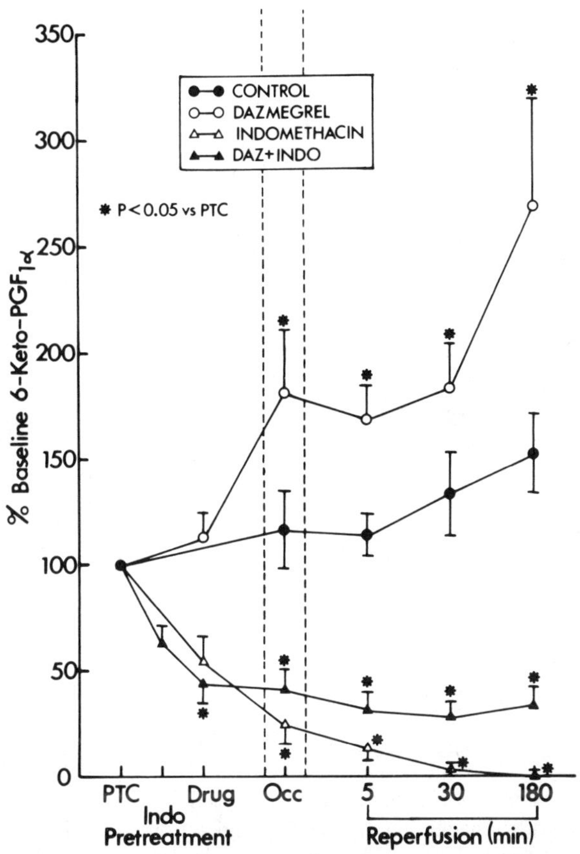

Figure 2 Coronary venous levels of prostacyclin as a percent of the pretreatment control (PTC), 10 minutes postindomethacin pretreatment, 10 minutes postdrug (Drug), coronary occlusion (Occ), and during reperfusion in control (saline); dazmegrel 3 mg/kg; indomethacin 5 mg/kg; and dazmegrel + indomethacin-treated dogs. *, Significant difference ($p < 0.05$) from the absolute levels measured at PTC. (Reprinted by permission from Farber and Gross, 1990.)

TxA_2 inhibitors have been shown to attenuate the loss of myocardial creatine kinase and nitrogenous compounds from the ischemic myocardium, attenuate the rise in plasma creatine kinase activity, and decrease the ischemia-induced ST-segment elevation after permanent coronary occlusions. Until recently, all studies with anti-TxA_2 drugs were performed in models of global ischemia and/or irreversible ischemic damage. It is of interest to note that in none of these previous studies were any drug effects on hemodynamics,

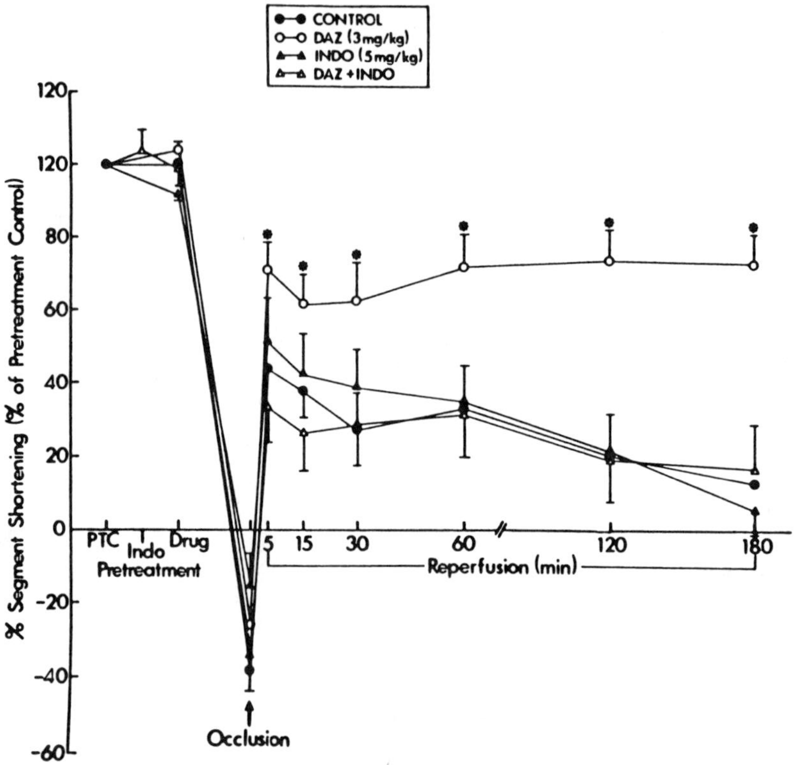

Figure 3 Percent segment shortening of pretreatment control (PTC) in the ischemic-reperfused area at PTC, postindomethacin pretreatment, 10 minutes postdrug (Drug), coronary occlusion, and during reperfusion. Time course curves for control, dazmegrel (DAZ), indomethacin (INDO), and DAZ + INDO groups. *, Significant difference ($p < 0.05$) versus control group. (Reprinted by permission from Farber and Gross, 1990.)

myocardial oxygen demand, or myocardial oxygen supply observed. Cardioprotective actions have been attributed to an attenuation of catecholamine release, an inhibition of TxA_2-mediated vasoconstriction, platelet aggregation, cellular lysis, or endoperoxide shunting to potentially beneficial prostanoids following the use of TxA_2 synthesis inhibitors.

A. Thromboxane A_2 (TxA_2) Synthetase Inhibition

The first truly selective inhibitor of TxA_2 synthetase was imidazole. Subsequently, other derivatives of imidazole (e.g., dazoxiben, dazmegrel) were found to be more potent inhibitors of TxA_2 synthetase. Earlier studies with TxA_2 synthetase inhibitors demonstrated efficacious responses in reducing certain indices of ischemic damage such as myocardial creatine kinase and amino-nitrogen loss (Hock and Lefer, 1986; Wargovich et al., 1987) in cats and rats after prolonged ischemic insults. Wargovich and colleagues (1987) observed a significant reduction in myocardial neutrophil accumulation in the infarcted myocardium following thromboxane synthetase inhibition. TxA_2 synthetase inhibition has also been shown to decrease infarct size in dogs by a platelet-dependent mechanism (Mullane and Fonabaio, 1988).

Functional recovery in the stunned myocardium has been shown to be dependent on the degree of coronary artery patency during early reperfusion and also on the coronary artery occluded, left anterior descending (LAD) versus left circumflex (Farber et al., 1987, 1988b). Using a model of myocardial stunning in which the LAD was occluded for 15 minutes and reperfusion was allowed into a critical stenosis in which reactive hyperemia was attenuated, the effect of TxA_2 synthesis inhibition on metabolic and functional recovery was investigated (Farber et al., 1988; Farber and Gross, 1990). Preocclusion treatment with dazmegrel completely attenuated the increase in TxA_2 release during reperfusion, which was observed in control conditions (see Fig. 1) and, in addition, markedly increased the synthesis of PGI_2 (see Fig. 2). This increase in PGI_2 synthesis after TxA_2 synthesis inhibition is known as endoperoxide shunting or steal (Aiken et al., 1981; Mullane and Fornabaio, 1988).

Inhibition of TxA_2 synthesis with dazmegrel markedly improved postischemic functional recovery in the stunned myocardium ($66 \pm 8\%$ vs. $12 \pm 11\%$) (see Fig. 3) in the absence of increases in regional blood flow or redistribution of flow to subendocardial layers. Enhanced functional recovery also occurred without changes in myocardial oxygen demand and without a reduction in the loss of systolic wall function during the ischemic period. TxA_2 synthesis inhibition with dazoxiben or dazmegrel has also been shown to be cardioprotective in terms of metabolism in the stunned myocardium (Pieper et al., 1988; Farber et al., 1988a). Both these agents preserved myocardial high-energy phosphate levels at 3 hours of reperfusion after brief coronary artery occlusions, suggesting a decrease in the release of inorganic phosphate during early reperfusion. These results are consistent with the observation that dazmegrel pretreatment has been shown to decrease the release of inorganic phosphate during early reperfusion. In a model utilizing multiple 3-minute ischemic periods, preocclusion treatment with dazmegrel decreased the release of inorganic phosphate, lactate, and potassium measured from coronary sinus blood during early reperfusion and reduced the oxygen debt required during ischemia (Hoeft et al., 1986). Beneficial effects were suggested to be due, in part, to enhanced flow to ischemic areas and to an increase in PGI_2. The results of these studies would seem to suggest that TxA_2

may play a role in the prolonged postischemic abnormalities in both function and metabolism following a transient ischemic insult in the absence of cell death. However, from the results of studies using TxA_2 synthetase inhibitors, one cannot exclude the possibility that the beneficial effects were not simply due to endoperoxide shunting and not specifically due to a decrease in TxA_2 per se. Herein lies a methodological problem in the sole use of thromboxane synthetase inhibitors to delineate the role of thromboxane in any given experimental or clinical study.

In clinical trials with TxA_2 synthetase inhibitors, single-dose studies have shown short-lived inhibition of TxA_2, little effect on platelet aggregation, and increased levels of PGI_2. In general, this class of drugs has been found to be ineffective in both chronic stable angina (Reuben et al., 1983) and vasospastic angina (Yui et al., 1986), although dosage regimens in these studies may have been inadequate to achieve sustained inhibition of TxA_2. Trials in which substantial inhibition of TxA_2 synthesis was obtained have shown moderate improvement in exercise-induced angina (Hutton et al., 1983). TxA_2 synthetase inhibition has been demonstrated to be efficacious in patients with unstable angina (Hutton et al., 1983) reducing episodes of silent ischemia and documented episodes of angina, and in 11 patients administered a TxA_2 synthetase inhibitor within 6 hours of onset of chest pain, plasma creatine kinase was reduced (Tada et al., 1985).

B. Thromboxane A_2 (TxA_2) Receptor Blockade

While inhibition of TxA_2 synthesis has been shown to have beneficial effects in many models of experimental ischemia, blockade of TxA_2 receptors may offer a potential theoretical advantage since these agents also antagonize prostaglandin endoperoxides and possibly $PGF_{2\alpha}$, which are thought to have overlapping activity at the same receptors. Pretreatment with a TxA_2 receptor antagonist, but not a synthesis inhibitor, was protective in a thrombotic model of sudden death (Lefer and Darius, 1987). Another potential advantage to TxA_2 receptor blockers over synthesis inhibitors is that TxA_2 receptor antagonists, in contrast to synthesis inhibitors, do not generate bisenoic prostaglandins, which may be deterimental in certain situations. A TxA_2 receptor antagonist would be expected to inhibit many of the postulated pathogenic effects of TxA_2 such as local vasoconstriction, bronchoconstriction, platelet aggregation, and membrane labilization. Moreover, blockade of TxA_2 receptors has been shown to inhibit cyclical reductions in blood flow in concentrically narrowed arteries and reduce the incidence and severity of both ischemia and reperfusion-induced arrhythmias. TxA_2 receptor blockers have consistently proven to be efficacious in decreasing infarct size and limiting ischemic damage during prolonged coronary artery occlusions in rats, cats, and dogs (Bhat et al., 1989; Grover and Schumacher, 1988). As stated earlier, the pathophysiological importance of thromboxane release from the postischemic myocardium in mediating the prolonged postischemic dysfunction in the stunned myocardium, although suggested by the studies with dazmegrel, does not definitively elucidate the role of thromboxane in this model.

The effects of BM 13.505, a potent TxA_2 receptor antagonist, were recently studied in the stunned canine myocardium (Farber et al., 1988a; Farber and Gross, 1990). BM 13.505 was administered at either 0.5 or 10 mg/kg, doses that significantly attenuated increases in aortic systolic and diastolic pressures produced by the TxA_2 analog, U46619. BM 13.505 had no effect on levels of TxA_2 or PGI_2 during occlusion or reperfusion, while the control group showed significant increases in TxA_2 concentrations in coronary venous blood by 3 hours of reperfusion. Preocclusion treatment with BM 13.505 did not affect hemodynamics, regional myocardial blood flow, or myocardial oxygen demand. In contrast to results with TxA_2 synthetase inhibition, TxA_2 receptor blockade with BM 13.505 did not alter the severity of the ischemic insult. There were no beneficial effects on postischemic myocardial contractile function (Fig. 4), nor were there any beneficial effects on myocardial content of adenine nucleotides in the stunned myocardium. Also, increased postischemic tissue edema, which was significantly reduced by dazmegrel (Farber et al., 1988a) was not affected by BM 13.505 treatment.

Thus, if TxA_2 were involved in myocardial stunning, pretreatment with BM 13.505 would be expected to have blocked all TxA_2-mediated effects and enhance functional and/or metabolic recovery. The results of these studies by Farber and colleagues (1988a, 1990) are not in agreement with those of Grover and Fulmor (1988), who found that a different TxA_2 receptor antagonist, SQ 29,548, enhanced the recovery of regional segment shortening (60% vs. 25%) in stunned myocardium of dogs subjected to 15 minutes of coronary artery occlusion followed by 5 hours of reperfusion (Fig. 5). In the study of Grover and Fulmor (1988) it was not determined if TxA_2 was elevated at any time during ischemia or reperfusion, and effects on myocardial metabolism by the receptor blocker were not addressed in that study. Grover and Fulmor (1988) observed beneficial effects by TxA_2 receptor blockade on functional recovery when the drug was given 15 minutes prior to coronary occlusion or immediately prior to reperfusion. It is interesting to note that functional recovery as a percent of baseline was greater at 5 hours of reperfusion when the drug was given immediately prior to reperfusion as compared to preocclusion treatment (80% vs. 60%). The beneficial effects of SQ 29,548 when given during reperfusion were not consistent throughout reperfusion as functional recovery was enhanced early, then returned to control levels and again significantly increased by 3 hours of reperfusion. SQ 29,548 had no beneficial effect on myocardial oxygen supply/consumption balance and

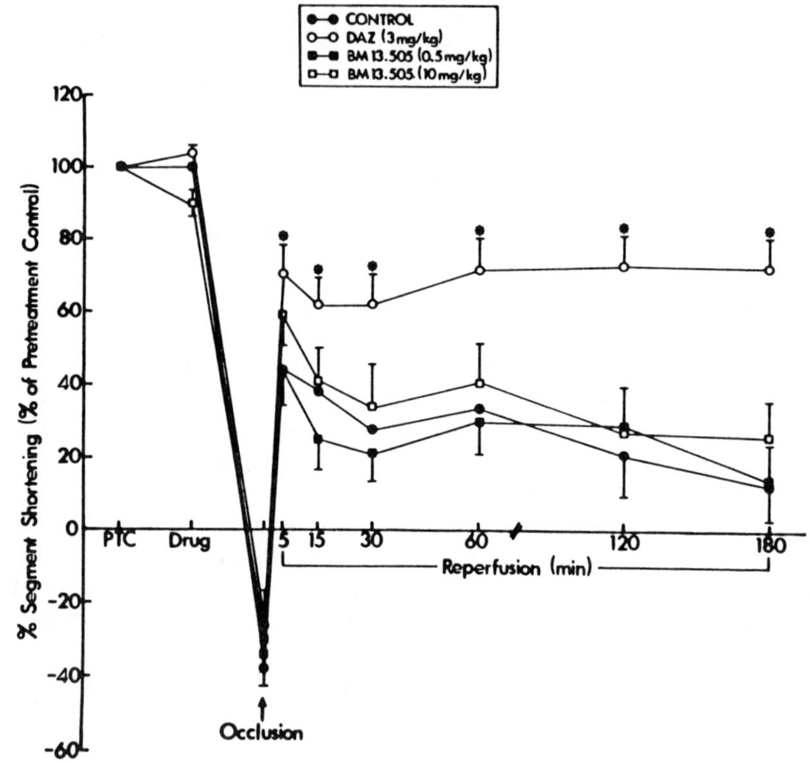

Figure 4 Percent segment shortening of pretreatment control (PTC) in the ischemic-reperfused area at PTC, 10 minutes postdrug (Drug), coronary occlusion, and during reperfusion. Time course curves for control, dazmegrel (DAZ), and BM 13.505 are shown. *, Significant difference ($p < 0.05$) versus control group. (Reprinted by permission from Farber and Gross, 1990.)

was postulated to be cardioprotective by virtue of its ability to block TxA_2 receptors and perhaps by attenuating an effect of TxA_2 on neutrophil activation or chemotaxis (Grover and Fulmor, 1988). While TxA_2 is known to be released from neutrophils, the effect of TxA_2 on neutrophils in reversible myocardial ischemia has not been investigated. Recently, Ito and coworkers (1989) showed that intracoronary administration of C5a produced increases in TxA_2 production in addition to leukocyte trapping and a reduction in blood flow and regional contractile function. Cyclooxygenase blockade decreased TxA_2 production but did not alter changes in flow, function, or neutrophil accumulation, suggesting that neutrophil accumulation, at least in their model, was not TxA_2-mediated.

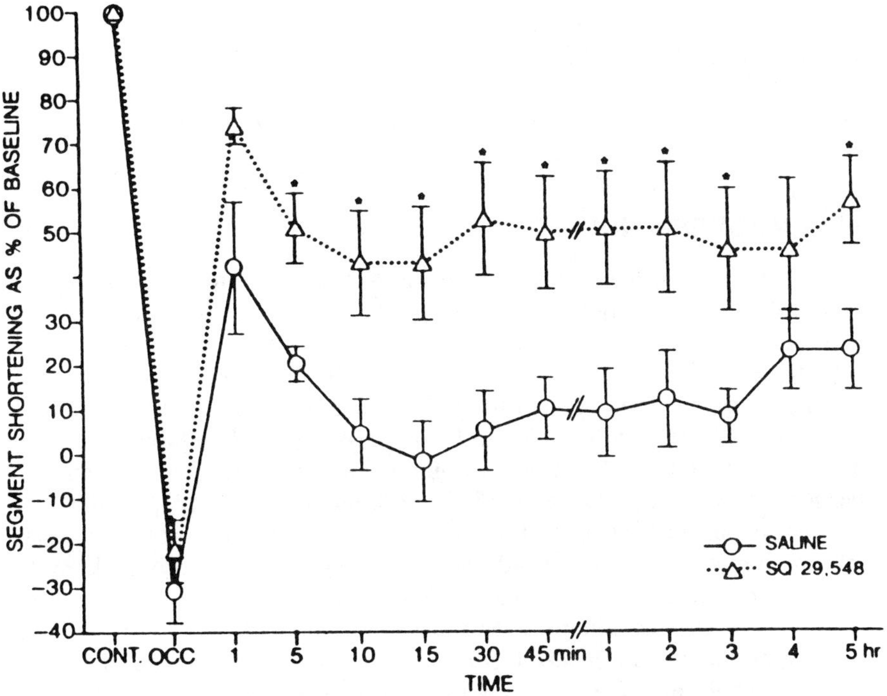

Figure 5 Effect of thromboxane receptor blockade with i.v. SQ 29,548 (0.20 mg/kg + 0.20 mg/kg/hr) versus saline on percent segment shortening (of preocclusion values) in the ischemic-reperfused region at control (CONT), during LAD occlusion (OCC), and during 5 hours of reperfusion. *, Significant difference ($p < 0.05$) versus saline group. (Reprinted by permission from Grover and Fulmor, 1988.)

Reasons for the differences in results between the study of Grover and Fulmor (1988) and that of Farber and Gross (1990) are not readily apparent but may be related to the experimental model (stenosis model used by Farber and Gross) or to differences in the properties of the receptor antagonists studied. However, both these agents have been shown to significantly block TxA_2 receptors in vitro, and both have been demonstrated to decrease infarct size in experimental models (Bhat et al., 1989; Grover and Schumacher, 1988). SQ 29,548 has also been found to reduce ST-segment elevation during pacing-induced ischemia perhaps in part by improving subendocardial blood flow (Grover and Parham, 1989). These findings are in contrast to those of clinical studies with TxA_2 receptor antagonists suggesting that there is no benefit in patients with exercise-induced angina (De Bono et al., 1986). In other models of cardiovascular disease, BM 13.177, the less potent precursor of BM 13.505, has proven beneficial in preventing restenosis after angioplasty and occlusion of coronary artery bypass grafts (Ludwig et al., 1987; Torka et al., 1988). Based on results using TxA_2 receptor antagonists it is clear that TxA_2 may well play a role as a mediator in irreversible myocardial ischemic damage, however, its role as a mediator in myocardial stunning has not been clearly defined.

IV. ENDOPEROXIDE STEAL

It has been well documented that while a TxA_2 synthetase inhibitor selectively blocks the transformation of cyclic endoperoxides into TxA_2, it also results in a reorientation of these endoperoxides and increased formation of prostaglandins $F_{2\alpha}$, E_2, D_2, and I_2 (Aiken et al., 1981). Therefore, a TxA_2 synthetase inhibitor may be expected to show effects that are possibly more detrimental or beneficial than would be observed by solely inhibiting TxA_2, depending upon the type of prostaglandins that are increased and their effects on the system being observed. The accumulation of endoperoxide intermediates in the platelet and neutrophil that occurs with TxA_2 synthesis inhibition may be donated to endothelial PGI_2 synthase by a process known as "endoperoxide steal." Endoperoxide steal has been shown to occur in a variety of species including rats, rabbits, dogs, and humans.

Also, an increase in the production of these prostanoids, as well as prostacyclin, would be possible in endothelium or leukocytes by conversion of endoperoxides released from platelets or from arachidonic acid released from tissues as a result of membrane damage. Prostacyclin could potentially inhibit many thromboxane-mediated events, such as vasoconstriction, platelet aggregation, cell membrane destabilization, catecholamine release, and profibrillatory action. By altering the ratio of thromboxane-prostacyclin in favor of the vasodilatory prostacyclin, myocardial perfusion at the microcirculatory level may be enhanced. On the other hand, the endoperoxides (PGG_2 and PGH_2) that accumulate have a profile of action similar to that of TxA_2 and may theoretically worsen a given disease state if TxA_2 is indeed a mediator. The effects of $PGF_{2\alpha}$, PGD_2, and PGE_2 on the functional recovery of the stunned myocardium are unknown.

To eliminate the possibility of confounding effects due to the endoperoxide steal phenomenon and to more clearly delineate the role of TxA_2 in myocardial stunning, Farber and Gross (1990) studied a group of dogs that were pretreated with indomethacin (5 mg/kg) to prevent endogenous prostanoid effects and then given the TxA_2 synthetase inhibitor dazmegrel prior to coronary artery occlusion. Coronary venous TxA_2 concentrations were significantly decreased prior to and during occlusion and throughout reperfusion (see Fig. 1). However, in contrast to dazmegrel treatment alone where a significant endoperoxide shunting to PGI_2 occurred, treatment with indomethacin + dazmegrel abolished the endoperoxide steal and PGI_2 levels were significantly depressed throughout the experiment (see Fig. 2). There were no effects observed after indomethacin and dazmegrel treatment in terms of oxygen supply (regional myocardial blood flow) during occlusion or reperfusion, and changes in myocardial oxygen demand were not significant. Importantly, while pretreatment with indomethacin significantly prevented the dazmegrel-induced increase in PGI_2, it also completely inhibited the beneficial effects of dazmegrel on both postischemic function (see Fig. 3) and metabolism in the stunned myocardium. It was felt that these results, along with those of BM 13.505, provide conclusive evidence that TxA_2 does not act as a mediator of myocardial stunning and that the cardioprotection exhibited during TxA_2 synthetase inhibition was due to the endoperoxide steal phenomenon (most likely the increase in PGI_2), and not directly due to the inhibition of TxA_2 (Farber and Gross, 1990).

While the finding that the beneficial action of a TxA_2 synthetase inhibitor in the stunned myocardium is via an increase in PGI_2 is a relatively recent development, previous studies have shown similar mechanisms in other models. Aiken and colleagues (1981) showed that endogenous PGI_2 was responsible for inhibiting coronary artery thrombosis following TxA_2 synthetase inhibition. The inhibition of superoxide production by human neutrophils after TxA_2 synthetase inhibition was found to be platelet dependent and most likely via an increase in PGI_2 (Mehta et al., 1988). Finally, Mullane and Fornabaio (1988) described a platelet-dependent mechanism in infarct size reduction by TxA_2 synthesis inhibition. This reduction in infarct size was also aspirin sensitive, showing definitively that the effect was mediated by endoperoxide shunting.

If the hypothesis that endogenous PGI_2 mediates the beneficial effects observed in the stunned myocardium after TxA_2 synthetase inhibition is correct, this should predict that exogenous administration of PGI_2 or a PGI_2 analog should mimic these cardioprotective actions. Indeed, Farber and coworkers (1988c) have shown that the PGI_2 analog iloprost significantly enhances functional and metabolic recovery in the stunned canine myocardium. The mechanism for the beneficial effects were postulated to be due, in part, to an inhibition of neutrophil-derived oxygen free radicals. Also, the vasodilatory prostanoid, PGE_1, was found to have similar cardioprotective actions in the stunned myocardium (Farber and Gross, 1989). The treatment of the stunned myocardium with prostaglandins will be discussed more fully in Chapter 13.

V. CONCLUSION

The inhibition of arachidonic acid metabolism through the cyclooxygenase pathway by the NSAID indomethacin provided no beneficial effect on func-

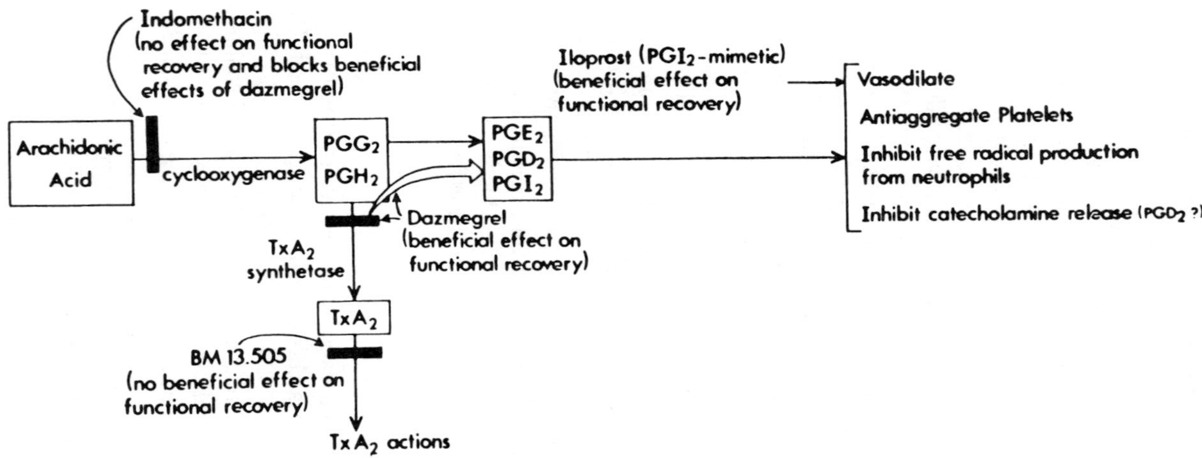

Figure 6 Schematic representation of the drugs used in blocking the formation or action of thromboxane A_2 (TxA_2), the pharmacological actions of the drugs, and the effects on postischemic functional recovery in the stunned myocardium. Possible prostaglandin-mediated beneficial mechanisms are also presented. (Reprinted by permission from Farber and Gross, 1990.)

tional or metabolic recovery during myocardial stunning. However, blockade of cyclooxygenase also decreases the production of the vasodilatory and cardioprotective prostanoid PGI_2. The TxA_2 receptor antagonist BM 13.505 provided no cardioprotective effects on regional postischemic function or metabolism although SQ 29,548, another TxA_2 receptor blocker, has been shown to have beneficial effects on functional recovery during reperfusion.

The TxA_2 synthetase inhibitor dazmegrel was cardioprotective in the stunned myocardium leading to greater postischemic myocardial function in addition to preservation of adenine nucleotides. Dazmegrel reduced coronary venous TxA_2 levels and also markedly increased PGI_2 levels, presumably by endoperoxide steal. When dogs were pretreated with indomethacin to block the dazmegrel-induced rise in PGI_2, the beneficial effects on function and metabolism were also abolished.

Thus, unlike in other models of ischemic injury, TxA_2 does not appear to be involved in reversible postischemic dysfunction, and inhibition of TxA_2 synthesis significantly attenuates postischemic dysfunction in the stunned myocardium only in the presence of enhanced prostacyclin production. Based on these conclusions, manipulating the TxA_2/PGI_2 balance would only be beneficial if PGI_2 levels were elevated exogenously or endogenously.

There remains a need for further studies investigating products of both the cyclooxygenase and lipoxygenase pathways in reversible myocardial ischemic injury. For example, experiments defining the role of other prostaglandins or the effect of combined TxA_2 synthetase inhibition and receptor blockade that would eliminate deleterious effects of cyclic endoperoxides are needed (Fig. 6)

Obviously, extrapolation of these findings to clinical situations must be extremely cautious; interventions to improve postischemic recovery in patients with acute ischemic heart disease and absent or minimal tissue necrosis may need to focus on increasing prostacyclin levels endogenously or exogenously, unless a specific model of cardiovascular disease is demonstrated to be mediated by TxA_2. Clinically, the increase in endoperoxides after TxA_2 synthetase inhibition as well as inadequate dosing regimens have yielded some disappointing results. Further large-scale investigations with both TxA_2 synthetase inhibitors and TxA_2 receptor antagonists are needed to more fully delineate the clinical potential of these agents.

REFERENCES

Aiken, J. W., Shebuski, R. J., Miller, O. V., and Gorman, R. R. (1981). Endogenous prostacyclin contributes to the efficacy of a thromboxane synthetase inhibitor for preventing coronary artery thrombosis. *J. Pharmacol. Exp. Ther. 219*: 299.

Bhat, A. M., Sacks, H. S., Osborne, J. A., and Lefer, A. M. (1989). Protective effect of the specific thromboxane receptor antagonist, BM-13.505, in reperfusion injury following acute myocardial ischemia in cats. *Am. Heart J. 117*: 799.

De Bono, D. P., Lumley, P., Been, M., Keery, R., Ince, S. E., and Woodings, D. E. (1986). Effect of the specific thromboxane receptor blocking drug AH23848 in patients with angina pectoris. *Br. Heart J. 56*: 509.

Farber, N. E., Pieper, G. M., and Gross, G. J. (1987). Regional differences in postischemic recovery in the stunned canine myocardium. *Am. Heart J. 114*: 1086.

Farber, N. E., Pieper, G. M., and Gross, G. J. (1988a). Lack of involvement of thromboxane A2 in postischemic recovery of stunned canine myocardium. *Circulation 78*: 450.

Farber, N. E., Pieper, G. M., and Gross, G. J. (1988b). Postischemic recovery with stunned myocardium after reperfusion in the presence or absence of a flow-limiting coronary artery stenosis. *Am. Heart J. 116*: 407.

Farber, N. E., Pieper, G. M., Thomas, J. P., and Gross, G. J. (1988c). Beneficial effects of iloprost in the stunned canine myocardium. *Circ. Res. 62*: 204.

Farber, N. E., and Gross, G. J. (1989). Prostaglandin E1 attenuates postischemic contractile dysfunction after brief coronary occlusion and reperfusion. *Am. Heart J. 118*: 17.

Farber, N. E., and Gross, G. J. (1990). Prostaglandin redirection by thromboxane synthetase inhibition. Attenuation of myocardial stunning in canine heart. *Circulation 81*: 369.

FitzGerald, G. A., Healy, C., and Daugherty, J. (1987). Thromboxane A_2 biosynthesis in human disease. *Federation Proc. 46*: 154.

Grover, G. J., and Fulmor, I. E. (1988). Thromboxane A_2 antagonist and diltiazem-induced enhancement of contractile function: The effect of timing of treatment. *J. Pharmacol. & Exp. Ther. 247*: 445.

Grover, G. J., and Schumacher, W. A. (1988). Effect of the thromboxane receptor antagonist SQ 29,548 on myocardial infarct size in dogs. *J. Cardiovasc. Pharmacol. 11*: 29.

Grover, G. J., and Parham, C. S. (1989). Role of thromboxane A_2 in the control of myocardial O_2 supply/consumption balance and severity of ischemia during pacing-induced ischemia. *Circ. Res. 64*: 575.

Hock, C. E., and Lefer, A. M. (1986). CGS-12970, a thromboxane synthetase inhibitor, limits ischemic damage following coronary artery occlusion. *Res. Comm. Path. Pharmacol. 52*: 285.

Hoeft, A., Korb, H., Bock, J., Wolpers, H. G., Wober, W., and Hellige, G. (1986). Preservation of myocardium in transient ischemia by the thromboxane synthetase inhibitor UK 38.485. *Res. Exp. Med. 186*: 35.

Hutton, I., Tweddel, A. C., Rankin, A. C., Walker, I. D., and Davidson, J. F. (1983). Effect of dazoxiben on transcardiac thromboxane levels and haemodynamics in coronary heart disease. *Br. J. Clin. Pharmacol. 15*: 79S.

Ito, B. R., Roth, D. M., Chenoweth, D. E., Lefer, A. M., and Engler, R. L. (1989). Thromboxane is produced in response to intracoronary infusion of complement C5a in pigs. Cyclooxygenase blockade does not reduce the myocardial ischemia and leukocyte accumulation. *Circ. Res. 65*: 1220.

Jolly, S. R. and Lucchesi, B. R. (1983). Effect of BW755C in an occlusion-reperfusion model of ischemic myocardial injury. *Am. Heart J. 106*: 8.

Jugdutt, B. I., Hutchins, G. M., Bulkley, B. H., Pitt, B., and Becker, L. C. (1979). Effect of indomethacin on collateral blood flow and infarct size in the conscious dog. *Circulation 59*: 734.

Karmazyn, M. (1983). Reduction of enzyme release from reperfused ischemic hearts by steroidal and nonsteroidal prostaglandin synthesis inhibitors. *Prost. Leuk. Med. 11*: 299.

Kirlin, P. C., Romson, J. L., Pitt, B., Abrams, G. D., Schork, M. A., and Lucchesi, B. R. (1982). Ibuprofen-mediated infarct size reduction: Effects on regional myocardial function in canine myocardial infarction. *Am. J. Cardiol. 50*: 849.

Lefer, A. M., and Darius, H. (1987). A pharmacological approach to thromboxane receptor antagonism. *Fed. Proc. 46*: 144.

Lepran, I., Koltai, M., and Szekeres, L. (1981). Effect of non-steroid anti-inflammatory drugs in experimental myocardial infarction in rats. *Eur. J. Pharmacol. 69*: 235.

Lewis, H. D. Jr., Davis, J. W., Archibald, D. G., Steinke, W. E., Smitherman, T. C., Doherty, J. E., Schnaper, H. W., LeWinter, M. M., Linares, E., Pouget, J. M., Sabharwal, S. C., Chesler, E., and De Mots, H. (1983). Protective effects of aspirin against acute myocardial infarction and death in men with unstable angina. Results of a Veterans Administration Cooperative Study. *N. Engl. J. Med. 309*: 396.

Ludwig, B., Hofling, B., Stablein, A., and von Arnim, T. (1987). Thromboxane-antagonist BM 13.177 compared to aspirin in preventing restenosis after PTCA (abstract). *Eur. Heart J. 8*: 225.

Mehta, P., and Mehta, J. (1979). Platelet function studies in coronary artery disease. V. Evidence for enhanced platelet microthrombus formation activity in acute myocardial infarction. *Am. J. Cardiol. 43*: 757.

Mehta, J. L., Lawson, D., and Mehta, P. (1988). Modulation of human neutrophil superoxide production by selective thromboxane synthetase inhibitor U63,557A. *Life Sciences 43*: 923.

Mullane, K. M., and McGiff, J. C. (1985). Platelet depletion and infarct size in an occlusion-reperfusion model of myocardial ischemia in anesthetized dogs. *J. Cardiovasc. Pharmacol. 7*: 733.

Mullane, K. M., and Fornabaio, D. (1988). Thromboxane synthetase inhibitors reduce infarct size by a platelet-dependent, aspirin-sensitive mechanism. *Circ. Res. 62*: 668.

Ogletree, M. L. (1987). Overview of physiological and pathophysiological effects of thromboxane A_2. *Federation Proc. 46*: 133.

Pieper, G. M., Farber, N. E., and Gross, G. J. (1988). Metabolic protection of the reperfused canine endocardium by the thromboxane synthetase inhibitor, dazoxiben. *Prost. Leuk. Essential Fatty Acids 33*: 13.

Reuben, S. R., Kuan, P., Cairns, T., and Gysle, O. H. (1983). Effects of dazoxiben and exercise performance in chronic stable angina. *Br. J. Clin. Pharmacol. 15*: 83S.

Sobel, M., Salzman, E. W., Davies, G. C., Handin, R. I., Sweeney, J., Ploetz, J., and Kurland, G. (1981). Circulating platelet products in unstable angina pectoris. *Circulation 63*: 300.

Tada, M., Hoshida, S., Kuzuya, T., Inoue, M., Minamino, T., and Abe, H. (1985). Augmented thromboxane A_2 generation and efficacy of its blockade in acute myocardial infarction. *Int. J. Cardiol. 8*: 301.

Torka, M. C., Hacker, R. W., Yukseltan, I., Pohlmann, V., Meier, P., Zimmerman, T., Etti, H., Bulitta, M., and Kondor, P. (1988). Reduction of the vein graft occlusion rate after coronary artery bypass surgery by treatment with a thromboxane receptor antagonist. *Eur. Heart. J. 9*: 325 (Abstract).

Wargovich, T. J., Mehta, J., Nichols, W. W., Ward, M. B., Lawson, D., Franzini, D., and Conti, C. R. (1987). Reduction in myocardial neutrophil accumulation and infarct size following administration of thromboxane inhibitor U-63,557A. *Am. Heart J. 114*: 1078.

Yui, Y., Hattori, R., Takatsu, Y., and Kawai, C. (1986). Selective thromboxane A_2 synthetase inhibition in vasospastic angina pectoris. *J. Am. Coll. Cardiol. 7*: 25.

11

Other Theories

Myths, Fads, or Facts?

Karin Przyklenk and Peter Whittaker

Hospital of the Good Samaritan and University of Southern California, Los Angeles, California

I. INTRODUCTION

Experimental evidence obtained by numerous investigators during the past 5 years strongly supports the hypotheses that production of oxygen-derived free radicals, abnormal calcium homeostasis, and alterations in the cyclooxygenase pathway all play a prominent role in the pathogenesis of the stunned myocardium. Even more recently, popular opinion favors the concept of a "unifying hypothesis": that is, the belief that any or all of these three mechanisms are interrelated. However, it must be recognized that these were by no means the first—or the only—mechanisms that have been proposed to explain the enigma of postischemic contractile dysfunction. In fact, explanations for the stunned myocardium have not been confined to the myocyte: perturbations in virtually every component of the heart (including the vasculature, the conduction pathway, and the collagen framework) have been implicated as potential causes of this postischemic dysfunction. Our objective in this chapter is to review these "other" mechanisms for the stunned myocardium, how and why these theories were proposed, and the subsequent evidence that, in many cases, has lead to their demise.

II. METABOLIC PERTURBATIONS

The stunned myocardium is characterized both by depressed contractile function and partial depletion of adenosine triphosphate (ATP) and adenosine diphosphate (ADP) stores. For example, subendocardial ATP content following 15 minutes of transient coronary artery occlusion in the canine model remains significantly depressed at 80% of baseline values for at least the initial 3 days of reflow (DeBoer et al., 1980). In addition, recovery of function following reperfusion was initially shown by some investigators to parallel recovery of ATP content (Ellis et al., 1983; Kloner et al., 1983). As myocardial contractility is clearly dependent upon adequate energy supply, it is tempting to speculate a cause-and-effect relationship between abnormalities in high-energy phosphate metabolism and postischemic contractile dysfunction. In fact, the stunned myocardium could theoretically be a consequence of three interrelated metabolic perturbations: impaired mitochondrial function, depleted energy stores, and/or abnormal energy utilization.

A. Impaired Mitochondrial Function

Although myocardial ATP stores remain depressed for prolonged periods following reperfusion, creatine phosphate (CP) content in the stunned tissue rapidly rebounds to 120–150% of normal, preocclusion values following reflow (DeBoer et al., 1980; Reimer et al., 1981; Swain et al., 1982; Ellis et al., 1983; Przyklenk and Kloner, 1989a; 1989b). As CP can only be produced by the phosphorylation of creatine by ATP, this "over-shoot" in CP to supranormal values indicates that oxidative phosphorylation is rapidly resumed upon restoration of blood flow to the stunned tissue (Greenfield and Swain, 1987). In addition, Ambrosio et al. (1987) have demonstrated that the rate of ATP turnover in isolated hearts stunned by a brief episode of global ischemia can be increased to match the increased energy demand caused by inotropic stimulation with isoproterenol. These data suggest that mitochondrial function is not impaired in the stunned myocardium.

B. Depletion of Energy Stores

1. Adenosine Triphosphate

While oxidative phosphorylation may resume upon restoration of blood flow to the stunned tissue, the fact remains that ATP concentrations remain significantly depressed during the initial days following reperfusion. Considerable evidence indicates that this slow recovery of myocardial ATP content is a consequence of the washout of nucleotide precursors from the ischemic myocardium at the time of reflow (Humphrey et al., 1985). That is, the stunned myocytes lack the necessary substrates for rapid resynthesis of ATP via the "salvage pathway" and must therefore produce ATP by the slower "de novo" pathway (DeBoer et al., 1980; Reimer et al., 1981; Swain et al., 1982). Given the apparent temporal relationship between recovery of contractile function and restoration of normal ATP stores, it is not surprising that depletion of ATP became one of the first factors that showed promise as a potential explanation for the stunned myocardium (Braunwald and Kloner, 1982).

Experimental evidence *has not*, however, supported this initially tempting hypothesis. In fact, four independent lines of evidence argue against this concept. As reviewed in detail in Chapter 13, a host of laboratories have demonstrated that the stunned myocardium can be forced to contract at normal—or even supranormal—levels for a sustained period of time by infusion of inotropic agents such as dopamine, isoproterenol, epinephrine, and hydralazine (Ellis et al., 1984; Bolli et al., 1985; Arnold et al., 1985; Becker et al., 1986; Ambrosio et al., 1987; Przyklenk and Kloner, 1989a). Furthermore, this recruitment was not accompanied by a further decrease in ATP content (Arnold et al., 1985; Ambrosio et al., 1987; Przyklenk and Kloner, 1989a), indicating that energy production and stores in the stunned postischemic tissue are sufficient to maintain normal contraction. Second, repletion of ATP stores in stunned myocardium by administration of exogenous adenine nucleotide precursors does not result in enhanced contractile function. For example, administration of adenosine following 20 minutes of global ischemia in isolated rat hearts increased ATP content from 65% of baseline at the time of reflow to 85% of normal at 2 hours following reperfusion. However, developed pressure in hearts treated with adenosine remained unchanged at 70–80% of normal throughout reperfusion (Fig. 1) (Ambrosio et al., 1989). Similar results have also been obtained in anesthetized open-chest dogs subjected to 45 minutes of transient coronary artery occlusion: adenosine given during reperfusion increased ATP content of the previously ischemic tissue, but had no effect on segment shortening (Hoffmeister et al., 1985). Third, depleting total ATP content (Kupriyanov et al., 1987) or the adenine nucleotide pool (Zucchi et al., 1990) in the absence of ischemia to values lower than those observed in stunned, previously ischemic tissue did not compromise the contractile performance of isolated perfused rat hearts. Finally, paired measurement of high-energy phosphate stores and contractile function in both in vivo and in vitro models of transient ischemia have revealed that ATP content of the stunned tissue does not correlate with or "predict" its function during the initial hours following reflow (Fig. 2) (Neely and Grotyohann, 1984; Taegtmeyer et al., 1985; Glower et al., 1987; Przyklenk and Kloner, 1989b).

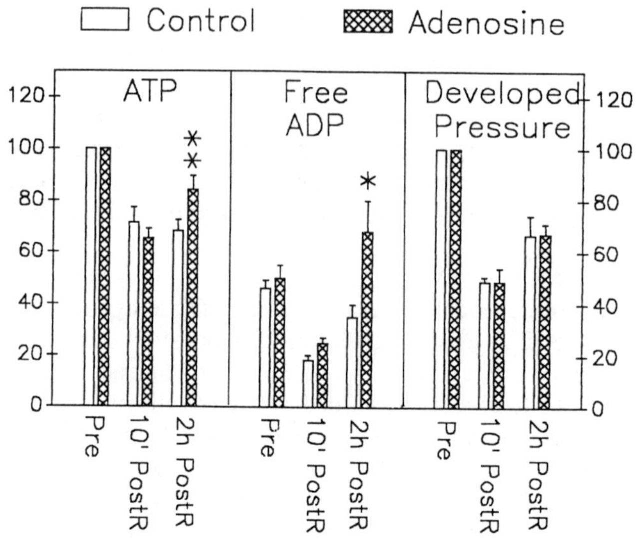

Figure 1 Effect of adenosine administration on recovery of ATP content (% of baseline), free ADP concentration (mM), and developed pressure (% of baseline) in isolated perfused rabbit hearts subjected to 20 minutes of global ischemia and 2 hours of reperfusion. Pre = preischemia baseline; R = reperfusion. $*p < 0.01$ vs. control; $**p < 0.001$ vs. 10 minutes postreperfusion by paired t-test. (Adapted with permission from Ambrosio et al., 1989.)

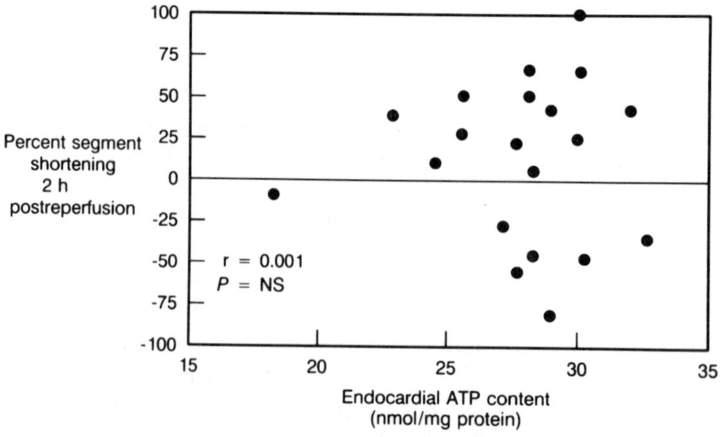

Figure 2 Adenosine triphosphate content versus contractile function postreperfusion. Segment shortening measured after reperfusion as a function of endocardial ATP content in canine myocardium stunned by 15 minutes of coronary artery occlusion. (Reprinted with permission from Przyklenk and Kloner, 1989b.)

2. Adenosine Diphosphate

The stunned myocardium also exhibits reduced concentrations of free ADP, which serves as a substrate for ATP regeneration at the myofibrils via the creatine kinase reaction (Greenfield and Swain, 1987; Ambrosio et al., 1989). Moreover, it has been suggested that the concentration of free cytosolic ADP may control mitochondrial respiration (Jacobus, 1985; Clarke et al., 1987). Using isolated guinea pig hearts stunned by 2.43 minutes of global ischemia, Clarke et al. (1987) further concluded that the "cytosolic phosphorylation potential" (i.e., [ATP]/[ADP]x[inorganic phosphate]) is the crucial metabolic factor in the control of myocardial contraction, perhaps by acting as the link between mitochondrial ATP synthesis and its utilization at the site of the contractile proteins. Ambrosio and colleagues (1989) found that administration of adenosine, in addition to increasing ATP content, also resulted in complete restoration of free ADP in the stunned rabbit hearts. However, as discussed previously, restoration of ATP and ADP stores failed to elicit a concomitant improvement in developed pressure of the stunned ventricles (see Fig. 1).

These data demonstrate that the depressed ATP stores characteristic of the stunned myocardium are due to a limited supply of the substrates (such as nucleotide precursors and ADP) needed for rapid resynthesis. However, the overwhelming evidence of a dissociation between recovery of contractile function and recovery of ATP and ADP content clearly lays to rest the theory that the stunned myocardium is a consequence of depleted or limited energy supply.

C. Abnormal Energy Utilization

While ATP depletion per se does not represent the mechanism for the stunned myocardium, this does not preclude the possibility that other metabolic perturbations triggered by transient ischemia may play a role in mediating postischemic contractile dysfunction. For example, Greenfield and Swain (1987) logically proposed that impaired transduction, or utilization of the available ATP by the contractile units, could also lead to the impaired mechanical function of the stunned myocardium.

By analyzing tissue samples from canine myocardium subjected to 15 minutes of coronary artery occlusion and 15 minutes of reflow, Greenfield and Swain (1987) observed two factors that could contribute to disruption of energy utilization: an estimated 50% reduction (based on mathematical calculation) in free ADP concentration, the substrate needed for rephosphorylation of ADP to ATP at the contraction site by the creatine kinase pathway, and a 17% reduction in the concentration to creatine kinase bound to the myofilaments. More recently, however, Krause (1990) found that the concentration of creatine kinase bound to myofilaments (determined by assay) was not altered in isolated rabbit hearts stunned by 15 minutes of global ischemia when compared with normally perfused controls. Furthermore, myofibrillar ATPase activity, which, coupled to creatine kinase, is an essential component in the resynthesis of ATP, did not differ between stunned vs. control hearts (Krause, 1990). That is, Krause convincingly demonstrated using continuous assay techniques that the kinetics of ATP transduction at the site of the contractile proteins via myosin-bound creatine kinase was normal in the stunned myocardium.

III. CIRCULATORY PERTURBATIONS

A. Low Reflow

Reperfusion of viable, previously ischemic myocardium does not ensure restoration of normal blood flow to the reversibly injured tissue. Rather, measurement of regional myocardial blood flow by injection of radiolabeled microspheres has revealed that perfusion of the stunned, previously ischemic tissue is often mildly depressed at 60–80% of normal. This phenomenon, termed low reflow, has been observed in myocardium stunned by a brief ischemic insult (Heyndrickx et al., 1978; Przyklenk and Kloner, 1989b; Bolli et al., 1990), and in viable subepicardium salvaged following prolonged coronary occlusion (Kloner and Alker, 1984). In fact, in their seminal reports of stunned myocardium following brief transient ischemia, Heyndrickx et al. (1975, 1978) suggested that the contractile dysfunction observed following reperfusion may be explained in part by this mild residual depression in blood flow.

Does low reflow represent a tenable mechanism for the stunned myocardium? The magnitude of flow reduction as detected by the radioactive microsphere technique (i.e., in the relatively large 1-g blocks of tissue used for analysis) is clearly not sufficient to compromise contractile function. That is, ongoing regional ischemia following removal of the coronary artery obstruction clearly is not an issue. In addition, retrospective regression analysis of data from four previous studies in our laboratory convincingly demonstrates that myocardial blood flow measured 2–2.5 hours following reperfusion does not correlate with or predict recovery of contractile function of canine myocardium stunned by 15 minutes of coronary artery occlusion (Przyklenk and Kloner, 1989b) (Fig. 3).

B. Role of the Neutrophil

While low reflow per se cannot account for the persistent hypokinesis observed following reperfusion, one of the potential culprits of low reflow—the neutrophil—has been implicated as an important mediator of the stunned

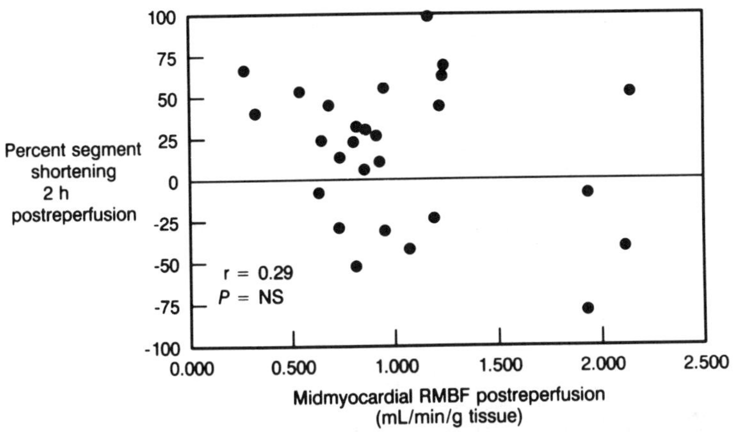

Figure 3 Myocardial blood flow postreperfusion versus contractile function postreperfusion. Segment shortening measured after reperfusion as a function of midmyocardial blood flow at 2–2.5 hours following reflow in canine myocardium stunned by 15 minutes of coronary artery occlusion. (Reprinted with permission from Przyklenk and Kloner, 1989b.)

myocardium. The first evidence that the neutrophil may contribute to postischemic dysfunction was provided by Engler and Covell (1987), who reported that removal of granulocytes from the coronary blood supply by extracorporeal perfusion through leukocyte filters essentially ablated postischemic contractile dysfunction in anesthetized dogs subjected to 15 minutes of coronary occlusion and 60 minutes of reperfusion (Fig. 4). Similar results were obtained by Westlin and Mullane (1989): Using the same canine model, extracorporeal filtration of blood entering the coronary vascular bed at the time of reperfusion restored segment shortening to 60–80% of preocclusion values, as compared with values of 10–30% observed following reflow in dogs perfused with whole blood. Furthermore, a subsequent return of leukocytes into the extracorporeal circuit during 3 hours of reperfusion was associated with deterioration in contractile function of the stunned tissue. These results lead both groups of investigators to speculate that the neutrophil may cause postischemic dysfunction by acting as a source of cytotoxic metabolites (including oxygen-derived free radicals, platelet activating factor, metabolites of arachidonic acid, and proteolytic enzymes), or by obstructing capillaries and thereby causing discrete foci of ischemia, which may contribute to the low reflow phenomenon (Engler and Covell, 1987; Westlin and Mullane, 1989). The investigators did, however, raise the possibility that additional nonspecific effects of neutrophil filtration (such as reduction in

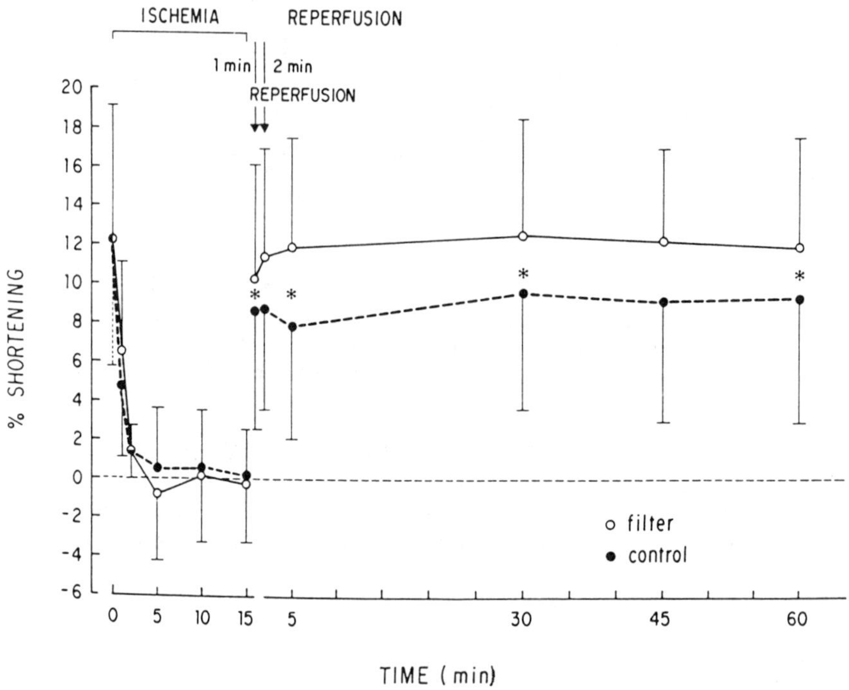

Figure 4 Segment shortening in the anterior ischemic area before ischemia (time = 0), during 15 minutes of ischemia, and during 60 minutes of reperfusion during agranulocytic perfusion (filter) and after filter removal in same dogs (control). $*p < 0.05$ vs. preischemia. (Reprinted from Engler and Covell, 1987, with permission of the American Heart Association.)

blood viscosity and/or activation of the complement system by the filters, resulting in release of adenosine from erythrocytes) may also in part contribute to the enhanced recovery of function (Engler and Covell, 1987; Westlin and Mullane, 1989).

In contrast, numerous other observations argue against the concept that the neutrophil plays a role in postischemic dysfunction following brief transient ischemia. For example, removal of neutrophils in this same canine model by either filtration of blood entering the ischemic/reperfused myocardium, by systemic administration of neutrophil antiserum, or by administration of $F(ab')_2$ fragments of anti-Mo1 monoclonal antibodies has, in the hands of other investigators, failed to enhance contractile function of the stunned myocardium (Fig. 5) (Jeremy and Becker, 1989; O'Neill et al., 1989; Schott et al., 1989). While there is no doubt that reperfusion following prolonged

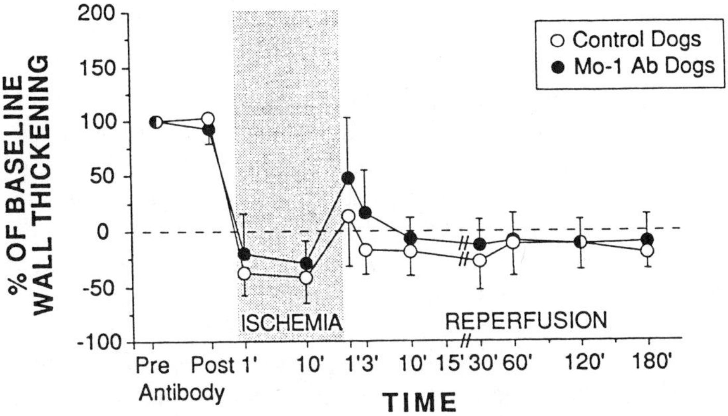

Figure 5 Relative changes in wall thickening in the ischemic myocardium during 15 minutes of coronary artery occlusion and 3 hours of reperfusion in control dogs and those that received $F(ab')_2$ fragments of anti-Mo1 monoclonal antibodies. (Reprinted from Schott et al., 1989, with permission of the American Heart Association.)

(>1 hour) coronary artery occlusion results in a rapid and massive influx of neutrophils into the previously ischemic tissue (Kloner and Alker, 1984), there is no evidence of appreciable neutrophil accumulation (assessed by histological and electron microscopic evaluation, indium labeling, and measurement of myeloperoxidase activity) following relief of a brief, 12- to 15-minute episode of transient ischemia (Kloner et al., 1974; Go et al., 1988; Schott et al., 1989). Furthermore, as described in Chapters 6, 9, and 14, there is no doubt that postischemic contractile dysfunction occurs in the absence of neutrophils in isolated buffer-perfused heart preparations stunned by global ischemia or hypoxia. These data do not preclude the possibility that neutrophils may mediate contractile dysfunction of viable subepicardium following prolonged ischemia/reperfusion—an issue that, to date, has not been specifically addressed. However, these results raise important doubts as to the role of the neutrophil as a primary mediator of the stunned myocardium.

IV. ELECTROPHYSIOLOGICAL ABNORMALITIES

There is no question that normal, synchronous myocardial contraction is dependent upon normal excitation-contraction coupling. In the in vivo canine model, the characteristic ST-segment shifts associated with myocardial ischemia are resolved within 1 minute following reperfusion of reversibly injured tissue (Heyndrickx et al., 1975, 1978). However, two clinical case reports have described parallel improvement in wall motion abnormalities and disappearance of Q waves in patients with angina but without evidence of infarction, implying a transient electrical abnormality of the stunned myocytes (Bashour et al., 1983; Bateman et al., 1983). In fact, experimental evidence obtained by Levine and colleagues (1987) suggested that transient ischemia/reperfusion resulted in profound cellular electrophysiological abnormalities: the resting potential, the action potential amplitude, the rate of depolarization, and the action potential duration were all significantly reduced in previously ischemic vs. normally perfused epicardial tissue harvested from dogs that had undergone 15 minutes of coronary artery occlusion and 20 minutes of reflow. In addition, the stunned tissue exhibited a slower, nonuniform conduction velocity and decreased space constant (i.e., a more rapid decrease in the amplitude of the electronic response as a function of increasing distance from the site of stimulation) when compared with normal myocardial samples. These data suggest that the stunned myocytes exhibited alterations in both active and passive membrane properties and impaired cell coupling and led Levine and colleagues to propose that the abnormalities in the action potentials, depolarization, and conduction may contribute to the impaired contractile function of the stunned myocardium.

In contrast to many of the other mechanisms for postischemic contractile dysfunction that have been proposed, the role of electrophysiological perturbations in the stunned myocardium has not been rigorously pursued. However, in vivo evidence obtained by Hanich et al. (1989) indicates that canine myocardium stunned by 15 minutes of coronary artery occlusion *is not* associated with electrophysiological abnormalities. That is, despite the expected contractile dysfunction observed at 20 minutes following reflow in the canine model, the action potential duration, refractory period, and conduction velocity had returned to normal, baseline values by this time (Hanich et al., 1989). These latter results raise the possibility that the electrophysiological measurements made by Levine et al. (1987) were confounded by isolation and handling of the tissue samples and cast doubt on the causal role of cellular electrophysiological abnormalities in the pathogenesis of the stunned myocardium.

V. IMPAIRED SYMPATHETIC NEURAL RESPONSIVENESS

Despite the overwhelming evidence that the stunned myocardium can be forced or recruited to contract by exogenous administration of inotropic agents, Ciuffo and colleagues (1985) have suggested that postischemic contractile dysfunction may be due to a disruption in the responsiveness of the myocardium to endogenous sympathetic nervous stimulation. Specifically, Ciuffo et al. (1985) found that canine myocardium stunned by 25 minutes of coronary artery occlusion could be recruited to contract at near-normal values by systemic administration of norepinephrine. In contrast, direct stimulation of the left ansa subclavia nerve following reflow failed to increase segment shortening of the stunned tissue. Although the reason for the selective loss of responsiveness to endogenous sympathetic stimulation was not determined, it could not be explained by regional sympathectomy due to surgical preparation or by depletion of norepinephrine from the nerve terminals (Ciuffo et al., 1985).

While the results of Ciuffo and colleagues are intriguing, it must be acknowledged that this is an isolated report based on a sample size of eight animals. This apparent ability of stunned myocytes to recognize—and respond differently to—exogenous vs. endogenous inotropic stimulation is difficult to reconcile and has, to date, neither been confirmed nor discredited. Thus, the decreased responsiveness of stunned myocardium to sympathetic neural stimulation can, at most, be considered an observation: whether this represents a cause or mechanism for postischemic contractile dysfunction awaits further investigation.

VI. MYOCARDIAL COLLAGEN DEGRADATION

Perhaps the most novel mechanism for the stunned myocardium was proposed by Zhao and colleagues (1987), who suggested that damage to the extracellular collagen matrix of the heart by brief ischemia/reperfusion may be responsible for postischemic contractile dysfunction. In fact, the nature and organization of the myocardial collagen network provides a reasonable basis for the concept that damage to the collagen might produce contractile dysfunction. Hearts contain an extensive and highly organized collagen network, which appears to provide—through connections between both individual myocytes and bundles of myocytes—mechanical coupling between and scaffolding for muscle fibers (Robinson et al., 1983). The inherent strength and stiffness of collagen adds credence to the concept that collagen provides a structural framework for the myocytes. Furthermore, disturbances of the myocardial collagen network have been shown to have functional consequences: for example, the increase in collagen content seen in hypertrophic hearts is at least partly responsible for their abnormal function (Weber and Brilla, 1991). Thus, as collagen has been shown to be damaged during ischemia (Sato et al., 1983; Cannon et al., 1983), it was proposed that if the integrity of the collagen matrix was compromised, then the coupling between myocytes and myocyte bundles would also be compromised, and hence contractility would decrease.

To examine this hypothesis, Zhao et al. (1987) subjected anesthetized open-chest dogs to 12 episodes of repeated ischemia (each consisting of 5 minutes of coronary occlusion and 10 minutes of reperfusion), followed by 90 minutes of uninterrupted reflow. At the end of the protocol the percent systolic shortening, measured using sonomicrometry, averaged only 35% of baseline preocclusion values. In addition, the collagen network, qualitatively examined using electron microscopy, appeared to be damaged: many of the collagen connections between myocytes were broken, and, in places, the collagen network appeared to have been completely degraded. Zhao et al. (1987) concluded from these data that the reduction in contractile function was mediated by this disruption of the collagen network.

However, this relationship between collagen damage and the stunned myocardium is difficult to reconcile with other experiments. For example, the improved contractile function obtained when verapamil (Przyklenk and Kloner, 1988) or nifedipine (Przyklenk et al., 1989) was given *after* reperfusion (i.e., after the collagen damage would have occurred) is difficult to explain in terms of this hypothesis. It is unlikely that these agents can reassemble the collagen network.

In addition, the model of stunning that Zhao et al. (1987) used—that of multiple repeated occlusions—appeared to have a greater potential for producing collagen damage than a single 15-minute occlusion. To investigate this possibility, we examined tissue obtained from canine hearts stunned by either repeated occlusion or single coronary occlusion (Whittaker et al., 1991). Although we found a similar degree of contractile dysfunction in both models (segment shortening was reduced to 37% of baseline in the repeated occlusion model versus 32% of baseline in the single occlusion model), the appearance of the collagen network in the two groups was different. Using polarized light microscopy, we found broken collagen fibers and changes in the optical properties of collagen in five of six dogs that underwent repeated occlusion and reperfusion. In contrast, no such damage was seen in dogs that underwent a single, 15-minute occlusion: in fact, the collagen network in myocardium subjected to the single episode of ischemia appeared the same as that in nonischemic control hearts (Whittaker et al., 1991).

Thus, although our results are consistent with those of Zhao et al. (1987), the interpretation of the results is different. The repeated occlusion experiments confirm that myocardial collagen is vulnerable to ischemia, a finding that could have important consequences in patients with angina. However, the lack of collagen damage following a single short period of ischemia suggests that disruption of the myocardial collagen matrix is not a primary mechanism of postischemic stunning.

VII. SUMMARY

While there is no question that the stunned myocardium is characterized by a transient depression in adenine nucleotides, ATP, and ADP stores, a wealth of experimental data now indicates that postischemic contractile dysfunction is clearly not a consequence of abnormalities in energy production or depletion of energy stores. Furthermore, utilization of ATP at the site of the contractile proteins does not appear to be compromised in the stunned myocardium. These data demonstrate that a cause-and-effect relationship between high-energy phosphate metabolism and myocardial stunning, although initially tempting, was a fad that has now been conclusively disproven. Similar conclusions can be drawn concerning both the role of the neutrophil and the role of electrophysiological abnormalities: despite initial results that implicated both of these factors as important mediators of postischemic contractile dysfunction, subsequent studies have failed to substantiate these concepts. In contrast, the role of myocardial collagen matrix as a mediator of postischemic contractile dysfunction remains a complex issue: degradation of the collagen fibroskeleton may play a crucial role in instances of repeated ischemia but cannot account for postischemic dysfunction in myocardium stunned by a single episode of ischemia. It is therefore unlikely that collagen degradation per se represents a fundamental mechanism for the stunned myocardium.

Although the other mechanisms discussed in this chapter have, for the most part, fallen out of favor, they represent a valuable lesson in our continued search for the mechanisms of postischemic dysfunction. The current popular theories that oxygen radicals, abnormal calcium homeostasis, and alterations in the cyclooxygenase pathway contribute to the pathogenesis of the stunned myocardium—now taken by most of us as dogma—may just as quickly fall from favor if, as with the other theories, evidence to the contrary appears in next month's scientific literature.

REFERENCES

Ambrosio, G., Jacobus, W. E., Bergman, C. A., Weisman, H. F., and Becker, L. C. (1987). Preserved high energy phosphate metabolic reserve in globally "stunned" hearts despite reduction of basal ATP content and contractility. *J. Mol. Cell. Cardiol. 19*: 953.

Ambrosio, G., Jacobus, W. E., Mitchell, M. C., Litt, M. R., and Becker, L. C. (1989). Effects of ATP precursors on ATP and free ADP content and functional recovery of postischemic hearts. *Am. J. Physiol. 256*: H560.

Arnold, J. M. O., Braunwald, E., Sandor, T., and Kloner, R. A. (1985). Inotropic stimulation of reperfused myocardium: effects on infarct size and myocardial function. *J. Am. Coll. Cardiol. 6*: 1026.

Bashour, T. T., Kabbani, S. S., Brewster, H. P., Wald, S. H., Hanna, E. S., and Cheng, T. O. (1983). Transient Q waves and reversible cardiac failure during myocardial ischemia: Electrical and mechanical stunning of the heart. *Am. Heart J. 106*: 780.

Bateman, T. M., Czer, L. C. S., Gray, R. J., Maddahi, J., Raymond, M. J., Geft, I. L., Ganz, W., Shah, P. K., and Berman, D. S. (1983). Transient pathologic Q waves during acute ischemic events: an electrocardiographic correlate of stunned but viable myocardium. *Am. Heart J. 106*: 1421.

Becker, L. C., Levine, J. H., DiPaula, A. F., Guarnieri, T., and Anversano, T. (1986). Reversal of dysfunction in postischemic stunned myocardium by epinephrine and postextrasystolic potentiation. *J. Am. Coll. Cardiol. 7*: 580.

Bolli, R., Zhu, W. X., Myers, M. L., Hartley, C. J., and Roberts, R. (1985). Beta-adrenergic stimulation reverses postischemic myocardial dysfunction without producing subsequent deterioration. *Am. J. Cardiol. 56*: 964.

Bolli, R., Triana, J. F., and Jeroudi, M. O. (1990). Prolonged impairment of coronary vasodilation after reversible ischemia: Evidence for microvascular stunning. *Circ. Res. 67*: 332.

Braunwald, E., and Kloner, R. A. (1982). The stunned myocardium: prolonged ischemic ventricular dysfunction. *Circulation 66*: 1146.

Cannon, R. O., Butany, J. W., McManus, B. M., Spier, E., Kravitz, A. B., Bolli, R., and Ferrans, V. (1983). Early degradation of collagen after acute myocardial infarction in the rat. *Am. J. Cardiol. 52*: 390.

Ciuffo, A. A., Ouyang, P., Becker, L. C., Levin, L., and Weisfeldt, M. L. (1985). Reduction of sympathetic inotropic response after ischemia in dogs: Contributor to stunned myocardium. *J. Clin. Invest. 75*: 1504.

Clarke, K., O'Connor, A. J., and Willis, R. J. (1987). Temporal relation between energy metabolism and myocardial function during ischemia and reperfusion. *Am. J. Physiol. 253*: H412.

DeBoer, L. V. W., Ingwall, J. S., Kloner, R. A., and Braunwald, E. (1980). Prolonged derangements of canine myocardial purine metabolism after a brief coronary artery occlusion not associated with anatomic evidence of necrosis. *Proc. Natl. Acad. Sci. USA 77*: 5471.

Ellis, S. G., Henschke, C. I., Sandor, T., Wynne, J., Braunwald, E., and Kloner, R. A. (1983). Time course of functional and biochemical recovery of myocardium salvaged by reperfusion. *J. Am. Coll. Cardiol. 1*: 1047.

Ellis, S. G., Wynne, J., Braunwald, E., Henschke, C. I., Sandor, T., and Kloner, R. A. (1984). Response of reperfusion-salvaged, stunned myocardium to inotropic stimulation. *Am. Heart J. 107*: 13.

Engler, R., and Covell, J. W. (1987). Granulocytes cause reperfusion ventricular dysfunction after 15-minute ischemia in the dog. *Circ. Res. 61*: 20.

Glower, G. G., Spratt, J. A., Newton, J. R., Wolfe, J. A., Rankin, J. S. and Swain, J. L. (1987). Dissociation between early recovery of regional function and prime nucleotide content in postischemic myocardium in the conscious dog. *Cardiovasc. Res. 21*: 328.

Go, L. O., Murry, C. E., Richard, V. J., Weischedel, G. R., Jennings, R. B., and Reimer, K. A. (1988). Myocardial neutrophil accumulation during reperfusion after reversible or irreversible ischemic injury. *Am. J. Physiol. 255*: H1188.

Greenfield, R. A., and Swain, J. L. (1987). Disruption of myofibrillar energy use: dual mechanisms that may contribute to postischemic dysfunction in stunned myocardium. *Circ. Res. 60*: 283.

Hanich, R. F., Levine, J. H., Prood, C., Spear, J. F., and Moore, E. N. (1989). Stunned myocardium: a forme fruste of electromechanical dissociation? *J. Am. Coll. Cardiol.* *13*: 90A (Abstract).

Heyndrickx, G. R., Millard, R. W., McRitchie, R. J., Maroko, P. R., and Vatner, S. F. (1975). Regional myocardial function and electrophysiological alterations after brief coronary artery occlusion in conscious dogs. *J. Clin. Invest.* *56*: 978.

Heyndrickx, G. R., Baig, H., Nellens, P., Leusen, I., Fishbein, M. C., and Vatner, S. F. (1978). Depression of regional blood flow and wall thickening after brief coronary occlusions. *Am. J. Physiol.* *234*: H653.

Hoffmeister, H. M., Mauser, M. M., and Schaper, W. (1985). Effect of adenosine and AICAribose on ATP content and regional contractile function in reperfused canine myocardium. *Basic Res. Cardiol.* *80*: 445.

Jacobus, W. E. (1985). Respiratory control and the integration of heart high energy phosphate metabolism by mitochondrial creatine kinase. *Ann. Rev. Physiol.* *47*: 707.

Jeremy, R. W., and Becker, L. C. (1989). Neutrophil depletion does not prevent myocardial dysfunction after brief coronary occlusion. *J. Am. Coll. Cardiol.* *13*: 1155.

Kloner, R. A., Ellis, S. G., Lange, R., and Braunwald, E. (1983). Studies of experimental coronary artery reperfusion: Effects on infarct size, myocardial function, biochemistry, ultrastructure and microvascular damage. *Circulation* *68*(Suppl. I): 1-8.

Kloner, R. A., and Alker, K. J. (1984). Effect of streptokinase on intramyocardial hemorrhage, infarct size and the no-reflow phenomenon during coronary reperfusion. *Circulation* *70*: 513.

Krause, S. M. (1990). Effect of global myocardial stunning on Ca^{2+}-sensitive myofibrillar ATPase activity and creatine kinase kinetics. *Am. J. Physiol.* *259*: H813.

Kupriyanov, V. V., Lakomkin, V. L., Kapelko, V. I., Steinschneider, A. Y., Ruuge, E. K., and Saks, V. A. (1987). Dissociation of adenosine triphosphate levels and contractile function in isovolumic hearts perfused with 2-deoxyglucose. *J. Mol. Cell. Cardiol.* *19*: 729.

Levine, J. H., Moore, E. N., Weisman, H. F., Kadish, A. H., Becker, L. C., and Spear, J. F. (1987). Depression of action potential characteristics and a decreased space content are present in postischemic, reperfused myocardium. *J. Clin. Invest.* *79*: 107.

Neely, J. R., and Grotyohann, L. W. (1984). Role of glycolytic products in damage to ischemic myocardium. Dissociation of adenosine triphosphate levels and recovery of function of reperfused ischemic hearts. *Circ. Res.* *55*: 816.

O'Neill, P. G., Charlat, M. L., Michael, L. H., Roberts, R., and Bolli, R. (1989). Influence of neutrophil depletion on myocardial function and flow after reversible ischemia. *Am. J. Physiol.* *256*: H341.

Przyklenk, K., and Kloner, R. A. (1988). Effect of verapamil on postischemic "stunned" myocardium: Importance of the timing of treatment. *J. Am. Coll. Cardiol.* *11*: 614.

Przyklenk, K., and Kloner, R. A. (1989a). Is "stunned myocardium" a protective mechanism? Effect of acute recruitment and acute beta-blockade on recovery of contractile function and high energy phosphate stores at 1 day post reperfusion. *Am. Heart J.* *118*: 480.

Przyklenk, K., and Kloner, R. A. (1989b). What factors predict recovery of contractile function in the canine model of the stunned myocardium? *Am. J. Cardiol. 64*: 18F.

Przyklenk, K., Ghafari, G. B., Eitzman, D. T., and Kloner, R. A. (1989). Nifedipine administered after reperfusion ablates systolic contractile dysfunction of postischemic "stunned" myocardium. *J. Am. Coll. Cardiol. 13*: 1176.

Reimer, K. A., Hill, M. L., and Jennings, R. B. (1981). Prolonged depletion of ATP and of the adenine nucleotide pool due to delayed resynthesis of adenine nucelotide following reversible myocardial ischemia in dogs. *J. Mol. Cell. Cardiol. 13*: 229.

Robinson, T. F., Cohen-Gould, L., and Factor, S. M. (1983). Skeletal framework of mammalian heart muscle: arrangement of inter- and pericellular connective tissue structures. *Lab. Invest. 49*: 482.

Sato, S., Ashraf, M., Millard, R. W., Fujiwara, H., and Schwartz, A. (1983). Connective tissue changes in early ischemia of porcine myocardium: an ultrastructural study. *J. Mol. Cell. Cardiol. 15*: 261.

Schott, R. J., Nao, B. S., McClanahan, T. B., Simpson, P. J., Stirling, M. C., Todd, R. F., and Gallagher, K. P. (1989). $F(ab')_2$ fragments of anti-Mo1 (904) monoclonal antibodies do not prevent myocardial stunning. *Circ. Res. 65*: 1112.

Swain, J. L., Sabina, R. L., McHale, P. A., Greenfield, J. C., and Holmes, E. W. (1982). Prolonged myocardial nucleotide depletion after brief ischemia in open-chest dogs. *Am. J. Physiol. 242*: H818.

Taegtmeyer, H., Roberts, A. F. C., and Raine, A. E. G. (1985). Energy metabolism in reperfused heart muscle: metabolic correlates to return of function. *J. Am. Coll. Cardiol. 6*: 864.

Weber, K. T., and Brilla, C. G. (1991). Pathological hypertrophy and cardiac interstitium: fibrosis and the renin-angiotensin-aldosterone system. *Circulation 83*: 1849.

Westlin, W., and Mullane, K. M. (1989). Alleviation of myocardial stunning by leukocyte and platelet depletion. *Circulation 80*: 1828.

Whittaker, P., Boughner, D. R., Kloner, R. A., and Przyklenk, K. (1991). Stunned myocardium and myocardial collagen damage: Differential effects of single and repeated occlusions. *Am. Heart J. 121*: 434.

Zhao, M., Zhang, H., Robinson, T. F., Factor, S. M., Sonnenblick, E. H., and Eng, C. (1987). Profound structural alterations of the extracellular collagen matrix in postischemic dysfunctional ("stunned") but viable myocardium. *J. Am. Coll. Cardiol. 10*: 1322.

Zucchi, R., Limbruno, U., di Vincenzo, A., Mariani, M., and Ronca, G. (1990). Adenine nucleotide depletion and contractile dysfunction in the "stunned" myocardium. *Cardiovasc. Res. 24*: 440.

12

The Stunned Myocardium

A Complex Phenomenon Demands an Integrated Explanation

Winifred G. Nayler

University of Melbourne, Heidelberg, Victoria, Australia

I. INTRODUCTION

The ischemic myocardium undoubtedly presents investigators and cardiologists with a problem. If the ischemic episode is not severe, but is sustained, then the myocardium may "hibernate"—a condition characterized by a state of impaired but reversible contractile dysfunction associated with a sustained reduction in coronary blood flow (Rahimtoola, 1989). Restitution of coronary perfusion under these conditions promotes a rapid recovery of function, without evidence of sustained injury to either the myocardium or its vasculature. The hibernating myocardium, however, is only one of the possible sequelae of inadequate coronary perfusion. Others include infarction—characterized by irreversible loss of structure and function—and stunning (Braunwald and Kloner, 1982; Kloner and Przyklenk, 1991). When applied to the mammalian heart, the process of stunning is essentially a postischemic event. It is characterized by the depressed functioning of potentially jeopardized myocardium that has been salvaged by reperfusion before the ischemic episode has had time to cause irreversible injury. The state can persist for hours or even days, but ultimately full contractile activity is restored (Braunwald and Kloner, 1982; Kloner et al., 1989; Bolli, 1990).

Although first observed as a laboratory phenomenon, evidence of the natural occurrence of myocardial stunning is not difficult to find. Conditions under which it is believed to occur include exercise-induced angina (Camici et al., 1986), unstable angina (Nixon et al., 1982), reperfusion for the treatment of evolving myocardial infarction (Christian et al., 1990), coronary bypass surgery (Briesblatt et al., 1990), and coronary vasospasm (Mathias et al., 1987). Precipitating factors include aggregates of thrombi (Davies, 1990), fracturing of atherogenic plaques (Fuster et al., 1990), intermittent coronary spasm (Luscher, 1991) and a sudden but temporary reduction in perfusion pressure.

Stunning is not the prerogative of in situ hearts. In fact there are almost as many animal models of myocardial stunning as there are clinical conditions that give rise to it. Some of these models are listed in Table 1. Even this limited list allows certain conclusions to be drawn concerning the conditions under which this postischemic loss of contractile function becomes evident. Thus, it cannot be species specific, since it has been detected in experiments relating to ferret, rabbit, rat, dog, and pig hearts—and of course it occurs in humans. Moreover, it cannot depend upon the presence of formed elements of the blood (including platelets and neutrophils) since it occurs in crystalloid-perfused hearts (Nayler et al., 1988) and neutrophil-depletion does not prevent its occurrence (Jeremy et al., 1989). Nor can the presence of the peripheral circulation or innervation be of great consequence as far as this phenomenon is concerned, otherwise it would not occur in isolated

Table 1 Animal Models of Myocardial Stunning

Model	Ref.
Isolated hearts (global ischemia and reperfusion)	
Ferret	Kusuoka et al., 1990
Rabbit	Krause, 1990
Rat	Nayler et al., 1988
	Limbruno et al., 1989
In situ hearts (acute regional ischemia and reperfusion)	
Anesthetized animals	
Dogs	Swain et al., 1984
	Reimer et al., 1986
	Bolli et al., 1989
	Przyklenk et al., 1989
Pigs	Buchwald et al., 1989
Conscious animals	
Dogs	Heyndrickx et al., 1975
	Thaulow et al., 1989
	Hittinger et al., 1990

hearts. Similarly, preexisting injury cannot be a prerequisite, otherwise it would not be possible to induce this condition in freshly isolated but otherwise healthy hearts.

II. PROPERTIES OF THE STUNNED MYOCARDIUM

Stunning of the myocardium is, as already mentioned, the condition that results from the restoration of coronary perfusion after short (10–15 minutes) periods of ischemia and that is characterized by prolonged contractile dysfunction without evidence of significant tissue injury. Prior to the expression of this stunned state, the myocardium exhibits changes directly attributable to the inadequacy of the coronary perfusion. This prestunned state is characterized by:

1. A rapid decline in peak developed tension, which, if the interruption in coronary flow persists, may progress to mechanical quiescence.
2. A substantial fall in the tissue reserves of adenosine triphosphate (ATP), a reduction in the total adenylate charge, and a precipitous fall in creatine phosphate (CP) (Jennings et al., 1990).
3. An increase in inorganic phosphate (P_i) (Jennings et al., 1985).
4. An increase in H^+ concentration and in cytosolic Mg^{2+} and cytosolic Ca^{2+} (Figs. 1,2) (Marban et al., 1987; Nayler, 1991a).
5. Relatively minor and fully reversible changes in ultrastructure, including some margination of the nuclear chromatin, disappearance of the glycogen granules, and relaxation of the myofibrils (Jennings et al., 1990).

Despite these changes, electrical activity persists, and provided that the ischemic episode has not been prolonged, there is a rapid recovery (Fig. 3) of contractile function, so much so that in the first 1 or 2 minutes of reperfusion the active tension-generating activity of the myocardium reaches, or even exceeds, its preischemic state. This is where the trouble starts, however, because peak developed tension then declines and may remain suppressed for hours or even days.

Despite this decline in contractile function, reperfusion after these relatively short periods of ischemia is accompanied by a relatively prompt restoration (see Fig. 1) of normal intracellular pH, P_i, and Mg^{2+}, and the tissue reserves of ATP and CP are rapidly replenished—or, as is the case with CP, there may be a considerable overshoot. Cytosolic Ca^{2+}, however, remains elevated, reaching levels higher than that caused by the initial ischemic event.

III. MECHANISMS

From a purely *theoretical* point of view, mechanisms that might contribute to the loss of contractile function that is so characteristic of the stunning condition include:

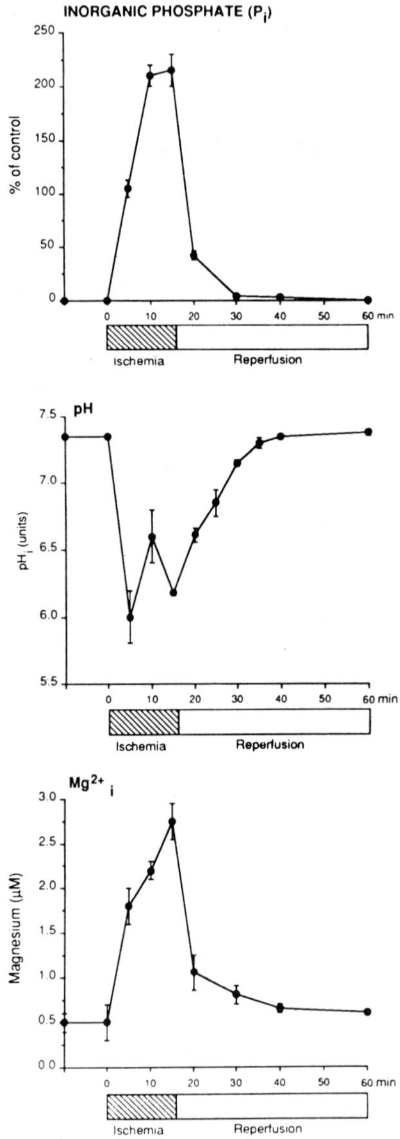

Figure 1 Effect of 15 minutes of global ischemia followed by reperfusion on inorganic phosphate (P_i), intracellular pH (pH_i), and intracellular Mg^{2+} ($Mg^{2+}{}_i$) in isolated rat hearts. Global ischemia was at 37 °C. P_i, pH_i, and $Mg^{2+}{}_i$ were measured by NMR spectroscopy. Each value is mean ± SEM of six experiments. (From Nayler, 1991b.)

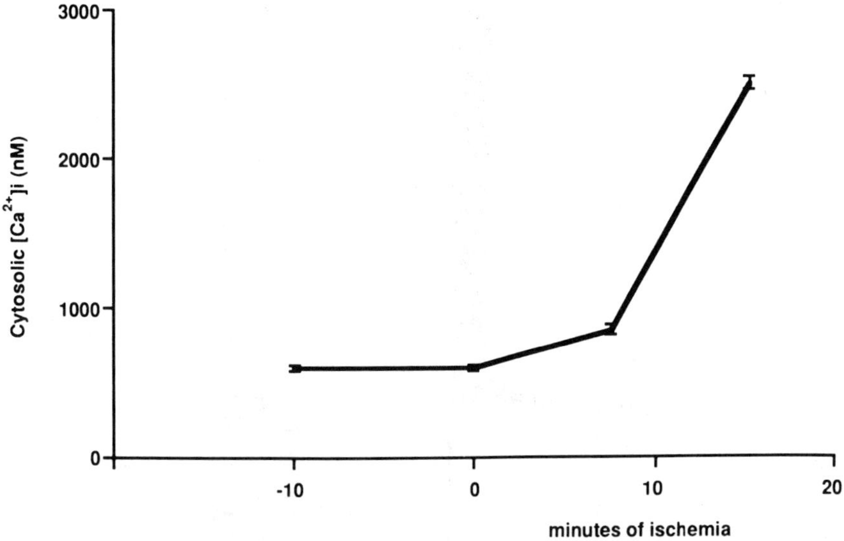

Figure 2 Effect of global ischemia on cytosolic Ca^{2+} in an isolated rat heart. Global ischemia was at 37 °C. Cytosolic Ca^{2+} was measured by NMR spectroscopy, using F-BAPTA.

1. Abnormal energy production
2. Impaired energy utilization
3. Subtle changes in the heart's ultrastructure not readily identifiable by electron microscopy
4. Impaired myocardial perfusion
5. Abnormal Ca^{2+} flux
6. Oxyradical-mediated injury
7. Abnormal functioning of the sarcoplasmic reticulum
8. A decreased sensitivity of the myofibrils to Ca^{2+}

A. Abnormal Energy Production

This can probably be discounted as a primary mechanism because the ATP levels of the stunned myocardium do not parallel the full return of contractile activity (Glower et al., 1987) and, in any case, the CP content of these hearts is either normal or supranormal, indicating that the phosphorylating activity of the mitochondria is well preserved. Moreover, manipulations of metabolic pathways to stimulate ATP regeneration does not hasten their recovery

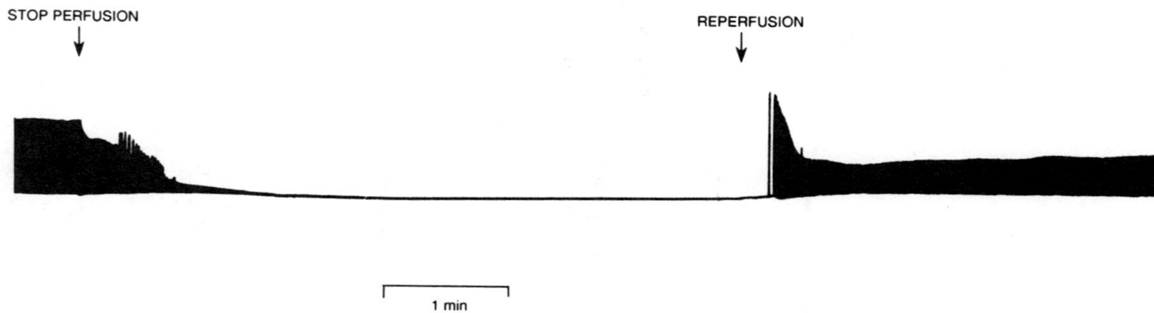

Figure 3 Effect of 10 minutes of global ischemia followed by reperfusion on the recovery of the tension-generating activity of an isolated rat heart. Note that after a relatively short period of ischemia, reperfusion resulted in full functional recovery after which the tension-generating activity of the heart declined and remained suppressed for some time.

(Hoffmeister et al., 1985). Perhaps the final nail in the coffin relating to the hypothesis that inadequate energy in the form of ATP is responsible for the state of contractile dysfunction so characteristic of these hearts is that they are capable of responding to a wide variety of inotropic stimuli, including additional Ca^{2+} (Ito et al., 1987), paired pacing (Becker et al., 1986), adrenaline (Przyklenk and Kloner, 1987), beta-adrenergic stimuli in general (Bolli et al., 1985), and pyruvate (Mentzer et al., 1989).

B. Energy Utilization

Again, this is an improbable explanation, because such a wide variety of inotropic interventions are capable of evoking a positive inotropic response, indicating that the myofibrils must be capable of utilizing ATP, albeit inefficiently (Stahl et al., 1988).

C. Impaired Perfusion

Incomplete coronary perfusion is also an improbable explanation, because the stunned hearts show little evidence of a no-reflow condition (Nayler et al., 1990). Moreover, they retain their full coronary reserve (Jeremy et al., 1989).

D. Abnormal Ca^{2+} Flux

Since cytosolic Ca^{2+} rises during the first few minutes of ischemia (see Fig. 1) and further upon reperfusion (Marban, 1991), it is difficult to account for the impaired contractile state of the myocardium in terms of an inadequate availability of Ca^{2+}. To the contrary, it may be this increased availability of Ca^{2+} that is responsible for the depressed contractile state, since Ca^{2+} has a desensitizing effect on the myofibrils (Kitakaze et al., 1987; Kusuoka et al., 1990). The precise cause of this desensitization is unknown, but since recovery is slow, it presumably involves structural damage caused by the activation of a Ca^{2+}-dependent process.

At this stage it may be relevant to consider why the stunned heart develops a raised cytosolic Ca^{2+}, which occurs in the absence of an increase in total tissue Ca^{2+} and which persists, and may be exacerbated, upon reperfusion (Marban, 1991). There are at least four potential sources of this Ca^{2+}:

1. Entry by way of the L-type Ca^{2+} channels, accompanied by downregulation of the Ca^{2+} extrusion mechanisms
2. Entry in exchange for Na^+
3. H^+ ion-induced displacement of protein-bound Ca^{2+}

4. Ca^{2+} leakage from the intracellular storage sites housed within the sarcoplasmic reticulum

Of these possibilities, leakage from the sarcoplasmic reticulum would seem to be the most likely, because Ca^{2+} efflux through the Ca^{2+} release channels of the sarcoplasmic reticulum is augmented under these conditions (Krause et al., 1989), and the activity of the Ca^{2+}-stimulated, Mg^{2+}-dependent ATPase enzyme responsible for pumping Ca^{2+} from the cytosol into the lumen of the reticulum is depressed (Limbruno et al., 1989).

E. Oxy- and Hydroxyradicals

There are many reasons for arguing that oxy- and hydroxyradicals may contribute to the occurrence of myocardial stunning caused by reperfusion after relatively brief episodes of ischemia:

1. Oxy- and hydroxyradicals are produced in limited amounts during periods of inadequate perfusion, and there is a burst of oxyradical production upon reperfusion (Bolli, 1990).
2. They interfere with many of the systems that either directly or indirectly regulate cytosolic Ca^{2+}. For example, they inhibit the Ca^{2+}-retrieval capacity of the sarcoplasmic reticulum (Rowe et al., 1983), possibly by inhibiting its Ca^{2+} ATPase activity (Thompson and Hess, 1986); they have an inhibitory effect on the Ca^{2+}-ATPase of the sarcolemma, leading inevitably to Ca^{2+} retention within the cytosol (Kaneko et al., 1989); and they have an inhibitory effect on the Na^+:K^+ ATPase enzyme (Xie et al., 1990), thereby facilitating the accumulation of Ca^{2+} in exchange for Na^+.
3. Oxy- and hydroxyradicals have a direct inhibitory effect on myofibrillar tension-generating activity (Przyklenk et al., 1990).
4. Inhibition of oxy- and hydroxyradical generation, and the addition of free radical scavengers, attenuate or prevent the depressed contractile state that is so characteristic of the stunned hearts (Bolli, 1990).

F. Damage to the Ultrastructure

Although minor changes in cardiac ultrastructure do occur during short episodes of ischemia that predispose the heart towards stunning and not irreversible injury, it is difficult to account for the occurrence of stunning in such terms. Thus, glycogen depletion does not necessarily result in contractile dysfunction, and although the myofibrils of the stunned heart are relaxed with prominent I bands, they resume their normal appearance early during reperfusion. Another potential cause that can be discounted relates to the suggestion that damage to the collagen scaffolding of the myocardium may be responsible for the contractile dysfunction of the stunned heart (Zhao et al., 1987). This, at one stage, provided an attractive hypothesis, since myocardial collagen is thought to provide the mechanical coupling between adjacent myocytes needed for efficient contraction, and repeated episodes of relatively short periods of ischemia can result in significant changes in myocardial collagen content (Zhao et al., 1987). This hypothesis has had to be discarded, however, because collagen damage cannot be detected after a brief but single period of ischemia of sufficient duration to stun the myocardium (Whittaker et al., 1991).

In general, therefore, the etiology of the stunned myocardium as it occurs during reperfusion after a relatively short period of ischemia is complex. While the depressed contractile state of the myocardium is the most obvious expression of this condition, the predominant causative factors would seem to involve a raised cytosolic Ca^{2+} and the generation of free radicals. These two events may be interrelated (Fig. 4).

IV. IS STUNNING BENEFICIAL TO THE REPERFUSED MYOCARDIUM?

Early investigations into the pathophysiology of myocardial stunning provided evidence suggesting that this process might be of benefit, in that it preconditioned the myocardium against damage caused by subsequent brief episodes of ischemia—as might occur, for example, if the coronary vasculature underwent repeated vasospastic episodes. This hypothesis was based on the following observations:

1. Repetitive short episodes of ischemia do *not* result in a cumulative loss of adenine nucleotides. This is well illustrated by the behavior of the canine myocardium when subjected to brief but repetitive 10-minute episodes of circumflex artery occlusion. Under these conditions the initial 10-minute episode of occlusion causes a 61% loss of adenosine triphosphate content and a 41% loss of adenine nucleotides (Reimer et al., 1986). Reperfusion after such a 10-minute ischemic episode results in some repletion of the adenine nucleotides, but now additional successive but brief episodes of ischemia fail to cause any further adenine nucleotide loss. This contrasts with the condition that results from continuous episodes of ischemia where there is a profound and additive depletion of the nucleotides. Thus stunning, it seemed, was having a protective effect against loss of nucleotides caused by subsequent, brief ischemic episodes (Reimer et al., 1986).
2. Ischemia-induced depression of cardiac contractility provided further evidence of apparent protection provided the ischemic episodes were short lived and interrupted by reperfusion. For example, whereas a prolonged episode of ischemia results in sustained loss of contractile function, one

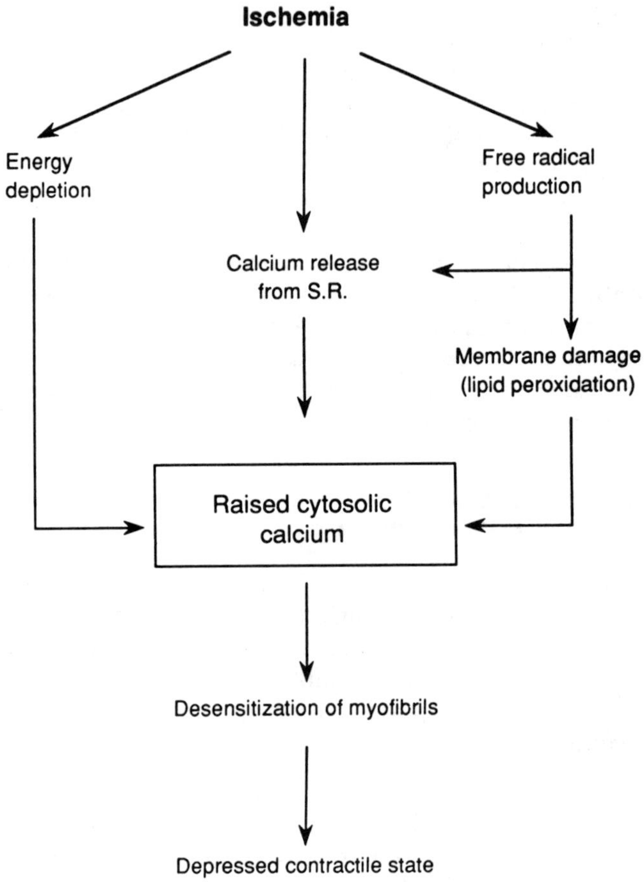

Figure 4 Schematic representation of the events involved in stunning of the myocardium. S.R., sarcoplasmic reticulum. (From Nayler, 1991b.)

> 10-minute period of ischemia followed by reperfusion protects against an equivalent loss of function during a second, third, or fourth period of ischemia provided the ischemic episodes are short and discontinuous (Heyndrickx et al., 1975).

These two observations—the absence of a cumulative loss of adenine nucleotides, and the failure of the myocardium to exhibit an additive decline in recovery upon postischemic reperfusion—gave rise to the hypothesis that stunning preconditions the heart so that it is more resilient to subsequent ischaemic episodes (Reimer et al., 1986). To some extent this conclusion is justified, but it only applies to brief ischemic episodes, and even so it is not the condition of stunning that is responsible for the preconditioning (Murry et al., 1991) because that cardioprotective effect that results from a preliminary but short-lived ischemic episode is lost during sustained reperfusion at a time when contractile function is still depressed and the myocardium is, therefore, still stunned. Hence it is not the process of stunning that preconditions the myocardium against the consequences of successive episodes of ischemia, but some other consequence of a short-lived ischemic episode.

V. THE SIGNIFICANCE OF MYOCARDIAL STUNNING

The question naturally arises whether the phenomenon of stunning as described here is of any physiological significance, and if it contributes to the myocardial dysfunction encountered during postischemic reperfusion. This is not an unreasonable question, since the introduction of thrombolytic therapy for the management of patients with acute myocardial infarction virtually ensures that some regions of the myocardium will be reperfused after a relatively brief period of ischemia, in which case the affected zone may well become stunned. Such an event does have considerable clinical significance, since it probably explains why, despite successful reperfusion and limitation of the infarct size, functional recovery in the affected area can be delayed for hours or even days. Under these conditions persistent wall motion abnormalities can be expected. The corollary to this is that the assessment of the success of any reperfusion technique cannot be made within a few hours of its introduction. An example of this is provided by the data collected by Stack et al. (1983), which shows that in patients with ischemic heart disease who are subjected to successful thrombolysis with intracoronary streptokinase, as long as 16 days is needed for a steady state to be reached with respect to functional recovery. Others have obtained similar results. For example, Reduto et al. (1981) found that at least 10 days was needed between the induction of streptokinase therapy and the expression of the maximum recovery as determined by the improvement in ejection fraction.

VI. THE SIGNIFICANCE OF THE LATENT CONTRACTILE ACTIVITY OF STUNNED MYOCARDIUM

Earlier in this chapter, mention was made of the fact that stunned myocardium retains its capacity to respond to a variety of inotropic stimuli, including additional Ca^{2+}, paired pacing, beta-adrenoceptor agonists, etc. Such a response may be clinically relevant under conditions in which successful reperfusion results in inadequate pump function. In other words, the introduction of a positive inotropic regime may allow the heart to support the circulation even though a significant proportion of the myocardium is stunned. Certainly there is data in the literature (Ballantyne et al., 1987) that supports this hypothesis.

VII. SUMMARY

In conclusion, hearts that are reperfused after a relatively short period of ischemia usually exhibit temporary contractile dysfunction. This condition may last for hours or days, but it is ultimately reversible. While stunned the myocardium retains its capacity to respond to a variety of inotropic stimuli but is not necessarily preconditioned against damage caused by subsequent ischemia episodes.

The phenomenon of stunning provides a challenge to those investigators who are interested in assessing the contractile state of the myocardium following reperfusion after a relatively short period of ischemia because when stunned the myocardium does not perform in accordance with its full contractile capacity.

The mechanisms responsible for myocardial stunning are complex. A raised cytosolic Ca^{2+} would seem to hold the key because of its effect on myofibrillar Ca^{2+} sensitivity. Excess free oxyradical production also seems to be involved, and indeed, these two factors—a raised cytosolic Ca^{2+} and excess free radical production—may be interdependent.

REFERENCES

Ballantyne, C. M., Verani, M. S., Short, H. K., Hyatt, C., and Noon, G. P. (1987). Delayed recovery of severely "stunned" myocardium with the support of a left ventricular assist device after coronary artery bypass surgery. *J. Am. Coll. Cardiol. 10*: 710.

Becker, L. C., Levine, J. H., Dipaula, A. T., Guarnieri, T., and Aversano, T. (1986). Reversal of dysfunction in postischaemic stunned myocardium by epinephine and postextrasystolic potentiation. *J. Am. Coll. Cardiol. 7*: 580.

Bolli, R. (1990). Mechanism of myocardial "stunning." *Circulation 82*: 723.

Bolli, R., Zhu, W-X., Myers, M. L., Hartley, C. J., and Roberts, R. (1985). Beta-adrenergic stimulation reverses post-ischemic myocardial dysfunction without producing subsequent functional deterioration. *Am. J. Cardiol. 56*: 964.

Bolli, R., Jeroudi, M. O., Patel, B. S., DuBose, C. M., Lai, E. K., Roberts, R., and McCay, P. B. (1989). Direct evidence that oxygen-derived free radicals contribute to postischemic myocardial dysfunction in the intact dog. *Proc. Natl. Acad. Sci. 86*: 4695.

Braunwald, E. and Kloner, R. A. (1982). The stunned myocardium: prolonged, post-ischemic ventricular dysfunction. *Circulation 66*: 1146.

Breisblatt, W. M., Stein, K. L., Wolfe, C. J., Follansbee, W. P., Capozzi, J., Armitage, J. M., and Hardesty, R. L. (1990). Acute myocardial dysfunction and recovery: A common occurrence after coronary bypass surgery. *J. Am. Coll. Cardiol. 15*: 1261.

Buchwald, A., Klein, H. H., Lindert, S., Pich, S., Nebendahl, K., Wiegand, V., and Kreuzer, H. (1989). Effect of intracoronary superoxide dismutase on regional function in stunned myocardium. *J. Cardiovasc. Pharmacol. 13*: 258.

Camici, P., Araujo, L. I., Spinks, T., Lammerstma, A. A., Kaski, J. C., Shea, M. J., Selwyn, A. P., Jones, T., and Maseri, A. (1986). Increased uptake of ^{18}F-fluorodeoxyglucose in postischemic myocardium of patients with exercise-induced angina. *Circulation 74*: 81.

Christian, T. F., Behrenbeck, T., Pellkia, P. A., Huber, K. C., Chesbero, J. H., and Gibbons, R. J. (1990). Mismatch of left ventricular function and infarct size demonstrated by technetium-99M isonitrile imaging after reperfusion therapy for acute myocardial infarction: Identification of myocardial stunning and hyperkinesia. *J. Am. Coll. Cardiol. 16*: 1632.

Davies, M. J. (1990). A macro and micro view of coronary vascular insult in ischemic heart disease. *Circulation 82(Suppl. II)*: II-38.

Fuster, V., Stein, B., Ambrose, J. A., Badimon, L., Badimon, J. J., and Chesbro, J. H. (1990). Atherosclerotic plaque rupture and thrombosis; evolving concepts. *Circulation 82(Suppl. II)*: II-47.

Glower, D. D., Spratt, J. A., Newton, J. R., Wolfe, J. A., Rankin, J. S., and Swain, J. L. (1987). Dissociation between early recovery of regional function and purine nucleotide content in postischaemic myocardium of conscious dogs. *Cardiovasc. Res. 21*: 328.

Hittinger, L., Shannon, R. P., Kohin, S., Manders, W. T., Kelly, P., and Vatner, S. F. (1990). Exercise-induced subendocardial dysfunction in dogs with left ventricular hypertrophy. *Circ. Res. 66*: 329.

Heyndrickx, G. R., Millard, R. W., McRitchie, R. J., Maroko, P., and Vatner, S. F. (1975). Regional myocardial function and electrophysiological alterations after brief coronary artery occlusion in conscious dogs. *J. Clin. Invest. 56*: 978.

Hoffmeister, H. M., Mauser, M., and Schaper, W. (1985), Effect of adenosine and AICaribinose on ATP content and regional contractile function in reperfused canine myocardium. *Basic Res. Cardiol. 80*: 445.

Ito, B. R., Tate, H., Kobayashi, M., and Schaper, W. (1987). Reversibly injured, post ischaemic canine myocardium retains normal contractile reserve. *Circ. Res. 61*: 834.

Jennings, R. B., Schaper, J., Hill, M. L., Steenbergen, C. Jr., and Reimer, K. A. (1985). Effect of reperfusion late in the phase of reversible ischemic injury. *Circ. Res. 56*: 262.

Jennings, R. B., Murry, C. E., Steenbergen, C., and Reimer, K. A. (1990). Development of cell injury in sustained acute ischemia. *Circulation 82* (*Suppl. II*): II-2.

Jeremy, R. W. and Becker, L. C. (1989). Neutrophil depletion does not prevent myocardial dysfunction after brief coronary occlusion. *J. Am. Coll. Cardiol. 13*: 1155.

Jeremy, R. W., Stahl, L., Gillinov, M., Litt, M., Aversano, T. R., and Becker, L. C. (1989). Preservation of coronary flow reserve in stunned myocardium. *Am. J. Physiol. 256*: H1303.

Kaneko, M., Beamish, R. E., and Dhalla, N. S. (1989). Depression of heart sarcolemmal Ca^{2+} pump activity by oxygen free radicals. *Am. J. Physiol.* 256: H368.

Kitakaze, M., Weisman, H. F., and Marban, E. (1987). Contractile dysfunction and

ATP depletion after transient calcium overload in perfused ferret hearts. *Circulation 77*: 685.

Kloner, R. A., Przyklenk, K., and Patel, B. (1989). Altered myocardial states: The stunned and hibernating myocardium. *Am. J. Med. 86 (Suppl.A)*: A14.

Kloner, R. A. and Przyklenk, K. (1991). Stunned and hibernating myocardium. *Annu. Rev. Med. 42*: 1.

Krause, S. M. (1990). Effect of global myocardial stunning on Ca^{2+}-sensitive myofibrillar ATPase activity and creatine kinase kinetics. *Am. J. Physiol. 259*: H813.

Kusuoka, H., Koretsune, Y., Chacko, V. P., Weisfeldt, M. L., and Marban, E. (1990). Excitation-contraction coupling in postischemic myocardium. *Circ. Res. 66*: 1268.

Limbruno, U., Zucchi, R., Ronca-Teston, S., Galbani, P., Ronca, G., and Mariani, M. (1989). Sarcoplasmic reticulum function in the "stunned" myocardium. *J. Mol. Cell. Cardiol. 21*: 1063.

Luscher, T. F. (1991). Endothelin: Key to coronary vasospasm, *Circulation 83*: 701.

Marban, E. (1991). Myocardial stunning and hibernation. The physiology behind the colloquialisms. *Circulation 83*: 681.

Marban, E., Kitakaze, M., Kusuoka, H. Porterfield, J. K., Yue, D. T., and Chacko, V. P. (1987). Intracellular free calcium concentration measured with ^{19}F NMR Spectroscopy in intact ferret hearts. *Proc. Natl. Acad. Sci. USA* 84: 6005.

Mathias, P., Kerin, N. Z., Blevins, R. D., Cascade, P., and Rubenfire, M. (1987). Coronary vasospasm as a cause of stunned myocardium. *Am. Heart J. 113*: 383.

Mentzer, R. M., Van Wylen, D. G. V., Sodhi, J., Weiss, R. J., Lasley, R. D., Willis, J., Bunger, R., Habil, D. R., and Fnint, L. M. (1989). Effect of pyruvate on regional ventricular function and stunned myocardium. *Ann. Surg. 209*: 629.

Murry, C. E., Richard, V. J., Jennings, R. B., and Reimer, K. A. (1991). Myocardial protection is lost before contractile function recovers from ischemic preconditioning. *Am. J. Physiol. 260*: H796.

Nayler, W. G. (1991a). The antiatherogenic effects of amlodipine: Promise of preclinical data. *Postgrad. Med. J.* in press.

Nayler, W. G. (1991b). *Second Generation of Calcium Antagonists.* Springer-Verlag, Heidelberg, in press.

Nayler, W. G., Elz, J. S., and Buckley, D. J. (1988). The stunned myocardium: effect of electrical and mechanical arrest and osmolarity. *Am. J. Physiol. 255*: H60.

Nayler, W. G., Buckley, D. J., and Leong, J. (1990). Calcium antagonists and the 'stunned myocardium.' *Cadioscience 1*: 61.

Nixon, J. V., Brown, C. N., and Smitherman, T. F. (1982). Identification of transient and persistent segmental wall motion abnormalities in patients with unstable angina by two-dimensional echocardiography. *Circulation 65*: 1497.

Przyklenk, K. and Kloner, R. A. (1987). Acute effects of hydralazine and enalapril on contractile function of postischemic 'stunned' myocardium. *Am. J. Cardiol. 60*: 934.

Przyklenk, K., Ghafari, G. B., Eitzman, D. T., and Kloner, R. A. (1989). Nifedipine administered after reperfusion ablates systolic contractile dysfunction of postischemic 'stunned' myocardium. *J. Am. Coll. Cardiol. 13*: 1176.

Przyklenk, K., Whittaker, P., and Kloner, R. A. (1990). In vivo infusion of oxygen free radical substrates caused myocardial systolic, but not diastolic dysfunction.

Am. Heart J. 119: 807.

Rahimtoola, S. H. (1989). The hibernating myocardium. *Am. Heart J. 117*: 211.

Reduto, L. A., Freund, G. C., Gaeta, J. M., Smalling, R. W., Lewis, B., and Gould, K. L. (1981). Coronary artery reperfusion in acute myocardial infarction: Beneficial effects of intracoronary streptokinase on left ventricular salvage and performance. *Am. Heart J. 102*: 1168.

Reimer, K. A., Murry, C. E., Yamasawa, I., Hill, M. L., and Jennings, R. B. (1986). Four brief periods of myocardial ischemia cause no cumulative ATP loss or necrosis. *Am. J. Physiol. 251*: H1306.

Rowe, G. T., Manson, N. H., Caplan, M., and Hess, M. L. (1983). Hydrogen peroxide and hydroxyl radical mediation of activated leucocyte depression of cardiac sarcoplasmic reticulum. Participation of the cyclooxygenase pathway. *Circ. Res. 53*: 584.

Stack, R. S., Phillips, H. R., Grierson, D. S., Behar, V. S., Kong, Y., Peter, R. H., Swain, J. L., and Greenfield, J. C., Jr. (1983). Functional improvement of jeopardized myocardium following intracoronary streptokinase infusion in acute myocardial infarction. *J. Clin. Invest.* 72: 84.

Stahl, L. D., Weiss, H. R., and Becker, L. C. (1988). Myocardial oxygen consumption, oxygen supply/demand heterogeneity and microvascular patency in regionally stunned myocardium. *Circulation 77*: 865.

Swain, J. L., Sabina, R. L., Hines, J. J., Greenfield, J. C., and Homes, E. W. (1984). Repetitive episodes of brief ischaemia (12 min) do not produce a cumulative depletion of high energy phosphate compounds. *Cardiovasc. Res.* 18: 264.

Thaulow, E., Goth, B. D., Heusch, G., Gilpin, E., Schulz, R., Kroeger, K., and Ross J. (1989). Characteristics of regional myocardial stunning after exercise in dogs with chronic coronary stenosis. *Am. J. Physiol. 257*: H113.

Thompson, J. A., and Hess, M. L. (1986). The oxygen free radicali system: A fundamental mechanism in the production of myocardial necrosis. *Prog. Cardiovasc. Dis. 28*: 449.

Whittaker, P., Boughner, D. R., Kloner, R. A., and Przyklenk, K. (1991). Stunned myocardium and myocardial collagen damage: differential effects of single and repeated occlusions. *Am. Heart J. 121*: 434.

Xie, Z., Wang, Y., Askari, A., Huang, W-H., Klaunig, J. E., and Askari, A. (1990). Studies on the specificity of the effects of oxygen metabolites on cardiac sodium pump. *J. Mol. Cell. Cardiol. 22*: 911.

Zhao, M., Zhang, H., Robinson, T. F., Factor, S. M., Sonnenblick, E. H., and Eng, G. (1987). Profound structural alterations of the extracellular collagen matrix in postischemic dysfunction ("stunned") but viable myocardium. *J. Am. Coll. Cardiol. 10*: 1322.

Part III

Treatment for the Stunned Myocardium

Most investigators, when confronted with the situation of postischemic contractile dysfunction, ask the obvious question: What can be done to improve contractile performance? Our objective in this section is to provide an overview of therapeutic interventions that have shown promise for the treatment of the stunned myocardium.

We began, in a sense, to address this issue in Part II: Mechanisms of Postischemic Dysfunction. For example, the free radical-scavenging agents superoxide dismutase and catalase, used experimentally to elucidate the pathophysiology of the stunned myocardium, attenuate contractile dysfunction. In this section, we expand our observations to include the effects of mainstream cardiovascular drugs—including inotropic agents, beta blockers, calcium channel antagonists, angiotensin converting enzyme inhibitors, prostacyclins, and steroids—on postischemic recovery of contractile function in ex vivo and in vivo models of ischemia followed by reperfusion. Initial efforts to assess these agents in clinical instances of coronary artery occlusion/reperfusion are also reviewed. Although we are not always certain how these drugs improve contractile performance, this section provides convincing evidence that the stunned myocardium is amenable to therapeutic intervention.

13

Inotropic Agents and Stimulation of Stunned Myocardium

Lewis C. Becker

Johns Hopkins University School of Medicine, Baltimore, Maryland

I. INTRODUCTION

Although much has been learned about the pathogenesis of stunned myocardium, the fundamental cellular abnormalities responsible for the contractile dysfunction remain elusive. As discussed in the preceding chapters, abnormal contraction may be related to, among other things, a deficiency of intracellular activator calcium, reduced calcium sensitivity of the contractile apparatus, abnormalities in the contractile proteins themselves, or, in some cases, to extracellular abnormalities in the collagen matrix, resulting in increased mechanical loading of the affected myocardium. Although we remain ignorant of the precise cellular defects responsible for the dysfunction of stunned myocardium, a considerable amount of information is available about how the contractile abnormality may be overcome, if only temporarily, by the use of inotropic agents. In this chapter we will first examine the extent to which diverse inotropic agents can stimulate the contractile function of stunned myocardium. We will then discuss the probable mechanisms involved and the implications regarding the underlying cellular defects in stunned myocardium. Finally, we will address certain clinical aspects relating to inotropic support of stunned myocardium.

II. EFFECT OF INOTROPIC AGENTS ON STUNNED MYOCARDIUM

A. Beta-Adrenergic Agonists

It has been known for over a decade that catecholamines with beta-adrenergic activity can enhance the function of depressed postischemic myocardium in canine models. Even before the concept of myocardial stunning as a prolonged but ultimately temporary dysfunction of postischemic myocardium was formulated (Braunwald and Kloner, 1982), Smith (1980) demonstrated that an intracoronary bolus of isoproterenol markedly increased the velocity of contraction of myocardium made dysfunctional by 10 minutes of coronary artery occlusion and 15 minutes of reperfusion. The effect on contractility was only transient, however, and function returned to the postischemic baseline by 10 minutes after treatment.

Mercier et al. (1982) reported that dopamine had no effect on segmental function *during* a 30-minute coronary artery occlusion, but markedly enhanced contractility of myocardium which remained depressed *after reperfusion*. Following a 3-hour occlusion, dopamine also increased contractility, but only when the myocardium had remained largely viable, as judged by tetrazolium staining. Ellis et al. (1984) extended this study by showing that dopamine increased myocardial contractility both at 1 and 24 hours after release of a 2-hour coronary occlusion. Systolic wall thickening (determined by echocardiography) fell from 44% at baseline to only 1% at 1 hr after reperfusion and increased to 15% with dopamine. At 24 hours, wall thickening increased from −6% (dyskinesia) to +6%. Dopamine clearly stimulated the noncontracting postischemic myocardium to contract, presumably through an effect on stunned or reversibly injured myocytes (and not the necrotic myocytes) within the wall.

Using a similar model, Arnold et al. (1985) reported that after a 2-hour occlusion and 45 minutes of reperfusion, dopamine (10 μg/kg/min infused continuously for 3 hours) produced a sustained augmentation of function without evidence of further myocardial necrosis or reduction in myocardial high-energy phosphate stores. After stopping the dopamine infusion, contractility returned to, but not below, the postischemic baseline.

In both the Ellis and Arnold studies, a 2-hour canine coronary occlusion model was used, resulting in a mixture of necrotic and reversibly injured (presumably stunned) myocytes. Other laboratories have done similar studies with beta-adrenergic agonists in pure models of stunned myocardium without necrosis. Bolli et al. (1985) reported that isoproterenol (0.1 μg/kg/min IV) increased the wall thickening of myocardium stunned by 15 minutes of occlusion and 4 hours of reperfusion to original baseline levels (i.e., 20.8% at baseline; 2.6% postischemia; 24.8% during isoproterenol). Becker et al. (1986)

demonstrated similar results when myocardium was stunned by 12 repetitive 5-minute coronary occlusions followed by 1 hour of reperfusion, and stimulated with IV epinephrine. In both studies, the inotropic effect of the catecholamine was sustained for the duration of the infusion (30 minutes in Bolli's study, 1 hour in Becker's), and in neither case did function fall below the postischemic (precatecholamine) baseline after discontinuing the infusion, implying that no further myocardial injury was sutained during inotropic stimulation.

Confirmatory results have been obtained in a model of globally stunned myocardium (Ambrosio et al., 1987). Following 20 minutes of zero flow ischemia, perfused rabbit hearts recovered about 75% of baseline developed pressure, concomitant with a 20% loss of ATP as detected by ^{31}P-NMR. Electron microscopy demonstrated mild reversible abnormalities, similar to those described for regionally stunned myocardium in intact animals. Infusion of isoproterenol (5×10^{-8} M) sufficient to raise developed pressure 34% above the preischemic baseline did not result in any further depression of tissue ATP, suggesting that ATP production was capable of keeping up with increased ATP demands (Ambrosio et al., 1987). Infusion of adenosine during reperfusion in this model resulted in a significant increase in postischemic tissue ATP, but not in functional improvement (Ambrosio et al., 1989). Hoffmeister et al. (1985) reported similar findings with adenosine in the regionally stunned canine heart.

These studies taken together appear to rule out the hypothesis that postischemic dysfunction is caused by a deficiency of cellular energy production or supply to the contractile apparatus. If energy deficiency were the underlying problem, catecholamines should have produced no inotropic response, or a short-lived one at best, similar to that observed in ischemic myocardium. In particular, the sustained inotropic response found with prolonged infusions is inconsistent with an energy deficiency hypothesis.

According to many previous reports, stunned myocardium is characterized by both reduced shortening during systole and increased shortening after the end of systole, as defined by the end of global left ventricular contraction. The significance of diastolic shortening has been uncertain and attributed variously to (1) impaired relaxation and altered diastolic properties of stunned myocardium (Przyklenk et al., 1987; Charlat et al., 1989), (2) delayed shortening of weakened myocardium trying to contract against an afterload created by contraction of normal myocardium (Takayama et al., 1988), or (3) delayed excitation-contraction coupling in stunned myocardium (Levine et al., 1987). The issue of whether postsystolic contraction represents an active contractile process or merely passive elastic recoil secondary to early systolic stretching has remained controversial (Takayama et al., 1988). Recently, Rivers et al. (1991) reported that isoproterenol not only increased systolic segment shortening of stunned myocardium in the dog, but also reduced the amount and duration of shortening occurring after end systole. The authors concluded that isoproterenol accelerated relaxation in stunned myocardium, since the time to peak postsystolic shortening was also reduced. Whether the effect of isoproterenol is on systolic contraction, diastolic relaxation, or both, the net result is more efficient myocardial function, since greater shortening occurs during left ventricular systolic ejection.

Although beta-adrenergic agonists can stimulate the stunned myocardium to contract normally, this does not imply that the dysfunction of stunned myocardium is caused by a deficiency or down-regulation of beta-adrenergic receptors. Using a canine microembolization model, Hori et al. (1989) showed that 24 hours after embolization, both systolic and diastolic function were depressed, the inotropic response to isoproterenol was preserved, but the response to forskolin, a substance that activates adenylate cyclase independently of the beta-adrenergic receptor, was markedly depressed. One week after embolization, resting systolic function had returned to normal and histological necrosis was absent, but myocardial relaxation remained abnormal and the inotropic response to forskolin was still markedly impaired. The density of beta-adrenergic receptors had increased by 48%, compensating for the impairment of contractility. When a 24-hour infusion of isoproterenol was administered, the beta-receptors downregulated and unmasked the latent systolic dysfunction still present in the stunned myocardium. These studies clearly show that the defect in stunned myocardium responsible for the contractile dysfunction lies distal to the beta-adrenergic receptor.

B. Cardiac Glycosides

Stunned myocardium may also be inotropically stimulated by non-beta-adrenergic means, such as by cardiac glycosides. In an unpublished study from my laboratory done in 1987, six anesthetized dogs underwent 25 minutes of occlusion of the anterior descending coronary artery followed by 30 minutes of reperfusion to produce anterior wall stunning. Regional myocardial function was measured in the anterior and posterior walls by sonomicrometry, using the load-independent end-systolic pressure-length relation, before and after administration of acetylstrophanthidin (20 μg/kg IV, repeated to toxicity). The end-systolic pressure-length relation shifted significantly leftward after acetylstrophanthidin in both stunned and control myocardial regions (10.0 $\pm$ 3.3% and 6.2 $\pm$ 1.5% shifts, respectively), indicating a positive inotropic effect.

C. Postextrasystolic Potentiation

Becker et al. (1986) showed that postextrasystolic potentiation (PESP) produced a marked inotropic effect in stunned myocardium. Stunning was created in the dog by 12 5-minute episodes of coronary artery occlusion followed by 1 hour of reperfusion. PESP was accomplished by programmed atrial stimulation, using the shortest A_1A_2 interval that did not produce AV block or arrhythmias. Before ischemia, PESP increased mean myocardial segment shortening from 21.8% to 31.1%. Following stunning, shortening of the same segments increased from 7.8% to 24.8%. Ito et al. (1987) reported similar results in a 15-minute coronary occlusion/30-minute reperfusion canine model. PESP increased segment shortening from 25% to 30% before stunning and from 12% to 19% afterwards.

D. Calcium

Ito et al. (1987) have also shown that intracoronary calcium chloride can reverse the dysfunction of stunned myocardium in the canine model. Calcium produced a dose-dependent increase in segment shortening in stunned myocardium, from 12% at baseline to 35% at the highest dose of 14.7 mg/min. Before stunning, segment shortening increased during calcium infusion over the same dose range from 25% to 36.6%. In the globally stunned perfused ferret heart (15 minutes of zero flow ischemia at 37°C, followed by 20–30 minutes of reperfusion), Kusuoka et al. (1987) reported that the functionally depressed myocardium was remarkably responsive to increases in perfusate calcium concentration. In nonischemic hearts, left ventricular developed pressure increased from 34 to 174 mmHg as external calcium concentration was raised from 0.5 to 7.5 mM. In stunned hearts, left ventricular developed pressure increased from 17 to 127 mmHg over the same range of perfusate calcium.

E. Myocardial Blood Flow

Augmentation of coronary blood flow above baseline levels can increase the function of stunned myocardium without the administration of an inotropic agent. Interestingly, the function of normal myocardium is not altered by increasing flow. In the canine model of regional stunning produced by repetitive 5-minute occlusions, Stahl et al. (1986) showed that increasing coronary flow with intravenous dipyridamole or papaverine produced significant increases in segment shortening (from 0.9% to 8.8%, and from 6.7% to 13.6%, respectively), while contraction was unchanged in the control region despite similar increases in blood flow (to 150% above baseline with dipyridamole, 80% above baseline with papaverine). The end-systolic pressure–length relationship was shifted leftward with both vasodilators, indicative of a true enhancement of contractile performance rather than an afterload effect on systolic shortening. Intravenous nitroglycerin also increased shortening of stunned myocardium, but did not alter the end-systolic pressure–length relationship or increase blood flow, suggesting that nitroglycerin improved function by decreasing afterload.

III. SIGNIFICANCE OF INOTROPIC RESPONSIVENESS

The fact that stunned myocardium is capable of inotropic stimulation, despite baseline dysfunction, carries certain pathophysiological implications. Myocardial contraction is controlled by depolarization-induced release of calcium from the sarcoplasmic reticulum, with subsequent binding to troponin C and activation of the contractile proteins. Relaxation involves dissociation of calcium from troponin C and reuptake by the sarcoplasmic reticulum.

All of the inotropic agents discussed above increase the cytoplasmic calcium concentration following cellular depolarization, leading to greater activation of the contractile proteins and more complete myocardial contraction. Beta-adrenergic agonists stimulate the activity of adenylate cyclase, which catalyzes the formation of cAMP, leading in turn to stimulation of cAMP-dependent protein kinase, increased calcium influx during the slow inward current and increased release of calcium from the sarcoplasmic reticulum (Ruegg, 1988). Diastolic relaxation is enhanced through more rapid uptake of calcium by the sarcoplasmic reticulum, mediated through cAMP-dependent protein kinase phosphorylation of phospholamban, a regulatory protein (Ruegg, 1988). Cardiac glycosides increase cytosolic calcium concentration by inhibiting the sarcolemmal Na-K ATPase, leading to reduced sodium extrusion and increased sodium/calcium exchange. The cytosolic calcium concentration is also increased when extracellular calcium concentration is raised to produce a greater transmembrane calcium gradient. Finally, PESP increases cytosolic activator calcium by means of enhanced sarcoplasmic reticulum uptake of calcium during the postextrasystolic pause, followed by increased release of calcium during cellular depolarization.

Since the dysfunction of stunned myocardium can be reversed by an increase in intracellular free calcium, it would appear that the defect in stunned myocardium involves either a deficiency of cytosolic calcium or an insensitivity of the contractile proteins for calcium, resulting in reduced responsiveness to a normal cytosolic calcium level. In the first case, the calcium-force relationship is normal, while in the second, it is shifted downward (Fig. 1). In either case, increasing cytosolic calcium results in movement up the respective calcium-force curve, and a restoration of myocardial function. Of course, functional improvement of stunned myocardium occurs only while the inotropic agent is being given; following withdrawal, cytosolic calcium concentration falls and function returns to its baseline (stunned) level. Un-

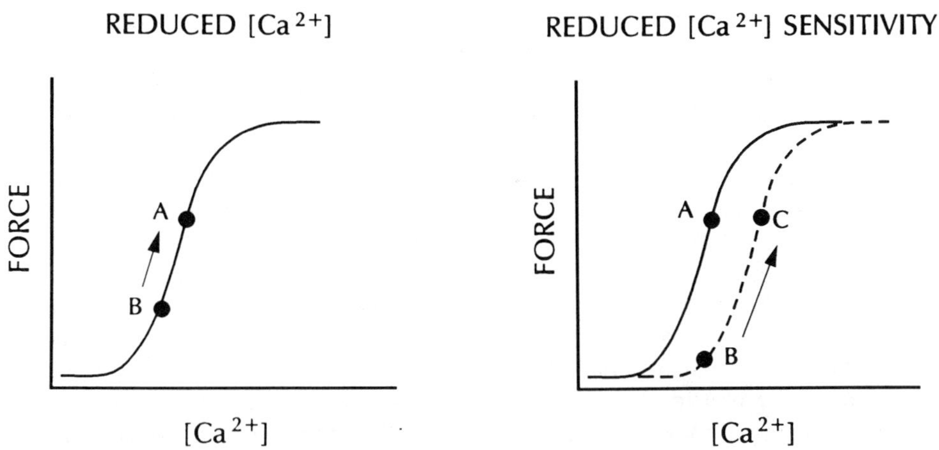

Figure 1 Possible alterations in the [Ca^{2+}]-myocardial force relationship in stunned myocardium. Point A represents normal preischemic values for force and [Ca^{2+}]. In the left panel, the [Ca^{2+}]-force relationship is normal in stunned myocardium, but the concentration of activator Ca^{2+} is reduced, causing a reduction in force to point B. Administration of an inotropic agent restores normal force by increasing [Ca^{2+}], causing the myocardium to move back up the normal [Ca^{2+}]-force relationship to point A. In the right panel, the contractile proteins in stunned myocardium are insensitive to a normal concentration of activator Ca^{2+}, causing a downward shift in the [Ca^{2+}]-force relationship and a decrease in force to point B. An inotropic agent restores normal force by increasing [Ca^{2+}], causing the myocardium to move up the depressed [Ca^{2+}]-force relationship to point C.

fortunately, the types of studies discussed above do not provide insight into whether the problem with stunned myocardium is a deficiency of activator calcium, reduced sensitivity of the contractile proteins, or both. However, as discussed in Chapter 9, studies measuring intracellular calcium concentration with ^{19}F NMR spectroscopy have demonstrated normal or increased levels of activator calcium in globally stunned ferret hearts, suggesting that the fundamental defect is altered calcium sensitivity of the contractile proteins (Kusuoka et al., 1990).

IV. CONTRACTILE RESERVE OF STUNNED MYOCARDIUM

An important unresolved issue is whether stunned myocardium possesses reduced contractile reserve in addition to impaired baseline function. A reduction in maximal contractile activity, if present, would implicate an abnormality of structure or function of the contractile proteins as a fundamental defect in stunned myocardium. As discussed above, a deficiency of activator calcium or a loss of sensitivity to calcium can be overcome by exposure of the stunned myocardium to higher concentrations of external calcium, but an abnormality of the contractile apparatus should not be correctable in this fashion.

The study by Ito et al. (1987) demonstrated that stepwise increases in intracoronary calcium concentration led to increases in segment shortening and that the maximal level achieved was not significantly different in stunned myocardium and normal myocardium (35.4% vs. 36.6%, respectively). PESP produced no additional increase in segment shortening at the highest calcium dose, consistent with the notion that contractile activity was already maximally stimulated by the calcium infusion. Calcium dose-response curves, obtained by plotting infused calcium dose against the change in segment shortening (percent of maximum), were virtually superimposable for stunned and normal myocardium, suggesting that stunning did not involve an alteration in calcium sensitivity of the contractile proteins (Fig. 2).

In contrast to these results, Kusuoka et al. (1987) reported that globally stunned ferret hearts demonstrated a 20% reduction in maximal calcium activated pressure (216 vs. 270 mmHg), measured during conditions under which contractile activation by calcium was likely to be maximal. This was achieved by producing tetani using rapid electrical stimulation after exposure to ryanodine, a substance that interferes with sarcoplasmic reticulum function (Marban et al., 1986). When developed pressure was expressed as a percent of maximal calcium-activated pressure and plotted against external calcium concentration (to yield curves of calcium sensitivity), stunned myocardium was found to have reduced responsiveness to calcium. The authors noted that this change could have reflected either diminished availability of activator calcium or a true reduction of calcium sensitivity of the contractile proteins.

The apparent contradictions between the Kusuoka and Ito studies may simply be a function of the models employed. It is quite possible that absence of flow in the perfused ferret heart for 15 minutes at 37°C produces greater myocardial injury than a 15-minute coronary artery occlusion in the dog with an intact collateral circulation. Alternatively, calcium activation was probably never truly maximal in Ito's study, which employed a nontetanized preparation with intact sarcoplasmic reticulum function. Additional studies in these and other models of myocardial stunning are needed to resolve the issue of whether maximal contractile activity is impaired.

V. CLINICAL ASPECTS OF INOTROPIC SUPPORT

Myocardial stunning appears to occur in patients following nonlethal episodes of myocardial ischemia, just as it does in the animal laboratory (see

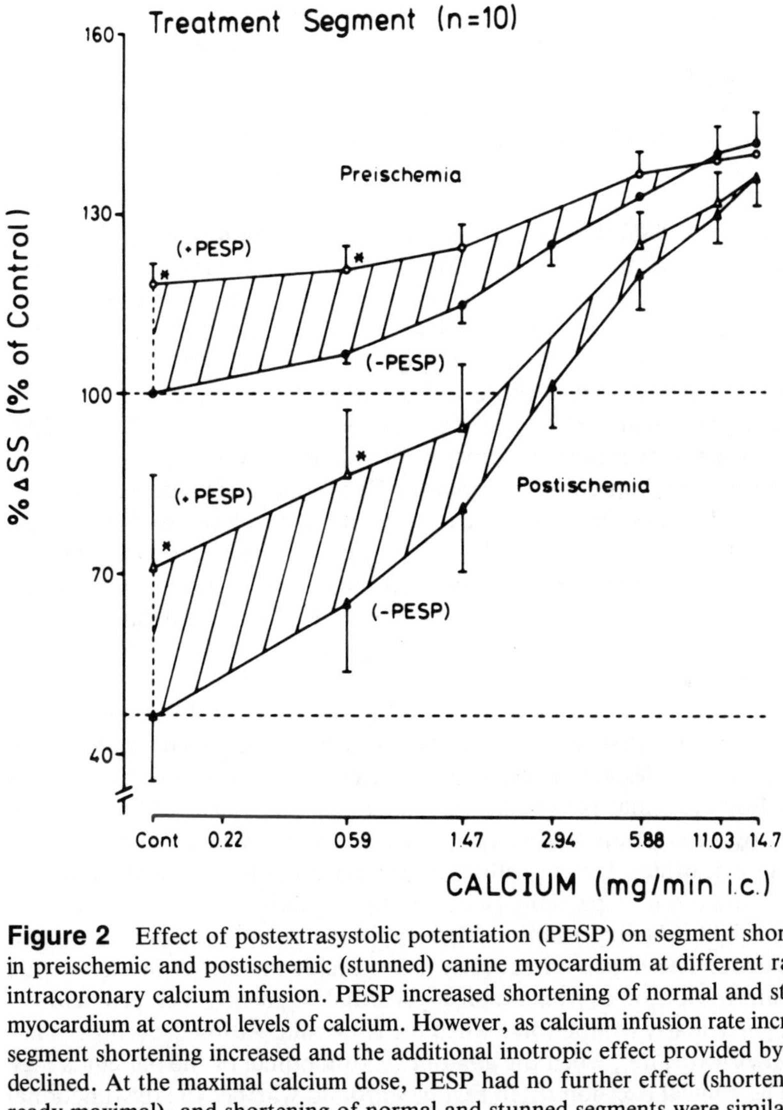

Figure 2 Effect of postextrasystolic potentiation (PESP) on segment shortening in preischemic and postischemic (stunned) canine myocardium at different rates of intracoronary calcium infusion. PESP increased shortening of normal and stunned myocardium at control levels of calcium. However, as calcium infusion rate increased, segment shortening increased and the additional inotropic effect provided by PESP declined. At the maximal calcium dose, PESP had no further effect (shortening already maximal), and shortening of normal and stunned segments were similar, suggesting that the contractile reserve of stunned myocardium was normal. (From Ito et al., 1987, by permission of the American Heart Association.)

Section IV). The response of stunned myocardium to inotropic agents provides a means for identifying stunning in patients. In addition, the response of dysfunctional myocardium to inotropic agents should permit a distinction between stunning and hibernation (chronic ischemia). While stunned myocardium responds readily to catecholamines, PESP, or calcium, ischemic myocardium cannot, or can only respond for a brief period of time (Vatner et al., 1976).

Satler et al. (1986) showed that left ventricular ejection fraction, measured by radionuclide ventriculography 2 weeks after an acute myocardial infarction, could be increased by intravenous isoproterenol in a group of patients that had been treated with streptokinase. The increase in ejection fraction during isoproterenol was significantly greater in patients with a patent infarct-related artery than in those with an occluded artery at the time of a predischarge coronary arteriogram. Sheehan et al. (1985) reported that PESP could increase contraction of segments with abnormal wall motion following acute myocardial infarction, and that the PESP response predicted improvement in wall motion in a subsequent study performed 8 or more days later. These postinfarct studies have been interpreted as showing contractile reserve in viable myocardium salvaged by thrombolytic therapy, which is dysfunctional (stunned) at the time of study but capable of significant recovery over time.

Other studies have shown that nitroglycerin (Helfant et al., 1974), PESP (Hamby et al., 1975), or catecholamines (Horn et al., 1974), can improve regional function in asynergic left ventricular segments in patients with chronic coronary artery disease. These results are consistent with the presence of stunned myocardium possessing contractile reserve, but could also be explained by a reduction in afterload, relief of silent ischemia, stimulation of normal myocardium present within the asynergic segment, or short-term inotropic stimulation of partially ischemic myocardium.

Why might it be important to identify stunned myocardium, assuming it can be done? The clinician frequently has to decide whether or not to attempt revascularization of dysfunctional myocardial segments. The problem becomes particularly troublesome when the revascularization procedure is not straightforward, i.e., when the anatomy is suboptimal or the patient is high risk. The clinical decision often revolves around whether the dysfunctional segment is largely alive (stunned or ischemic) or dead (necrotic or scarred). If it is alive, revascularization may be essential for the recovery of the patient, whereas if it is already dead, no improvement is expected. The presence of contractile reserve during catecholamine infusion or PESP would certainly support viability in the dysfunctional segment. An absence of contractile reserve, however, is not so easily interpreted, since it could be related to ongoing (often silent) ischemia of otherwise viable myocardium. Newer techniques, such as positron emission tomography or NMR spectroscopy, may eventually prove better than the presence of preserved contractile reserve for identifying viable postischemic myocardium, based on sufficient preservation of metabolic function.

The inotropic response of stunned myocardium may be important therapeutically as well as diagnostically. Following relief of ischemia in patients with acute coronary syndromes, function may remain depressed in one or more myocardial segments, leading to a clinically important depression in global left ventricular function. This is particularly a problem in patients with previous myocardial infarction and preexisting left ventricular damage. To the extent that postischemic dysfunction is caused by stunning, as opposed to necrosis, the myocardium can be supported by an inotropic intervention, usually a catacholamine infusion, until spontaneous recovery occurs. Judging from laboratory studies, this process may take days to weeks. The appropriate use of inotropic agents may keep patients with stunned myocardium out of cardiogenic shock and may avoid use of aortic counterpulsation. It should be cautioned, however, that the use of inotropic agents in patients with ongoing ischemia may lead to an extension of myocardial injury and ultimately to a worsening of left ventricular function. If the myocardium is stunned rather than ischemic, prolonged inotropic support should be possible, without functional depression or extension of damage following withdrawal of therapy.

Probably the most dramatic and well-documented case of prolonged support was reported by Ballantyne et al. (1987). Following coronary artery bypass surgery for unstable angina, a man developed profound functional depression of the left ventricle (ejection fraction = 6%; preoperative ejection fraction = 50%). The patient was treated with a left ventricular assist device for 7 days, an intraaortic balloon pump for 9 days, and intravenous inotropic agents (amrinone and dobutamine) for 12 days. On the eighth postoperative day, the ejection fraction had improved to 38%, and on the 17th postoperative day, it was 34% without any inotropic support. This case is a vivid reminder that some patients who appear to have suffered massive myocardial necrosis may actually have large amounts of reversibly stunned myocardium and can be maintained by inotropic support.

REFERENCES

Ambrosio, G., Jacobus, W. E., Bergman, C. A., Weisman, H. F., and Becker, L. C. (1987). Preserved high energy phosphate metabolic reserve in globally "stunned" hearts despite reduction of basal ATP content and contractility. *J. Mol. Cell Cardiol. 19*: 953.

Ambrosio, G., Jacobus, W. E., Mitchell, M. C., Litt, M. R., and Becker. L. C. (1989). Effects of ATP precursors on ATP and free ADP content and functional recovery of postischemic hearts. *Am. J. Physiol. 256*: H560.

Arnold, J. M. O., Braunwald, E., Sandor, T., and Kloner, R. A. (1985). Inotropic stimulation of reperfused myocardium with dopamine: Effects on infarct size and myocardial function. *J. Am. Coll. Cardiol. 6*: 1026.

Ballantyne, C. M., Verani, M. S., Short, H. D., Hyatt, C., and Noon, G. P. (1987). Delayed recovery of severely "stunned" myocardium with the support of a left ventricular assist device after coronary artery bypass graft surgery. *J. Am. Coll. cardiol. 10*: 710.

Becker, L. C., Levine, J. H., DiPaula, A. F., Guarnieri, T., and Aversano, T. (1986). Reversal of dysfunction in postischemic stunned myocardium by epinephrine and postextrasystolic potentiation. *J. Am. Coll. Cardiol. 7*: 580.

Bolli, R., Zhu, W.-X., Myers, M. L., Hartley, C. J., and Roberts, R. (1985). Beta-adrenergic stimulation reverses postischemic myocardial dysfunction without producing subsequent functional deterioration. *Am. J. Cardiol. 56*: 964.

Braunwald, E., and Kloner, R. A. (1982). The stunned myocardium: Prolonged, postischemic ventricular dysfunction. *Circulation 66*: 1146.

Charlat, M. L., O'Neill, P. G., Hartley, C. J., Roberts, R., and Bolli, R. (1989). Prolonged abnormalities of left ventricular diastolic wall thinning in the "stunned" myocardium in conscious dogs: Time course and relation to systolic function. *J. Am. Coll. Cardiol. 13*: 185.

Ellis, S. G., Wynne, J., Braunwald, E., Henschke, C. I., Sandor, T., and Kloner, R. A. (1984). Response of reperfusion-salvaged, stunned myocardium to inotropic stimulation. *Am. Heart J. 107*: 13.

Hamby, R., Aintablian, A., Wisoff, B. G., and Harstein, M. L. (1975). Response of the left ventricle in coronary artery disease to postextrasystolic potentiation. *Circulation 51*: 428.

Helfant, R. H., Pine, R., Meister, S. G., Feldman, M. S., Trout, R. G., and Banka, V. S. (1974). Nitroglycerin to unmask reversible asynergy. Correlation with post-coronary bypass ventriculography. *Circulation 50*: 108.

Hoffmeister, H. M., Mauser, M., and Schaper, W. (1985). Effect of adenosine and AICAR on ATP content and regional contractile function in reperfused canine myocardium. *Basic Res. Cardiol. 80*: 445.

Hori, M., Koretsune, Y., Kagiya, T., Watanabe, Y., Iwakura, K., Iwai, K., Kitabatake, A., Yoshida, H., Inoue, M., and Kamada, T. (1989). An increase in myocardial b-adrenoreceptors to compensate for postischemic dysfunction following coronary micro-embolisation in dogs. *Cardiovasc. Res. 23*: 424.

Horn, H. R., Teicholz, L. E., Cohn, P. F., Herman, M. V., and Gorlin, R. (1974). Augmentation of left ventricular contraction pattern in coronary artery disease by an inotropic catecholamine. The epinephrine ventriculogram. *Circulation 49*: 1063.

Ito, B. R., Tate, H., Kobayashi, M., and Schaper, W. (1987). Reversibly injured, postischemic canine myocardium retains normal contractile reserve. *Circ. Res. 61*: 834.

Kusuoka, H., Porterfield, J. K., Weisman, H. F., Weisfeldt, M. L., and Marban, E. (1987). Pathophysiology and pathogenesis of stunned myocardium. Depressed Ca^{2+} activation of contraction as a consequence of reperfusion-induced cellular calcium overload in ferret hearts. *J. Clin. Invest. 79*: 950.

Kusuoka, H., Koretsune, Y., Chacko, V. P., Weisfeldt, M. L., and Marban, E. (1990). Excitation-contraction coupling in postischemic myocardium. Does failure of activator Ca^{2+} transients underlie stunning? *Circ. Res. 66*: 1268.

Levine, J. H., Moore, E. N., Weisman, H. F., Kadish, A. H., Becker, L. C., and Spear, J. F. (1987). Depression of action potential characteristics and a decrease space constant are present in postischemic, reperfused myocardium. *J. Clin. Invest. 79*: 107.

Marban, E., Kusuoka, H., Yue, D. T., Weisfeldt, M. L., and Wier, G. (1986). Maximal Ca^{2+}-activated force elicited by tetanization of ferret papillary muscle and whole heart: Mechanism and characteristics of steady contractile activation in intact myocardium. *Circ. Res. 59*: 262.

Mercier, J. C., Lando, U., Kanmatsuse, K., Ninomiya, K., Meerbaum, S., Fishbein, M. C., Swan, H. J. C., and Ganz, W. (1982). Divergent effects of inotropic stimulation on the ischemic and severely depressed reperfused myocardium. *Circulation 66*: 397.

Przyklenk, K., Patel, B., and Kloner, R. A. (1987). Diastolic abnormalities of postischemic "stunned" myocardium. *Am. J. Cardiol. 60*: 1211.

Rivers, J. T., Norris, R. M., and Cross, D. B. (1991). Changes in systolic canine myocardium by isoproterenol or calcium. *Coronary Artery Dis. 2*: 101.

Ruegg, J. C. (1988). *Calcium in Muscle Activation. A Comparative Approach,* Springer-Verlag, Berlin.

Satler, L. F., Kent, K. M., Fox, L. M., Goldstein, H. A., Green, C. E., Rogers, W. J., Pallas, R. S., Del Negro, A. A., Pearle, D. L., and Rackley, C. E. (1986). The assessment of contractile reserve after thrombolytic therapy for acute myocardial infarction. *Am. Heart J. 111*: 821.

Sheehan, F. H., Mathey, D. G., Dodge, H. T., and Schofer, J. (1985). Postextrasystolic potentiation predicts recovery of LV function in patients reperfused late after infarction. *J. Am. Coll. Cardiol. 5*: 495 (Abstract).

Smith, H. J. (1980). Depressed contractile function in reperfused canine myocardium: Metabolism and response to pharmacological agents. *Cardiovasc. Res. 14*: 458.

Stahl, L. D., Aversano, T. R., and Becker, L. C. (1986). Selective enhancement of function of stunned myocardium by increased flow. *Circulation 74*: 843.

Takayama, M., Norris, R. M., Brown, M. A., Armiger, L. C., Rivers, J. T., and White, H. D. (1988). Postsystolic shortening of acutely ischemic canine myocardium predicts early and late recovery of function after coronary artery reperfusion. *Circulation 78*: 994.

Vatner, S. F., Millard, R. W., Patrick, T. A., and Heyndrickx, G. R. (1976). Effects of isoproterenol on regional myocardial function, electrocardiogram and blood flow in conscious dogs with myocardial ischemia. *J. Clin. Invest. 57*: 1261.

14

Calcium Antagonists as Treatment for the Stunned Myocardium

Karin Przyklenk and Robert A. Kloner

Hospital of the Good Samaritan and University of Southern California, Los Angeles, California

I. INTRODUCTION

Calcium antagonists—including verapamil, nifedipine, diltiazem, and the newer second-generation dihydropyridine derivatives such as amlodipine—are potent vasodilators which act by regulating the entry of calcium ions into myocytes and smooth muscle cells through the voltage-dependent calcium channels (Opie, 1990). In addition to the proven efficacy of these agents in the clinical management of hypertension and angina pectoris (Opie, 1990), the recent reports of altered calcium homeostasis in isolated perfused heart preparations stunned by brief episodes of ischemia (Kusuoka et al., 1987; Marban, 1991) and apparent oxygen free radical-scavenging properties of calcium antagonists (Shridi and Robak, 1988; Janero et al., 1988; Koller and Bergman, 1989; Mak and Weglicki, 1990) have raised interest in the possibility that these agents may, in theory, also provide a promising form of treatment for postischemic contractile dysfunction. Thus, the objectives of this chapter are to review our current knowledge of the effects of calcium antagonists in various experimental models of postischemic myocardial stunning, and attempt to explain *why* these agents enhance recovery of contractile function following transient ischemia/reperfusion. Several of the concepts addressed in this chapter have been discussed in other recent reviews (Przyklenk and Kloner, 1991a,b).

II. CALCIUM ANTAGONISTS IN MODELS OF GLOBAL ISCHEMIA

The first indication that calcium antagonists improve contractile function of stunned myocardium was observed in isolated perfused heart preparations subjected to global ischemia or hypoxia followed by reoxygenation. For example, Watts et al. (1986) assessed the effects of verapamil, diltiazem, and nifedipine on recovery of left ventricular function (defined as the product of peak systolic pressure and heart rate) and high-energy phosphate metabolism in isolated working rat hearts subjected to 27 minutes of ischemia and 30 minutes of reflow. As expected, function in untreated control hearts assessed 30 minutes after reperfusion was profoundly stunned, averaging only 20% of baseline values. In contrast, addition of verapamil, diltiazem, or nifedipine to the perfusate prior to ischemia was associated with a significant improvement in postischemic function to >80% of baseline values. In addition, adenosine triphosphate stores were in part preserved at 50-60% of normal, nonischemic values in all treatment groups. Similar results have also been obtained in experimental models of global ischemic arrest during cardiopulmonary bypass: addition of nifedipine, diltiazem, or verapamil to various cardioplegic solutions has been shown to enhance recovery of ventricular performance and preservation of high-energy phosphate stores following restoration of blood flow (Robb-Nicholson et al., 1978; Clark et al., 1980; Vouhe et al., 1980; Barner et al., 1981; Magovern et al., 1981; Allen et al., 1986; Rebeyka et al., 1990). In fact, numerous investigators have consistently reported that pretreatment with calcium antagonists significantly improves recovery of contractile function following global ischemia/reperfusion (Nayler, 1981; Bersohn and Shine, 1983; McGoon, 1985; Higgins and Blackburn, 1986; Ferrari et al., 1986; Kirkels et al., 1988).

III. CALCIUM ANTAGONISTS IN MODELS OF BRIEF REGIONAL ISCHEMIA

A. Recovery of Systolic Function

Considerable evidence indicates that calcium antagonists also enhance recovery of contractile function in models of brief, transient *regional* ischemia designed to mimic clinical instances of angina. For example, Nagao et al. (1980) first addressed this question more than a decade ago by assessing recovery of regional developed tension (measured using epicardial strain gauges) following 5-10 minutes of circumflex coronary occlusion in the canine model. In this very early study, the authors reported that diltiazem administered before and during ischemia enhanced recovery of developed tension when compared with controls. Nearly 8 years later, our laboratory addressed this same issue by evaluating the effects of verapamil on recovery of regional systolic and diastolic function in anesthetized open-chest dogs subjected to 15 minutes of coronary artery occlusion and 3 hours of reperfusion (Przyklenk and Kloner, 1988). Dogs were randomly assigned to one of four treatment groups: verapamil given 30 minutes before coronary occlusion; at the moment of reperfusion; 30 minutes after reflow had been established; or saline alone. Segment shortening in control animals remained stunned throughout reperfusion, averaging only 30% of baseline values following relief of ischemia. In contrast, verapamil given before coronary occlusion essentially ablated postischemic dysfunction: segment shortening was restored to 100% of normal, baseline values in dogs pretreated with verapamil (Fig. 1A).

Similar episodes of enhanced postischemic recovery of function have been observed when diltiazem (Fig. 2), amlodipine (Fig. 3), nifedipine, or the intracellular calcium antagonist KT-362 were given before coronary occlusion (Taylor et al., 1990; Dunlap et al., 1989; Lamping and Gross, 1985; Farber and Gross, 1989). For example, Taylor et al. (1990) reported that prophylactic administration of diltiazem significantly improved wall thickening in conscious dogs subjected to 15 minutes of transient ischemia. Furthermore, Taylor and colleagues concluded that the most ischemic myocardial segments—that is, those that exhibited paradoxical wall thinning during coronary occlusion—benefited the most from diltiazem pretreatment (Fig. 2). Even very small doses of nifedipine initiated prior to occlusion have been shown by Lamping and Gross (1985) to produce a small but significant improvement in postischemic function when compared with controls.

Although these data are important, pharmacological interventions given prior to or during ischemia do not always represent a feasible means of treatment. Thus, we were especially interested to find that verapamil administered *at or after* reperfusion also attenuated postischemic contractile dysfunction (Przyklenk and Kloner, 1988). Verapamil administered either at the moment of reflow or 30 minutes after reperfusion restored segment shortening to approximately 65% of baseline values—significantly greater than the value of 30% observed in the untreated controsl (Fig. 1A). Using this same canine model, we observed even more striking results when nifedipine was administered 30 minutes after reperfusion (Przyklenk et al., 1989): "delayed" treatment with nifedipine restored segment shortening to 90-100% of baseline vs. values of only 20% observed in the control group (Fig. 4A). Thus, although there are differences in efficacy among the various calcium antagonists, there is little doubt that these agents can attenuate—or even resolve—the systolic

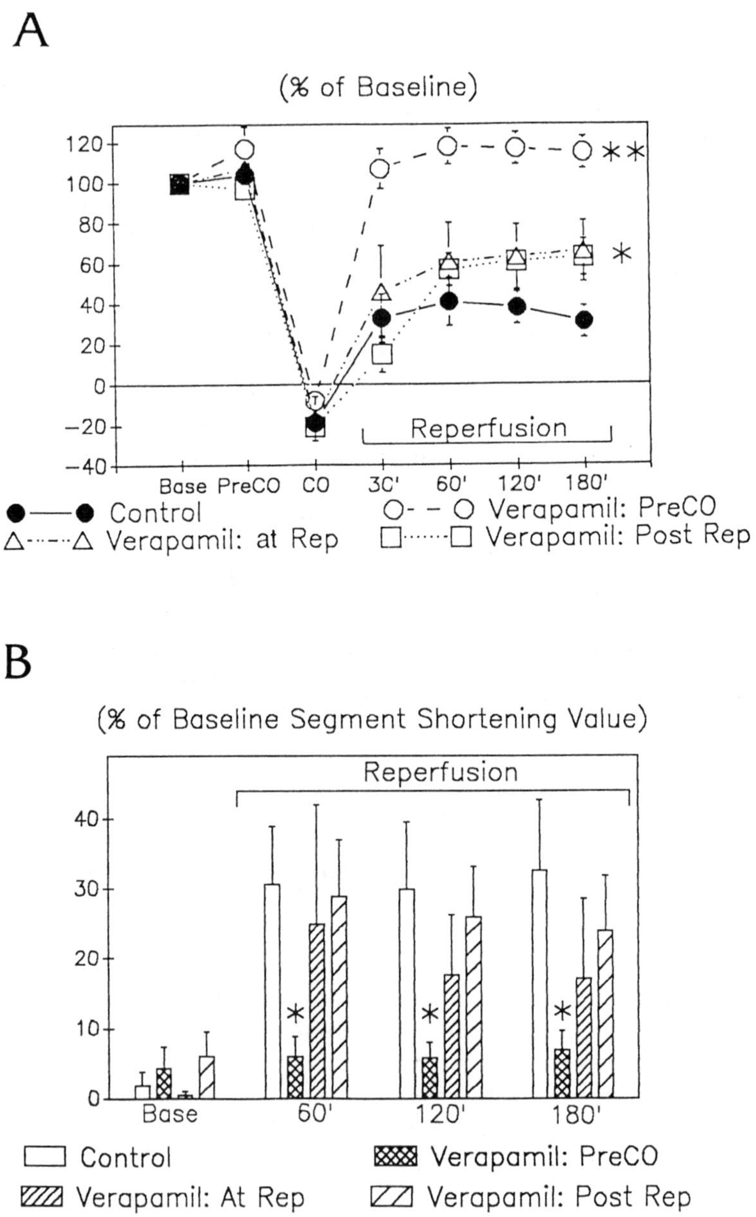

Figure 1 Effect of verapamil on recovery of: (A) segment shortening during systole (expressed as % of baseline, preocclusion values); and (B) paradoxical postsystolic shortening during early diastole (expressed as % of baseline segment shortening values) following a 15-minute episode of left anterior descending (LAD) coronary artery occlusion. CO = coronary occlusion; Rep = reperfusion. $^*p < 0.05$, $^{**}p < 0.01$ vs. control group. (Figure 1A adapted from Przyklenk and Kloner, 1988; Figure 1 reprinted with permission from Przyklenk and Kloner, 1991b.)

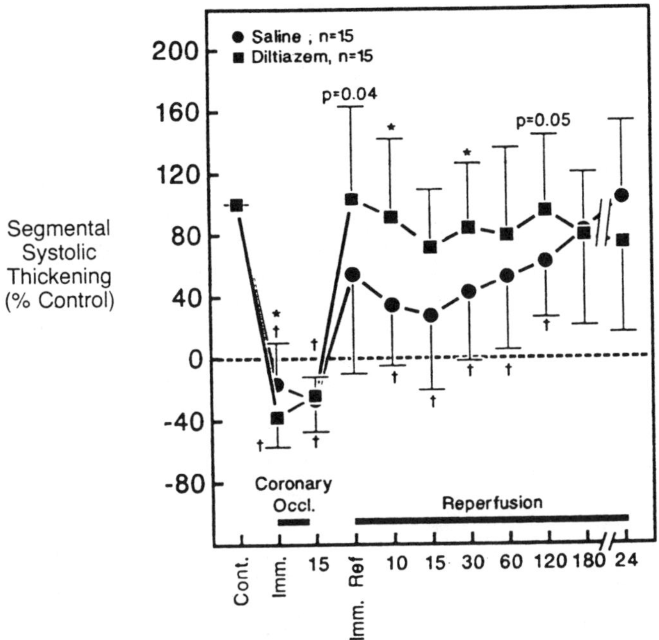

Figure 2 Segmental systolic thickening (as % of control) over time comparing treatment with saline solution and diltiazem for class 3 myocardial segments (those that exhibited systolic wall thinning during occlusion) during 15 minutes of coronary artery occlusion. Cont = control study; Imm = immediately after coronary artery occlusion; Imm Ref = at immediate reflow; Occl = occlusion. (From Taylor et al., 1990, with permission of the American College of Cardiology.)

contractile abnormalities of canine myocardium stunned by a brief episode of transient ischemia, even when treatment is initiated at or after reperfusion.

B. Recovery of Diastolic Function

In addition to well-documented depression in systolic contractile following brief but transient coronary occlusion, the stunned myocardium is also characterized by marked paradoxical shortening during what should be isovolumic diastole, and by prolonged diastolic relaxation time τ (Brown et al., 1987; Przyklenk et al., 1987a,b). We found that verapamil given before coronary occlusion in our canine model restored paradoxical postsystolic shortening to normal, near-zero values following reflow, as compared with the expected postsystolic shortening values of 30% observed throughout reperfusion in the control group (Przyklenk and Kloner, 1991b). In contrast, delayed treatment with verapamil did not resolve this abnormality in diastolic

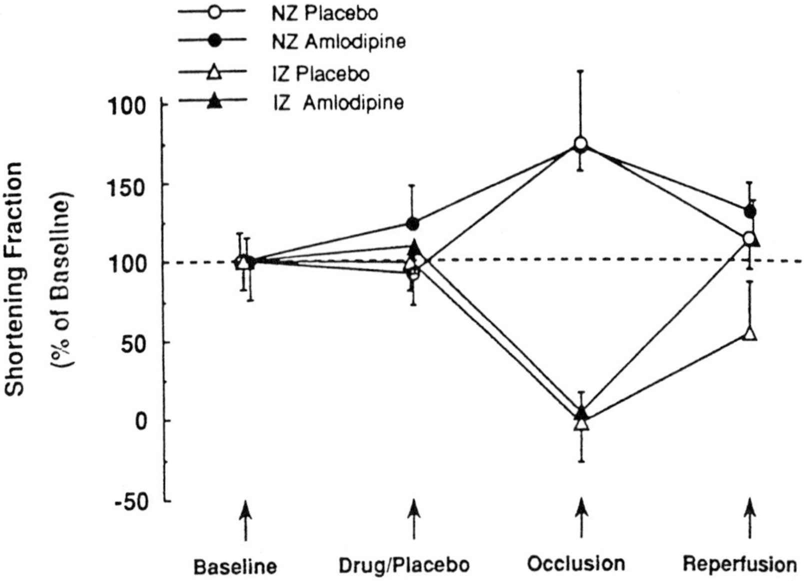

Figure 3 Effect of amlodipine (3 mg/kg) or placebo (3 ml saline solution) on percent change from baseline of systolic shortening fraction in ischemic zone (IZ) and normal zone (NZ) of canine myocardium. Shortening fraction before administration of drug/placebo, 10 minutes after intravenous drug/placebo administration, and at the end of 10 minutes of coronary occlusion, and after 60 minutes of reperfusion is plotted. (From Dunlap et al., 1989, with permission.)

relaxation: postsystolic shortening persisted at 20-30% in dogs that received verapamil at or after reperfusion (Fig. 1B) (Przyklenk et al., 1987a; Przyklenk and Kloner, 1991b). That is, although delayed treatment with verapamil enhanced recovery of systolic contraction following brief ischemia, verapamil given at or after reperfusion did not improve postischemic recovery of diastolic function.

Delayed treatment with nifedipine did, however, have beneficial effects on diastolic function following 15 minutes of transient coronary occlusion. At 10 minutes after reperfusion (that is, before randomization and treatment), postsystolic shortening was elevated at 30-45% in all dogs. Although paradoxical contraction during diastole persisted throughout reflow in the control group, we found that postsystolic shortening was restored to normal near-zero values following administration of nifedipine (Fig. 4B). Furthermore, nifedipine given after reperfusion also had a beneficial effect on diastolic relaxation time (Fig. 4C). In control animals, τ remained prolonged at 125%

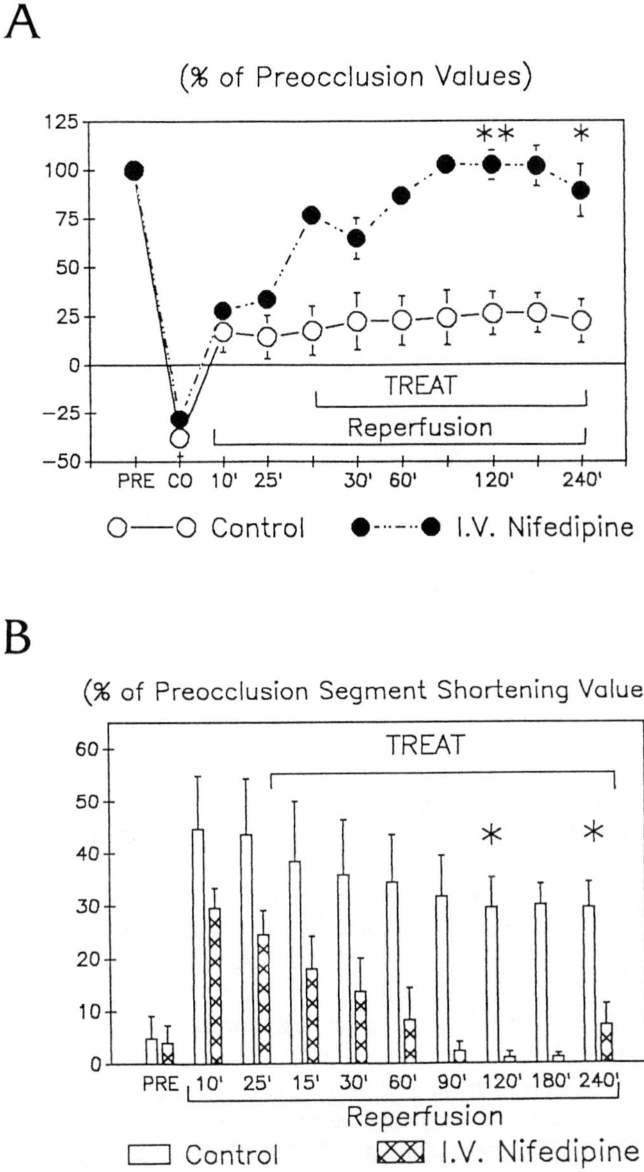

Figure 4 Effect of intravenous (IV) nifedipine, administered after reperfusion, on: (A) segment shortening during systole (expressed as % of baseline, preocclusion values); (B) paradoxical postsystolic shortening during early diastole (expressed as % of baseline segment shortening values); and (C) time constant of diastolic relaxation (expressed as % of preocclusion values) following a 15-minute episode of left anterior descending (LAD) coronary artery occlusion. CO = coronary occlusion. $*p < 0.03$; $**p < 0.003$ vs. control group. (Figure 4A adapted from Przyklenk et al., 1989. Figure 4 reprinted with permission from Przyklenk and Kloner, 1991b.)

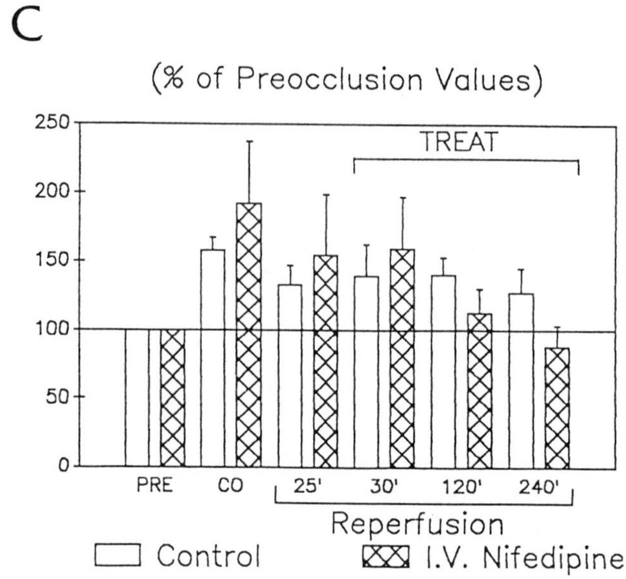

Figure 4 (Continued)

of preocclusion values throughout reperfusion, whereas T was restored to baseline values in the nifedipine-treated group (Przyklenk and Kloner, 1991).

Similar salutary results were also reported by Fujibayashi and colleagues (1985): nifedipine administered either during ischemia or following reperfusion enhanced the recovery of early diastolic velocity of luminal area change (an index of diastolic function assessed by echocardiography) following 1-2 minutes of coronary artery occlusion in the canine model. In other studies, however, nifedipine has failed to resolve diastolic abnormalities following a brief ischemic episode. For example, Applegate et al. (1987) found that a 30- to 60-second period of simultaneous left anterior descending and circumflex coronary occlusions in conscious dogs resulted in an increase in diastolic relaxation time τ both during ischemia and at 30-60 seconds following reperfusion. Nifedipine infused prior to and during ischemia did not, however, alter relaxation time when compared with untreated controls. In addition, Bourdillion et al. (1986) have reported that pretreatment with verapamil did not alter the upward shift in the left ventricular diastolic pressure-volume relationship following 3 minutes of pacing-induced ischemia in the canine model. Thus, while calcium antagonists clearly enhance recovery of systolic function following brief ischemia, the effects of these agents on the diastolic abnormalities of stunned myocardium remain less well defined.

IV. CALCIUM ANTAGONISTS IN MODELS OF PROLONGED BUT TRANSIENT CORONARY OCCLUSION

Do calcium antagonists have beneficial effects on salvaged, previously ischemic myocardium stunned by a prolonged (1-2 hour) period of coronary artery occlusion—that is, in models that mimic reperfusion for the treatment of acute myocardial infarction? In contrast to the consistent results obtained in the brief occlusion models, the effect of calcium antagonists on recovery of systolic contractile function following prolonged but transient ischemia have ranged from clearly significant improvements in function, acute but short-lived increases in contractility, improvements in function only during potentiated beats, and a complete lack of improvement in function. For example, pretreatment with amlodipine (Fig. 5) (Gross et al., 1989) and diltiazem

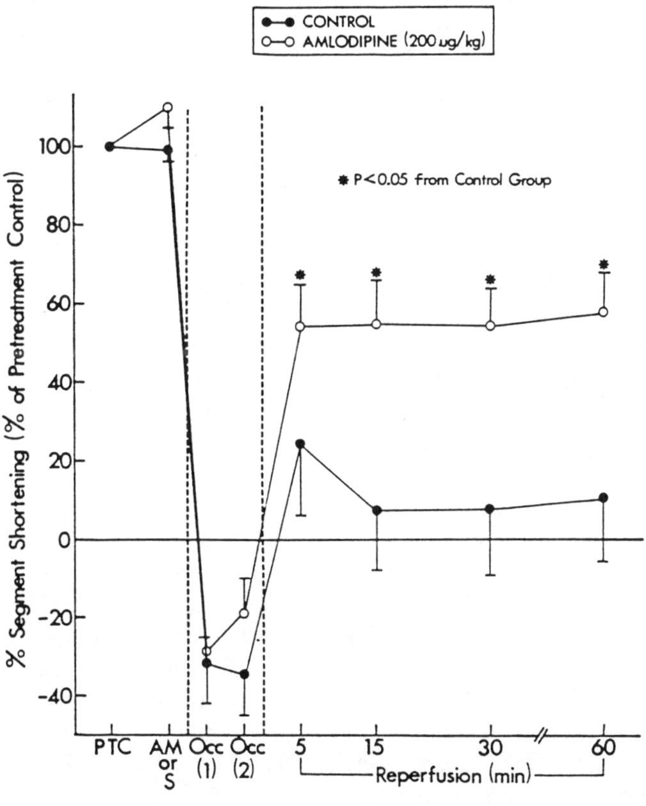

Figure 5 Percent segment shortening of the ischemic-reperfused area (% of control) in the saline (control) and amlodipine (AM)-treated groups before occlusion (PTC), during 45 minutes of occlusion (Occ 1,2) and at various times after reperfusion. (From Gross et al., 1989, with permission.)

(Higginson et al., 1991) have both been shown to enhance recovery of segment shortening of the presumably viable subepicardium in open-chest dogs subjected to 45-90 minutes of coronary artery occlusion and 1-4 hours of reperfusion. Although the beneficial results obtained with amlodipine may have solely been a consequence of the significant increase in collateral blood flow to the ischemic tissue associated with amlodipine treatment (i.e., a reduction in the severity of the ischemic insult) (Gross et al., 1989), the improvement in function with intracoronary infusion of diltiazem could not be attributed to alterations in either myocardial perfusion or hemodynamic parameters (Higginson et al., 1991). Using an anesthetized porcine model, Sullivan et al. (1991) found that the effects of verapamil pretreatment on recovery of postischemic function were dose-dependent: high doses of verapamil (resulting in a decrease in segment shortening prior to occlusion) were associated with superior recovery of function following reflow, whereas lower doses of verapamil (with no negative inotropic effect) failed to enhance postischemic contractile performance. In other studies in the canine model, diltiazem (van der Vusse et al., 1986) and KT-362 (Pelc et al., 1989) produced short-lived improvements in regional wall motion, which then deteriorated during the initial hours following reperfusion. In contrast, Sherman et al. (1981) found that pretreatment with verapamil had no effect on segment shortening of paced beats measured during 2 hours of occlusion and 1 hour of reperfusion, but significantly increased contractility during postextrasystolic potentiation when compared with controls. That is, verapamil appeared to enhance the *latent* capacity for contraction following prolonged ischemia.

Calcium antagonists given during occlusion or at the time of reperfusion have, in general, yielded disappointing results. For example, although pretreatment with diltiazem improved segmental wall motion following 90 minutes of coronary occlusion in the canine model, this agent was ineffective when treatment was initiated at the time of reperfusion (Higginson et al., 1991). Negative results have also been obtained using the porcine model of transient ischemia: Odom and colleagues (1988) found no difference in wall thickening following 1 hour of coronary occlusion and 2 hours of reflow in pigs treated with verapamil, nifedipine, or vehicle alone. Similarly, nifedipine failed to enhance recovery of segment shortening at 3-4 hours following thrombolysis in pigs that underwent 30 minutes of thrombotic occlusion (van der Giessen et al., 1988). In contrast, modest improvements in function were observed by Klein et al. (1989) at 3 days after reflow in the porcine model when diltiazem, nifedipine, or verapamil were given at the end of a 45-minute episode of coronary artery occlusion (Figure 6).

How can we reconcile the consistent improvement in systolic function with calcium antagonist treatment following brief ischemia vs. the mixed results

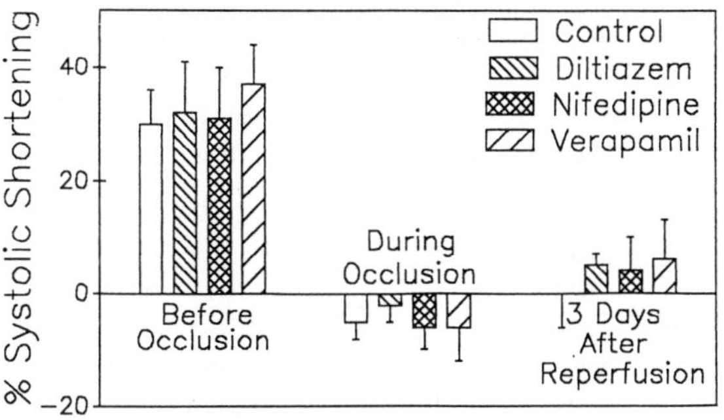

Figure 6 Regional systolic shortening in the ischemic/reperfused myocardium of pigs subjected to 45 minutes of coronary occlusion and 3 days of reperfusion. (Adapted with permission from Klein et al., 1989.)

that have been observed with the agents following prolonged coronary occlusion/reperfusion? In addition to the obvious differences in doses, routes of administration, durations of occlusion and reperfusion, and differences in the inotropic properties among the various calcium antagonists, three additional factors may play a role. First, despite the lack of an acute beneficial effect in some studies, the evidence of preserved latent contractility with verapamil reported by Sherman and colleagues (1981) suggests that calcium antagonists may accelerate the ultimate functional recovery of the tissue in the weeks following reperfusion. This hypothesis, however, remains to be tested. In addition, this apparent "discrepancy" may also reflect fundamental differences in the mechanism(s) of stunning following brief vs. prolonged ischemia (see Chapter 8). It is interesting to note that a difference in efficacy in models of brief vs. prolonged ischemia is not unique to calcium antagonist treatment: a similar "discrepancy" has been observed with the oxygen radical-scavenging agents superoxide dismutase + catalase, which consistently enhance recovery of contractile function following 15 minutes—but not following 90-120 minutes—of coronary artery occlusion (Kloner et al., 1989; Bolli, 1990). These data may also indicate that timely pharmacological intervention may improve recovery of function if the ischemic insult is brief and/or mild, but prolonged and severe ischemia may simply be beyond the therapeutic limits of these agents. Finally, some of these "discrepancies" may be due in part to inherent limitations in the measurement of contractile function in viable tissue overlying a subendocardial infarct. That is, in contrast to the brief occlusion models, measurement of function in following prolonged ischemia/reperfusion—especially measurement of wall thickening—is influenced both by the stunned subepicardium and the subendocardial necrosis. Measurement of contractile function in salvaged subepicardium may be further confounded by tethering of the stunned tissue to the adjacent infarct. These inherent limitations make interpretation of the effects of calcium antagonists (or any other treatment) on recovery of function following prolonged periods of ischemia complex and, as yet, unresolved.

V. MECHANISMS OF ACTION

Although the effects of calcium antagonists in models of prolonged regional ischemia have been inconclusive, there is little doubt that these agents enhance postischemic recovery of contractile function following either global ischemia or following brief but transient coronary artery occlusion. Furthermore, calcium antagonists enhance recovery of systolic function in models of brief transient ischemia even when treatment is delayed. The obvious question arising from these data is: What are the mechanism(s) of action of these agents in the setting of transient ischemia/reperfusion?

A. Role of Hemodynamics and High-Energy Phosphate Metabolism

Any intervention that reduces the severity of the ischemic insult will, not surprisingly, reduce the degree of injury and dysfunction following reperfusion (Opie, 1989). There is no doubt that calcium antagonists are potent systemic and coronary vasodilators (Opie, 1989). In addition, a host of ex vivo studies (Nayler, 1981; Bersohn and Shine, 1983; Ferrari et al., 1986; Watts et al., 1986; Kirkels et al., 1988) and in vivo studies (Lange et al., 1984; Przyklenk and Kloner, 1988) have found that calcium antagonists given before coronary occlusion in part preserve myocardial high-energy phosphate stores. Pretreatment with these agents may therefore improve function of stunned myocardium simply by reducing myocardial oxygen demand and increasing oxygen supply during occlusion, or by blunting the depletion of high-energy stores during the ischemic episode.

For example, we found in our canine model that ATP content in the previously ischemic subendocardium of control animals stunned by 15 minutes of coronary artery occlusion remained depressed at 3 hours following reflow, averaged only 75% of normal values (Przyklenk and Kloner, 1988). As expected, ATP content in dogs pretreated with verapamil was 90% of normal, significantly greater than the value of 75% observed in the control group (Przyklenk and Kloner, 1988). This partial preservation of ATP stores could, in theory, have contributed significantly to the enhanced recovery of function in the pretreated group. Verapamil did not, however, preserve ATP content of the stunned tissue when treatment was begun at or after reperfusion, yet both these delayed treatment groups exhibited improved recovery of systolic function to 65% of baseline values (Przyklenk and Kloner, 1989). Thus, the improved function associated with delayed verapamil treatment clearly was not a consequence of ATP preservation.

It is also not surprising that verapamil and nifedipine in our brief occlusion protocols were potent vasodilators (Przyklenk and Kloner, 1988; Przyklenk et al., 1989). For example, mean arterial pressure measured 2 hours following reperfusion and treatment averaged 84 mmHg in animals that received nifedipine vs. 122 mmHg in the control group. In addition, regional myocardial blood flow measured after reperfusion and treatment was doubled in the nifedipine-treated dogs when compared with controls (Przyklenk et al., 1989). Previous evidence indicates that contractile function of stunned myocardium may be sensitive to both reductions in afterload and increased myocardial blood flow (Stahl et al., 1986). Thus, it is possible that the improved recovery of function that we observed with systemic administration of nifedipine or verapamil may simply have been a nonspecific consequence of reduced afterload or enhanced coronary perfusion following reflow.

B. Direct Effect of Calcium Antagonists on Stunned Myocardium?

To further investigate the importance of these hemodynamic alterations on recovery of function with calcium antagonist treatment, we performed an additional series of experiments in which very small intracoronary doses of nifedipine were infused directly into the stunned region of the heart beginning 30 minutes after reperfusion (Przyklenk et al., 1989). Intracoronary infusions of 1-3 $\times$ 10^{-4} mg/kg/min had no effect on mean arterial pressure or myocardial blood flow. This small dose of nifedipine did, however, significantly enhance segment shortening to 75-90% of baseline values in the absence of any apparent hemodynamic effect (Fig. 7) (Przyklenk et al., 1989). These data provide strong evidence that calcium antagonists given after reperfusion did not enhance contractile function of stunned myocardium solely by reducing afterload or increasing coronary blood flow. Rather, these results suggest that nifedipine administered after reperfusion exerted a direct, beneficial effect on the stunned, previously ischemic tissue. This concept is further supported by the reports of improved recovery of function in isolated perfused heart preparations (i.e., models not confounded by peripheral hemodynamic effects) with calcium antagonist therapy. But the question still remains: What is the mechanism of this apparent direct effect of calcium antagonists on the stunned myocytes?

We do not yet have an answer to this question. However, the solution may lie in an apparent complex interrelationship that may exist between production

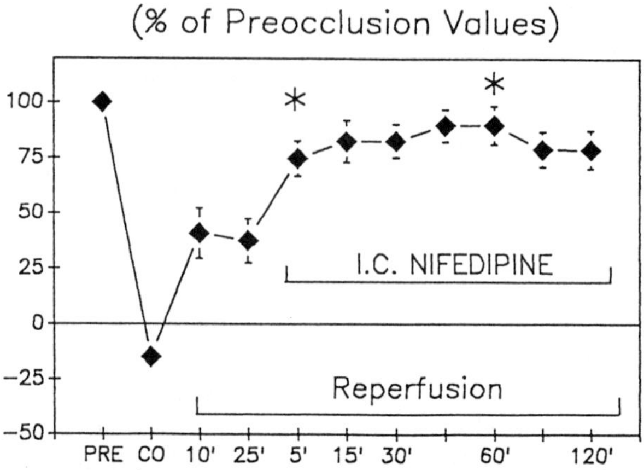

Figure 7 Segment shortening, expressed as % of baseline preocclusion values, for dogs that received intracoronary (IC) nifedipine beginning 30 minutes after reperfusion. CO = coronary occlusion; LAD = left anterior descending coronary artery. $*p < 0.03$ vs. 25 minutes after reperfusion. (Adapted from Przyklenk et al., 1989, and reprinted with permission from Przyklenk and Kloner, 1991b.)

of oxygen free radicals and altered calcium homeostasis (Fig. 8), both of which have been implicated as important mediators of postischemic contractile dysfunction (Kusuoka et al., 1987; Marban, 1991; Kloner et al., 1989; Bolli, 1990). The role of oxygen radicals and calcium homeostasis in the pathogenesis of the stunned myocardium have been reviewed in detail in Part II of this book. Briefly, there is little doubt that oxygen-derived free radicals (such as the superoxide anion and the hydroxyl radical) contribute to postischemic contractile dysfunction (Kloner et al., 1989; Bolli, 1990). In addition, an increase in the peak systolic intracellular calcium concentration and decrease in myofilament calcium responsiveness has been observed in isolated perfused heart preparations stunned by 15 minutes of global ischemia (Kusuoka et al., 1987; Marban, 1991). The third—and perhaps most important—component of this interrelationship is the apparent link between abnormal calcium flux and production of oxygen radicals. For example, exposure of isolated cardiac membranes to oxygen radicals has been shown to inhibit sarcolemmal calcium pump function and enhance membrane permeability to calcium (Levedev et al., 1982; Kaneko et al., 1989, 1990). Furthermore, exposure of intact myocytes to oxygen radicals in the absence of ischemia causes peroxidation of the membranes, abnormalities in calcium transients, and asynchronous contraction (Burton et al., 1990). It is also interesting to note that the calcium antagonists verapamil, nifedipine, and diltiazem have all been

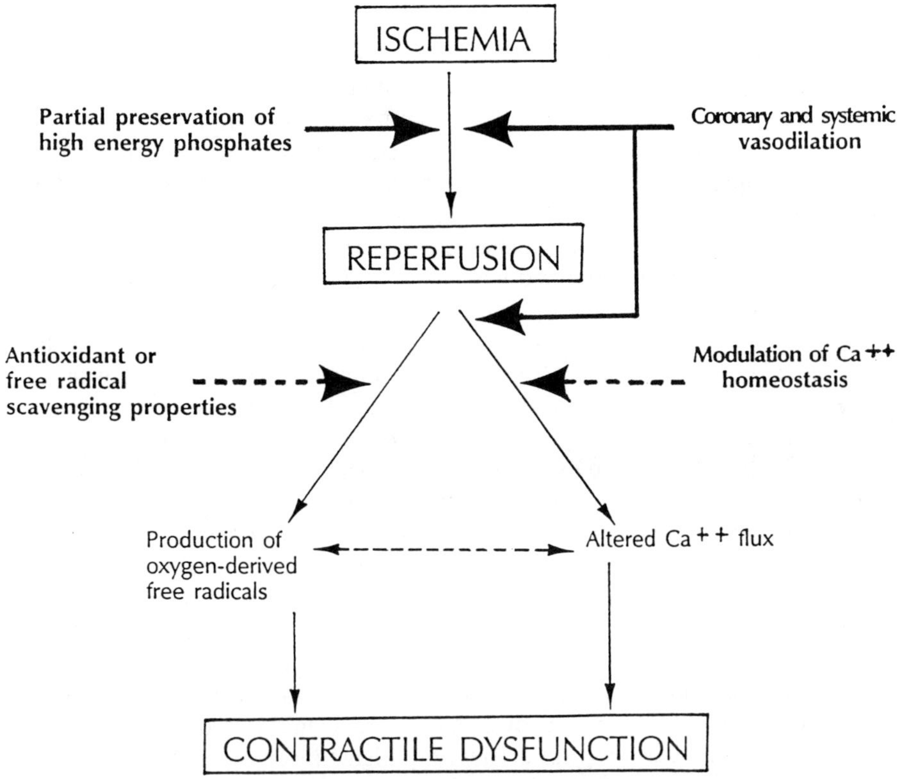

Figure 8 Possible mechanisms of action of calcium antagonists on stunned myocardium. In addition to their well-documented vasodilator and energy-sparing properties, calcium antagonists may also exert a direct, beneficial effect on the stunned myocytes by acting as antioxidants/oxygen radical scavengers, and/or by favorably modulating calcium homeostasis.

reported to have either direct, free radical-scavenging properties or inhibit peroxidation of membrane lipids (Shridi and Robak, 1988; Janero et al., 1988; Koller and Bergman, 1989; Mak and Weglicki, 1990). In fact, Adachi and colleagues (1990) have postulated that cardioprotection by verapamil may be contingent upon the presence of the enzyme xanthine oxidase, considered to be an important source of oxygen radicals in species such as the dog and rat, but present in only negligible amounts in rabbit and man. These various pieces of data raise the possibility that calcium antagonists, in addition to their well-documented hemodynamic effects, may favorably alter calcium homeostasis within the stunned myocytes, either directly or by acting as scavenging agents. This hypothesis, however, remains to be substantiated.

IV. SUMMARY AND CLINICAL IMPLICATIONS

Considerable experimental evidence indicates that calcium antagonists can attenuate postischemic contractile dysfunction of viable myocardium stunned by a transient episode of ischemia. When treatment is initiated prophylactically, calcium antagonists can enhance postischemic recovery of systolic and—in some cases—diastolic function, and in part preserve myocardial high-energy phosphate stores. It is especially interesting to note that delayed treatment does not preclude a beneficial effect: significant improvements in systolic function were obtained with these agents even when treatment was begun at or after reperfusion. Despite the wealth of experimental data that has been collected, the mechanisms of action of calcium antagonists in the setting of transient ischemia/reperfusion remains uncertain. In addition to the obvious and expected vasodilatory effects of these agents, evidence obtained from isolated heart preparations and from our in vivo intracoronary nifedipine protocol strongly suggests that calcium antagonists may exert a direct—but as yet unspecified—beneficial effect on the stunned myocytes.

These data obtained in various ex vivo and in vivo models raise the possibility that calcium antagonists may prove useful in the clinical management of stunned myocardium. In fact, the effects of calcium antagonists on recovery of contractile function following ischemia/reperfusion have been evaluated in a small number of randomized clinical trials. For example, addition of nifedipine to two different cardioplegic solutions resulted in a twofold greater postoperative improvement in cardiac index, stroke volume, and stroke work index when compared with patients receiving standard cardioplegia alone (Clark et al., 1983). Similarly, addition of diltiazem to crystalloid cardioplegia was shown to preserve myocardial high-energy phosphate stores and improve myocardial metabolism following coronary bypass (Christakis et al., 1986). These data are similar to the overwhelmingly positive results that have been obtained in experimental models of global ischemia/reperfusion (Robb-Nicholson et al., 1978; Clark et al., 1980; Vouhe et al., 1980; Barner et al., 1981; Magovern et al., 1981; Allen et al., 1986; Rebeyka et al., 1990). However, despite the salutary effects of diltiazem on postoperative recovery of myocardial metabolism, Christakis and colleagues (1986) stressed caution in the use of diltiazem with cardioplegia due to the potent negative inotropic properties of this agent.

Several clinical studies have assessed the effects of calcium antagonists in the setting of acute myocardial infarction—and obtained generally disappointing results (Held et al., 1989). The negative findings in these early studies may have been due in part to hypotension (resulting in a drop in coronary perfusion pressure) and reflex tachycardia caused by the relatively high doses of calcium channel antagonists used (Kloner and Przyklenk, 1991). In addition, most of these studies were done *before the era of thrombolysis*: there is considerably less data available on the effect of calcium antagonists as "adjuvant therapy" with reperfusion. Erbel et al. (1988) found that nifedipine, administered before, during, and after thrombolysis did not enhance recovery of global or regional left ventricular function at the time of hospital discharge. The negative results obtained in this study may be due, however, to the relatively late start of treatment: approximately 2.5 hours after the onset of symptoms. Although not evaluated in this protocol, Erbel and colleagues also raise the possibility that nifedipine may have in part preserved the latent capacity for contraction during postextrasystolic potentiation. In contrast, preliminary unpublished observations from our institution suggests that small doses of intracoronary nifedipine (approximately 30 μg) can enhance contractile function following reperfusion for the treatment of acute myocardial infarction. In the two patients studied, infusion of nifedipine was assoicated with a modest reduction in the number of abnormally contracting myocardial segments (assessed from left ventriculograms) following treatment, suggesting that contractile function of salvaged but stunned myocardium in these patients was somewhat enhanced by infusion of nifedipine. Further clinical trials are needed, however, in order to evaluate the potential role of calcium antagonists in the treatment of postischemic dysfunction following ischemia/reperfusion.

REFERENCES

Adachi, T., Miura, T., Noto, T., Ooiwa, H., Ogawa, T., Tsuchida, A., Iwamoto, T., Goto, M., and Iimura, O. (1990). Does verapamil limit infarct size in a heart deficient in xanthine oxidase? *Clin. Exper. Pharmacol. Physiol. 17*: 769.

Allen, B. S., Okamoto, F., Buckberg, G. D., Acar, C., Partington, M., Bugyi, H., and Leaf, J. (1986). Studies of controlled reperfusion after ischemia. IX. Reperfusate composition: benefits of marked hypocalcemia and diltiazem on regional recovery, *J. Thorac. Cardiovasc. Surg. 92*: 564.

Applegate, R. J., Walsh, R. A., and O'Rourke, R. A. (1987). Effects of nifedipine on diastolic function during brief periods of flow-limiting ischemia in the conscious dog. *Circulation 76*: 1409.

Barner, H. B., Jellinek, M., Standeven, J. W., Menz, L. J., and Hahn, J. W. (1982). Cold blood-diltiazem cardioplegia. *Ann. Thorac. Surg. 33*: 55.

Bersohn, M. M., and Shine, K. I. (1983). Verapamil protection of ischemic isolated rabbit heart: Dependence on pretreatment. *J. Mol. Cell. Cardiol. 15*: 659.

Bolli, R. (1990). Mechanisms of myocardial stunning. *Circulation 82*: 723.

Bourdillion, P. D., Paulus, W. J., Serizawa, T., and Grossman, W. (1986). Effects of verapamil on regional myocardial diastolic function in pacing-induced ischemia in dogs. *Am. J. Physiol. 251*: H834.

Brown, M. A., Norris, R. M., Takayama, M., and White, H. D. (1987). Post-systolic shortening: a marker of potential for early recovery of acutely ischemic myocardium in the dog. *Cardiovasc. Res. 21*: 803.

Burton, K. P., Morris, A. C., Massey, K. D., Buja, L. M., and Hagler, H. K. (1990). Free radicals alter ionic calcium levels and membrane phospholipids in cultured rat ventricular myocytes. *J. Mol. Cell. Cardiol. 22*: 1035.

Christakis, G. T., Fremes, S. E., Weisel, R. D., Tittley, J. G., Mickle, D. A. G., Ivanov, J., Madonik, M. M., Benak, A. M., McLaughlin, P. R., and Baird, R. J. (1986). Diltiazem cardioplegia: a balance of risk and benefit. *J. Thorac. Cardiovasc. Surg. 91*: 647.

Clark, R. E., Christlieb, I. Y., Spratt, J. A., Henry, P. D., Fischer, A. E., Williamson, J. R., and Sobel, B. E. (1981). Myocardial preservation with nifedipine: a comparative study at normothermia. *Ann. Thorac. Surg. 31*: 3.

Clark, R. E., Magovern, G. J., Christlieb, I. Y., and Boe, S. (1983). Nifedipine cardioplegia experience: Results of a 3 year cooperative clinical study. *Ann. Thorac. Surg. 36*: 654.

Dunlap, E. D., Matlib, M. A., and Millard, R. W. (1989). Protection of regional mechanics and mitochondrial oxidative phosphorylation by amlodipine in transiently ischemic myocardium. *Am. J. Cardiol. 64*: 841.

Erbel, R., Pop, T., Meinertz, T., Olshausen, C. V., Treese, N., Heinrichs, K. J., Schuster, C. J., Rupprecht, H. J., Schlurmann, W., and Meyer, J. (1988). Combination of calcium channel blocker and thrombolytic therapy in acute myocardial infarction. *Am. Heart J. 115*: 529.

Farber, N. E., and Gross, G. J. (1989). Cardioprotective effects of a new vascular intracellular calcium antagonist, KT-362, in the stunned myocardium. *J. Pharmacol. Exp. Ther. 248*: 39.

Ferrari, F., Albertini, A., Curello, S., Ceconi, C., Di Lisa, F., Raddino, R., and Visioli, O. (1986). Myocardial recovery during postischemic reperfusion: Effects of nifedipine, calcium and magnesium. *J. Mol. Cell. Cardiol. 18*: 487.

Fujibayashi, Y., Yamazaki, S., Chang, B. L., Rajagopalan, R. E., Meerbaum, S., and Corday, E. (1985). Comparative echocardiographic study of recovery of diastolic versus systolic function after brief periods of coronary occlusion: Differential effects of intravenous nifedipine administered before and during occlusion. *J. Am. Coll. Cardiol. 6*: 1289.

Gross, G. J., Farber, N. E., and Pieper, N. E. (1989). Effects of amlodipine on myocardial ischemia-reperfusion injury in dogs. *Am. J. Cardiol. 64*: 941.

Held, P. H., Yusuf, S., and Furberg, C. D. (1989). Calcium channel blockers in acute myocardial infarction and unstable angina: an overview. *Br. Med. J. 299*: 1187.

Higgins, A. J., and Blackburn, K. J. (1986). Prevention of reperfusion damage in working rat hearts by calcium antagonists and calmodulin antagonists. *J. Mol. Cell. Cardiol. 16*: 427.

Higginson, L., Tang, A., Knoll, G., and Calvin, J. (1991). Effect of intracoronary diltiazem on infarct size and regional myocardial function in the ischemic-reperfused canine heart. *J. Am. Coll. Cardiol., 18*: 867.

Janero, D. R., Burghardt, B., and Lopez, R. (1988). Protection of cardiac membrane phospholipid against oxidative injury by calcium antagonist. *Biochem. Pharmacol. 37*: 4197.

Kaneko, M., Beamish, R. E., and Dhalla, N. S. (1989). Depression of heart sarcolemmal Ca^{2+} pump activity by oxygen free radicals. *Am. J. Physiol. 256*: H368.

Kaneko, M., Singal, P. K., and Dhalla, N. S. (1990). Alterations in heart sarcolemmal Ca^{2+}-ATPase and Ca^{2+} binding activities due to oxygen free radicals. *Basic Res. Cardiol. 85*: 45.

Kirkels, J. H., Ruigrok, T. J. C., von Echtheld, C. J. A., and Meijler, F. L. (1988). Protective effect of pretreatment with the calcium antagonist anipamil on the ischemic-reperfused rat myocardium: A phosphorous-31 nuclear magnetic resonance study. *J. Am. Coll. Cardiol. 11*: 1087.

Klein, H. H., Pich, S., Lindert, S., Nebendahl, K., Warneke, G., and Kreuzer, H. (1989). Treatment of reperfusion injury with intracoronary calcium channel antagonists and reduced coronary free calcium concentration in regionally ischemic, reperfused porcine hearts. *J. Am. Coll. Cardiol. 13*: 1395.

Kloner, R. A., Przyklenk, K., and Whittaker, P. (1989). Deleterious effects of oxygen radicals in ischemia/reperfusion: Resolved and unresolved issues. *Circulation 80*: 1115.

Kloner, R. A., and Przyklenk, K. (1991). Experimental infarct size reduction with calcium channel blockers. *J. Am. Coll. Cardiol. 18*: 876.

Koller, P. T., and Bergmann, S. R. (1989). Reduction of lipid peroxidation in reperfused isolated rabbit hearts by diltiazem. *Circ. Res. 65*: 838.

Kusuoka, H., Porterfield, J. K., Weisman, H. F., Weisfeldt, M. L., and Marban, E. (1987). Pathophysiology and pathogenesis of stunned myocardium: Depressed Ca^{2+} activation of contraction as a consequence of reperfusion-induced cellular calcium overload in ferret hearts. *J. Clin. Invest. 79*: 950.

Lamping, K. A., and Gross, G. J. (1985). Improved recovery of myocardial segment function following a short coronary occlusion in dogs by nicorandil, a potential new antianginal agent, and nifedipine. *J. Cardiovasc. Pharmacol. 7*: 158.

Lange, R., Ingwall, J. S., Hale, S. L., Alker, K. J., and Kloner, R. A. (1984). Preservation of myocardial high energy phosphates by verapamil in reperfused myocardium. *Circulation 70*: 734.

Levedev, A. V., Levitsky, D. O., Loqinov, V. A., and Smirnov, V. O. N. (1982). The effect of primary products of lipid peroxidation on transmembrane transport of calcium ions. *J. Mol. Cell. Cardiol. 14* (Suppl. IV): 99.

Magovern, G. J., Dixon, C. M., and Burkholder, J. A. (1981). Improved myocardial protection with nifedipine and potassium-based cardioplegia. *J. Thorac. Cardiovasc. Surg. 82*: 239.

Mak, I. T., and Weglicki, W. B. (1990). Comparative antioxidant activities of propranolol, nifedipine, verapamil and diltiazem against sarcolemmal membrane lipid peroxidation. *Circ. Res. 66*: 1449.

Marban, E. (1991). Myocardial stunning and hibernation: The physiology behind the colloquialisms. *Circulation 83*: 681.

McGoon, D. G. (1985). The ongoing quest for ideal myocardial protection: A catalog of the recent english literature. *J. Thorac. Cardiovasc. Surg. 89*: 639.

Nagao, T., Matlib, M. A., Franklin, D., Millard, R. W., and Schwartz, A. (1980). Effects of diltiazem, a calcium antagonist, on regional myocardial function and mitochondria after brief coronary occlusion. *J. Mol. Cell. Cardiol. 12*: 29.

Nayler, W. G. (1981). The role of calcium in the ischemic myocardium. *Am. J. Pathol. 102*: 262.

Odom, H., Peng, C. F., Murphy, M. L., Davis, J. L., and Straub, K. D. (1988). Evaluation of biochemical functions and ventricular performance in regional ischemic-reperfused myocardium by afterload reduction: Differential effects of calcium blocking and non-calcium blocking vasodilators. *Int. J. Cardiol. 21*: 233.

Opie, L. H. (1989). Reperfusion injury and its pharmacologic modification. *Circulation 80*: 1049.

Opie, L. H. (1990). Calcium channel antagonists. Part I: Fundamental properties, mechanisms, classification, sites of action. *Clinical Use of Calcium Channel Antagonist Drugs, 2nd ed.* (L. H. Opie, ed.), Kluwar Academic Publishers, Boston, p. 28.

Pelc, L. R., Farber, N. E., Warltier, D. C., and Gross, G. J. (1989). Reduction of myocardial ischemia/reperfusion injury by KT-362, a new intracellular calcium antagonist in anesthetized dogs. *J. Cardiovasc. Pharmacol. 13*: 586.

Przyklenk, K., Patel, B., and Kloner, R. A. (1987a). Isovolumic relaxation and systolic contraction of postischemic stunned myocardium: divergent effects of verapamil. *J. Am. Coll. Cardiol. 9*: 93A (Abstract).

Przyklenk, K., Patel, B., and Kloner, R. A. (1987b). Diastolic abnormalities of postischemic stunned myocardium. *Am. J. Cardiol. 60*: 1211.

Przyklenk, K., and Kloner, R. A. (1988). Effect of verapamil on postischemic stunned myocardium: Importance of the timing of treatment. *J. Am. Coll. Cardiol. 11*: 614.

Przyklenk, K., Ghafari, G. B., Eitzman, D. T., and Kloner, R. A. (1989). Nifedipine administered after reperfusion ablates systolic contractile dysfunction of postischemic stunned myocardium. *J. Am. Coll. Cardiol. 13*: 1176.

Przyklenk, K., and Kloner, R. A. (1991a). Calcium antagonists and stunned myocardium; importance for clinicians? *Cardiovasc. Drugs Ther. 5*: 985.

Przyklenk, K., and Kloner, R. A. (1991b). Calcium antagonists and the stunned myocardium. *J. Cardiovasc. Pharmacol. 18* (Suppl. 10): S93.

Rebeyka, I. M., Axford-Gatley, R. A., Bush, B. G., del Nido, P. J., Mickle, D. A. G., Romanschin, A. D., and Wilson, G. J. (1990). Calcium paradox in an in vivo model of multidose cardioplegia and moderate hypothermia. *J. Thorac. Cardiovasc. Surg. 99*: 475.

Robb-Nicholson, C., Currie, W. D., and Wechsler, A. S. (1978). Effects of verapamil on myocardial tolerance to ischemic arrest: comparison to potassium arrest. *Circulation 58* (Suppl. I): 1-119.

Sherman, L. G., Liang, C. S., Boden, W. E., and Hood, W. B. Jr. (1981). The effect of verapamil on myocardial performance of acutely ischemic and reperfused myocardium in the conscious dog. *Circ. Res. 48*: 224.

Shridi, F., and Robak, J. (1988). The influence of calcium channel blockers on superoxide anions. *Pharmacol. Res. Comm. 20*: 13.

Stahl, L., Anversano, T., and Becker, L. C. (1986). Selective enhancement of function of stunned myocardium by increased flow. *Circulation 74*: 843.

Taylor, A. L., Golino, P., Eckels, R., Pastor, P., Buja, M., and Willerson, J. T. (1990). Differential enhancement of postischemic segmental systolic thickening by diltiazem. *J. Am. Coll. Cardiol. 15*: 737.

van der Giessen, W. J., Harmsen, E., de Tombe, P. P., Hugenholtz, P. G., and Verdow, P. D. (1988). Coronary thrombolysis with and without nifedipine in pigs. *Basic Res. Cardiol. 83*: 258.

van der Vusse, G. J., van der Veen, F. H., Prinzen, F. W., Coumans, W. A., van Bilsen, M., and Reneman, R. S. (1986). The effect of diltiazem on myocardial recovery after regional ischemia in dogs. *Eur. J. Pharmacol. 125*: 383.

Vouhe, P. R., Helias, J., and Grondin, C. M. (1980). Myocardial protection through cold cardioplegia using diltiazem, a calcium channel blocker. *Am. Thorac. Surg. 30*: 342.

Watts, J. A., Maiorano, L. J., and Maiorano, P. C. (1986). Comparison of the protective effects of verapamil, diltiazem, nifedipine and buffer containing low calcium upon global myocardial ischemic injury. *J. Mol. Cell. Cardiol. 18*: 255.

15

Beta Blockers

Garrett J. Gross

Medical College of Wisconsin, Milwaukee, Wisconsin

I. INTRODUCTION

Beta-adrenergic receptor blocking agents are commonly used in the treatment of myocardial ischemia and have been shown to be effective as antiarrhythmic and antianginal agents and to reduce the incidence of reinfarction and mortality in patients who have suffered a previous myocardial infarction (ISIS-1, 1986). In addition, these compounds have been shown to reduce myocardial infarct size in anesthetized dogs (Lange et al., 1983) and to enhance regional wall motion in conscious dogs subjected to exercise-induced ischemia (Guth et al., 1987). On the other hand, evidence in support of a positive effect of beta blockade to enhance recovery of postischemic contractile function in stunned myocardium is equivocal. Several studies in experimental animals suggest that beta blockade results in an enhanced recovery of regional wall motion in stunned myocardium (Lange et al., 1984; Al-Wathiqui et al., 1989), whereas other investigators have shown no effect of beta blockade (Przyklenk and Kloner, 1989; Kitakaze et al., 1991). Therefore, it is the goal of this review to summarize the available evidence for or against a positive effect of beta blockade on postischemic dysfunction in stunned myocardium and the possible clinical implications.

II. EFFECT OF PRETREATMENT WITH BETA BLOCKERS ON STUNNED MYOCARDIUM

A. Acute Pretreatment

Initial studies by Lange et al. (1984) demonstrated that an intravenous infusion of the short-acting beta receptor antagonist, esmolol, 1 hour prior to and during a 15-minute occlusion period, resulted in an enhanced recovery of regional wall motion during a subsequent 4-hour reperfusion period in anesthetized dogs. In another study (Lange et al., 1983), esmolol was infused intravenously into anesthetized dogs subjected to 3 hours of left anterior descending coronary artery occlusion followed by 3 hours of reperfusion. Esmolol was administered 15 minutes after the onset of occlusion and continued throughout reperfusion. As compared to nontreated control dogs, those treated with esmolol had a smaller area of tissue necrosis at 3 hours of reperfusion (48 ± 7 vs. 73 ± 6%) and less regional systolic wall bulging in stunned border segments adjacent to the infarcted zone. In both studies, there was a reduction in heart rate and left ventricular dP/dt during the ischemic period in the beta-blocked animals. Thus, it is likely that a reduction in the severity of ischemia during coronary artery occlusion as a result of the negative chronotropic and inotropic effects of esmolol may be at least partially responsible for the beneficial effects observed on postischemic dysfunction in these two studies.

In contrast, results from a more recent study of Kitakaze et al. (1991) in anesthetized dogs showed that an intracoronary infusion of propranolol into an area of the myocardium to be rendered ischemic for 15 minutes followed by 3 hours of reperfusion had no effect on the time course of recovery of regional systolic function. Propranolol was administered prior to the occlusion period and for the first 2 hours of reperfusion. These results suggest that acute treatment with beta blockers does not attenuate contractile dysfunction during reperfusion in stunned myocardium. Possible explanations for the differences observed in this study and those of Lange et al. (1983,1984) may be the result of the choice of beta blocker, the timing of treatment or the route of drug administration. Since esmolol has a very brief serum half-life of 9 minutes as compared to several hours for propranolol (Sum et al., 1983), any direct negative inotropic effects that continuous beta blockade may have on the stunned myocardium may not be as evident in esmolol-treated dogs as in those treated with propranolol. Also, in both studies of Lange et al. (1983, 1984), esmolol was present during the ischemic period, whereas in the study of Kitakaze et al. (1991) propranolol infusion was stopped during the 15-minute occlusion period. Thus, it is likely that for maximum benefit on stunned myocardium, the drug needs to be present during the ischemic episode. Finally, Kitakaze et al. (1991) administered propranolol directly into an already depressed ischemic-reperfused area for 2 hours following reperfusion. It seems probable that the direct negative inotropic effect of propranolol would mask any beneficial effect that pretreatment may have had to enhance the recovery of postischemic dysfunction following reperfusion in the absence of beta blockade. Thus, current evidence suggests that acute pretreatment or treatment with beta blockers during the ischemic period most likely results in an enhanced recovery of regional contractile function in the anesthetized dog. However, more well-controlled studies are needed with different beta receptor antagonists in both anesthetized as well as conscious, chronically instrumented dogs to more definitively answer the question as to the efficacy of acute beta blockade to attenuate postischemic dysfunction in stunned myocardium.

B. Chronic Pretreatment

Al-Wathiqui et al. (1989) recently investigated the effect that prior long-term pretreatment with propranolol (160 mg daily × 8 days) had on the recovery of regional systolic shortening in anesthetized dogs subjected to 15 minutes of coronary artery occlusion followed by 3 hours of reperfusion. As compared to the control group, propranolol-treated dogs had a significantly lower heart rate and rate-pressure product throughout the experiment. More importantly, dogs pretreated with propranolol demonstrated a marked improvement in the recovery of regional percent systolic shortening (%SS) in stunned myocardium following reperfusion as compared to controls (65 ± 7% vs. 11 ± 10%) (see Fig. 1). There was also an increase in regional myocardial blood flow to the subepicardium, midmyocardium, and subendocardium at 3 hours of reperfusion in the propranolol-treated group (Fig. 2). When heart rate was maintained at the control rate in another group of propranolol-treated dogs, the beneficial actions of propranolol on the recovery of %SS in stunned myocardium and the increase in reperfusion blood flow were completely abolished (see Figs. 1 and 2). These results are in agreement with and extend those of Lange et al. (1984) and suggest that pretreatment with beta blockers enhances the recovery of contractile function in postischemic, reperfused myocardium. This protective effect of beta blockade appears to be primarily related to the beta adrenergic blockade-induced reduction in heart rate since pacing eliminated these beneficial actions. In support of this hypothesis, Gross and Daemmgen (1986) have shown that pretreatment with two specific bradycardic agents, AQ-A39 and AQ-AH 208, that lack beta-blocking activity also enhanced the recovery of %SS in postischemic stunned myocardium of anesthetized dogs. These results suggest the importance of heart rate reduction per se as an important mechanism to enhance the recovery of postischemic dysfunction in the reversibly injured, stunned myocardium.

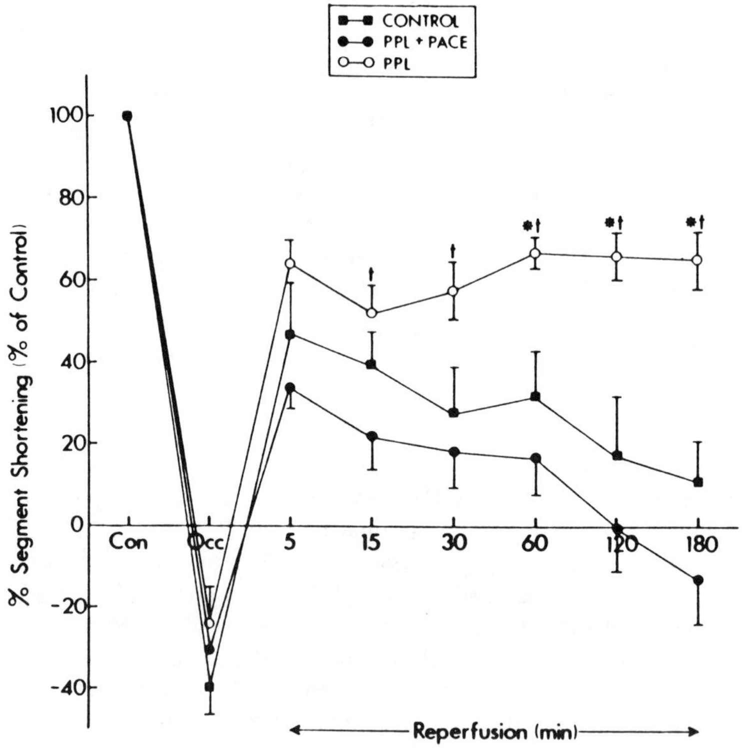

Figure 1 Percent segment shortening (%SS) in the ischemic left anterior descending region of control, propranolol, and propranolol + pacing groups. *, Significantly different from the control group ($p < 0.05$); †, Significantly different from the propranolol + pacing group ($p < 0.05$). CON = baseline; OCC = coronary artery occlusion. (From Al-Wathiqui et al., 1989, by permission from the *American Heart Journal*.)

III. EFFECT OF BETA BLOCKERS ADMINISTERED FOLLOWING REPERFUSION ON STUNNED MYOCARDIUM

Przyklenk and Kloner (1989) recently tested the hypothesis that myocardial stunning is a protective mechanism and that forcing the heart to contract more forcefully may have deleterious effects on the eventual recovery of regional wall thickening (WT) and adenosine triphosphate (ATP) content, whereas resting the heart might result in an enhanced or accelerated recovery of regional WT and ATP content. To test this hypothesis, Przyklenk and Kloner (1989) administered either hydralazine, an afterload reducing and

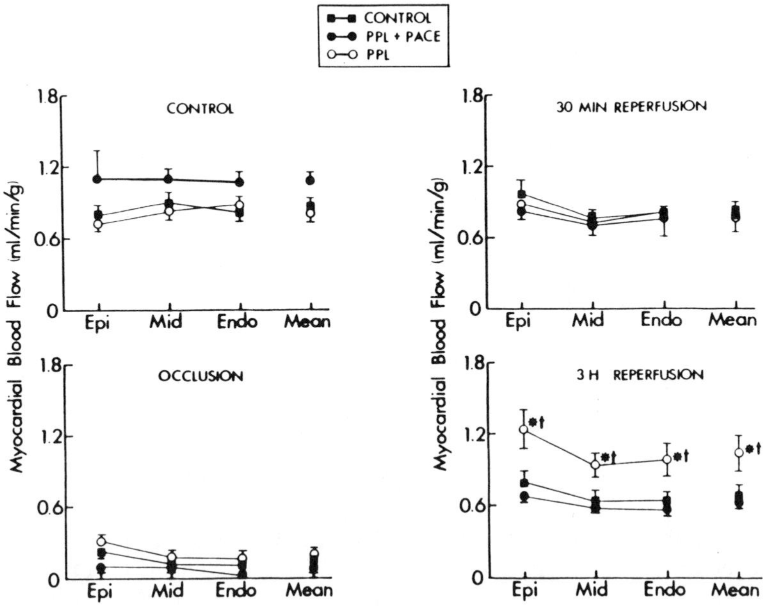

Figure 2 Myocardial blood flow in the ischemic left anterior descending region of control, propranolol, and propranolol + pacing groups in the subepicardial (Epi), midmyocardial (Mid), and subendocardial (Endo) layers during the control period, coronary artery occlusion and 30 minutes and 3 hours after reperfusion. Mean = transmural blood flows. *, Significantly different from the control group ($p < 0.05$); †, Significantly different from propranolol + pacing group ($p < 0.05$). (From Al-Wathiqui et al., 1989, by permission from the *American Heart Journal.*)

cardiostimulatory agent or the ultrashort-acting beta blocker, esmolol, for 2 hours starting at 30 minutes of reperfusion following a 15-minute episode of coronary artery occlusion. Subsequently, the recovery of contractile function and high energy phosphate content was measured at 1 day following reperfusion, which was well beyond the half-lives of hydralazine and esmolol. Acute beta blockade with esmolol had no effect on WT or endocardial ATP content during the 2 hours of infusion or 24 hours later (see Fig. 3). These results are different from those previously reported by Lange et al. (1983), where it was observed that pretreatment with similar doses of esmolol prior to and during a 15-minute period of coronary occlusion resulted in an enhanced recovery of regional wall motion in stunned myocardium during 4 hours of reperfusion. The most obvious reason for the discrepancy between the results of Lange et al. (1983) and those of Przyklenk and Kloner (1989) is the timing of the esmolol treatment. It appears that it is essential that es-

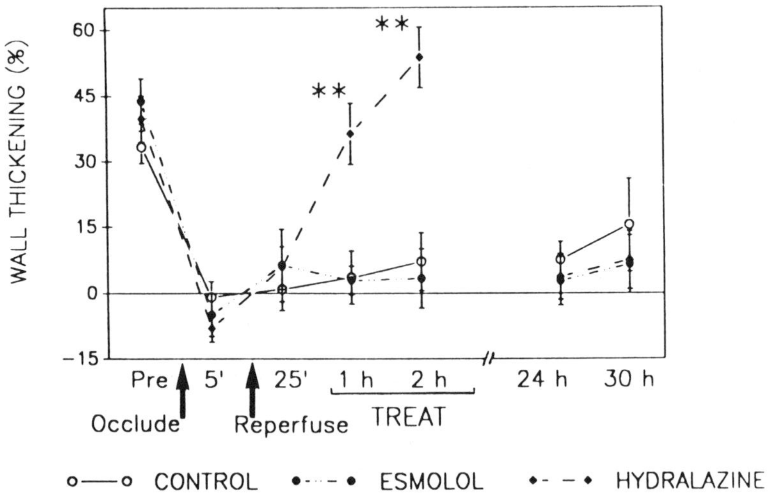

Figure 3 Regional left ventricular wall thickening in the central ischemic zone in control, esmolol, and hydralazine-treated animals. Wall thickening in all groups remained depressed, even at 30 hours after reperfusion and treatment, $**p < 0.01$ versus corresponding control values by ANOVA. (From Przyklenk and Kloner, 1988, by permission from the *American Heart Journal.*)

molol or other beta blockers be administered prior to or during the ischemic period instead of following reperfusion to exert a maximum beneficial effect on stunned myocardium. This agrees with previous results observed with the calcium antagonist verapamil (Przyklenk and Kloner, 1988), which is also more effective in stunned myocardium when administered prior to occlusion versus at reperfusion.

IV. CLINICAL IMPLICATIONS

These results with beta blockers in experimental animals may have important clinical implications. Based upon data thus far obtained, it appears that pretreatment with beta blockers would be necessary to observe a salutory effect on the recovery of postischemic function in patients with stunned myocardium since beta blockade following reperfusion is without benefit in experimental studies (Przyklenk and Kloner, 1989; Kitakaze et al., 1991). To avoid exacerbation of heart failure, severe sinus bradycardia, or heart block in patients subjected to acute myocardial ischemia and reperfusion, the use of an ultrashort-acting beta blocker such as esmolol where the dose can be carefully titrated, or perhaps the use of a beta blocker with intrinsic sympathomimetic activity (ISA) such as pindolol, may be preferable to using other long-acting beta blockers that lack ISA. Alternatively, a specific bradycardic agent (Indolfi et al., 1989) may also be preferable to a beta blocker in patients undergoing clinical procedures, which most likely will result in severe myocardial stunning such as transluminal coronary angioplasty or thrombolysis. Obviously, more experimental as well as clinical studies are necessary before the use of beta blockers in the treatment of stunned myocardium is well established.

REFERENCES

Al-Wathiqui, M., Farber, N., Pelc, L., Gross, G. J., Brooks, H. L., and Warltier, D. C. (1989). Improvement in functional recovery of stunned canine myocardium by long-term pretreatment with oral propranolol. *Am. Heart J. 117*: 791.

Gross, G. J., and Daemmgen, J. W. (1986). Beneficial effects of two specific bradycardic agents AQ-A39 (Falipamil) and AQ-AH 208 on reversible myocardial reperfusion damage in anesthetized dogs. *J. Pharmacol & Exp. Ther. 238*: 422.

Guth, B. D., Heusch, G., Seitelberger, R., and Ross, Jr. J. (1987). Mechanism of beneficial effect of b-adrenergic blockade on exercise-induced myocardial ischemia in conscious dogs. *Circulation 60*: 738.

Indolfi, C., Guth, B. D., Miura, T., Miyazaki, S., Schulz, R., and Ross, Jr., J. (1989). Mechanisms of improved ischemic regional dysfunction by bradycardia: Studies on UL-FS 49 in swine. *Circulation 80*: 983.

ISIS-1 (First International Study of Infarct Survival). (1986). Collaborative group randomized trial of intravenous atenolol among 16,027 cases of suspected acute myocardial infarction. *Lancet 2*: 57.

Kitakaze, M., Hori, M., Sato, H., Iwakura, K., Gotoh, K., Inoue, M., Kitakabe, A., and Kamada, T. (1991). Beneficial effects of a_1-adrenoceptor activity on myocardial stunning in dogs. *Circ. Res. 68*: 1322.

Lange, R., Kloner, R. A., and Braunwald, E. (1983). First ultra-short-acting beta adrenergic blocking agent: Its effect on size and segmental wall dynamics of reperfused myocardial infarcts in dogs. *Am. J. Cardiol. 51*: 1759.

Lange, R., Kloner, R. A., and Braunwald, E. (1984). Enhancement of functional recovery of "stunned" reperfused myocardium by a new ultrashort-acting beta blocker. *J. Am. Coll. Cardiol. 3*: 545.

Przyklenk, K., and Kloner, R. A. (1988). Effect of verapamil on postischemic "stunned" myocardium: importance of the timing of treatment. *J. Am. Coll. Cardiol. 11*: 614.

Przyklenk, K., and Kloner, R. A. (1989). Is "stunned myocardium" a protective mechanism? Effect of acute recruitment and acute b-blockade on recovery of contractile function and high-energy phosphate stores at 1 day post-reperfusion. *Am. Heart J. 118*: 480.

Sum, C. Y., Yacobi, A., Kartzinel, R., Stampfi, H., Davis, C. S., and Lai, C. M. (1983). Kinetics of esmolol, an ultra-short acting beta blocker, and of its metabolites. *Clin. Pharmacol. Ther. 34*: 427.

16

Prostacyclinmimetics and Steroids

Garrett J. Gross

Medical College of Wisconsin, Milwaukee, Wisconsin

I. PROSTACYCLINMIMETICS

A. Introduction

Prostacyclin (PGI_2) is a major biologically active substance produced from the metabolism of arachidonic acid (Johnson et al., 1976). PGI_2 is known to be a potent coronary vasodilator and to possess cytoprotective properties, which include an inhibition of platelet aggregation, stabilization of lysosomal membranes, and an inhibitory effect on oxygen free radical production by neutrophils (Lefer et al., 1978; Simpson et al., 1987). As a result of these favorable properties, PGI_2 has been shown to decrease the incidence of cardiac arrhythmias (Coker and Parratt, 1983) and to reduce myocardial infarct size (Simpson et al., 1987) in experimental animals. However, because of its short biological half-life (approximately 3 minutes), a number of stable analogs of PGI_2 such as iloprost (Schror et al., 1981) have been synthesized in an attempt to prolong the vasodilatory and/or cytoprotective actions for possible therapeutic benefit. Alternatively, another method to increase and prolong the effects of PGI_2 is to pharmacologically stimulate its endogenous synthesis. A compound that has been shown to produce such an effect is defibrotide, a single-stranded fraction of mammalian DNA (Niada et al., 1985). Thus, the major goal of the initial section of this chapter is to summarize the evidence that suggests that these novel approaches to increase the endogenous synthesis of or mimic the effects of PGI_2 with long-acting analogs exert a beneficial action on the stunned myocardium.

B. Effect of Prostacyclinmimetics on Stunned Myocardium

1. Iloprost

No reports have been published concerning the effects of PGI_2 per se on the recovery of postischemic function in the regionally ischemic, stunned myocardium of experimental animals. However, several recent studies have been performed with the stable PGI_2 analog iloprost. In the first study, van der Giessen et al. (1986) administered iloprost to anesthetized pigs that had been subjected to 20 minutes of coronary artery occlusion followed by 2 hours of reperfusion. Although iloprost did not prevent the loss of systolic wall function during ischemia, it resulted in an enhanced recovery of regional myocardial function during the 2-hour reperfusion period.

More recently, Farber et al. (1988) administered iloprost either before and during the occlusion period or only at reperfusion in anesthetized dogs subjected to 15 minutes of coronary artery occlusion followed by 3 hours of reperfusion. Iloprost produced a dose-dependent increase in regional myocardial segment shortening (%SS) as compared to the control group when administered prior to and during coronary occlusion (Fig. 1). Iloprost given at reperfusion also enhanced the recovery of %SS, however, the beneficial effect was not as great as when iloprost was administered prior to occlusion (Fig. 2). These beneficial actions of iloprost did not appear to be related to its effects on systemic hemodynamics, high-energy phosphates, or coronary collateral blood flow but may have partially been the result of its action to decrease superoxide anion production by activated neutrophils.

2. Defibrotide

To determine if an increase in endogenous PGI_2 formation is capable of attenuating myocardial stunning, Hohlfeld et al. (1991) administered defibrotide or vehicle to anesthetized minipigs which were subjected to 5 minutes of coronary artery occlusion followed by 120 minutes of reperfusion. Defibrotide treatment resulted in a significant increase in transcardiac PGI_2 formation and concurrently increased regional systolic wall thickening in the ischemic area throughout the reperfusion period as compared to the vehicle-treated control group (Fig. 3). Regional wall motion in the nonischemic area was not affected. Defibrotide also reduced platelet aggregation. These authors (Hohlfeld et al., 1991) concluded that the improvement in regional contrac-

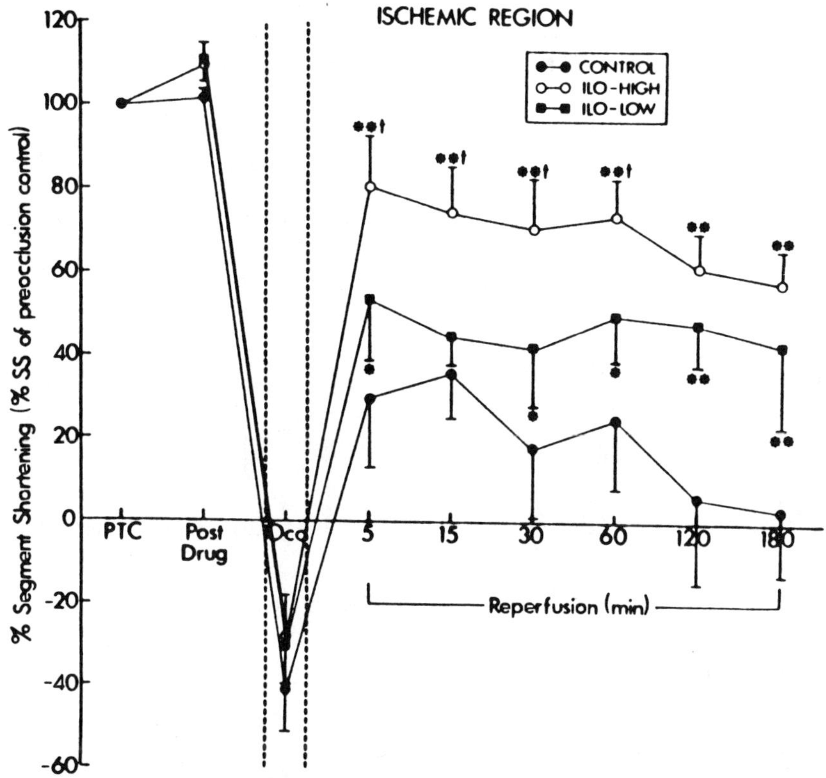

Figure 1 Percent segment shortening (%SS) expressed as a percent of the pretreatment control (PTC) value in the ischemic-reperfused area at various times. Time-course values for pretreatment infusions with vehicle (control, $n = 9$), iloprost at 0.1 μg/kg/min (ILO-HIGH, $n = 8$) and iloprost at 0.05 μg/kg/min (ILO-LOW, $n = 8$) are shown. Each point is the mean ± S.E.M. Significant differences from vehicle (CONTROL) are $*p < 0.05$ or $**p < 0.01$ and from ILO-LOW are $\dagger p < 0.05$. (Reprinted from Farber et al., 1988, by permission from the American Heart Association.)

tile function was most likely related to the defibrotide-induced inhibition of platelet aggregation or to the protection of cardiac cell membranes as a result of the enhanced transcardiac formation of PGI_2.

II. STEROIDS

A. Introduction

Many of the chemical mediators released during myocardial ischemia and/or reperfusion are similar to those released during the acute inflammatory re-

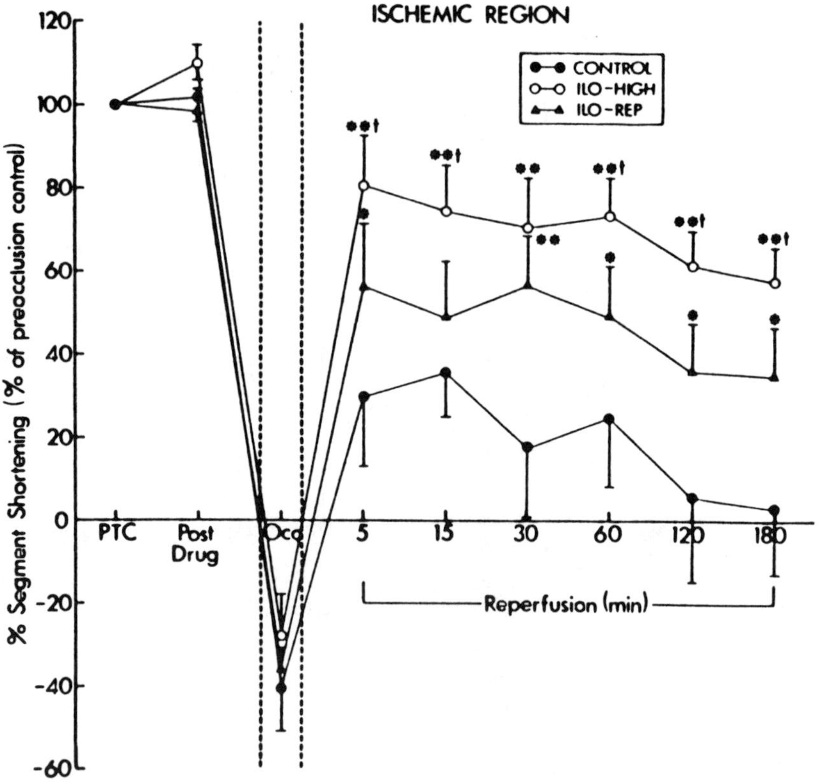

Figure 2 Percent segment shortening (%SS) expressed as a percent of the pretreatment control (PTC) value in the ischemic-reperfused area at various times. Time-course values for pretreatment infusions with vehicle (CONTROL, $n = 9$), iloprost at 0.1 μg/kg/min (ILO-HIGH, $n = 8$) and iloprost at 0.1 μg/kg/min given at reperfusion (ILO-REP, $n = 8$). Each point is the mean ± S.E.M. Significant differences from vehicle (CONTROL) are $*p < 0.05$ and $**p < 0.01$ and from ILO-REP are $\dagger p < 0.05$. (Reprinted from Farber et al., 1988, by permission from the American Heart Association.)

sponse in other tissues (Wynsen et al., 1988). Even brief periods (less than 15 minutes) of myocardial ischemia have been associated with oxygen free radical production and membrane lipid peroxidation (Rao et al., 1983) and activation of phospholipases, which may result in the generation of cyclooxygenase and lipoxygenase products. All of these processes are detrimental to the heart and may produce myocardial cell damage during ischemia and reperfusion. Since glucocorticoids are known to reduce the inflammatory

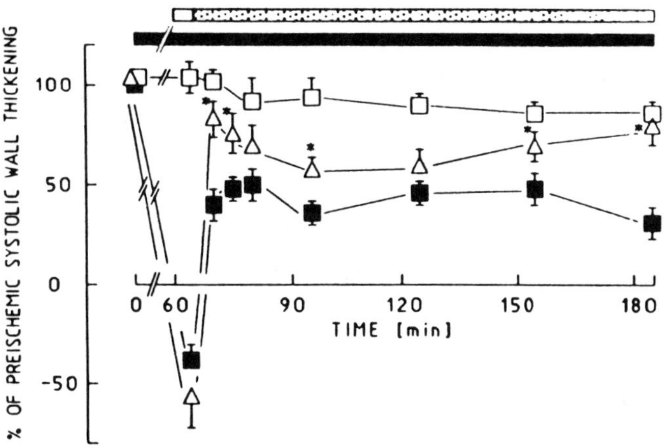

Figure 3 Systolic wall thickening in pigs subjected to LAD occlusion (5 min) and reperfusion (120 min). Animals were treated with vehicle (solid squares, $n = 6$) or defibrotide (open triangles, $n = 7$) and compared with sham-operated vehicle controls (open squares, $n = 4$). The black bar represents the period of defibrotile infusion, the open bar represents the duration of ischemia, and the stripped bar represents the period of reperfusion. Data are the mean ± S.E.M. $^*p < 0.05$ versus the vehicle-treated group. (Reprinted from Hohlfeld et al., 1991, by permission from the *Journal of Cardiovascular Pharmacology*.)

response and have been shown to decrease myocardial infarct size (Bernauer, 1985), there is a rationale for studying these compounds in stunned myocardium. The available evidence concerning a potential beneficial effect in this model is summarized in the following section.

B. Effect of Steroids on Stunned Myocardium

1. Methylprednisolone

Recently, Wynsen et al. (1988) studied the effect of methylprednisolone sodium succinate (MSS) on the recovery of regional systolic shortening (%SS) in conscious, chronically instrumented dogs subjected to 15 minutes of coronary artery occlusion and a 5-hour period of reperfusion. Animals receiving MSS 90 minutes prior to occlusion showed a marked improvement in the recovery of %SS in the ischemic-reperfused region throughout the entire reperfusion period (Fig. 4), whereas dogs given MSS at reperfusion demonstrated a delayed but marked improvement in %SS at 3, 4, and 5 hours postreperfusion (Fig. 5). Methylprednisolone given 15 minutes postreperfusion had no beneficial effect. In addition, sodium succinate administration 90 minutes prior

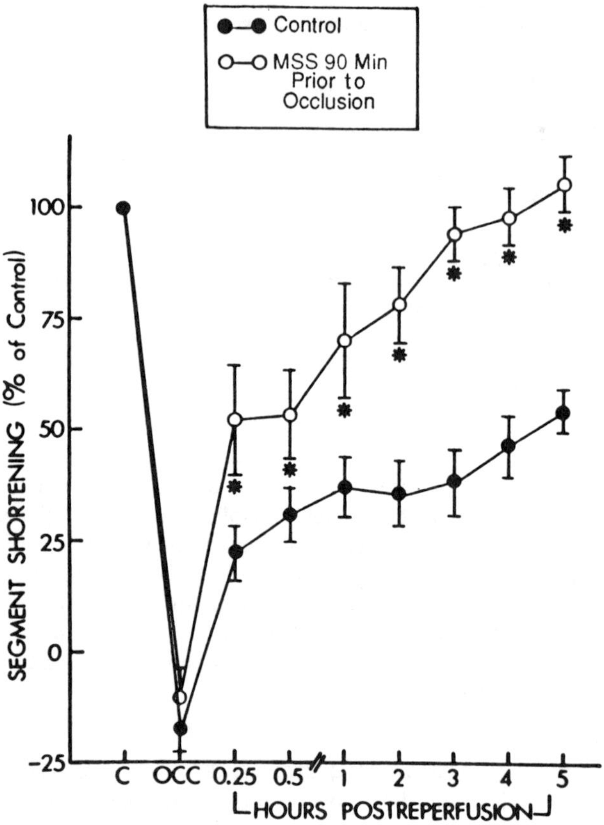

Figure 4 Time course of recovery of segment shortening (% of control) in postischemic, reperfused myocardium over time. Open circles represent the group treated with methylprednisolone sodium succinate (MSS) (20 mg/kg/i.v.) 90 minutes prior to coronary artery occlusion (OCC, $n = 6$). Closed circles represent the control group ($n = 8$). All values are the mean ± S.E.M. $*p < 0.05$ compared to control group. (Reprinted from Wynsen et al., 1988, by permission from the *American Heart Journal*.)

to occlusion also had no effect. These results could not be attributed to any hemodynamic effects of the steroid but were postulated to be the result of a steroid-induced increase in the release and/or synthesis of a phospholipase A_2 inhibitory protein. However, no direct evidence for such an effect was obtained.

2. Lazeroids

Recently, a novel group of 21-aminosteroids that lack glucocorticoid activity have been synthesized and have been termed lazeroids (Braughler et al., 1987).

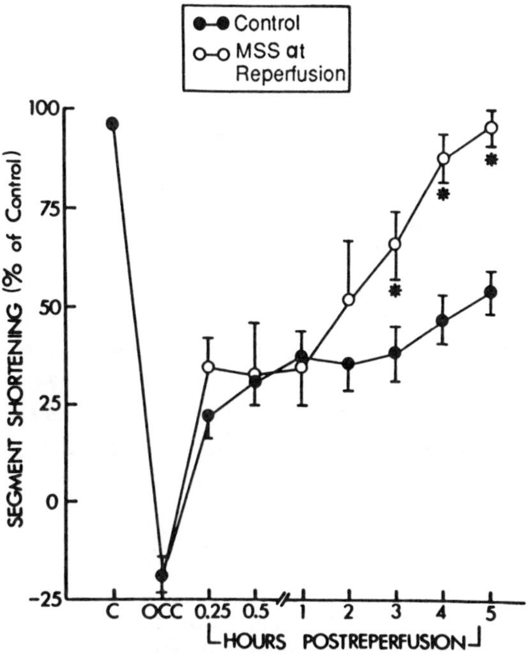

Figure 5 Time course of recovery of segment shortening (% of control) in postischemic, reperfused myocardium over time. Open circles represent the group treated with methylprednisolone sodium succinate (MSS) (20 mg/kg, i.v.) immediately prior to reperfusion ($n = 6$). Closed circles represent the control group ($n = 8$). All values are the mean ± S.E.M. $*p < 0.05$ compared to control group. (Reprinted from Wynsen et al., 1988, by permission from the *American Heart Journal.*)

These compounds have been shown to be potent inhibitors of iron-dependent lipid peroxidation and to have protective effects in several models of cerebral trauma or ischemia (Hall et al., 1988; Hall and Travis, 1988). Since free radical-induced injury has been shown to be important in the pathogenesis of stunned myocardium (Bolli, 1991), Holzgrefe and co-workers (1990) examined the efficacy of the 21-aminosteroid, U 74006F, on the recovery of percent wall thickening (%WT) in anesthetized dogs subjected to 15 minutes of coronary artery occlusion followed by 3 hours of reperfusion. In U 74006F-treated animals, %WT in the ischemic-reperfused area recovered to a greater extent than in vehicle-treated dogs throughout reperfusion. These effects of U 74006F could not be related to changes in hemodynamics or collateral blood flow, and it was concluded that its beneficial actions were the result of its ability to inhibit free radical-induced lipid peroxidation in the myocardium.

III. CLINICAL IMPLICATIONS

A. Prostacyclinmimetics

Several clinical studies suggest that PGI_2 or other similar vasodilatory prostaglandins such as iloprost or PGE_1 may exert beneficial actions on postischemic myocardial dysfunction. PGI_2 has been shown to increase left ventricular ejection fraction in patients (Auinger et al., 1989), and iloprost has been shown to increase exercise capacity in patients with stable angina pectoris (Bugiardini et al., 1986). Sharma et al. (1986) found that administration of PGE_1 plus streptokinase in patients with an acute myocardial infarction resulted in an improvement in left ventricular regional and global function. Similar improvements in regional wall motion were also obtained with PGE_1 in anesthetized dogs that were stunned by 15 minutes of coronary artery occlusion (Farber and Gross, 1989). These results obtained in experimental animals and man are promising and suggest that by mimicking or enhancing the effects of PGI_2, an improvement in postischemic function may result in clinical situations of myocardial stunning.

B. Steroids

Although the results obtained with methylprednisolone in dogs are intriguing, there are no clear-cut clinical results available that suggest that corticosteroids are of benefit in stunned myocardium in humans. The results obtained with the new 21-aminosteroid U 74006F are very exciting and suggest that these types of compounds, which lack the side effects commonly associated with glucocorticoids, may be potentially useful as new adjunctive therapy in myocardial reperfusion injury in humans.

REFERENCES

Auinger, C., Virgolini, I., Weissel, M., Bergmann, H., and Sinzinger, H. (1989). Prostacyclin I_2 (PGI_2) increases left ventricular ejection fraction (LVEF). *Prostagl. Leucotr. Med. 36*: 149.

Bernauer, W. (1985). Inhibiting effect of dexamethasone on evolving myocardial necrosis in coronary-ligated rats with and without reperfusion. *Pharmacology 31*: 328.

Bolli, R. (1991). Oxygen-derived free radicals and myocardial reperfusion injury: An overview. *Cardiovasc. Drugs Ther. 5*: 249.

Braughler, J. M., Pregenzer, J. F., Chase, R. L., Duncan, L. A., Jacobsen, E. J., and McCall, J. M. (1987). Novel 21-aminosteroids as potent inhibitors of iron-dependent lipid peroxidation. *J. Biol. Chem. 262*: 10438.

Bugiardini, R., Galvani, M., Ferrini, D., Gridelli, C., Mari, L., Puddu, P., and Lenzi, S. (1986). Effects of iloprost, a stable prostacyclin analogue, on exercise capacity and platelet aggregation in stable angina pectoris. *Am. J. Cardiol. 58*: 453.

Coker, S. J., and Parratt, J. R. (1983). Prostacyclin-antiarrhythmic or arrhythmogenic? Comparison of the effects of intravenous prostacyclin and ZK 36374 during coronary artery occlusion and reperfusion in anesthetized greyhounds, *J. Cardiovasc. Pharmacol. 5*: 557.

Farber, N. E., Pieper, G. M., Thomas, J. P., and Gross, G. J. (1988). Beneficial effects of iloprost in the stunned canine myocardium. *Circ. Res. 62*: 204.

Farber, N. E., and Gross, G. J. (1989). Prostaglandin E_1 attenuates postischemic contractile function after brief coronary occlusion and reperfusion. *Am. Heart J. 118*: 17.

Hall, E. D., and Travis, M. A. (1988). Effects of the nonglucocorticoid 21-aminosteroid, U 74006F, on acute cerebral hypoperfusion following experimental subarachnoid hemorrhage. *Exp. Neurol. 102*: 244.

Hall, E. D., Yonkers, P. A., McCall, J. M., and Braughler, J. M. (1988). Effects of the 21-aminosteroid, U 74006F, on experimental head injury in mice. *J. Neurosurg. 68*: 456.

Hohlfeld, T., Strobach, H., and Schror, K. (1991). Stimulation of prostacyclin synthesis by defibrotide: improved contractile recovery from myocardial "stunning." *J. Cardiovasc. Pharmacol. 17*: 108.

Holzgrefe, H. H., Buchanan, L. V., and Gibson, J. K. (1990). Effects of U 74006F, a novel inhibitor of lipid peroxidation, in stunned reperfused canine myocardium. *J. Cardiovasc. Pharmacol. 15*: 239.

Johnson, R. A., Morton, D. R., Kinner, J. H., Gorman, R. R., McGuire, J. C., Sun, F. F., Whittaker, N., Bunting, S., Salmon, J. A., Moncada, S., and Vane, J. R. (1976). The chemical characterization of prostaglandin x (prostacyclin). *Prostaglandins 12*: 915.

Lefer, A. M., Ogletree, M. L., Smith, J. B., Silver, M. J., Nicolau, K. C., Barnette, W. E., and Gasic, G. P. (1978). Prostacyclin: A potentially valuable agent for preserving myocardial tissue in acute myocardial ischemia. *Science 200*: 52.

Niada, R., Porta, R., Pescador, R., Mantovani, M., and Prino, G. (1985). Cardioprotective effects of defibrotide in acute myocardial ischemia in the cat. *Throm. Res. 38*: 71.

Rao, P. S., Cohen, M. V., and Mueller, H. S. (1983). Production of free radicals and lipid peroxides in early experimental myocardial ischemia. *J. Mol. Cell. Cardiol. 15*: 713.

Schror, K., Darius, H., Matzky, R., and Ohlendorf, R. (1981). The antiplatelet and cardiovascular actions of a new carbacyclin derivative (ZK 36374)-equipotent to PGI_2 *in vitro. Nauyn Schmiedebergs Arch. Pharmacol. 316*: 252.

Sharma, B., Wyeth, R. P., Gimenez, H. P., and Franciosa, J. A. (1986). Intracoronary prostaglandin E_1 plus streptokinase in acute myocardial infarction. *Am. J. Cardiol. 58*: 1161.

Simpson, P. J., Mitsos, S. E., Ventura, A., Gallagher, K. P., Fantone, J. C., Abrams, G. D., Schork, M. A., and Lucchesi, B. R. (1987). Prostacyclin protects ischemic reperfused myocardium in the dog by inhibition of neutrophil activation. *Am. Heart J. 113*: 129.

Van der Giessen, W. J., Schoutsen, B., Tijssen, J. G. P., and Verdouw, P. D. (1986). Iloprost (ZK 36374) enhances recovery of regional myocardial function during reperfusion after coronary artery occlusion in the pig. *Br. J. Pharmacol. 87*: 23.

Wynsen, J. C., Preuss, K. C., Gross, G. J., Brooks, H. L., and Warltier, D. C. (1988). Steroid-induced enhancement of functional recovery of postischemic, reperfused myocardium in conscious dogs. *Am. Heart J. 116*: 915.

17

Angiotensin Converting Enzyme Inhibitors

Karin Przyklenk

Hospital of the Good Samaritan and University of Southern California, Los Angeles, California

I. INTRODUCTION

The renin-angiotensin system plays a crucial role in regulating cardiovascular homeostasis. Perturbations in this complex endocrine/autocrine/paracrine system have been shown to contribute to the pathogenesis of various cardiovascular disease states including hypertension, congestive heart failure, and cardiac hypertrophy (Dzau, 1988; Gavras and Gavras, 1991). In addition, coronary artery occlusion also perturbs the renin-angiotensin system and results in the production of angiotensin II (Ertl et al., 1983; McAlpine et al., 1988), a potent vasoconstrictor and positive inotropic agent (Hock et al., 1985).

Angiotensin converting enzyme (ACE) inhibitors, although a structurally diverse class of compounds (Ondetti, 1988), all by definition blunt the conversion of angiotensin I to angiotensin II. Thus, it is not surprising that the salutary effects of captopril, enalapril, and other ACE inhibitors in studies of hypertension, congestive heart failure, and experimental myocardial infarction have traditionally been attributed to the well-documented hemodynamic consequences (i.e., reductions in afterload and preload, reduction in coronary vascular resistance, and increase in myocardial blood flow) associated with the blunting of angiotensin II formation. ACE inhibitors also, however, exert a variety of *direct*, protective effects on the heart—including inhibition of bradykinin metabolism and increased prostaglandin production—the nature and efficacy of which appear to be dependent upon the specific molecular structure of each agent (Cushman and Ondetti, 1980; Schwartz and Williams, 1982). In particular, recent evidence has suggested that the cardioprotective effects of ACE inhibitors that contain a sulfhydryl (SH) group (i.e., captopril and zofenopril) may be due to the apparent antioxidant or oxygen radical-scavenging properties imparted on these compounds by the SH moiety (Westlin and Mullane, 1988; Weglicki et al., 1990; McMurray and Chopra, 1991).

These reports of free radical-scavenging properties of sulfhydryl-containing ACE inhibitors raised the intriguing possibility that these agents may be useful in the treatment of oxygen radical-mediated disorders, and thereby sparked a recent flurry of investigation of SH- and non-SH-containing ACE inhibitors in the setting of ischemia/reperfusion. This chapter summarizes our current understanding of the effects of ACE inhibitors on the recovery of contractile function in experimental models of the stunned myocardium, the potential mechanisms of action of these various agents in models of brief transient ischemia, and the initial attempts to use ACE inhibitors as adjuvant therapy in patients reperfused for the treatment of acute myocardial infarction.

II. ACE INHIBITORS IN THE ISOLATED PERFUSED HEART PREPARATION

Our knowledge of the effects of ACE inhibitors in the isolated perfused heart model can be largely attributed to the numerous studies performed during the past decade by van Gilst, de Graeff, Kingma, and their colleagues (summarized by de Graeff, 1989). For example, van Gilst et al. (1984) demonstrated that addition of captopril to the coronary perfusate enhanced the recovery of left ventricular (LV) developed pressure and dP/dt in isolated perfused rat hearts subjected to 15 minutes of regional ischemia and 30 minutes of reperfusion. Furthermore, this improvement in function proved to be dose-dependent: LV pressure at 30 minutes following reflow recovered to 35% of preischemic values in untreated control hearts vs. 95%, 103%, and 116% of preischemic values in hearts perfused with 1, 10, and 80 μg/l of captopril, respectively (de Graeff et al., 1986) (Fig. 1). Captopril added to the perfusate also reduced the overflow of adenosine, inosine, hypoxanthine, and xanthine in the coronary effluent during the initial minutes following reperfusion, providing indirect evidence that captopril in part preserved myocardial adenosine triphosphate (ATP) stores during the brief ischemic insult (van Gilst

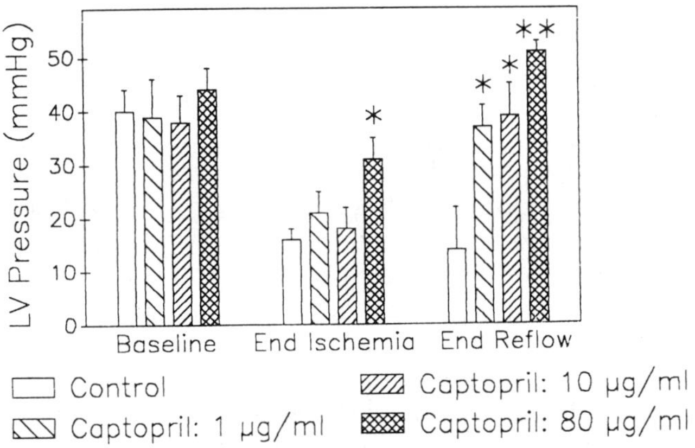

Figure 1 Dose-dependent effects of captopril on left ventricular (LV)-developed pressure in the isolated rat heart during 15 minutes of regional ischemia and 30 minutes of reperfusion. $*p < 0.05$, $**p < 0.01$ vs. control group. (Adapted with permission from de Graeff et al., 1986.)

et al., 1984, 1986; de Graeff et al., 1986). This was subsequently confirmed by nuclear magnetic resonance spectroscopy: ATP concentrations following reperfusion were slightly (but significantly) higher in captopril-treated hearts vs. control hearts (Rahusen et al., 1988). Addition of enalapril (8 μg/l) to the perfusate in this same ex vivo model of ischemia/reperfusion also blunted purine overflow in the coronary effluent, but myocardial contractility (in this case, the rate-pressure product) did not differ between treated and control hearts at 30 minutes after reflow (van Gilst et al., 1986).

Grover and colleagues (1991) recently compared the effects of seven ACE inhibitors (captopril, enalapril, zofenopril, fosinopril, ceranapril, lisinopril, and ramipril) on recovery of postischemic contractile function in isolated rat hearts subjected to 25 minutes of global ischemia and 30 minutes of reoxygenation. Rate-pressure product assessed following reperfusion was significantly greater in hearts perfused with the SH-containing agents captopril and zofenopril, whereas enalapril and the other four agents failed to improve function when compared with control hearts perfused with vehicle alone. Similarly, Fleetwood et al. (1991) found no difference in recovery of LV-developed pressure between control and enalapril-treated hearts subjected to a more prolonged 40-minute episode of global ischemia and 1 hour of reperfusion. Fleetwood and colleagues (1991) further concluded that angiotensin II, although produced in the ischemic/reperfused rat heart, is not an important mediator of mechanical function in this ex vivo model. Somewhat different results have been reported by Li and Chen (1987), who observed a greater force of contraction following 20 minutes of global ischemia and 30 minutes of reflow when enalapril was administered to rats before sacrifice. In contrast, captopril added to the coronary perfusate did not, in the model of Li and Chen (1987), enhance the force of contraction measured following ischemia/reperfusion.

Thus, in most of these ex vivo protocols, postischemic contractile dysfunction could be attenuated by addition of ACE inhibitors (particularly captopril) to the perfusate. These data are important, in that they demonstrate that ACE inhibitors can exert a cardioprotective effect in the absence of afterload reduction, neurohumoral effects, or the presence of cellular blood elements. However, interpretation of these data is confounded by the fact that in all protocols the agents were added to the perfusate prior to the ischemic insult. Thus, it is difficult to determine whether the improvement in postischemic function is due to an anti-ischemic effect of ACE inhibitors (such as the partial preservation of ATP stores reported in some studies) or whether the improved function reflects a direct effect of ACE inhibitors on the stunned, postischemic myocytes.

III. ACE INHIBITORS IN IN VIVO MODELS OF THE STUNNED MYOCARDIUM

A. Brief Ischemia/Reperfusion

Our first in vivo experience with ACE inhibitors and the stunned myocardium was obtained in 1987: we found that high doses of enalapril (2 mg/kg bolus + 2 mg/kg/h infusion), initiated 45 minutes after reperfusion, significantly enhanced regional wall motion in anesthetized open-chest dogs subjected to 15 minutes of coronary artery occlusion. Specifically, segment shortening during the 2.5 hours following treatment was restored to 50-60% of baseline values in enalapril-treated animals vs. 20% of baseline in the control group (Przyklenk and Kloner, 1987). Similarly, Bittar et al. (1991) reported that captopril administered before and during coronary occlusion in this same canine model improved segment shortening measured 2-3 hours following reperfusion. However, these results may be influenced by the significant reductions in mean arterial pressure (Przyklenk and Kloner, 1987) or rate-pressure product (Bittar et al., 1991) associated with ACE inhibitor treatment in these two studies. As contractile function of the stunned myocardium may be sensitive to alternatives in afterload (Stahl et al., 1986), we cannot distinguish whether the improved function in these two protocols was simply a consequence of the reduction in arterial pressure, or whether enalapril or captopril exerted some sort of direct beneficial effect on the ischemic/reperfused tissue.

This issue was more rigorously pursued by Westlin and Mullane (1988), who assessed the effects of both captopril and enalaprilat on recovery of contractile function in this same canine model of the stunned myocardium. Captopril (5 mg/kg) administered either before coronary occlusion or 2 minutes prior to reflow significantly attenuated postischemic dysfunction: segment shortening during the initial 3 hours following reflow averaged 50-60% of baseline values in the captopril-treated groups vs. 10% of baseline in the control groups (Fig. 2). Furthermore, this improvement in function was not accompanied by alterations in arterial pressures. In contrast, pretreatment with enalaprilat (1-2 mg/kg) failed to improve segment shortening of the stunned tissue. In fact, contractile dysfunction was exacerbated in the enalaprilat-treated animals, both during the ischemic insult and following reperfusion (Westlin and Mullane, 1988) (Fig. 2).

Evidence obtained from our laboratory further confirmed that ACE inhibitors could improve recovery of contractile function in canine myocardium stunned by a brief, 15-minute episode of coronary occlusion. Zofenopril (5 mg/kg) given at the moment of reperfusion had no effect on systemic hemo-

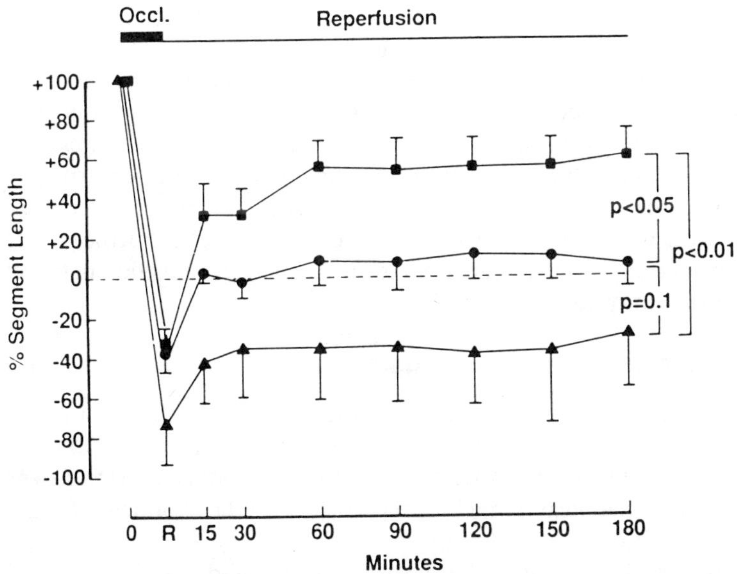

Figure 2 Segment shortening, expressed as percent of preocclusion values, for captopril (squares), enalaprilat (triangles), and control (circles) groups. Drugs were administered 15 minutes before the 15-minute episode of coronary artery occlusion. (Reprinted from Westlin and Mullane, 1988, with permission of the American Heart Association.)

dynamic parameters or myocardial blood flow in this model, yet segment shortening during the initial 3 hours of reflow was restored to 50-75% of baseline values in zofenopril-treated animals vs. 0-20% of baseline in untreated controls (Przyklenk et al., 1989; Przyklenk and Kloner, 1991) (Fig. 3). These data are in good agreement with the previous ex vivo and in vivo reports of improved recovery of function following treatment with an SH-containing ACE inhibitor. However, in marked contrast to the results obtained by Westlin and Mullane (1988), we found that enalaprilat (1.5 mg/kg given at the time of reflow) also improved recovery of function in the stunned tissue—in this case, to 70-80% of baseline values (Przyklenk and Kloner, 1991). That is, in our hands, both zofenopril and enalaprilat were equally effective in attenuating postischemic dysfunction (Przyklenk and Kloner, 1991). The reasons for this discrepancy between our results and those of Westlin and Mullane (1988) are difficult to reconcile, but may be due to differences in the anesthesia used in the two protocols, or due to the difference in the timing of drug treatment (before occlusion vs. at the time of reperfusion). More importantly, the exacerbated dysfunction observed by Westlin and Mullane (1988) may indicate that the enalaprilat-treated animals were more ischemic during occlusion than the control group. However, as myocardial blood flow was not assessed by Westlin and Mullane (1988), this argument remains speculative.

Although the effects of enalapril on the stunned myocardium remain inconclusive, data from these various studies provide convincing evidence that captopril and zofenopril enhance recovery of contractile function following a 15-minute episode of coronary artery occlusion. The beneficial effects of ACE inhibitor treatment in this canine model cannot be attributed to an anti-ischemic effect, as improvements in function were obtained even when the agents were administered at the time of reperfusion. Furthermore, these improvements in function are not mediated solely by reduction in blood pressure or coronary vasodilation.

B. Prolonged Ischemia/Reperfusion

All discussion to this point has focused on the effects of ACE inhibitors in models of brief ischemia not associated with myocardial necrosis. Do these agents also enhance recovery of function following prolonged but transient ischemia—that is, in models mimicking reperfusion for the treatment of acute myocardial infarction?

Numerous experimental and clinical studies have found that chronic ACE inhibitor treatment attenuates left ventricular dilitation and hypertrophy following *permanent* coronary artery occlusion, and thereby improves left ventricular function postinfarction (Pfeffer et al., 1985, 1988; Gay, 1990; Pinto et al., 1991; Shoemaker et al., 1991; Sharpe et al., 1988, 1991). Sur-

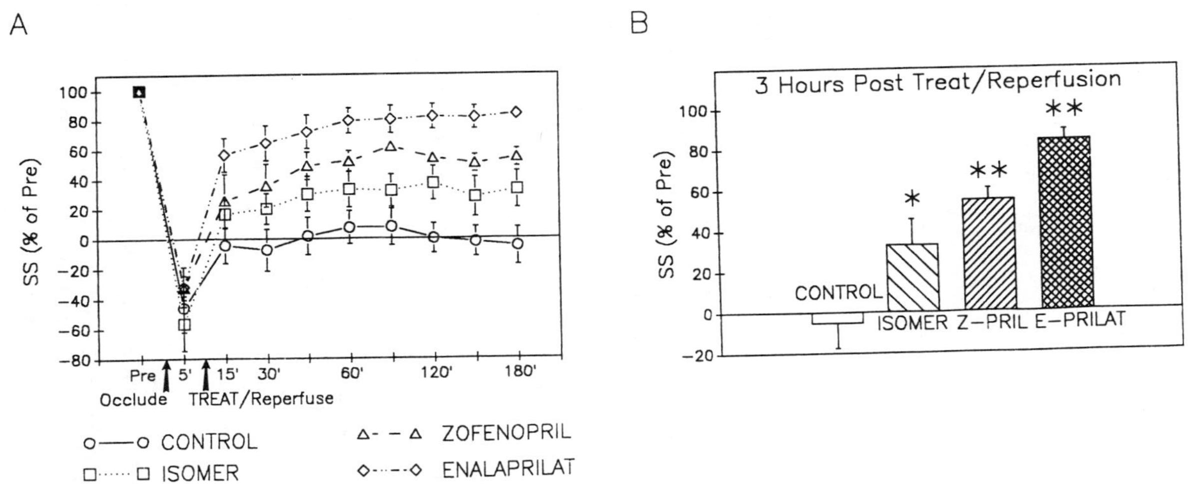

Figure 3 Segment shortening [SS: % of baseline, preocclusion (Pre) values] for the control, zofenopril (Z-pril)-, enalaprilat (E-prilat)-, and isomer-treated groups. All agents were administered at the time of reperfusion. (A) Data obtained during 15-minute period of occlusion and throughout initial 3 hours following treatment/reperfusion. (B) Recovery of contractile function at 3 hours after reflow. $*p < 0.05$; $**p < 0.01$ vs. control by analysis of variance. (Reprinted with permission from Przyklenk and Kloner, 1991.)

prisingly, however, the effects of these agents on contractile function of viable but stunned myocardium following prolonged ischemia/reperfusion are virtually unknown. In a recent preliminary report, Xu and Liu (1991) addressed this question in isolated rabbit hearts subjected to 3 hours of hypothermic ischemic arrest followed by normothermic reperfusion. Addition of captopril to the cardioplegic solution resulted in a doubling of cardiac output and stroke volume following reflow to 227% and 225% of values measured in untreated control hearts. Despite the fact that treatment was administered during ischemia, the superior recovery of contractile performance in the captopril-treated hearts was attributed at least in part to an improvement in contractility of the ischemic/reperfused tissue (Xu and Liu, 1991). Similar beneficial effects of enalapril treatment have also been described by Liu et al. (1987) in an in vivo canine model of ischemia/reperfusion: although details concerning the severity of ischemia are sketchy, Liu and colleagues reported improved segmental shortening following 60 minutes of coronary occlusion in dogs pretreated with enalapril. In contrast, de Graeff and colleagues (1987) found that pretreatment with captopril did not improve cardiac output or stroke volume in anesthetized pigs subjected to 1 hour of coronary occlusion and 2 hours of reflow. Thus, the question of whether ACE inhibitor treatment can enhance contractile function of peri-infarct tissue stunned by prolonged ischemia/reperfusion remains unresolved and clearly demands further investigation.

IV. MECHANISMS OF ACTION OF ACE INHIBITORS: CRUCIAL ROLE OF THE SULFHYDRYL GROUP?

Most recent studies investigating the effects of ACE inhibitors in models of ischemia/reperfusion were initiated in response to in vitro data obtained by Westlin and Mullane (1988), which suggested that SH-containing ACE inhibitors acted as scavengers of cytotoxic, oxygen-derived free radicals. For example, auto-oxidation of epinephrine to adrenochrome, a reaction thought to be mediated by the superoxide anion, was inhibited by captopril, zofenopril, and SQ 14,534 (a stereoisomer of captopril that contains the SH moiety but has essentially no ACE inhibitor properties). In contrast, neither enalaprilat nor teprotide (which do not contain the SH group) inhibited this reaction (Westlin and Mullane, 1988). These data raised the possibility that SH-containing ACE inhibitors may prove useful in the treatment of the stunned myocardium and other free radical-mediated disorders. (A detailed review of the role of oxygen radicals in the pathophysiology of the stunned myocardium is provided in Chapter 8.) Furthermore, these results lead investigators to speculate that an agent that both inhibits ACE *and* scavenges oxygen radicals may provide superior protection against ischemia/reperfusion-induced injury and dysfunction than either an ACE inhibitor or a free radical scavenger alone.

Any compound that contains an SH (or thiol) group will, in theory, spare tissue from oxidation by free radicals by acting as an electron acceptor. However, in contrast to the results obtained by Westlin and Mullane, thiol compounds are generally considered to be scavengers of hydroxyl radicals (Weglicki et al., 1990). Numerous subsequent studies using a variety of in vitro models have confirmed that the SH-containing ACE inhibitors captopril and zofenopril are potent scavengers of hydroxyl radicals (Bagchi et al., 1989; Mak et al., 1990; Aruoma et al., 1991), hypochlorous acid (Bagchi et al., 1989; Aruoma et al., 1991), or other "nonspecific" radical species (Chopra et al., 1989; McMurray et al., 1990a; Kukreja et al., 1990), but failed to find any inhibitory effect of these agents on superoxide anion production (Mak et al., 1990; Chopra et al., 1989; Kukreja et al., 1990; Mehta et al., 1990; Aruoma et al., 1991). Thus, although SH-containing ACE inhibitors probably do not scavenge superoxide anions, they clearly scavenge hydroxyl radicals and/or have general antioxidant properties.

Any extrapolation of these data must be tempered by the fact that the in vitro systems involve incubation of membranes and cells with relatively high (micromolar) concentrations of the drugs being tested (Weglicki et al., 1990). The obvious question is: do these SH-containing ACE inhibitors have significant free radical-scavenging properties at the lower, therapeutic plasma concentrations than would be achieved in vivo? Aruoma and colleagues (1991) were pessimistic in this regard: although they reported that captopril reacted rapidly with the hydroxyl radical, they concluded that captopril in lower, in vivo concentrations would be unlikely to compete with most biological molecules in this reaction. In addition, SH-containing agents may have deleterious consequences: some thiol compounds enhance neutrophil activity and may thereby exacerbate ischemia/reperfusion injury (McMurray and Chopra, 1991; Mitsos et al., 1986), and reaction of thiols with hydroxyl radicals can, in some cases, lead to the generation of toxic sulfur-containing radicals (Auroma et al., 1991).

The first steps toward answering this question were provided by Pi and Chen (1989), who assessed the effects of the ACE inhibitors captopril and ramiprilat in isolated working rat hearts in which oxygen radicals were generated by electrolysis of the perfusate. Although captopril did not scavenge superoxide anions directly, this agent did protect against free radical-mediated injury and dysfunction. More interestingly, ramiprilat was equally protective in this model. Furthermore, the beneficial effects of ramiprilat were abolished by co-administration of indomethacin. That is, although ramiprilat does not contain the protective antioxidant SH group, this agent attenuated free radical-mediated injury and dysfunction by stimulating prostaglandin synthesis (Pi and Chen, 1989).

Our laboratory further pursued this question in the in vivo setting by comparing the efficacy of zofenopril, enalaprilat, and the SH-containing isomer SQ 14,534 with negligible ACE inhibitor properties on recovery of contractile function of canine myocardium stunned by 15 minutes of transient ischemia (Przyklenk and Kloner, 1991). As mentioned previously, we found that both zofenopril and enalaprilat given at the time of reperfusion restored segment shortening in the ischemic/reperfused tissue to 60-80% of baseline values. Furthermore, SQ 14,543 also improved function of the stunned tissue to approximately 35% of baseline values (Fig. 3). We further found that the enhanced contractile function associated with enalaprilat treatment was essentially reversed when indomethacin was infused at 2 hours following reflow (Fig. 4). Interestingly, these data are similar to the results obtained with ramiprilat and indomethacin in the ex vivo model of free radical-mediated dysfunction (Pi and Chen, 1989). In contrast, infusion of indomethacin had no effect on the improved contractile function in dogs that had been treated with zofenopril (Fig. 4) (Przyklenk and Kloner, 1991).

The improved function obtained with SQ 14,543 observed both in our study and by Westlin and Mullane (1988) confirm that the SH moiety per se can confer a protective effect in the setting of transient ischemia/reperfusion, probably due to the well-documented free radical-scavenging or antioxidant properties common to all thiol compounds. The beneficial effects of zofenopril are also likely due, at least in part, to the presence of the SH group. However, the differential improvement in function with zofenopril vs. SQ 14,534 would suggest that other, as yet unidentified factors also play a role. Although one preliminary report suggests that enalaprilat may inhibit peroxidation of membrane lipids (Kedziora et al., 1991), the improved function associated with enalaprilat treatment cannot be attributed to direct free radical-scavenging properties. Rather, the beneficial effects of enalaprilat treatments in this model appear to be a consequence of increased prostaglandin synthesis.

These data obtained from a host of in vitro and in vivo experiments clearly demonstrate that ACE inhibitors that contain the SH group do have free radical-scavenging or antioxidant properties. However, the mechanisms of action of both SH- and non-SH-containing ACE inhibitors in the setting of ischemia/reperfusion are complex and multifactorial. Although there remain discrepancies among the studies, our results strongly suggest that the SH group does not play a crucial role in mediating the efficacy of ACE inhibitor treatment in canine myocardium stunned by brief transient ischemia.

V. CLINICAL USE OF ACE INHIBITORS IN ISCHEMIA/REPERFUSION: THE FIRST ATTEMPTS

Increases in plasma levels of renin and angiotensin II have been documented in patients following coronary artery occlusion (McAlpine et al., 1988). In

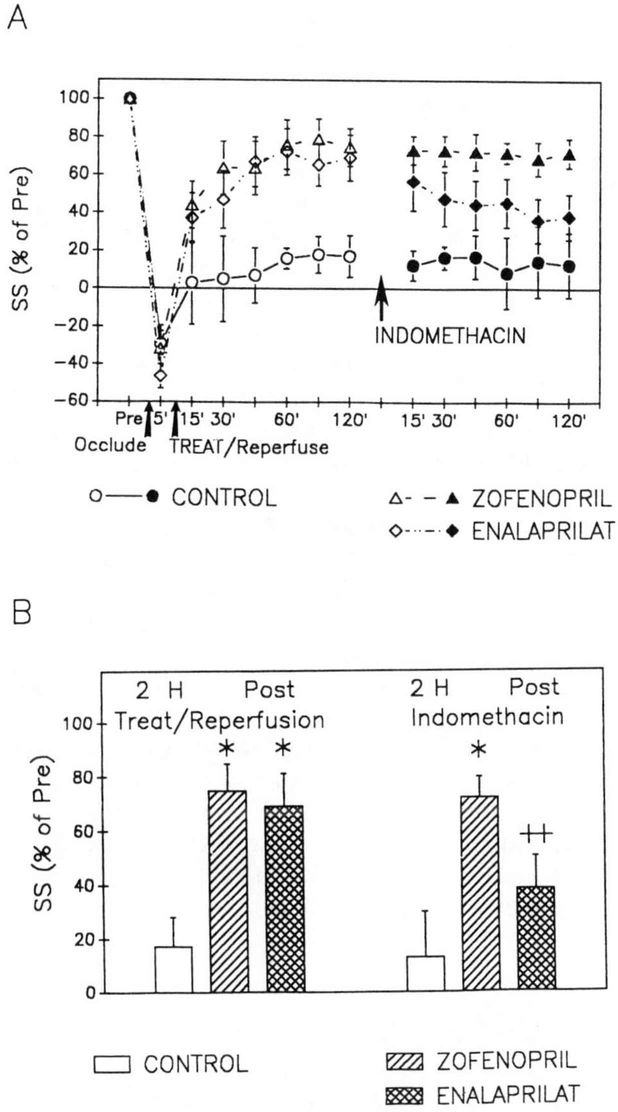

Figure 4 Segment shortening [SS: % of baseline, preocclusion (Pre) values] for control, zofenopril- and enalaprilat-treated groups. All groups then received indomethacin at 2 hours after reflow. (A) Data obtained during the 15-minute period of occlusion, during the initial 2 hours following treatment/reperfusion, and for 2 hours following infusion of indomethacin. (B) Recovery of contractile function at 2 hours after treatment/reperfusion and at 2 hours after indomethacin. $*p < 0.05$ vs. control by analysis of variance; $^{++}p < 0.01$ vs. 2 hours after treatment/reperfusion by paired *t*-test. (Reprinted with permission from Przyklenk and Kloner, 1991.)

addition, indirect evidence of myocardial oxidative injury has recently been reported by McMurray et al. (1990b) in patients with coronary artery disease. These observations, combined with the interest in the free radical-scavenging properties of SH-containing ACE inhibitors and the promising results obtained with these agents in some experimental models of ischemia/reperfusion, has prompted the clinical evaluation of captopril as adjuvant therapy with thrombolysis (Ertl, 1988; Kingma et al., 1989, 1990; di Pasquale et al., 1990; Nabel et al., 1991).

Does captopril enhance contractile function of salvaged but stunned myocardium in patients successfully reperfused for the treatment of acute myocardial infarction? As with any clinical assessment of adjuvant therapy, this will prove to be a difficult question to answer (Popma and Topol, 1991). Initial studies assessing the effects of intravenous captopril administered with streptokinase were confounded by profound hypotension (Ertl, 1988; Kingma et al., 1989). Oral captopril therapy has, however, been better tolerated, and has been associated with significant reductions in the incidence of early and late arrhythmias (di Pasquale et al., 1990) and lower catacholamine levels (Kingma et al., 1990) following reperfusion. In addition, Nabel and colleagues (1991) found that captopril (2-10 mg intravenous given with t-PA, followed by oral doses of 25-100 mg/day for 3 months) significantly attenuated the progressive left ventricular dilitation and enlargement observed in control patients that received t-PA alone. Adjuvant therapy with captopril did not, however, enhance left ventricular ejection fraction assessed at 7 days following treatment (Nabel et al., 1991). To date, the effects of early captopril treatment administered with thrombolysis on indices of regional wall motion in the infarct-related area have not been reported. Thus, although these studies have demonstrated the feasibility of adjuvant therapy with captopril, the specific question of whether captopril improves function of stunned myocardium in clinical instances of ischemia/reperfusion remains unanswered.

IV. SUMMARY

There is no doubt that ACE inhibitors acutely enhance contractile function of myocardium stunned by a brief episode of transient ischemia. However, the mechanisms of action of this structurally diverse class of drugs in the setting of ischemia/reperfusion are complex. Although there is no question that ACE inhibitors have profound hemodynamic and anti-ischemic effects, improvement in contractile performance with these agents is not dependent upon systemic or coronary vasodilation. Furthermore, these agents effectively attenuate postischemic dysfunction even when administered at the time of reperfusion. The SH-containing agents captopril and zofenopril have consistently been shown to improve function of stunned myocardium, due at least in part to the free radical or antioxidant properties shared by all thiol compounds. While the SH group appears to be cardioprotective, ACE inhibitors that do not contain the SH group (such as enalapril) have, in some models, proven equally effective in attenuating postischemic dysfunction, but the beneficial effects of these agents appear to be largely a consequence of enhanced prostaglandin synthesis. It must be stressed that virtually all evidence of improved function with ACE inhibitor treatment has been derived from ex vivo models or from in vivo models of brief ischemia not associated with subendocardial necrosis. In addition, most studies have used high doses of these agents. The effects of lower, more clinically relevant doses of ACE inhibitors on contractile performance of peri-infarct tissue stunned by prolonged ischemia/reperfusion awaits further investigation in both the experimental laboratory and in the clinical setting.

REFERENCES

Aruoma, O., Akanmu, D., Cecchini, R., and Halliwell, B. (1991). Evaluation of the ability of the angiotensin-converting enzyme inhibitor captopril to scavenge reactive oxygen species. *Chem. Biol. Interactions 77*: 303.

Bagchi, D., Prasad, R., and Das, D. K. (1989). Direct scavenging of free radicals by captopril, an angiotensin converting enzyme inhibitor. *Biochem. Biophys. Res. Comm. 158*: 52.

Bittar, N., Zheng, H. N., and Nwosu, E. A. (1991). Captopril is more effective than dipyridamole or labetolol in attenuating myocardial stunning in the dog. *Proceedings of the Second International Symposium on ACE Inhibition,* London UK, p. P-179 (Abstract).

Chopra, M., Scott, N., McMurray, J., McLay, J., Bridges, A., Smith, W. E., and Belch, J. J. F. (1989). Captopril: A free radical scavenger. *Br. J. Pharmacol. 27*: 396.

Cushman, D. W., and Ondetti, M. A. (1980). Inhibitors of angiotensin converting enzyme. *Prog. Med. Chem. 17*: 41.

de Graeff, P. A., van Gilst, W. H., de Langen, C. D. J., Kingma, J. H., and Wesseling, H. (1986). Concentration-dependent protection of captopril against ischemia-reperfusion injury in the isolated rat heart. *Arch. Int. Pharmacodynam. Ther. 280*: 181.

de Graeff, P. A., van Gilst, W. H., Bel, K., de Langen, C. D. J., Kingma, J. H., and Wesseling, H. (1987). Concentration-dependent protection by captopril against myocardial damage during ischemia and reperfusion in a closed-chest pig model. *J. Cardiovasc. Pharmacol. 9* (Suppl. 2): S31.

de Graeff, P. A. (1989). *Effects of Captopril on the Heart: Mechanisms and Therapeutic Potentials.* Drukkerij van Denderen B. V., Groningen, The Netherlands.

di Pasquale, P., Barone, G., Paterna, S., Cannizzaro, S., and Giubilato, A. (1990). Efficacy of captopril before thrombolysis in acute myocardial infarction: preliminary findings. *Drugs Exp. Clin. Res. 16*: 581.

Dzau, V. J. (1988). Tissue renin-angiotensin system: physiologic and pharmacologic implications. *Circulation 77* (Suppl. I): I-1.

Ertl, G., Alexander, R. W., and Braunwald, E. (1983). Interaction between coronary occlusion and the renin-angiotensin system in the dog. *Basic Res. Cardiol. 78*: 518.

Ertl, G. (1988). Angiotensin converting enzyme inhibitors in ischemic heart disease. *Eur. Heart J. 9*: 716.

Fleetwood, G., Boutinet, S., Meier, M., and Wood, J. M. (1991). Involvement of the renin-angiotensin system in ischemic damage and reperfusion arrhythmias in the isolated perfused rat heart. *J. Cardiovasc. Pharmacol. 17*: 351.

Gavras, H., and Gavras, I. (1991). Cardioprotective potential of angiotensin converting enzyme inhibitors. *J. Hypertension 9*: 385.

Gay, R. G. (1990). Early and late effects of captopril treatment after large myocardial infarction in rats. *J. Am. Coll. Cardiol. 16*: 967.

Grover, G. J., Steph, P. G., Dzwonczyk, S., Wang, P., Fung, W., Tobias, D., and Cushman, D. W. (1991). Effects of different angiotensin converting enzyme (ACE) inhibitors on ischemic isolated rat hearts: relationship between cardiac ACE inhibition and cardioprotection. *J. Pharmacol. Exp. Ther. 257*: 919.

Hock, C. E., Ribeiro, L. G. T., and Lefer, A. M. (1985). Preservation of ischemic myocardium by a new converting enzyme inhibitor, enalaprilic acid, in acute myocardial infarction. *Am. Heart J. 109*: 222.

Kedziora, J., Ikaczewski, W., Blaszcyk, J., Buczynski, A., Ryniec, A., and Dziekanski, S. (1991). Effect of enalapril on lipid peroxidation and adenine nucleotides in patients with unstable angina. *Proceedings of the Second International Symposium on ACE Inhibition*, London UK, p. P-158 (Abstract).

Kingma, J. H., van Gilst, W. H., de Graeff, P. A., Louwerenburg, H. W., Six, A. J., and Wesseling, H. (1989). Captopril during thrombolysis in acute myocardial infarction: Feasibility, tolerance and beneficial neurohumoral effects. In *Current Advances in ACE Inhibition* (G. A., MacGregor and P. S. Sever, eds.), Churchill Livingstone, New York, p. 291.

Kingma, J. H., van Gilst, W. H., Peels, C. H., Jaarsma, W., and Verheugt, F. W. (1990). Converting enzyme inhibition during thrombolytic therapy in acute myocardial infarction. *Circulation 82* (Suppl. III): III-666 (Abstract).

Kukreja, R. C., Kontos, H. A., and Hess, M. L. (1990). Captopril and enalaprilat do not scavenge the superoxide anion. *Am. J. Cardiol. 65*: 241.

Li, K., and Chen, X. (1987). Protective effects of captopril and enalapril on myocardial ischemia and reperfusion damage of rat. *J. Mol. Cell. Cardiol. 19*: 909.

Liu, L. Y., Chen, X., Li, K., and Wu, H. J. (1987). Beneficial effects of enalapril on reperfusion arrhythmia and segmental contraction in anesthetized dogs. *Acta Pharmacol. Sin 43*: 434.

Mak, I. T., Freedman, A. M., Dickens, B. F., and Weglicki, W. B. (1990). Protective effects of sulfhydryl-containing angiotensin converting enzyme inhibitors against free radical injury in endothelial cells. *Biochem. Pharmacol. 40*: 2169.

McAlpine, H. M., Morton, J. J., Leckie, B., Ramley, A., Gillen, G., and Dargie, H. J. (1988). Neuroendocrine activation after acute myocardial infarction. *Br. Heart J. 60*: 117.

McMurray, J., Chopra, M., Smith, W. E., and Dargie, H. J. (1990a). Free radical scavenging: A potentially beneficial action of -SH containing ACE inhibitors? *Circulation 82* (Suppl. III): III-264 (Abstract).

McMurray, J., Chopra, M., Smith, W. E., and Dargie, H. (1990b). Free radical activity in chronic heart failure: Evidence for trans-myocardial oxidative stress. *Circulation 82* (Suppl. III): III-566 (Abstract).

McMurray, J., and Chopra, M. (1991). Influence of ACE inhibitors on free radicals and reperfusion injury: Pharmacological curiosity or therapeutic hope? *Br. J. Clin. Pharmacol. 31*: 373.

Mehta, J. L., Nicolini, F. A., and Lawson, D. L. (1990). Sulfhydryl group in angiotensin converting enzyme inhibitors and superoxide radical formation. *J. Cardiovasc. Pharmacol. 16*: 847.

Mitsos, S. E., Fantone, J. C., Gallagher, K. P., Walden, K. M., Simpson, P. J., Abrams, G. D., Shork, M. A., and Lucchesi, B. R. (1986). Canine myocardial reperfusion injury: protection by a free radical scavenger N-2-mercaptopropionylglycine. *J. Cardiovasc. Pharmacol. 8*: 1978.

Nabel, E. G., Topol, E. J., Galeana, A., Ellis, S. G., Bates, E. R., Werns, S. W., Walton, J. A., Muller, D. W., Schwaiger, M., and Pitt, B. (1991). A randomized placebo-controlled trial of combined early intravenous captopril and recombinant tissue-type plasminogen activator therapy in acute myocardial infarction. *J. Am. Coll. Cardiol. 17*: 467.

Ondetti, M. A. (1988). Structural relationships of angiotensin-converting enzyme inhibitors to pharmacologic activity. *Circulation 77* (Suppl. I): I-74.

Pfeffer, M. A., Pfeffer, J. M., and Braunwald, E. (1985). Influence of chronic captopril therapy on the infarcted left ventricle of the rat. *Circ. Res. 57*: 84.

Pfeffer, M. A., Lamas, G. A., Vaughan, D. E., Parisi, A. F., and Braunwald, E. (1988). Effect of captopril on progressive ventricular dilitation after anterior myocardial infarction. *N. Engl. J. Med. 319*: 80.

Pi, X. J., and Chen, X. (1989). Captopril and ramiprilat protect against free radical injury in isolated working hearts. *J. Mol. Cell. Cardiol. 21*: 1261.

Pinto, Y. M., van Wijngaarden, J., van Gilst, W. H., de Graeff, P. A., and Wesseling, H. (1991). The effects of short and long-term treatment with an ACE inhibitor in rats with myocardial infarction. In *Pharmacology of Cardiac and Vascular Remodelling.* (J. F. M. Smits, ed.), Steinkopff Verlag, Darmstadt, 1991, p. 165.

Popma, J. J., and Topol, E. J. (1991). Adjuncts to thrombolysis for myocardial reperfusion. *Ann. Int. Med. 115*: 34.

Przyklenk, K., and Kloner, R. A. (1987). Acute effects of hydralazine and enalapril on contractile function of postischemic "stunned" myocardium. *Am. J. Cardiol. 60*: 934.

Przyklenk, K., Whittaker, P., and Kloner, R. R. (1989). Zofenopril, a newly developed sulfhydryl-containing angiotensin converting enzyme inhibitor, enhances contractile function of "stunned" myocardium. *Current Advances in ACE Inhibition* (G. A. MacGregor and P. S. Sever, eds.), Churchill Livingstone, New York, p. 279.

Przyklenk, K., and Kloner, R. A. (1991). Angiotensin converting enzyme inhibitors improve contractile function of stunned myocardium by different mechanisms of action. *Am. Heart J. 121*: 1319.

Rahusen, F. D., van Gilst, W. H., Robillard, G. T., Dijkstra, K., and Wildevurr, C. R. H. (1988). Captopril improves recovery of adenosine triphosphate during reperfusion of the ischemic isolated rat heart: a 31-phosphorus-nuclear magnetic resonance study. *Basic Res. Cardiol. 83*: 540.

Schwartz, S. L., and Williams, G. H. (1982). Angiotensin converting enzyme inhibition and prostaglandins. *Am. J. Cardiol. 49*: 1405.

Sharpe, N., Murphy, J., Smith, H., and Hannan, S. (1988). Treatment of patients with symptomless left ventricular dysfunction after myocardial infarction. *Lancet 1*: 255.

Sharpe, N., Smith, H., Murphy, J., Greaves, S., Hart, H., and Gamble, G. (1991). Early prevention of left ventricular dysfunction after myocardial infarction with angiotensin converting enzyme inhibition. *Lancet 337*: 872.

Shoemaker, R. G., Debets, J. J. M., Struyker-Boudier, H. A. J., and Smits, J. F. M. (1991). Delayed but not immediate captopril therapy improves cardiac function in conscious rats following myocardial infarction. *J. Mol. Cell. Cardiol. 23*: 187.

Stahl, L., Anversano, T., and Becker, L. C. (1986). Selective enhancement of function of stunned myocardium by increased flow. *Circulation 74*: 843.

van Gilst, W. H., de Graeff, P. A., Kingma, J. H., Wesseling, H., and de Langen, C. D. J. (1984). Captopril reduces purine loss and reperfusion arrhythmias in the rat heart after coronary occlusion. *Eur. J. Pharmacol. 100*: 113.

van Gilst, W. H., de Graeff, P. A., Wesseling, H., and de Langen, C. D. J. (1986). Reduction of reperfusion arrhythmias in the ischemic isolated rat heart by angiotensin converting enzyme inhibition. A comparison of captopril, enalapril and HOE 498. *J. Cardiovasc. Pharmacol. 8*: 722.

Weglicki, W. B., Mak, I. T., and Simic, M. G. (1990). Mechanisms of cardiovascular drugs as antioxidants. *J. Mol. Cell. Cardiol. 22*: 1199.

Westlin, W., and Mullane, K. (1988). Does captopril attenuate reperfusion-induced myocardial dysfunction by scavenging free radicals? *Circulation 77* (Suppl. I): I-30.

Xu, S. C., and Liu, F. M. (1991). The myocardial protective effect of captopril cardioplegia against ischemia in the isolated working rabbit heart: Study on the cardiac function. *Proceedings of the Second International Symposium on ACE Inhibition*, London UK, p. P-172 (Abstract).

Part IV

Stunned Myocardium and the Clinician

While the current concepts of stunned myocardium largely originated in the experimental animal laboratory, there has been increasing awareness of stunned myocardium in the clinical realm. Evidence that stunned myocardium occurs in patients is derived from a number of clinical reports. The purpose of Part IV is to review some of these clinical reports as well as to provide opinions of the importance of stunned myocardium to the clinician.

The 1980s ushered in the era of thrombolytic therapy for acute myocardial infarction, and it is likely that this form of therapy will be with us for some time. Dr. Kloner will review studies that suggest that stunned myocardium may occur in humans following thrombolytic therapy. Two chapters review evidence that stunned myocardium may occur in humans following brief episodes of ischemia (no infarction): Drs. Murphy, Wijns, and Serruys describe increased ventricular stiffness following brief periods of ischemia induced by coronary angioplasty procedures, while Drs. Allen and Kloner discuss studies that suggest that stunned myocardium occurs in patients following brief episodes of exercise-induced ischemia. Another clinical situation in which stunned myocardium has been appreciated is the period following cardiac surgery. Patients who have undergone cardiopulmonary bypass procedures may exhibit depressed left ventricular function requiring inotropic support for hours to days following the procedure. This concept is discussed by Drs. Wilson and Gardner.

Identification of the stunned myocardium may be made by observing a gradual improvement in postischemic regional function over time. Alternate techniques for early identification of stunned myocardium would be desirable. Drs. Schelbert and Buxton examine the potential role of positron emission tomography in the identification of stunned myocardium.

The final two chapters provide opinions as to the importance of stunned myocardium in cardiovascular surgery and clinical cardiology. Dr. Kay and associates review the surgical approach to the concept of stunning including some recent advances in trying to prevent the development of this complication following cardiopulmonary bypass. Dr. Braunwald then reviews our existing knowledge regarding the role of stunning in the clinical practice of medicine and discusses whether this phenomenon is important for the practitioner.

18

Stunned Myocardium in Patients Reperfused for the Treatment of Acute Myocardial Infarction

Robert A. Kloner

Hospital of the Good Samaritan and University of Southern California, Los Angeles, California

I. BACKGROUND

Thrombolytic therapy for acute myocardial infarction has become routine in most medical centers worldwide. Timely thrombolysis with agents such as streptokinase, tissue plasminogen activator, or anisoylated plasminogen streptokinase activator complex has been shown to lyse acute occlusive coronary thrombi, decrease myocardial infarct size, improve survival, and enhance long-term recovery of left ventricular function with a reduction in congestive heart failure (Grines and DeMaria, 1990). One area where the concept of stunned myocardium appears to be particularly relevant to clinical medicine is in the field of thrombolysis (Patel et al., 1988; Kloner et al., 1990).

As described in Part I of this book, reperfusion in experimental models of acute myocardial infarction can reduce the extent of necrosis, but does not result in the immediate restoration of normal ventricular function. For example, Ellis et al. (1983) observed in a canine model that reperfusion following 2 hours of coronary artery occlusion resulted in subendocardial necrosis but significant salvage in the overlying subepicardium. In contrast, if the proximal coronary artery was occluded permanently (i.e., not reperfused), then the myocardial infarction was, in many cases, virtually transmural.

Two-dimensional echocardiography was used by Ellis et al. to compare the return of left ventricular function in animals with versus without reperfusion. Within the central ischemic zone, reperfusion resulted in an early reduction in the degree of paradoxical wall thinning. However, active systolic contraction was not observed until 48 hours after restoration of flow. This was followed by a further gradual improvement in contraction during the initial 14 days postreperfusion. In contrast, in animals that did not receive reperfusion as a therapy, there was an initial worsening of function during the first several hours of ischemia and no restoration of active contraction during the 2-week protocol.

Thus, although timely reperfusion enhanced the return of regional wall motion, recovery was slow, presumably due to stunning of the myocardium. As thrombolytic therapy for acute myocardial infarction became accepted, numerous clinical studies have analyzed the effect of thrombolysis on regional wall motion in patients. The following discussion summarizes the clinical evidence, which suggests that stunned myocardium occurs following timely restoration of blood flow to ischemic tissue.

II. CLINICAL TRIALS WITH THROMBOLYTIC AGENTS

Anderson et al. (1983) were some of the first investigators to monitor the return of left ventricular function in patients who had received intracoronary streptokinase for acute myocardial infarction. Using a two-dimensional echocardiographic wall motion score, they described a modest improvement in wall motion between pretreatment and 1 day after reperfusion. Between 1 and 10 days after thrombolysis, there was further gradual improvement in wall motion. Stack et al. (1983) utilized left ventricular angiography to follow the return of cardiac function following intracoronary streptokinase therapy. The percent radial shortening of infarct-related segments was 8% on admission and remained unchanged at 24 hours following treatment. That is, there was no immediate or dramatic improvement in regional wall motion within the first day of thrombolytic therapy. However, by 16 days after reperfusion, radial shortening had increased significantly to 18% in the infarct-related zone. Similarly, Reduto et al. (1981) described a lack of immediate improvement in global left ventricular ejection fraction (measured by radionuclide ventriculography) after intracoronary streptokinase (46% vs. 44% pretreatment), but a substantial increase in global ejection fraction (to 56%) at 10 days posttreatment. In fact, review of data from some of the major streptokinase trials performed during the 1980s (Patel and Kloner, 1987) revealed that improvements in global left ventricular ejection fraction and regional wall motion abnormalities occurred late after thrombolysis (usually near the time of hospital discharge). However, improvement in function was, in most studies, dependent on success of reperfusion: patients who did not develop successful reperfusion had the same, or even worse, LV function at the time of hospital discharge.

Further support for the concept that stunned myocardium may occur following thrombolysis comes from a study by Satler et al. (1986), who evaluated the potential of postischemic reperfused myocardium to respond to inotropic intervention. Following streptokinase therapy and successful reperfusion, they observed that a brief infusion of isoproterenol improved regional wall motion and ejection fraction to a greater extent in patients who were successfully reperfused when compared with those patients in whom thrombolysis was unsuccessful. These observations are analogous to experimental animal studies which have shown that the viable but stunned myocardium maintains a latent capacity for contraction and can be stimulated to contract with inotropic interventions (Ellis et al., 1984; Arnold et al., 1985).

Sheehan et al. (1991) recently reported that intravenous streptokinase therapy may have some early benefit on left ventricular function. Left ventricular angiography was performed and the centerline method of wall motion analysis used to monitor return of regional wall motion following thrombolysis. Studies 1-4 days after therapy showed less hypokinesis in the streptokinase-treated group when compared with controls who received no thrombolytic therapy. At 5 weeks, regional function in the streptokinase group was further improved, and there was a significant increase in global ejection fraction in the streptokinase group (49%) compared with controls (40%). In another study, Sheehan et al. (1988) demonstrated that patients with sustained coronary reperfusion following thrombolysis had continued improvement in left ventricular function between 3 days and 6 months following reflow (Fig. 1). Similarly, Voth et al. (1990) showed that improvements in left ventricular function observed with intravenous streptokinase at 1 month persisted at 7 months after treatment. In particular, anterior wall infarctions and those that received thrombolysis within the first 3 hours showed the most impressive improvement in function.

Evidence of stunned myocardium has also been reported following successful administration of other thrombolytic agents. One of the first studies suggesting that tissue plasminogen activator (t-PA) improved recovery of function after infarction was reported by Guerci et al. (1987), who studied the change in left ventricular global ejection fraction in patients receiving either placebo or the lytic agent. Patients receiving t-PA had a significant increase in ejection fraction between day 1 and day 10 after thrombolysis (+ 3.6%), while global ejection fraction usually deteriorated during this time in patients who received placebo (−4.7%). Of note, patients receiving tissue plasminogen activator had a lower incidence of clinical congestive heart failure than the placebo group. Similarly, Armstrong et al. (1989) demonstrated improved

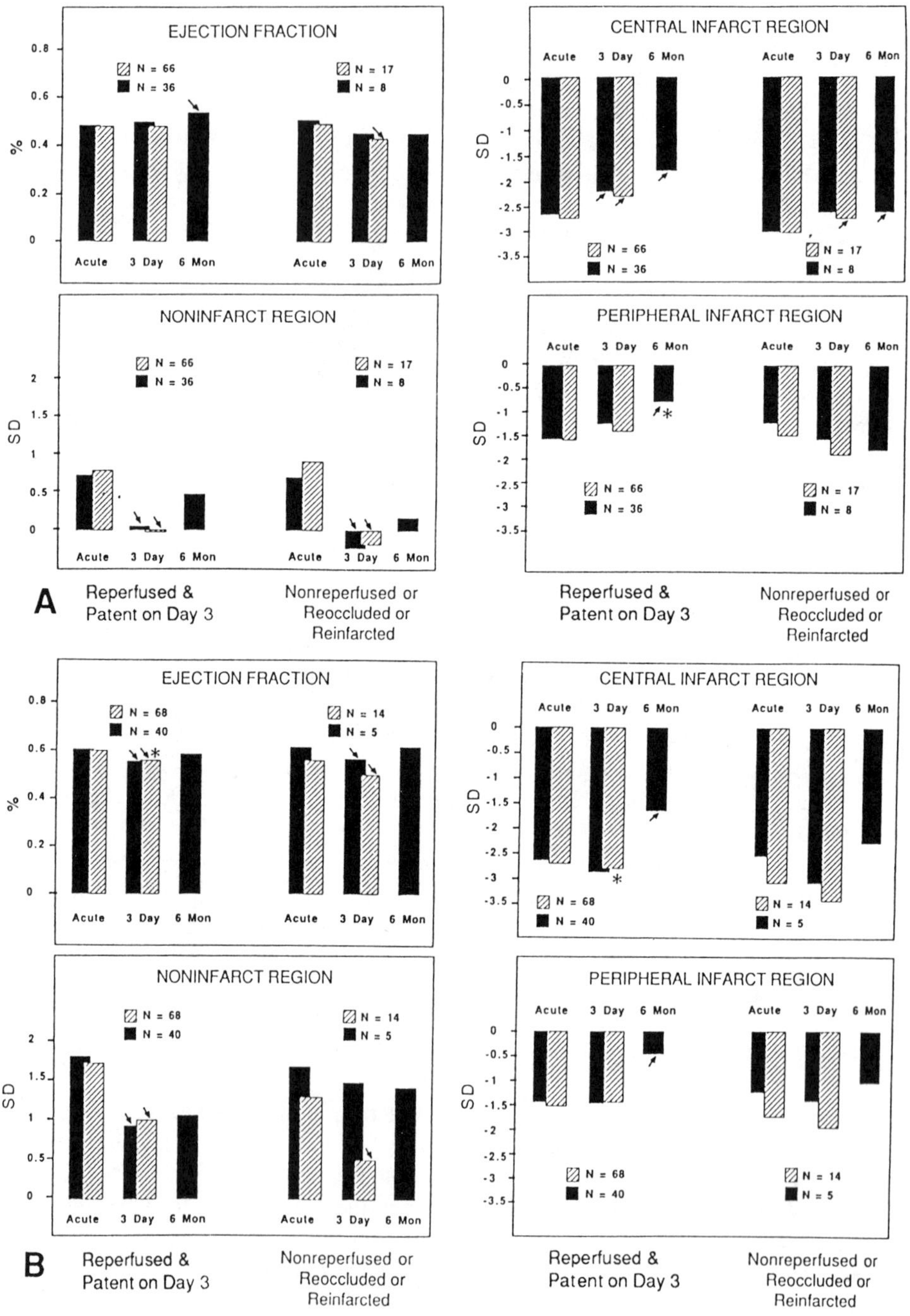
EJECTION FRACTION
%
N = 66
N = 36
N = 17
N = 8
Acute 3 Day 6 Mon
CENTRAL INFARCT REGION
SD
NONINFARCT REGION
PERIPHERAL INFARCT REGION
A
Reperfused & Patent on Day 3
Nonreperfused or Reoccluded or Reinfarcted
EJECTION FRACTION
N = 68
N = 40
N = 14
N = 5
CENTRAL INFARCT REGION
NONINFARCT REGION
PERIPHERAL INFARCT REGION
B
Reperfused & Patent on Day 3
Nonreperfused or Reoccluded or Reinfarcted

regional function in the infarct zone at or near hospital discharge in patients treated with t-PA. Pfisterer et al. (1991) observed delayed recovery of function after treatment with this agent; left ventricular ejection fraction increased from hospital discharge to 3-6 months after treatment.

While many of the studies described above used left ventricular angiography or radionuclide ventriculography to assess left ventricular function, a number of recent studies have used two-dimensional echocardiography to quantify regional wall motion abnormalities following thrombolytic therapy. The advantages of two-dimensional echocardiography include its portability to coronary care units, its noninvasive nature, the fact that no radionuclide substances need to be injected, its relative ease in obtaining repeated measurements, and, finally, its relatively low cost. An additional advantage of this technique is its ability to detect concomitant mechanical complications of acute myocardial infarction (such as ventricular septal rupture and rupture of the papillary muscles). For example Touchstone et al. (1989) used two-dimensional echocardiography to monitor recovery of left ventricular function over a course of 45 days following intravenous streptokinase therapy. While 45% of patients with a patent infarct-related artery showed eventual improvement in regional wall motion, this improvement did not occur during the first few days after treatment. Rather, the improvement in contractile function occurred 3-10 days following reperfusion (Fig. 2). Some patients exhibited further improvement in regional function between days 10 and 45. In contrast, some two-dimensional echocardiography studies have

Figure 1 Serial changes in regional and global left ventricular function in patients who underwent contrast ventriculography in the acute period and at 3 days ($n = 165$) and 6 months after treatment ($n = 89$). (A) Anterior infarction; (B) inferior infarction. The improvement measured at 3 days is a fraction of the total recovery seen at 6 months. The changes seen at 3 days are comparable in the groups with (black bars) versus those without (hatched bars) 6-month data. Arrows indicate significant change in left ventricular function from the acute study; asterisks indicate that left ventricular function at that time point differs significantly between patients with sustained reperfusion and patients with nonreperfusion, reocclusion, or infarction. Note that for anterior infarcts in the central infarct region reperfused infarcts have some improved function at three days with further improvement in regional function at six months. This may represent both early and later recovery of function of the stunned myocardium. Improvement in function in the peripheral infarct region is also evident. For inferior infarcts the most striking improvement in function in both central and peripheral regions occurred between days 3 and 6. Again, this may represent gradual return of function of stunned myocardium. (Reprinted from Sheehan et al., 1988, with permission of the American College of Cardiology.)

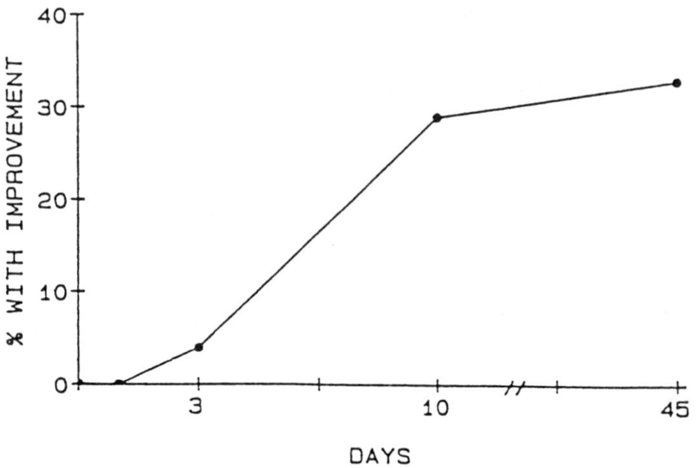

Figure 2 Percent of patients showing time-related improvement in regional left ventricular function after intravenous streptokinase. One-third of all the patients receiving this therapy showed improvement in function. Most of the improvement occurred between days 3 and 10 after streptokinase infusion. (Reprinted from Touchstone et al., 1989, with permission of the American College of Cardiology.)

demonstrated some very early improvement in regional function after thrombolysis followed by continued improvement over the course of several days. Using a semiquantitive scoring system ranging from 4+ (denoting severe hypokinesis) to 1+ (normal function), Bourdillon et al. (1989) found that wall motion improved from a mean score of 1.78 to 1.56 in the first day following reperfusion by either thrombolysis or angioplasty, and further improved to 1.48 at 3-7 days following reflow. This was accompanied by a gradual improvement in the percentage of myocardium that functioned normally, from 53% at 6 hours, to 62% at 1 day, and 67% at 3-7 days posttreatment. Otto et al. (1990) also utilized two-dimensional echocardiography to assess the effects of thrombolysis with t-PA on left ventricular function following reperfusion. The wall motion score index improved from early (11 hours) to late (13 weeks) readings. Furthermore, improvement in regional wall function was associated with early reperfusion (within 2 hours of chest pain) and evidence of successful reperfusion at coronary angiography.

III. ANGIOPLASTY FOR ACUTE MYOCARDIAL INFARCTION

Restoration of blood flow in acute infarction patients by angioplasty results in improvement in myocardial function, but detailed assessment of stunning is lacking. Brodie et al. (1991) studied 383 patients with acute myocardial infarction who were treated with coronary angioplasty without prior thrombolytic therapy. Improvement in left ventricular ejection fraction assessed at 6 months was +10.5% in patients who received angioplasty, with the most marked improvements in ejection fraction observed in patients with anterior wall infarction. In addition, Lee et al. (1991) have shown better survival of patients with acute myocardial infarction and cardiogenic shock in those patients undergoing primary angioplasty than in those not undergoing this procedure.

These data suggest that some patients exhibiting severe contractile dysfunction at the time of reperfusion who may have been thought to have fully completed infarcts in fact had some areas of viable myocardium that were either stunned or hibernating. Angioplasty, by removing the coronary artery stenosis rather than just lysing a thrombus overlying a stenosis, might in theory further enhance reflow and thereby improve the rate of recovery of stunned myocardium. However, in contrast to the studies described above, combination of immediate angioplasty during thrombolytic therapy with tissue plasminogen activator was shown by Arnold et al. (1991) *not* to improve function. This apparent discrepancy may be a consequence of a greater proportion of high-risk patients in the invasive treatment group. That is, the invasive treatment group may have been more prone towards reocclusion, reinfarction, or both. It is also possible that combination of thrombolysis with angioplasty may exacerbate plaque hemorrhage and coronary artery dissection.

IV. SUMMARY AND CLINICAL IMPLICATIONS

In summary, most, but not all (Kennedy et al. 1985) thrombolytic trials have described some gradual increase in regional (and/or global) left ventricular function during the initial 1-2 weeks following successful reperfusion. In some studies, the improvement in function was not immediate or dramatic in the first few days of reperfusion; in others, there was some early improvement in function during the first day or so followed by further improvement at 10-16 days postreflow. These results are important in that they indicate that the absence of an early dramatic improvement in left ventricular function following reperfusion should not be interpreted as a sign of failed reperfusion. Rather, these clinical data are similar to numerous experimental results that indicate that the postischemic, salvaged reperfused myocardium may require several days before recovering function. Cautious use of inotropes may overcome this postischemic dysfunction if needed (as may be the case in patients who have been successfully reperfused but remain in severe heart failure or borderline cardiogenic shock; see Part III). However, care must be taken to ensure that ischemia is not ongoing, as inotropic stimulation of ischemic myocardium could potentially exacerbate myocardial injury.

It is also important to note that in evaluating the return of function of the stunned myocardium, regional wall motion (rather than simply global ejection fraction) should be assessed. For example, global measurements of function during the early days postreperfusion are determined both by the stunned, hypokinetic myocardium and the compensatory hyperkinesis of the noninfarcted tissue, making detection and interpretation of stunned myocardium difficult. Another factor that confounds global measurements of left ventricular function after an acute myocardial infarction is the concomitant topographic shape changes of the left ventricle including infarct expansion and dilation and hypertrophy of the noninfarct zone (Pfeffer and Braunwald, 1990). It is now appreciated that reperfusion that is too late to salvage ischemic myocardium may nevertheless limit infarct expansion and left ventricular dilation (Hochman and Choo, 1987; Hale and Kloner, 1988). Thus, some studies that reported early improvements in global ejection fraction following reperfusion may have in fact detected an attenuation of early infarct expansion rather than improvement in function of stunned myocardium per se. Thus, when assessing stunned myocardium in patients, techniques that assess regional wall motion of the infarct-related area (such as two-dimensional echocardiography or centerline left ventricular angiography) will yield the most useful and reliable data.

REFERENCES

Anderson, J. L., Marshall, H. W., Bray, B. E., Lutz, J. R., Frederick, P. R., Yanowitz, F. G., Datz, F. L., Klausner, S. C., and Hagan, A. D. (1983). A randomized trial of intracoronary streptokinase in the treatment of acute myocardial infarction. *N. Engl. J. Med. 308*: 1313.

Armstrong, P. W., Baigrie, R. S., Daly, P. A., Haq, A., Gent, M., Roberts, R. S., Freeman, M. R., Burns, R., Liu, P., and Morgan, C. D. (1989). Tissue plasminogen activator: Toronto (TPAT) placebo-controlled randomized trial in acute myocardial infarction. *J. Am. Coll. Cardiol. 13*: 1469.

Arnold, J. M. O., Braunwald, E., Sandor, T., and Kloner, R. A. (1985). Inotropic stimulation of reperfused myocardium with dopamine: effects on infarct size and myocardial function. *J. Am. Coll. Cardiol. 6*: 1026.

Arnold, A. E., Serruys, P. W., Rutsch, W., Simoons, M. L., deBono, D. P., Tijssen, J. G., Lubsen, J., and Verstraete, M. (1991). Reasons for the lack of benefits of immediate angioplasty during recombinant tissue plasminogen activator therapy for acute myocardial infarction: A regional wall motion analysis. European Cooperactive Study Group. *J. Am. Coll. Cardiol.* 17: 11.

Bourdillon, P., Broderick, T. M., Williams, E. S., Davis, C., Dillon, J. C., Armstrong, W. F., Fineberg, N., Ryan, T., and Feigenbaum, H. (1989). Early recovery of regional left ventricular function after reperfusion in acute myocardial infarction assessed by serial two-dimensional echocardiography. *Am. J. Cardiol. 63*: 641.

Brodie, B. R., Weintraub, R. A., Stuckey, T. D., LeBauer, E. J., Katz, J. D., Kelly, T. A., and Hansen, C. J. (1991). Outcomes of direct coronary angioplasty for acute myocardial infarction in candidates and non-candidates for thrombolytic therapy. *Am. J. Cardiol. 67*: 7.

Ellis, S. G., Henschke, C. I., Sandor, T., Wynne, J. A., Braunwald, E., and Kloner, R. A. (1983). Time course of functional and biochemical recovery of myocardium salvaged by reperfusion. *J. Am. Coll. Cardiol. 1*: 1047.

Ellis, S. G., Wynne, J., Braunwald, E., Henschke, C. I., Sandor, T., and Kloner, R. A. (1984). Response of reperfusion—salvaged, stunned myocardium to inotropic stimulation. *Am. Heart J. 107*: 13.

Grines, C. L., and DeMaria, A. N. (1990). Optimal utilization of thrombolytic therapy for acute myocardial infarction: concepts and controversies. *J. Am. Coll. Cardiol. 16*: 223.

Guerci, A. D., Gerstenblith, G., Brinker, J. A., Chandra, N. C., Gottlieb, S. O., Bahr, R. D., Weiss, J. L., Shapiro, E. P., Flaherty, J. T., Bush, D. E., Chew, P. H., Gottlieb, S. H., Halperin, H. R., Ouyang, P., Walford, G. D., Bell, W. R., Fatterpaker, A. K., Llewellyn, M., Topol, E. J., Healy, B., Siu, C. O., Becker, L. C., and Weisfeldt, M. L. (1987). A randomized trial of intravenous tissue plasminogen activator for acute myocardial infarction with subsequent randomization to elective coronary angioplasty. *N. Engl. J. Med. 317*: 1613.

Hale, S. L., and Kloner, R. A. (1988). Left ventricular topographic alterations in the completely healed rat infarct caused by early and late coronary reperfusion. *Am Heart J. 116*: 1508.

Hochman, J. S., and Choo, H. (1987). Limitation of myocardial infarct expansion by reperfusion independent of myocardial salvage. *Circulation 75*: 299.

Kennedy, J. W., Ritchie, J. L., Davis, K. B., Stadius, M. L., Maynard, C., and Fritz, J. K. (1985). Western Washington randomized trial of intracoronary streptokinase in acute myocardial infarction: A 12-month follow-up report. *N. Engl. J. Med. 312*: 1985.

Kloner, R. A., Przyklenk, K., Rahimtoola, S. H., and Braunwauld, E. (1990). Myocardial stunning and hibernation: Mechanisms and clinical implications. In *Heart Disease Update* (E. Braunwald, ed.), Saunders, Philadelphia, p. 241.

Lee, L., Erbel, R., Brown, T. M., Laufer, N., Meyer, J., and O'Neill, W. W. (1991). Multicenter registry of angioplasty therapy of cardiogenic shock: Initial and long-term survival. *J. Am. Coll. Cardiol. 17*: 599.

Otto, C. M., Stratton, J. R., Maynard, C., Althouse, R., Johannessen, K. A., and Kennedy, J. W. (1990). Echocardiographic evaluation of segmental wall motion early and late after thrombolytic therapy in acute myocardial infarction: The Western Washington Tissue Plasminogen Activator Emergency Room Trial. *Am. J. Cardiol. 65*: 132.

Patel, B., and Kloner, R. A., (1987). Analysis of reported randomized trials of streptokinase therapy for acute myocardial infarction in the 1980's. *Am. J. Cardiol. 59*: 501.

Patel, B., Kloner, R. A., Przyklenk, K., and Braunwald, E. (1988). Postischemic myocardial "stunning:" A clinically relevant phenomenon. *Ann. Intern. Med. 108*: 626.

Pfeffer, M. A., and Braunwald, E. (1990). Ventricular remodeling after myocardial infarction. Experimental observations and clinical implications. *Circulation 81*: 1161.

Pfisterer, M., Zuber, M., Wenzel, R., and Burkart, F. (1991). Prolonged myocardial stunning after thrombolysis: Can left ventricular function be assessed definitely at hospital discharge? *Eur. Heart J. 12*: 214.

Reduto, L. A., Freund, G. C., Gaeta, J. M., Smalling, R. W., Lewis, B., and Gould, K. L. (1981). Coronary artery reperfusion in acute myocardial infarction: Beneficial effects of intracoronary streptokinase on left ventricular salvage and performance. *Am. Heart. J. 102*: 1168.

Satler, L. F., Kent, K. M., Fox, L. M., Goldstein, H. A., Green, C. E., Rogers, W. J., Pallas, R. S., DelNegro, A. A., Pearle, D. L., and Rackley, C. E. (1986). The assessment of contractile reserve after thrombolytic therapy for acute myocardial infarction. *Am. Heart J. 111*: 821.

Sheehan, F. H., Doerr, R., Schmidt, W. G., Bolson, E. L., Uebis, R., Von Essen, R., Effert, S., and Dodge, H. T. (1988). Early recovery of left ventricular function after thrombolytic therapy for acute myocardial infarction: An important determinant of survival. *J. Am. Coll. Cardiol. 12*: 289.

Sheehan, F. H., Thery, C., Durand, P., Bertrand, M. E., and Bolson, E. L. (1991). Early beneficial effect of streptokinase on left ventricular function in acute myocardial infarction. *Am. J. Cardiol. 69*: 555.

Stack, R. S., Phillips, H. R., Grierson, D. S., Behar, V. S., Kong, Y., Peter, R. H., Swain, J. S., and Greenfield, J. C. (1983). Functional improvement of jeopardized myocardium following intracoronary streptokinase infusion in acute myocardial infarction. *J. Clin. Invest. 72*: 84.

Touchstone, D. A., Beller, G. A., Nygaard, T. W., Tedesco, C., and Kaul, S. (1989). Effects of successful intravenous reperfusion therapy on regional myocardial function and geometry in humans: A tomographic assessment using two-dimensional echocardiography. *J. Am. Coll. Cardiol. 13*: 1506.

Voth, E., Tebbe, V., Schicha, H., Neumann, P., Schroder, R., Neuhaus, K. L., and Emrich, D. (1990). Intravenous streptokinase in acute myocardial infarction (I.S.A.M.): Assessment of left ventricular function 1 and 7 months after infarction by radionuclide ventriculography. *Eur. Heart J. 11*: 885.

Wackers, F. J., Terrin, M. L., Kayden, D. S., Knatterud, G., Furman, S., Braunwald, E., and Zaret, B. L. (1989). Quantitative radionuclide assessment of regional ventricular function after thrombolytic therapy for acute myocardial infarction: Results of phase I Thrombolysis in Myocardial Infarction (TIMI) trial. *J. Am. Coll. Cardiol. 13*: 998.

19

Stunned Myocardium in Angioplasty

Edward S. Murphy

Oregon Health Sciences University and Veterans Administration Hospital, Portland, Oregon

William Wijns

University of Louvain Medical School, Brussels, Belgium

Patrick W. Serruys

Erasmus University, Rotterdam, The Netherlands

I. INTRODUCTION

Percutaneous transluminal coronary angioplasty (PTCA) is not only an effective method of myocardial revascularization, but also a valuable tool for the investigation of ischemia induced by the transient interruption of epicardial coronary blood flow (Serruys et al., 1984, McDonald et al., 1986; Myler et al., 1990). The electrocardiographic, hemodynamic, coronary, metabolic, and ventricular effects during and following PTCA will be reviewed in this chapter, with an emphasis on the effects of PTCA on diastolic ventricular function. We will review the evidence of myocardial stunning following angioplasty, with myocardial stunning defined as the mechanical dysfunction that persists after reperfusion despite the absence of irreversible myocardial damage (Braunwald and Kloner, 1982).

Research regarding the effects of PTCA on myocardial function has largely been reported only in clinically stable patients with localized single vessel coronary disease and normal left ventricular ejection fraction. The extent of the ischemic response during PTCA will vary among patients, and with repeated occlusions in the same patient (Deutsch et al., 1990). Factors contributing to these variations include amount of myocardium at risk and degree of collateralization to the vessel dilated. Also for clinical and ethical reasons the duration of interruption of coronary blood flow has been a maximum of 90 seconds, and the number of interruptions fewer than five per patient. The impact of longer interruptions, clinical instability, compromised hemodynamic state, multivessel disease, or reduced left ventricular function are essentially unknown.

II. ELECTROCARDIOGRAPHIC EFFECTS OF BALLOON-INDUCED CORONARY OCCLUSION

Anterior electrocardiographic ST-segment elevation develops within 30 seconds in the majority of left anterior descending (LAD) angioplasties (Hauser et al., 1985; McDonald et al., 1986; Wohlgelernter et al., 1986; Berry et al., 1989), while precordial segment depression is more common than elevation during left circumflex occlusion (Berry et al., 1989). The electrocardiographic changes resolve rapidly and are back to baseline by 60 seconds (often less than 30 seconds) after balloon deflation. Persistence of ECG changes implies persistently impaired coronary blood flow.

III. EFFECTS OF PTCA ON CORONARY BLOOD FLOW

Great cardiac vein flow decreases by 30% with balloon occlusion of the LAD. With deflation, reactive hyperemia develops, with an increase in great cardiac vein flow of about 50 to 91% over baseline values. Larger increases are noted after more prolonged inflations and less residual stenosis. The duration of the hyperemic response is generally less than 1 minute (Rothman et al., 1982; Feldman et al., 1983; Serruys et al., 1984). Proximal coronary sinus blood flow changes to a lesser degree, with blood flow from nonoccluded arteries not changing significantly. Coronary sinus flow and great cardiac vein flow return to control values by 5 minutes after angioplasty (Rothman et al., 1982; Feldman et al., 1983; Serruys et al., 1984).

Intracoronary doppler blood flow velocity measurements demonstrate an increase in both resting and hyperemic velocities (Serruys et al., 1988). With serial inflations there is a major increase in resting velocity (100-200%) from the low predilatation velocities. Reactive hyperemia is maximal within 21-33 seconds after deflation and usually lasts less than 1 minute (Serruys et al., 1988).

Coronary flow reserve as measured by intracoronary doppler or radiography increases substantially in the dilated vessel but does not return to normal immediately after dilitation (O'Neill et al., 1984; Bates et al., 1985; Hodgson et al., 1987; Wilson et al., 1988; Zijlstra et al., 1988). This abnormal response is restricted to the myocardium supplied by the dilated coronary artery (Hodgson et al., 1987) and, we believe, is due to a persistent reduction in cross-sectional area of the artery, although other pathophysiological mechanisms might also contribute (Zijlstra et al., 1988). In the absence of restenosis, this abnormality is resolved by 3-5 months after PTCA (Johnson et al., 1986; Wilson et al., 1988; Zijlstra et al., 1988).

IV. METABOLIC EFFECTS OF PTCA

Studies of the metabolic effects of PTCA have been restricted to sampling coronary venous blood at the time of the PTCA. Techniques based upon magnetic resonance or using ion-sensitive indicators are not sufficiently developed. Great cardiac vein oxygen saturation transiently decreases (from a control value of 53% to 49%) and, on release of occlusion, transiently increases (to 62%) during reactive hyperemia before returning to normal (Rothman et al., 1982). Arteriovenous lactate differences have not been demonstrated to change significantly during PTCA, but the number of measurements has been small (Serruys et al., 1984). After occlusions of only 10-15 seconds duration, a brief washout of both potassium and hydrogen has been observed (Webb et al., 1987; Crake et al. 1987).

Hypoxanthine, a marker of myocardial ATP breakdown, also peaks with hyperemia after deflation of balloon occlusion (Serruys et al., 1989). Importantly, after the third or fourth serial inflation, hypoxanthine release was not significantly different from the values obtained after the first or second coronary occlusion. Coronary sinus urate, a potential marker of xanthine oxidoreductase activity and generation of superoxide and hydroxyl radicals, is transiently increased after PTCA (de Jong et al., 1990).

In recent years, an increasing number of studies have provided indirect evidence that postischemic myocardial dysfunction may be mediated in part by the generation of reactive oxygen species, such as the superoxide radical (O_2^-), hydrogen peroxide (H_2O_2), and the hydroxyl radical ($^{\bullet}OH$). Direct evidence of injury by free radicals has yet to be shown in the human heart, but many studies in experimental models have linked reactive oxygen metabolites with myocardial injury and dysfunction. The potential sources of oxygen radicals in the setting of ischemia/reperfusion and role of reactive oxygen species in postischemic dysfunction have been summarized by Bolli (1990) and are reviewed in detail in Chapter 8.

We demonstrated that repeated episodes of LAD occlusion during a PTCA procedure leads to a significant increase in great cardiac vein-arterial (VA) concentration gradients of hypoxanthine and uric acid (unpublished observation). Increased concentrations of malondialdehyde, a breakdown product resulting from the peroxidation of membrane lipids, were also detected following repeated balloon inflations (unpublished observation). While hypoxanthine A-V differences were maximal following the second or third inflation, the A-V difference in malondialdehyde showed a progressive increase, which peaked at 5 minutes after the last inflation. On average, the changes in uric acid A-V difference paralleled those of malondialdehyde, but regression analysis revealed a poor correlation between the two variables (r = 0.34 p = NS). These abnormalities were transient, however, and had been resolved by 15 minutes following completion of the procedure.

Although malondialdehyde is only one of many products of lipid peroxidation and the assay for malondialdehyde lacks specificity, this byproduct is produced in relatively constant proportion to the rate of lipid peroxidation (Aust, 1985). Thus, when all samples from one patient are assayed simultaneously, the results should reflect temporal changes in the degree of lipid peroxidation. These data are especially interesting in light of recent suggestions that the enzyme xanthine oxidase is not present in human myocardium (Muxfeldt and Schaper, 1987; Downey et al., 1988): the parallel production of both uric acid and malondialdehyde during repeated balloon inflations suggests that the xanthine oxidase pathway of oxygen radical production may in fact be important in human ischemic myocardium and may play a role in persistent regional left ventricular dysfunction following reperfusion.

In summary, metabolic disturbances induced by repeated PTCA are quickly reversible, provided the inflations are of short (<90 seconds) duration and the total occlusion time is less than 190 seconds. Additional work is needed, however, in order to fully characterize these derangements in subcellular metabolism.

V. LEFT VENTRICULAR FUNCTION DURING PTCA

Left ventricular (LV) function during and after PTCA has been studied using echocardiography, doppler, cineangiography, and hemodynamic parameters as well as epicardial markers (Das et al., 1983; Serruys et al., 1984; Jaski et al., 1985; Hauser et al., 1985; Wohlgelernter et al., 1987; Deutsch et al., 1990). Left ventricular systolic and diastolic function are markedly altered shortly after balloon occlusion. Stroke volume and ejection fraction decrease, largely due to an increase in end-systolic volume. Left ventricular end systolic pressure increases and left ventricular relaxation is delayed (Wijns et al., 1986). There is a tendency for both chamber and myocardial stiffness to increase, indicating a reduction in left ventricular compliance (Wijns et al., 1986). In addition, there is an upward shift in the diastolic pressure-volume relationship during angioplasty. The following paragraphs provide a detailed summary of the specific changes in LV function and geometry during PTCA.

A. Regional Wall Motion

Six to eight seconds after the onset of balloon inflation, wall shortening in the region of occlusion is reduced while velocity of shortening is initially maintained (Serruys et al., 1984). After 40 seconds of ischemia, despite paradoxic lengthening throughout systole and an outward displacement of the ischemic segment, early diastolic shortening still occurs. This is consistent with a markedly diminished (yet persistent) tension becoming manifest only after a decline in the load imposed upon the region by the remainder of the effectively contracting ventricle (Serruys et al., 1984; Wijns et al., 1986). The moment of maximum wall displacement for the anterior wall occurs at end diastole (Serruys et al., 1984; Hauser et al., 1985; Wohlgelernter et al., 1986). By 3 minutes after occlusion, however, regional wall motion is similar to that observed at the onset of occlusion (Serruys et al., 1984; Hauser et al., 1985; Wohlgelernter et al., 1986). Augmented wall motion can occasionally be demonstrated in the nonischemic, normally perfused region of the heart (Serruys et al., 1984).

B. Left Ventricular Filling and Geometry

Five to six seconds after LAD occlusion, left ventricular geometry and filling begin to change. The duration of isovolumetric relaxation lengthens, and, at 12 seconds, the negative dP/dt becomes notched on its ascending limb, which coincides with asynchrony of the anteroseptal wall (Serruys et al., 1984). The LV diastolic pressure curve changes, and the lowest diastolic point moves to the middle of diastole. Rapid filling is reduced by the diastolic late relaxation and rigidity of the anteroseptal wall (Serruys et al., 1984). In addition, when LV rapid filling does occur, the anteroseptal wall is still contracting, thus further impeding normal filling.

After 25-30 seconds of occlusion, the pattern of LV filling deteriorates even more. The anteroseptal wall becomes stiff, the LV end-diastole volume tends to increase slightly (by 6%), the LV pressure-volume curve is shifted upward and to the right, and LV filling pressure increases. The end-systolic volume increases markedly (by 100%), resulting in a reduced ejection fraction. With this impairment of rapid LV filling, the contribution of atrial contraction to terminal filling increases from 26 to 57% (Serruys et al., 1984).

C. Diastolic Relaxation

Within 10 seconds of occlusion, a deformation appears in the ascending limb of the negative dP/dt curve. During the next 10 seconds, this deformation gradually increases such that the irregularity in the negative dP/dt curve reaches the same height as peak negative dP/dt, which has progressively decreased to its nadir. In the next 20-50 seconds, peak negative dP/dt begins to return toward control levels with a resolution of the irregularity in the ascending limb (Serruys et al., 1984; Wijns et al., 1986). At 50 seconds of occlusion, peak negative dP/dt is back to 77% of the preocclusion value, and the deformity is no longer present (Serruys et al., 1984; Wijns et al., 1986). This transient deformation in dP/dt indicates that the time course of LV pressure decay deviates substantially from the monoexponential model, and that asynchronous contraction or relaxation may be involved at the very beginning of the occlusion.

The time constants of LV relaxation Tau 1 (during the first 40 msec of relaxation) and Tau 2 (after 40 msec) both rapidly increase and are maximally prolonged at 20-25 seconds after balloon inflation. This prolongation of the time constants of diastolic relaxation is the earliest hemodynamic marker of ischemia, but both Tau 1 and Tau 2 return to control values after 40-50 seconds of occlusion. In parallel to the prolongation of Tau 1 and Tau 2, the isovolumic relaxation period is increased at 20 seconds but not following 50 seconds of occlusion. The mean rate of volume inflow from the mitral opening to minimal diastolic pressure also declines significantly. Although the LV volumes at lowest diastolic pressure and at end diastole do not change significantly during and after angioplasty, the lowest diastolic and end-diastolic *pressures* are increased after 50 seconds of LAD occlusion (Serruys et al., 1984; Wijns et al., 1986; Grbic and Sigwart, 1990). This increase in pressure relative to volume during PTCA results in an upward shift of the entire pressure-volume relationship (Wijns et al., 1986).

VI. POSTISCHEMIC DIASTOLIC ABNORMALITIES: CLINICAL EXPERIENCE

To further characterize the changes in diastolic function induced by coronary occlusion in conscious humans, we sought to determine (1) whether an upward shift in the diastolic pressure-volume relation in fact occurred during PTCA and (2) whether this increase in chamber stiffness, if any, was reversible and could be ascribed to an increased regional stiffness of the ischemic zone. Details concerning our clinical study have been published previously (Wijns et al., 1986) and are summarized below.

A. Protocol and Methods

Our study consisted of nine patients with normal LV function and wall motion at rest who underwent PTCA of a proximal and isolated left anterior descending coronary stenosis. We obtained simultaneous left ventricular pressure and volume measurements by contrast ventriculography before the angioplasty procedure was started ($n = 9$), after a median occlusion of 20 seconds during the second dilation ($n = 9$), after a median occlusion of 48 seconds during the fourth dilation ($n = 5$), and after a median time of 12 minutes after the end of the angioplasty procedure ($n = 9$).

A total of 3-10 occlusions were performed; the duration of each balloon inflation ranged from 15 to 75 seconds. No investigational occlusions were carried out after completion of a technically successful dilation. In four patients, this result was achieved after three dilations, so that angiographic data after 48 seconds (fourth occlusion) are available only in five of nine patients. These sequential angiograms were made only after the return to baseline of the end-diastolic pressure and of the left ventricular pressure-derived isovolumic variables of contractility and relaxation.

Frame-by-frame LV volumes and the corresponding pressures were simultaneously obtained from the complete cardiac cycle as previously described (Meester et al., 1975). The LV pressure decay during the isovolumic relaxation was quantified using a biexponential model (Serruys et al., 1984), where Tau represents the time constant of early relaxation (during the first 40 msec after peak negative dP/dt. To detect the ventricular contours and analyze the segmental wall motion, the previously described "endocardial landmark model" (Slager et al., 1984) was used. The length of the 20 segmental radii defined by our previously described model was measured frame by frame, and, among them, we selected for analysis 6 radii located in the core of the ischemic segment (anterior, anterolateral, and apical radii) or in the nonischemic segment (anterobasal and posterobasal radii), as well as the inferior radius immediately adjacent to the ischemic segment (Fig. 1).

For evaluation of global chamber stiffness, the LV pressure (P) and volume (V) data obtained every 20 msec starting at the lowest diastolic pressure and ending at the end-diastolic pressure were fitted by a simple elastic model: $P = a\,e^{BV} + C$, where a = intercept (mmHg), B = constant of elastic chamber stiffness, C = baseline pressure (mmHg), and e is the base of the natural logarithm. The three constants of this equation (A, B, and C) were determined using an iteration procedure until the best nonlinear curve fit was obtained (Hess et al., 1979). For the evaluation of regional chamber stiffness, the LV pressure and the segment radius length (L) data were fitted in a similar way for each of the six analyzed segmental radii to the relationship: $P = a_n e^{B_n L} + C_n$, where B_n represents the regional elastic stiffness constant for a given radius (Theroux et al., 1974; Hess et al., 1979). Further specific details concerning our methods of data acquisition and analysis can be found in our original published manuscript (Wijns, 1986).

B. Global Pressure-Volume Relations

The left ventricular volume at the lowest diastolic pressure as well as at end diastole did not change significantly during and after angioplasty, whereas

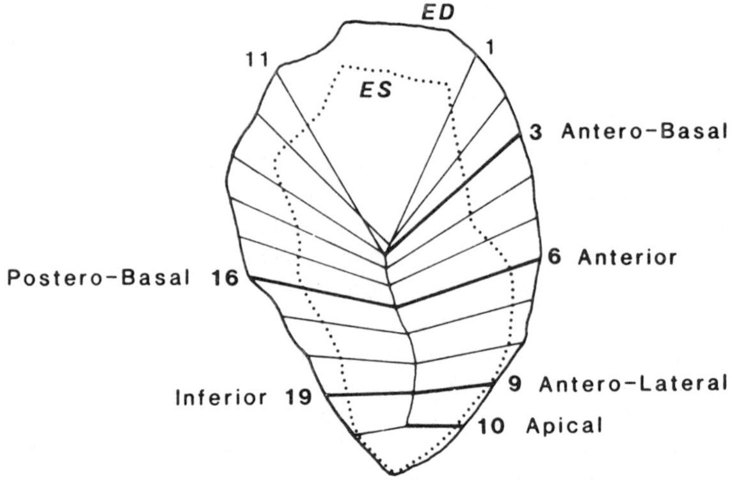

Figure 1 The end-diastolic (ED) and end-systolic (ES) contours of a left ventriculogram during transluminal occlusion are displayed with the system of 20 radii along which regional wall displacement was determined. For the analysis of regional diastolic function, we selected radii, 6, 9, and 10 within the ischemic zone, radii 3 and 16 within the nonischemic zone, as well as radius 19 in the adjacent inferior zone. (Reprinted from Wijns et al., 1986, with permission of the American College of Cardiology.)

the end-systolic volume and Tau had increased markedly after 20 seconds of occlusion. The lowest diastolic and the end-diastolic pressures were increased in the subgroup of patients studied after 50 seconds of occlusion. After completion of the procedure, all the hemodynamic variables returned toward control values. The increase in pressure relative to volume during transluminal occlusion resulted in an upward shift of the entire pressure-volume relation, as shown in Figure 2 for two representative patients. In only two instances did we observe a shift downward and to the right of the pressure-volume relation. The calculated variables of global chamber stiffness showed a similarly increased constant of elastic stiffness (B) after 20 seconds as well as after 50 seconds of occlusion.

The baseline pressure (C) increased significantly only after 50 seconds of coronary occlusion. No change in the intercept (a) was observed. All patients except one showed an increase in chamber stiffness during coronary occlusion, which, after the procedure, returned to values not significantly different from the preangioplasty value. However, the postangioplasty elastic constant remained higher than the control value in five instances. This is further illustrated in Figure 2: the pressure-volume relation obtained after the

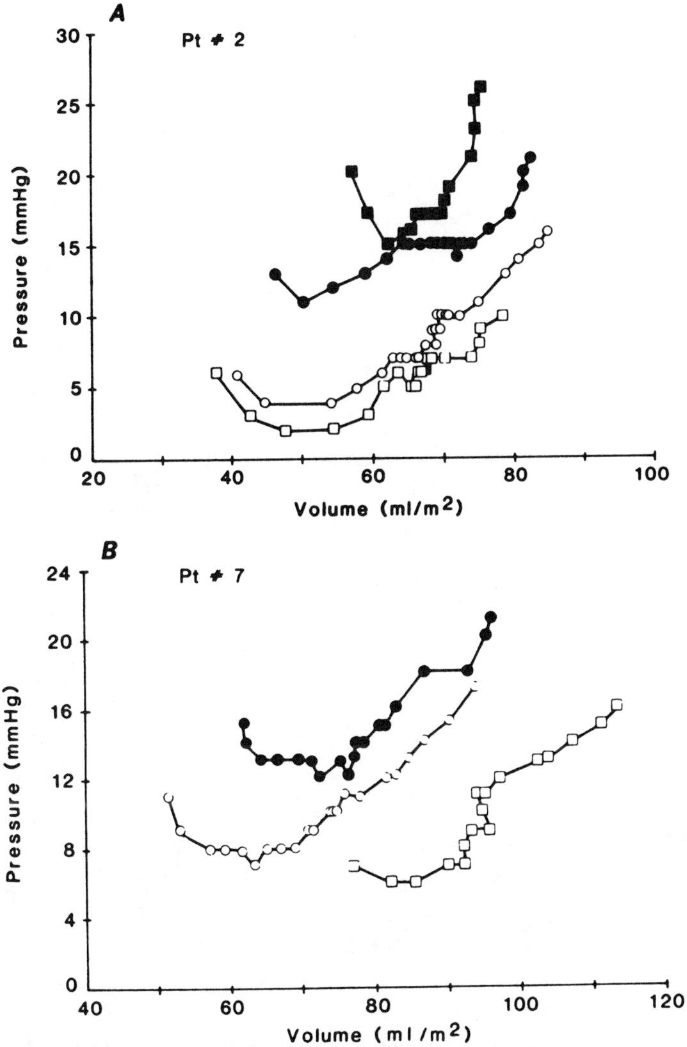

Figure 2 Diastolic pressure-volume relation in two representative patients. Note the upward shift of the relation during coronary occlusion. (A) In patient 2, the post-angioplasty relation returned toward control, whereas it remained shifted upward in patient 7. (B) Open squares = preangioplasty; closed circles = 20-sec occlusion; closed squares = 50-sec occlusion; open circles = postangioplasty. (Reprinted from Wijns et al., 1986, with permission of the American College of Cardiology.)

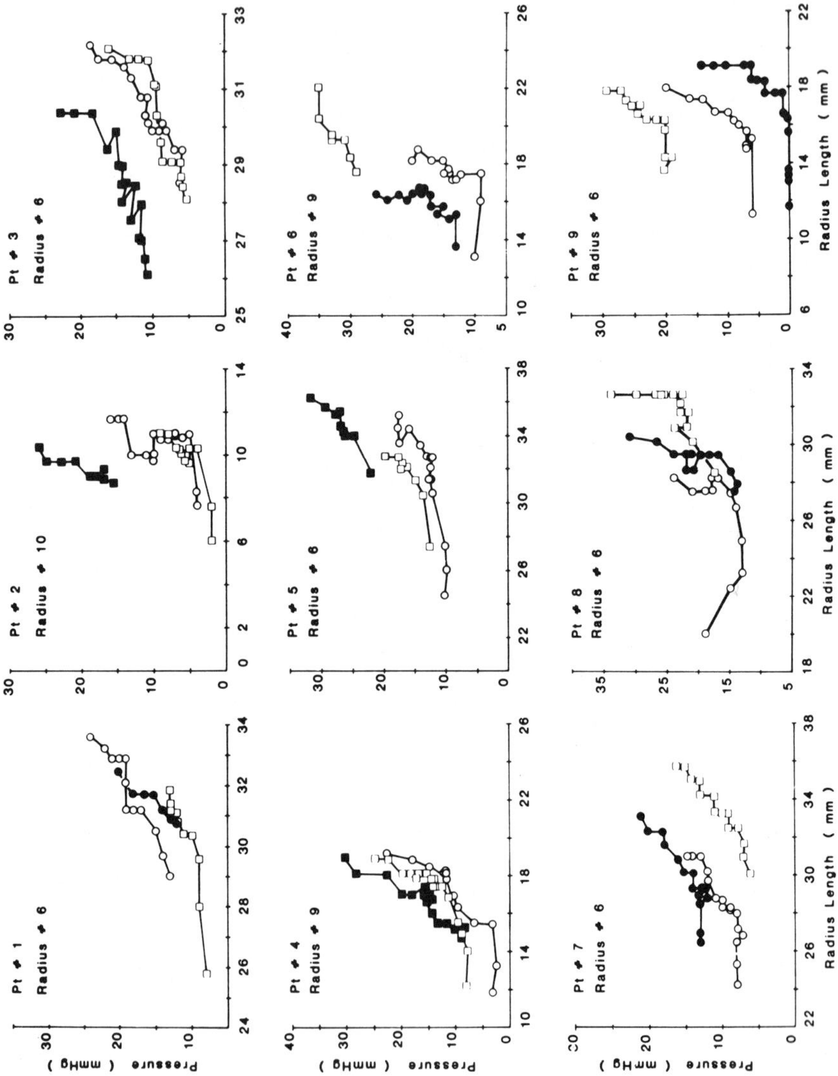
Pt # 1
Radius # 6
Pt # 2
Radius # 10
Pt # 3
Radius # 6
Pt # 4
Radius # 9
Pt # 5
Radius # 6
Pt # 6
Radius # 9
Pt # 7
Radius # 6
Pt # 8
Radius # 6
Pt # 9
Radius # 6
Pressure (mmHg)
Radius Length (mm)

procedure is nearly superimposed on the control curve in patient 2 (Figure 2A), whereas the postangioplasty curve remains shifted upward in patient 7 (Figure 2B).

C. Regional Pressure-Radius Length Relations

There was no significant difference during the procedure in the length at end diastole of the various segmental radii. Plots of the left ventricular pressure against a representative radius within the ischemic segment are shown in Figure 3. During occlusion, the slope of the pressure-radius length relation increased; this was often accompanied by an upward shift. The postangioplasty curves either showed a return toward the control relation or remained parallel to the curves during occlusion. The latter instance was mainly observed in patients 4, 6, 7, and 9, all of whom exhibited a persistent increase in chamber stiffness after the procedure.

These relations were fitted with the same elastic model used for calculation of the global chamber stiffness. The changes in the constant of regional chamber stiffness (B_n) showed a marked and persistent increased stiffness in the ischemic segment as well as in the adjacent inferior segment (radius 19). The regional stiffness in the nonischemic segments was not significantly affected by the coronary occlusions. There were also no significant changes in the nonlinear elastic constant (a_n). Similar shifts in the baseline pressure (C) and global diastolic function were observed because the same left ventricular pressure data were used for calculations of both global and regional chamber stiffness.

D. Interpretation and Significance of Diastolic Dysfunction Post-PTCA

There is general agreement that the global and regional systolic performance fully recovers within 100 seconds after balloon deflations. Studies performed 10-15 minutes after the end of the entire procedure involving repeated occlusions and multiple intracoronary contrast injections have shown return of

Figure 3 Plots of left ventricular pressure versus radius length in the ischemic zone in the nine patients. During occlusion the slope of this relationship increased as compared with slope before angioplasty. The increased slope was mostly accompanied by an upward shift. The postangioplasty curves either showed a return toward the control relation or remained parallel to the curves observed during occlusion (cases 4, 6, 7, and 9). Symbols as in Figure 2. Radius number refers to specific radius in Figure 1. (Reprinted from Wijns et al., 1986, with permission of the American College of Cardiology.)

all measured variables to control values (including relaxation parameters) (Serruys et al., 1984; Carlson et al., 1987).

While systolic function is restored immediately after PTCA, our data (Wijns et al., 1986) and those of Carlson and co-workers (1987) suggest that recovery of normal diastolic function is delayed. For example, Carlson et al. (1987) found that, after 60 seconds of reperfusion, the pressure-volume relationship remained abnormal despite normalization of systolic function within 20 seconds of reperfusion. Our data obtained on average 12 minutes after completion of PTCA revealed that, in half of the patients, there were persistent regional postischemic abnormalities while complete recovery of systolic function and relaxation parameters had already occurred.

Sustained abnormalities in diastolic filling also have been reported by other investigators after PTCA. For example, Wind et al. (1987) studied diastolic filling by pulsed doppler echocardiography at 24 hours after successful angioplasty and found no improvement. Similar findings were reported by Lewis and colleagues (1985) with radionuclide angiography performed 2-5 days after PTCA. They also observed that peak filling rate was unchanged at rest but improved during exercise (supporting a postischemic rather than ischemic effect) (Lewis et al., 1985).

Thus, although postischemic left ventricular dysfunction (or stunning) is usually thought of as a systolic phenomenon, these clinical data demonstrated delayed recovery of diastolic function following PTCA. These results are similar to experimental data obtained in dogs after a single 15-minute left anterior descending coronary artery occlusion, which indicated that not only systolic, but also diastolic derangements persisted for hours after reperfusion (Piscione et al., 1987). A time course study comparing systolic thickening and the rate of diastolic thinning in the postischemic area showed, however, that the recovery towards baseline of both systolic and diastolic parameters was parallel in the canine model (Charlat et al., 1989).

The major finding of our clinical study (Wijns et al., 1986) was that ischemia induced by complete occlusion of the left anterior descending coronary artery increased the regional chamber stiffness of the ischemic anterior wall, even during an occlusion as short as 20 seconds. Parallel to that increase in regional stiffness, the global stiffness of the left ventricle increased significantly. In experimental studies (Hess et al., 1979, 1980, 1983; Paulus et al., 1985), an increase in global chamber stiffness was seen only when the area rendered ischemic was large, such as during acute occlusion of the left anterior descending coronary artery.

Twelve minutes after the end of the procedure, the variables of global and regional systolic function were back to normal, as shown by the indices of isovolumic contraction, relaxation, and segment wall motion (Serruys et al., 1984). In contrast, the variables of regional diastolic function were still abnormal, and the constant of global chamber stiffness and the baseline pressure remained slightly elevated. This suggests the persistence of postischemic diastolic abnormalities, while complete recovery of systolic function and relaxation had already occurred.

1. Significance of the Upward Shift in Pressure-Volume and Pressure-Radius Relations

As indicated in our original publication (Wijns et al., 1986), the significance of the upward shift in the pressure-volume and/or pressure-radius length relation is still the subject of controversy. In previous studies, this shift was attributed to any or all of the following factors: changes in intrinsic diastolic myocardial stiffness, delayed left ventricular relaxation, loss of elastic recoil due to ventricular asynergy, changes in right ventricular loading conditions, effects of the pericardium, and coronary perfusion (Shirato et al., 1978; Hess et al., 1979, 1980, 1983; Sasyama et al., 1985; Grossman et al., 1980; Serizawa et al., 1980; Bourdillon et al., 1983; Paulus et al., 1985). A limitation of current study is that these specific issues are not addressed. For instance, fitting of the pressure volume relation by a simple elastic model does not allow one to infer that the intrinsic diastolic properties of the myocardium were affected by acute coronary occlusion, as this would require analysis of left ventricular stress and strain (Glantz and Parmley, 1978). For this purpose, regional wall thickness measurements are needed, which cannot be obtained accurately at 20-msec intervals from the left ventricular angiograms. Also, the strain data should be normalized for a reference unloaded muscle length (i.e., at a transmural pressure of 0 mmHg), which cannot be obtained easily during cardiac catheterization in humans. As far as extrinsic factors are concerned, we believe that coronary perfusion, or the so-called erectile effect, is not likely to account for the increased stiffness in the core of the ischemic segment. During occlusion of the left anterior descending coronary artery, inflation of the dilation balloon results, on average, in a 44% decrease in regional blood flow (Serruys et al., 1983), thereby decreasing the myocardial wall blood volume. Similarly, the postangioplasty measurements were obtained at a time when any increased myocardial turgor due to reactive hyperemia had worn off (Serruys et al., 1983). Interestingly, the increase in regional stiffness observed in the adjacent inferior segment could be related to an increased turgor, as the collateral flow to that area might increase during left anterior descending artery occlusion (Wahr et al., 1985).

2. Comparison with Animal Models of Acute Low-Flow Ischemia

Coronary angioplasty mimics experimental coronary occlusion in the animal laboratory and induces transient acute low-flow ischemia. In their animal model, Hess et al. (1983) showed that "myocardial wall stiffness is increased during complete coronary occlusion when there is systolic thinning of the ischemic wall." In their conscious chronically instrumented dogs, the ischemic alteration in the intrinsic diastolic properties of the muscle resulted in an upward shift of the pressure volume control curve. Hess et al. (1983) observed an average 27% increase in diastolic wall stiffness, which compares well with the 35% increase in global chamber stiffness after 50 seconds of left anterior descending coronary artery occlusion in our data (Wijns et al., 1986). It is worth mentioning that in the animal study, the upward shift of the pressure volume curve was prevented by inferior vena cava obstruction. This emphasizes the modulating role of right ventricular loading conditions and the ventricular interaction, which can offset the increase in pressure. Thus, the observed changes in global and regional diastolic chamber stiffness are in accordance with previous experimental studies (Theroux et al., 1974; Hess et al., 1980, 1983) demonstrating an increase in myocardial stiffness during coronary occlusion.

3. Mechanism of Increased Myocardial Stiffness

As discussed in our original publication (Wijns et al., 1986), the mechanism by which ischemia causes myocardial stiffness remains speculative and may depend on the pathophysiology (Paulus et al., 1985) and the duration (Jaski et al., 1985) of a given ischemic condition. In the acute coronary occlusion model (Hess et al., 1980, 1983), systolic overstretch of the akinetic muscle fibers by adjacent nonischemic myocardium was thought to be responsible for the diastolic thinning of the ischemic wall and the increase in muscle length at rest. This "creep" effect causes the ischemic myocardium to operate at a higher point on the pressure-sarcomere length relation and therefore at an increased stiffness level. Although we observed no significant changes in end-diastolic volume throughout the procedure, it cannot be excluded that creep actually occurred. Echocardiographic evidence of wall thinning during angioplasty and during attacks of variant angina supports this hypothesis (Das et al., 1983; Distante et al., 1984).

The other major mechanism refers to the concept of residual diastolic actinmyosin interaction (Nayler and Williams, 1978). An increase in cytosolic ionic calcium and a decrease in adenosine triphosphate available for cross-bridge dissociation could result in the presence of an abnormal myocardial "tone." This mechanism is unlikely after prolonged occlusion because the ischemic segment becomes akinetic or dyskinetic, and systolic cross-bridge formation is probably minimal or absent. However, after 20 seconds of occlusion, we observed asynchrony and late shortening of the ischemic wall (Serruys et al., 1984; Jaski et al., 1985), which have been shown to affect the stiffness of rat heart trabeculae (Wiegner et al., 1978). Also, the persistent abnormalities in diastolic function observed after the procedure could be related to an abnormal myocardial tone despite normalization of the rate of relaxation. As was reported by Sasyama et al. (1985) and Paulus et al. (1985), such failure of complete myofilament inactivation implies a decreased extent of relaxation that is not necessarily synonymous with a decreased rate of relaxation as measured from the time constant of isovolumic left ventricular pressure decay.

Finally, it should be realized that the increase in calculated stiffness constant could also be related to an increased resistance to early filling. It has been shown in humans (Carroll et al., 1983) that early diastolic filling can be kept normal during ischemia despite delayed relaxation and loss of elastic recoil (increase in end-systolic volume) by increasing the left atrial driving pressure. Under these conditions, the diastolic properties of the myocardium would be better characterized by a viscoelastic model rather than by a simple elastic stress-strain relation (Rankin et al., 1977; Pouleur et al., 1979). We used a simple elastic model because the present angiocardiographic data did not allow proper quantitation of the strain rates, which are essential for determining diastolic viscous effects. Therefore, our calculated stiffness constant includes both elastic and viscous forces.

VII. SUMMARY

Repeated occlusions of the left anterior descending coronary artery in conscious humans are associated with profound alterations in diastolic chamber stiffness that persist well after restoration of myocardial blood flow and normal systolic function. Further study is needed to document the time course of the recovery to a normal regional diastolic function and to elucidate the derangement of subcellar metabolism responsible for these abnormalities. Additional studies, including continuous measurement of both functional and metabolic parameters (rather than "snapshot" observations), and acquisition of data in patients with more complex coronary artery disease, would provide a better understanding of postischemic diastolic dysfunction. We therefore recommend that the term "diastolic stunning" (Patel et al., 1988) be used with caution until this phenomenon is further clarified.

From the clinical point of view, many factors have contributed to increase the extent and severity of ischemia during angioplasty: longer balloon inflation time, dilation of multiple lesions during a single setting, and inclusion of patients with unstable angina or impaired left ventricular function. This has prompted studies attempting to modify ischemic changes induced by balloon inflation by various means of intervention (Serruys et al., 1984; Jaski et al., 1985). Data presented in this chapter suggest that the analysis of diastolic function may prove to be a sensitive tool in assessing the possibly deleterious effects of repeated coronary occlusion during angioplasty and could be a useful end point in evaluating the efficacy of cardioprotective interventions. Furthermore, analysis of diastolic function during PTCA may provide additional insight into myocardial stunning.

REFERENCES

Aust, S. D. (1985). Lipid perioxidation. In *CRC Handbook of Methods for Oxygen Radical Research* (R. A. Greenwald, ed.), CRC Press, London, p. 203.

Bates, E. R., Aueron, F. M., Legrand, V., LeFree, M. T., Mancini, G. B. J., Hodgson, J. M., and Vogel, R. A. (1985). Comparative long-term effects of coronary artery bypass graft surgery and percutaneous transluminal coronary angioplasty on regional flow reserve. *Circulation 72*: 833.

Berry, C., Zalweski, A., Kovach, R., Savage, M., and Goldberg, S. (1989). Surface electrocardiogram in the detection of transmural myocardial ischemia during coronary artery occlusion. *Am. J. Cardiol. 63*: 21.

Bolli, R. (1990). Mechanism of myocardial stunning. *Circulation 82*: 723.

Bourdillion, P. D., Lorell, B. H., Mirsky, I., Paulus, W. J., Wynne, J., and Grossman, W. (1983). Increased regional myocardial stiffness of the left ventricle during pacing-induced angina in man. *Circulation 67*: 316.

Braunwald, E., and Kloner, R. A. (1982). The stunned myocardium: Prolonged postischemic ventricular dysfunction. *Circulation 66*: 1146.

Carlson, E. B., Hinohara, T., and Morris, K. (1987). Recovery of systolic and diastolic left ventricular function after a 60-second coronary arterial occlusion during percutaneous transluminal coronary angioplasty for angina pectoris. *Am. J. Cardiol. 60*: 460.

Carroll, J. D., Hess, O. M., Hirzel, H. O., and Krayenbueh, H. P. (1983). Dynamics of left ventricular filling at rest and during exercise. *Circulation 68*: 59.

Charlat, M. L., O'Neill, P. G., Hartley, C. J., Roberts, R., and Bolli, R. (1989). Prolonged abnormalities of left ventricular diastolic wall thinning in the stunned myocardium in conscious dogs: time course and relation to systolic function. *J. Am. Coll. Cardiol. 13*: 185.

Crake, T., Cream, P. A., Shapiro, L. M., Rickards, A. F., and Poole-Wilson, P. A. (1987). Coronary sinus pH during percutaneous transluminal coronary angioplasty: early development of acidosis during myocardial ischemia in man. *Br. Heart J. 58*: 110.

Das, S. K., Serruys, P. W., van den Brand, J., Domenicucci, S., Vletter, W. B., and Roelandt, J. (1983). Acute echocardiographic changes during percutaneous coronary angioplasty and their relationship to coronary blood flow. *J. Cardiovasc. Ultrasound 2*: 269.

de Jong, J. W., Huizer, T., Nelson, J. A., Czarneckt, W., Bonnier, J., and Serruys, P. W. (1990). Myocardial release of hypoxanthine and urate during angioplasty. *PTCA An Investigational Tool and Non Operative Treatment of Acute Ischemia* (P. W. Serruys, R. Simon, and K. J. Beatt, eds.), Kluwer Academic Publishers, Boston, p. 143.

Deutsch, E., Berger, M., Kussmaul, W. G., Hirschfeld, J. W., Hermann, H. C., and Laskey, W. K. (1990). Adaption to ischemia during percutaneous transluminal angioplasty. *Circulation 82*: 2044.

Distante, A., Roval, D., and Picano, E. (1984). Transient changes in the left ventricular mechanics during attacks of Prinzmetal's angina. *Am. Heart J. 107*: 465.

Downey, J. M., Hearse, D. J., and Yellow, D. M. (1988). The role of xanthine oxidase during myocardial ischemia in several species including man. *J. Mol. Cell. Cardiol. 20 (Suppl II)*: 55.

Feldman, R. L., Conti, C. R., and Pepine, C. J. (1983). Regional coronary venous flow responses to transient coronary artery occlusion in human beings. *J. Am. Coll. Cardiol. 2*: 1.

Glantz, S. A., and Parmley, W. W. (1978). Factors which effect the diastolic pressure-volume curve. *Circ. Res. 42*: 171.

Grbic, M., and Sigwart, U. (1990). Left ventricular filling during ischemia. In *PTCA: An Investigational tool and Non Operative Treatment of Acute Ischemia* (P. W. Serruys, R. Simon, and K. J. Beatt, eds.), Kluwer Academic Publishers, Boston, p. 167.

Grossman, W., Serizawa, T., and Carabello, B. A. (1980). Studies on the mechanism of altered left ventricular diastolic pressure-volume relations during ischemia. *Eur. Heart J. (Suppl A)*: 141.

Hauser, A. M., Gangadharan, V., Ramos, R. G., Gordon, S., Timmis, G. C., and Dudleto, P. (1985). Sequence of mechanical electrocardiographic and clinical effects of repeated coronary artery occlusion in human beings: echocardiographic observations during coronary angioplasty. *J. Am. Coll. Cardiol. 5*: 193.

Hess, O. M., Grimm, J., and Krayenbuehl, H. P. (1979). Diastolic simple elastic and viscoelastic properties of the left ventricle in man. *Circulation 59*: 1178.

Hess, O. M., Koch, R., Bamert, C., and Krayenbuehl, H. P. (1980). Regional wall stiffness during acute myocardial ischemia in the canine left ventricle. *Eur. Heart J. 1*: 435.

Hess, O. M., Osakada, G., Lavelle, J. F., Gallagher, K. P., Kemper, W. S., and Ross, J., Jr. (1983). Diastolic myocardial wall stiffness and ventricular relaxation during partial and complete coronary occlusion in the conscious dog. *Circ. Res. 52*: 387.

Hodgson, J. M., Riley, R., Most, A. S., and Williams, D. O. (1987). Assessment of coronary flow reserve using digital angiography before and after successful percutaneous transluminal coronary angioplasty. *Am. J. Cardiol. 60*: 61.

Jaski, B. E., Serruys, P. W., ten Katen, H., and Meij, S. (1985). Epicardial wall motion and left ventricular function during coronary graft angioplasty in humans. *J. Am. Coll. Cardiol. 6*: 695.

Johnson, M. R., Brayden, G. P., Ericksen, E. E., Collins, S. M., Skorton, D. J., Harrison, D. G., Marcus, M. L., and White, C. W. (1986). Changes in cross-sectional area of the coronary lumen in the six months after angioplasty: a quantitative analysis of the variable response to percutaneous transluminal angioplasty. *Circulation 73*: 467.

Lewis, J. F., Verani, M. S., Poliner, L. R., Lewis, J. M., and Raizner, A. E. (1985). Effects of transluminal coronary angioplasty on left ventricular systolic and diastolic function at rest and during exercise. *Am. Heart J. 109*: 792.

McDonald, R. G., Hill, J. A., and Feldman, R. L. (1986). ST segment response to acute coronary occlusion: coronary hemodynamic and angiographic determinants of direction of ST segment shift. *Circulation 74*: 973.

Meester, G. T., Bernard, N., Zeelenberg, G., Brower, R. W., and Hugenholtz, P. G. (1975). A computer system for real time analysis of cardiac catheterization data. *Cathet. Cardiovasc. Diagn. 1*: 112.

Muxfeldt, M., and Schaper, W. (1987). The activity of xanthine oxidase in heart of pigs, guinea pigs, rabbits, rats and humans. *Basic Res. Cardiol. 82*: 486.

Myler, R. K., Stretzer, S. H., Cumberland, D. C., Webb, J. G., and Shaw, R. T. (1990). Coronary angioplasty: Indications contraindications, and limitations. *J. Intervent. Cardiol. 2*: 179.

Nayler, W. G., and Williams, A. (1978). Relaxation in heart muscle: some morphological and biochemical considerations. *Eur. J. Cardiol. 7 (Suppl)*: 35.

O'Neill, W. W., Walton, J. A., Bates, E. R., Colter, H. T., Aueron, F. M., LeFree, M. T., Pitt, B., and Vogel, R. A. (1984). Criteria for successful coronary vasodilatory reserve. *J. Am. Coll. Cardiol. 3*: 1382.

Patel, B., Kloner, R. A., Przyklenk, K., and Braunwald, E. (1988). Postischemic myocardial "stunning": A clinical relevant phenomenon. *Ann. Int. Med. 108*: 626.

Paulus, W. J., Grossman, W., Serizawa, T., Bourdillon, P. D., Pasipoularides, A., and Mirsky, I. (1985). Different effects of two types of ischemia on myocardial systolic and diastolic functions. *Am. J. Physiol. 248*: H719.

Piscione, F., Hugenholtz, P. G., and Serruys, P. W. (1987). Impaired left ventricular filling dynamics during percutaneous transluminal angioplasty for coronary artery disease. *Am. J. Cardiol. 59*: 29.

Pouleur, H., Karliner, J. S., LeWinter, M. M., and Covell, J. W. (1979). Diastolic viscous properties of the intact canine left ventricle. *Circ. Res. 45*: 410.

Rankin, J. S., Arntzen, C. F., McHale, P. A., Ling, D., and Anderson R. W. (1972). Viscoelastic properties of the diastolic left ventricle in the conscious dog. *Circ. Res. 41*: 37.

Rothman, M. T., Balm, D. S., Simpson, J. B., and Harrison, D. C. (1982). Coronary hemodynamics during percutaneous transluminal coronary angioplasty. *Am. J. Cardiol. 49*: 1615.

Sasyama, S., Nonogi, H., and Migazaki, S. (1985). Changes in diastolic properties of the regional myocardium during pacing-induced ischemia in human subjects. *J. Am. Coll. Cardiol. 5*: 599.

Serizawa, T., Carabello, B. A., and Grossman, W. (1980). Effect of pacing-induced ischemia on left ventricular diastolic pressure-volume relations in dogs with coronary stenoses. *Circ. Res. 46*: 430.

Serruys, P. W., van den Brand, M., Brower, R. W., and Hugenholtz, P. G. (1983). Regional cardioplegia and cardioprotection during transluminal angioplasty: Which role for nifedipine? *Eur. Heat J. 4 (Suppl C)*: 115.

Serruys, P. W., Wijns, W., van den Brand, M., Meij, S., Slager, C., Schuurbiers, J. C. H., Hugenholtz, P. G., and Brower, R. W. (1984). Left ventricular performance, regional blood flow, wall motion, and lactate metabolism during transluminal angioplasty. *Circulation 70*: 25.

Serruys, P. W., Julliere, Y., Zijlstra, F., Beatt, K. J., de Feyter, P. J., Suryapranata, H., van den Brand, M., and Roelandt, J. (1988). Coronary blood flow velocity during percutaneous transluminal coronary angioplasty as a guide for assessment of the functional result. *Am. J. Cardiol. 61*: 253.

Serruys, P. W., Suryapranata, H., Piscione, F., Harmsen, E., van den Brand, M., de Feyter, P., Hugenholtz, P., and de Jong, J. W. (1989). Myocardial release of hypoxanthine and lactate during percutaneous transluminal coronary angioplasty. *Am. J. Cardiol. 63*: 45E.

Shirato, K., Shabetai, R., Bhargava, V., Franklin, D., and Ross, J., Jr. (1978). Alteration of the left ventricular diastolic pressure segment-length relation produced by the pericardium: Effects of cardiac distension and afterload reduction in conscious dogs. *Circulation 57*: 1191.

Slager, C. J., Hooghouldt, T. E. H., Reiber, J. H. C., Booman, F., and Meester, G. T. (1980). Left ventricular contour segmentation from anatomical landmark trajectories and its application to wall motion analysis. Computer in Cardiology, IEEE Computer Society, Los Angeles, California, pp. 347-350.

Slager, C. J., Hooghoudt, T. E. H., Reiber, J. H. C., Schuurbiers, J. C. H., Verdouw, P. D., and Hugenholtz, P. G. (1984). Left ventricular wall motion as derived from endocardially implanted radiopaque markers and from contrast angiograms. In *Ventricular Wall Motion* (U. Sigwart and P. H. Heitzen, eds.), Thieme-Stratton, New York, p. 149.

Theroux, P., Franklin, D., Ross, J., Jr., and Kemper, W. S. (1974). Regional myocardial function during acute coronary artery occlusions and its modification by pharmacologic agents in the dog. *Circ. Res. 35*: 896.

Wahr, D. W., Ports, J. A., and Botvinick, E. H. (1985). The effects of coronary angioplasty and reperfusion on distribution of myocardial flow. *Circulation 72*: 334.

Webb, S. C., Canepa-Anson, R., Rickards, A. F., and Poole-Wilson, P. (1987). Myocardial potassium loss after acute coronary occlusion in humans. *J. Am. Coll. Cardiol. 9*: 1230.

Wiegner, A. W., Allen, G. J., and Bing, O. H. L. (1978). Weak and strong myocardium in series: implications for segmental dysfunction, *Am. J. Physiol. 235*: H776.

Wijns, W., Serruys, P. W., Slager, C. J., Grimm, J., Krayenbuehl, H., Hugenhotz, P. G., and Hess, O. (1986). Effect of coronary occlusion during percutaneous transluminal angioplasty in humans on left ventricular chamber stiffness and regional diastolic pressure-radius relations. *J. Am. Coll. Cardiol. 7*: 455.

Wilson, R. F., Johnson, M. R., Marcus, M. L., Aylward, P. E. G., Skorton, D. J., Collins, S., and White, C. W. (1988). The effect of coronary angioplasty on coronary flow reserve. *Circulation 77*: 873.

Wind, B. E., Snider, R., Buda, A. J., O'Neill, W. W., Topol, E. J., and Dilworth, L. R. (1987). Pulsed doppler assessment of left ventricular diastolic filling in coronary artery disease before and immediately after coronary angioplasty. *Am. J. Cardiol. 59*: 1041.

Wohlgelernter, D., Cleman, M., Highman, H. A., Fetterman, R. C., Duncan, J. S., Zaret, B. L., and Jaffee, C. C. (1986). Regional myocardial dysfunction during angioplasty: Evaluation by two dimensional echocardiography and 12 lead electrocardiography. *J. Am. Coll. Cardiol. 7*: 1245.

Zijlstra, F., Reiber, J. H. V., Juilliere, Y., and Serruys, P. W. (1988). Normalization of coronary flow reserve by percutaneous transluminal coronary angioplasty. *Am. J. Cardiol. 61*: 55.

20

Stunned Myocardium Postexercise

Robert A. Kloner and John W. Allen

Hospital of the Good Samaritan and University of Southern California, Los Angeles, California

I. BACKGROUND

Stunned myocardium was initially described in models of ischemia induced by total coronary artery occlusion followed by reperfusion. Now there is evidence that stunning may also occur following myocardial ischemia induced with partial coronary artery stenosis plus exercise. As described earlier, Homans et al. (1986,1989) noted that dogs subjected to coronary artery stenosis plus treadmill exercise developed regional wall motion abnormalities that persisted for at least 60–120 minutes after exercise. Three repetitive episodes of myocardial ischemia induced by partial stenosis and exercise caused progressive deterioration in segmental function (Homans et al., 1989). Thaulow et al. (1989) described a persistent depression in regional function in the canine heart which lasted at least 30 minutes following exercise. The obvious question to follow from these experimental data is: Does this phenomenon occur in patients with coronary artery disease who undergo exercise stress testing?

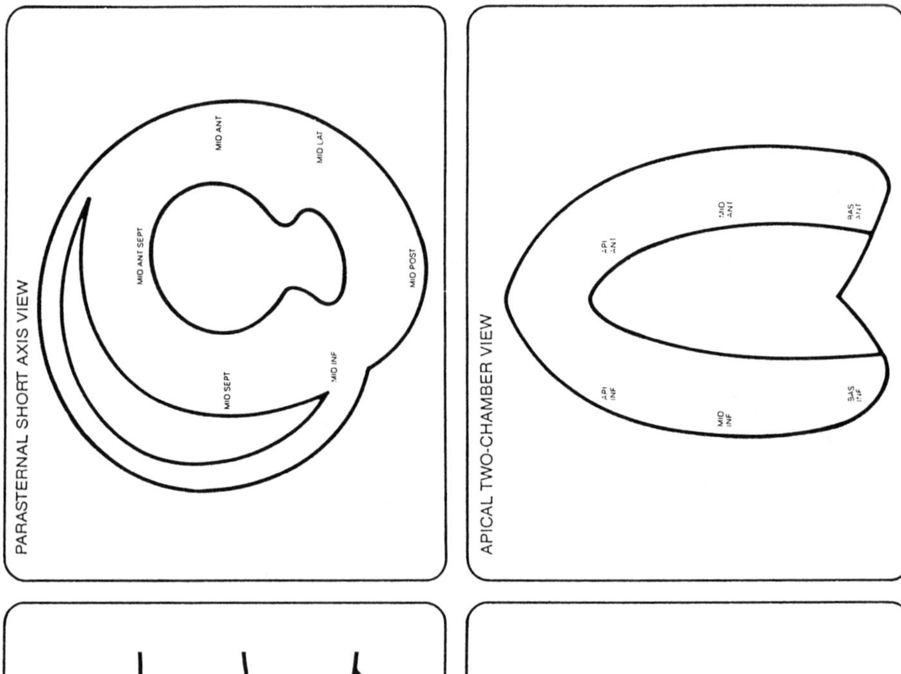
PARASTERNAL SHORT AXIS VIEW
MID ANT
MID LAT
MID ANT SEPT
MID POST
MID SEPT
MID INF
APICAL TWO-CHAMBER VIEW
PARASTERNAL LONG AXIS VIEW
BAS ANT SEPT
BAS POST
MID ANT SEPT
MID POST
APICAL FOUR-CHAMBER VIEW

II. CLINICAL EVIDENCE FOR STUNNING FOLLOWING EXERCISE IN PATIENTS WITH CORONARY ARTERY DISEASE

A. Systolic Dysfunction

A study by Robertson et al. (1983) suggested that persistent regional wall motion abnormalities occur in patients with multivessel coronary artery disease for at least 30 minutes after treadmill testing. In patients referred for suspected or known coronary artery disease, they studied two-dimensional echocardiograms obtained at rest, immediately after exercise, and at 12 minutes and 30 minutes after treadmill testing. In 13 of 20 patients (65%), function measured at 30 minutes postexercise was the same as at rest—any new exercise-induced regional wall motion abnormality had returned to normal. In 7 of 20 patients (35%), a wall motion abnormality that developed during exercise persisted at 30 minutes. Four out of eight (50%) patients with double-vessel disease (documented by coronary angiography) and two out of two (100%) patients with triple-vessel disease had a persistent wall motion abnormality at 30 minutes; no patients with single-vessel disease showed this abnormality. One patient without coronary artery disease showed a persistent wall motion abnormality and was thought to have a cardiomyopathy. In several cases the exercise-induced wall motion abnormalities were observed on the following day during left ventricular angiography. While the authors did not call their observation "stunned myocardium," it is likely that they were observing the stunning phenomenon. Their results paralleled to some extent those of Homans et al. (1986, 1989) and Thaulow et al. (1989) in the dog model.

To further investigate the phenomenon of contractile dysfunction postexercise in a systematic and semi-quantitative manner, Kloner et al. (1991) assessed regional wall motion utilizing two-dimensional echocardiography in patients with either known or suspected coronary artery disease. Patients performed either a standard or modified low-level Bruce protocol exercise test. Echocardiograms were obtained at rest, immediately after exercise, and at 15 and/or 30 minutes postexercise. Four echocardiographic views of the heart were attempted (parasternal long axis, short axis, apical 4-chamber, and 2-chamber views) in order to assess 16 regions of the left ventricle (Fig. 1). A semi-quantitative scoring system was used to grade regional wall motion,

Figure 1 Schematic representation of the four echocardiographic views obtained. BAS = basal anterior septum; BP = basal posterior; MAS = midanterior septum; MA = midanterior; ML = midlateral; MP = midposterior; MI = midinferior; MS = midseptum; BS = basal septum; AS = apical septum; AL = apical lateral; BL = basal lateral; BI = basal inferior; AI = apical inferior; AA = apical anterior; BA = basal anterior. (Diagram courtesy of J. T. Freeland. Reprinted with permission from Kloner et al., 1991.)

where Grade 1 = normal contraction, Grade 2 = hypokinesis, Grade 3 = akinesis, Grade 4 = dyskinesis. Eight normal volunteers without a history of coronary artery disease were studied as the control group.

As expected, all eight control patients in the normal volunteer group had normal wall motion at rest, immediately postexercise, and at 15 and 30 minutes after exercise. However, 16 of 22 (73%) of the coronary artery disease patients developed new wall motion abnormalities immediately after exercise. In addition, 18 of 19 (95%) patients exhibited new wall motion abnormalities 15 minutes after exercise compared to the measurement obtained at rest, while 19 of 21 patients (90%) had new wall motion abnormalities at 30 minutes postexercise. On average, 6 of 16 left ventricular regions that were normal at rest demonstrated a significant worsening of the wall motion score. The midanterior septum increased its score at 30 minutes compared to the results obtained at rest (from 1.0 to 1.6; $p < 0.002$); the midinferior wall from 1.0 to 1.7 ($p < 0.001$); the midportion of the septum from 1.0 to 1.6 ($p < 0.004$); the apical septum from 1.0 to 1.5 ($p < 0.03$); the apical lateral wall from 1.0 to 1.4 ($p < 0.03$); and basal inferior wall from 1.0 to 1.9 ($p < 0.01$). Examples of echocardiographic evidence for stunning from this study and pilot studies are shown in Figures 2–4.

In general, patients with left anterior descending coronary artery disease primarily exhibited regional wall motion abnormalities in the left ventricular septum, followed by abnormalities in the anterior wall and apex. Atherosclerotic narrowing of the right coronary artery and circumflex arteries correlated best with abnormal wall motion in the inferior and/or posterior walls. There was only a moderate correlation between circumflex disease and lateral wall motion abnormalities.

These data demonstrate that ischemia induced by a partially stenosed coronary artery in association with exercise treadmill testing may result in relatively prolonged derangement of regional contraction, and this observation supports the concept that stunned myocardium can occur in humans. The length of time required for full resolution of exercise-induced wall motion abnormalities remains, however, to be determined. We have observed persistence of these abnormalities in some patients for up to at least 45 minutes postexercise. Ambrosio et al. (1991) showed similar findings.

B. Diastolic Dysfunction

Diastolic stunning of the myocardium may also occur in humans following exercise stress testing. Fragasso et al. (1991) studied 15 patients with angiographically documented coronary artery disease who underwent exercise testing with radionuclide ventriculograms obtained at rest, peak exercise, during early recovery from exercise, and at 2 and 7 days postexercise. Functional analysis of the left ventricle included both ejection fraction and peak

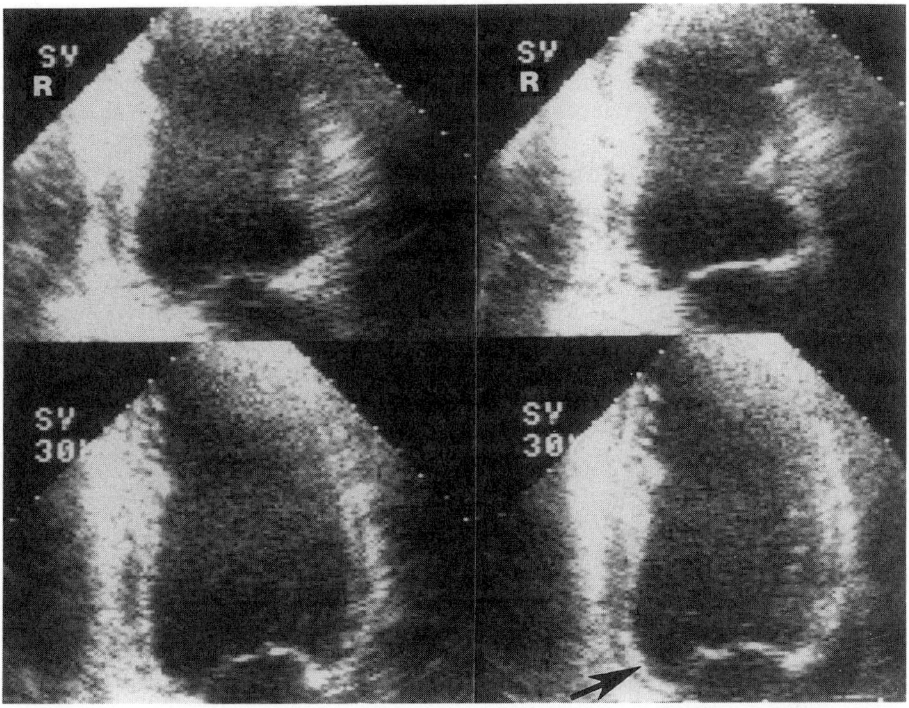

Figure 2 Echocardiographic example of stunned myocardium in a patient with coronary artery disease. Top row: apical two-chamber views of the left ventricle (LV) at rest (R)—end diastole on left; end systole on right. The inferior wall thickens, and there is shortening of the LV diameter from end diastole to end systole. Bottom row: 30 minutes after exercise when the patient is asymptomatic. The inferior basal portion of the LV paradoxically bulges (arrow) at end systole and there is less shortening of the LV diameter compared to at rest.

filling and emptying rates. Nine age-matched controls with a history of atypical chest pain but normal coronary arteries were also studied.

In the coronary artery disease patients, global ejection fraction fell from 57 at rest to 51 at peak exercise ($p < 0.02$) but recovered to 53, 54, and 55 (p = NS vs. rest) at 14 minutes, 48 hours, and 7 days postexercise, respectively. Peak emptying rates were significantly reduced at peak exercise, but also recovered early following exercise. In contrast, peak left ventricular filling rates (a parameter of ventricular diastolic function) fell from 1.8 (end-diastolic volume per second) to 1.4 ($p < 0.002$) during the early recovery phase, and remained depressed at 1.6 even at 48 hours postexercise ($p < 0.02$ vs. rest values). By 7 days, the peak LV filling rate had returned to normal. Of

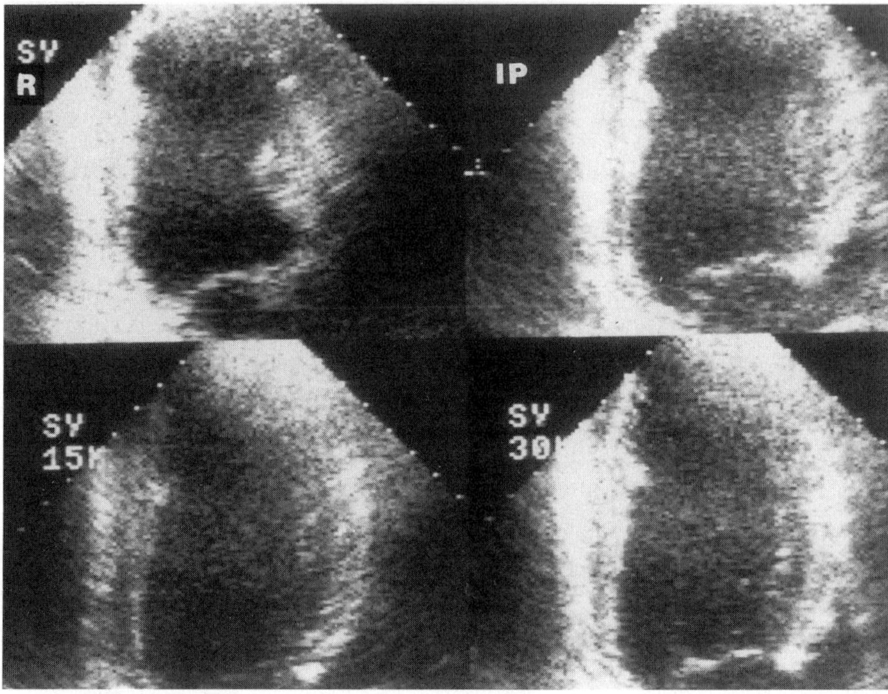

Figure 3 Same patient as in Figure 2 showing end-systolic frames at rest (R) (upper left); immediately post (IP) exercise (upper right); 15 minutes postexercise (bottom left); 30 minutes postexercise (bottom right). LV appears dilated immediately post-exercise, 15 and 30 minutes postexercise. There is paradoxical bulging of inferior basal portion of the LV after exercise, which persists for at least 30 minutes.

note, while global left ventricular ejection fraction returned towards normal during the early phase of recovery (i.e., on average 14 minutes postexercise), four regional segments in two patients demonstrated depressed systolic function at this time but recovered by 48 hours.

C. Metabolic Abnormalities

The studies by Robertson et al. (1983), Fragasso et al. (1991), and our group (Kloner et al., 1991) all support the concept that exercise-induced ischemia in humans can result in stunned myocardium manifest by abnormalities in systolic and/or diastolic function. Positron emission tomography studies also suggest that exercise-induced ischemia in humans is associated with a prolonged alteration in cardiac metabolism. Camici et al. (1986) used ru-

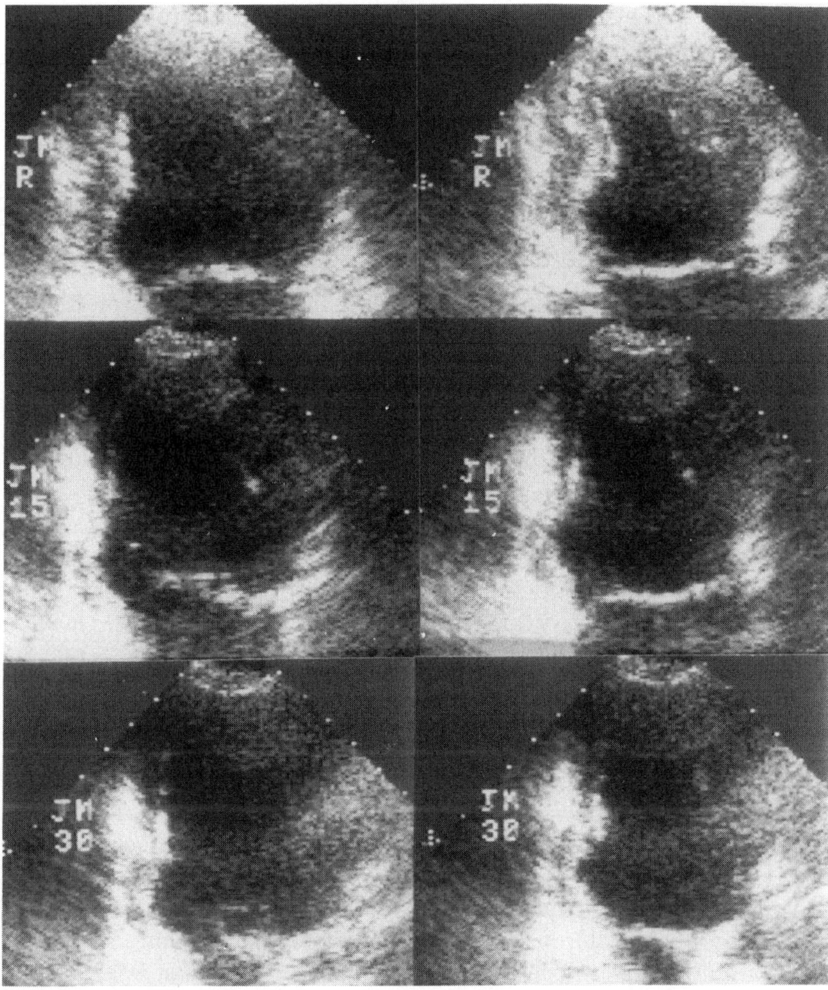

Figure 4 Apical two-chamber views of a patient at rest (R; top row), 15 minutes after exercise (middle row), and 30 minutes after exercise (bottom row). Photographs at left represent end diastole; at right, end systole. The inferior apical and anterior walls thicken normally at rest with a reduction in LV diameter. By 30 minutes post-exercise there is less thickening toward the apical half of the ventricle and the LV diameter appears wider than at rest (compare lower right with upper right figures). (Reprinted with permission from Kloner et al., 1991.)

bidium-82 as a marker of myocardial blood flow and fluorodeoxyglucose as a marker of glucose uptake in coronary artery disease patients who were undergoing exercise treadmill testing. At peak exercise there were areas of reduced rubidium uptake (indicative of ischemia), which recovered to control levels by 5-14 minutes following exercise. Uptake of fluorodeoxyglucose, injected when all hemodynamic values and rubidium uptake had returned to normal, was increased in those regions of reduced rubidium uptake during exercise. This increase in glucose uptake was present for at least one hour in some patients. Therefore, exercise-induced ischemia in man is associated with both a relatively prolonged abnormality in function and a prolonged alteration in cardiac metabolism.

III. IMPLICATIONS OF EXERCISE-INDUCED STUNNING

What are the implications of the observation that exercise-induced ischemia in humans may lead to stunned myocardium? Fragasso et al. (1991) questioned whether maximal exercise testing is advisable in patients with known severe coronary artery disease, and implied that perhaps lower-level exercise tests should be utilized for such patients. Some patients who complain of fatigue for a day or so after exercise stress testing may be experiencing symptoms due to stunned myocardium. Multiple episodes of exercise-induced ischemia could lead to progressive deterioration of cardiac function as suggested by at least one experimental report by Homans et al. (1989). It is conceivable that the syndrome of ischemic cardiomyopathy may be due in part to repetitive episodes of ischemia followed by stunning. Finally, if ischemia can be avoided by proper anti-ischemic regimens (nitrates, beta blockers, calcium blockers), then the sequelae of ischemia such as stunning could also be avoided.

Two important additional implications arise from these data. First, resting wall motion abnormalities may represent myocardial stunning from previous episodes of symptomatic or silent ischemia rather than infarction or hibernating myocardium. Second, stunning may occur in areas of the myocardium that do not show evidence of ischemia immediately post exercise. These two possibilities imply that the routine stress test with imaging before, at peak, or immediately after exercise gives an incomplete picture of the degree of abnormality. Delayed imaging may be required in selected patients with coronary artery disease to correctly identify their degree of abnormality.

REFERENCES

Ambrosio, G., Betocchi, S., Pace, L., Ciarmiello, A., Salvatore, C., Salvatore, M., Chiariello, M. (1991). Prolonged impairment of regional left ventricular systolic function after exercise in patients with stable angina. *Circulation* (Suppl. II) *84*: II-475.

Camici, P., Araujo, L. I., Spinks, T., Lammertsma, A. A., Kaski, J. C., Shea, M. J., Selwyn, A. P., Jones, T. J., and Maseri, A. (1986). Increased uptake of 18-F-fluorodeoxyglucose in postischemic myocardium of patients with exercise-induced angina. *Circulation 74*: 81.

Fragasso, G., Benti, R., Sciammarella, M., Rossetti, E., Savi, A., Gerundini, P., and Chierchia, S. L., (1991). Symptom-limited exercise testing causes sustained diastolic dysfunction in patients with coronary disease and low effort tolerance. *J. Am. Coll. Cardiol. 17*: 1251.

Homans, D. C., Sublett, E., Dai, X. Z., and Bache, R. J. (1986). Persistence of regional left ventricular dysfunction after exercise induced ischemia. *J. Clin. Invest. 77*: 66.

Homans, D. C., Laxson, D. D., Sublett, E., Lindstrom, P., and Bache, R. J. (1989). Cumulative deterioration of myocardial function after repeated episodes of exercise-induced ischemia. *Am. J. Physiol. 256*: H1462.

Kloner, R. A., Allen, J., Cox, T. A., Zheng, Y., and Ruiz, C. E. (1991). Stunned left ventricular myocardium following exercise treadmill testing in coronary artery disease. *Am. J. Cardiol. 68*: 329.

Robertson, W. S., Feigenbaum, H., Armstrong, W. F., Dillon, J. C., O'Donnel, J., and McHenry, P. W. (1983). Exercise echocardiography: A clinically practical addition in evaluation of coronary artery disease. *J. Am. Coll. Cardiol. 2*: 1085.

Thaulow, E., Guth, B. D., Heusch, G., Gilpin, E., Schultz, R., Kroeger, K., and Ross, J., Jr. (1989). Characteristics of regional myocardial stunning after exercise in dogs with chronic coronary stenosis. *Am. J. Physiol. 257*: H113.

21

Stunned Myocardium in Cardiac Surgery

Ian C. Wilson and Timothy J. Gardner

Johns Hopkins University School of Medicine, Baltimore, Maryland

I. INTRODUCTION

Open heart surgery requires the achievement of a still, bloodless field for precise formation of anastomoses and intracardiac repairs. This surgical exposure is most commonly accomplished at the expense of a period of global myocardial ischemia requiring the use of extracorporeal circulation and oxygenation. Such intervention results in exposure of the myocardium to possible ischemia/reperfusion injury (Hearse, 1977) and the initiation of a systemic inflammatory reaction when blood elements are exposed to the cardiopulmonary bypass circuit (Kirklin et al., 1987).

Myocardial ischemia and subsequent reperfusion results in reversible or irreversible myocellular damage, the relative extent of which is dependent upon the severity of the ischemic insult. However, the controlled induction of ischemia during cardiac surgery allows manipulation of the myocardial environment during aortic cross clamping and early reperfusion, affording "myocardial protection." Alteration of myocardial energy requirements, optimizing conditions of coronary reperfusion, and pharmacological enhancement of myocardial tolerance to ischemia and reperfusion are means by which the duration of ischemia can be prolonged without producing irreversible myocardial damage. Nonetheless, the consequences of extending the ischemic interval prior to irreversible myocyte injury and the contribution of inflammatory mediators from extracorporeal circulation are poorly understood and may produce considerable modification of the myocardial injury previously described in other models of ischemia.

II. NATURE OF MYOCARDIAL INJURY FOLLOWING CARDIAC SURGERY

Myocardial injury during cardiac surgery is heterogeneous in nature and contains elements of both reversible and irreversible damage. The reversible extent of the injury can be quantitated by anatomical and functional measures.

A. Anatomic Indices

Anatomical evidence of irreversible injury has been documented by studies showing uptake of indium-111 monoclonal antimyosin antibody (van Vlies et al., 1990), a sensitive indicator of myocyte necrosis, as well as the release of creatine kinase MB (Roberts et al., 1981) in the majority of patients undergoing routine coronary artery surgery. However, electron microscopic analysis reveals predominantly reversible myocardial damage postoperatively (Schaper et al., 1986) in which myocytes with severe ultrastructural changes at the end of ischemia undergo structural reconstitution during reperfusion (Schaper et al., 1977).

B. Functional Indices

Postischemic ventricular dysfunction after cardiac surgery is common (Breisblatt et al., 1990). Stunned myocardium represents the prolonged but reversible depression of ventricular function (Braunwald and Kloner, 1982) that occurs postoperatively, which is out of proportion to the degree of myocyte necrosis. However, the reversible component of ventricular dysfunction is difficult to establish accurately.

Animal preparations simulating cardiac surgical conditions have usually been short term, nonsurvival procedures with accurate assessment of ventricular performance, using Langendorff or support animal models, but thereby not allowing assessment of the reversibility of postischemic ventricular dysfunction. Moreover, in the clinical setting measurement of left ventricular function is imprecise. Most indices of systolic ventricular function used in patients are dependent upon preload or cardiac volume, in both preejection and ejection phases. Use of the relatively *load-independent* indices of function, such as the end-systolic pressure-volume relationship and preload recruitable stroke work, requires accurate measurement of ventricular volume:

there exists no simple, reproducible, noninvasive technique to measure this in humans.

Therefore the heterogeneous nature of the myocardial injury, the complexity of in vivo models, and the insensitivity of clinical methods in assessing left ventricular function preclude analysis of pure myocardial stunning following cardiac surgery, but rather allow evaluation of postoperative ventricular dysfunction following a combination of reversible and irreversible myocardial damage. However, the major contributing factor to ventricular dysfunction following routine uneventful cardiac surgery appears to be myocardial stunning (Gray et al., 1979; Roberts et al., 1981).

III. ETIOLOGY OF POSTOPERATIVE VENTRICULAR DYSFUNCTION

The etiology of postischemic ventricular dysfunction following cardiopulmonary bypass is likely to be multifactorial. In addition to the modified ischemia/reperfusion injury during cardiac surgery, residual depression of myocyte metabolism can result from hypothermia (Czer et al., 1983; Greene et al., 1989) and from direct trauma to the myocardium due to manipulation of the heart. However, the predominant factor is undoubtedly ischemia/reperfusion injury.

Global myocardial ischemia during cardiac surgery results in a rapid reduction of intramyocardial oxygen tension to extremely low levels (Gardner et al., 1971); these low levels quickly revert to normal after release of the aortic cross clamp. Following reoxygenation the myocardium demonstrates a reduced ability to extract oxygen from the reperfusate (Kanter et al., 1981), the etiology of which is unclear. Elevation of cytosolic calcium during ischemia and early reperfusion (Steenberg et al., 1987), reduction of myocardial ATP levels during ischemia and reperfusion (Miller et al., 1991), and production of oxygen free radicals (Weisel et al., 1989) have all been demonstrated in surgical models of global ischemia. However, the relative roles of oxyradical generation, abnormal energy transduction, sarcoplasmic reticular dysfunction, sarcolemmal injury, and capillary no-reflow in inducing postischemic ventricular dysfunction following cardiac surgery are unknown.

The importance of acute inflammatory mediators in producing postoperative ventricular dysfunction is also unclear, although the initiation of an acute inflammatory reaction during cardiac surgery has been well demonstrated (van Oeveren et al., 1985; Kirklin et al., 1987). Exposure of blood elements to the cardiopulmonary bypass circuit results in activation of complement (Chenoweth et al., 1981), kallikrein, clotting, and fibrinolytic cascades (Westaby, 1987). C5a induces neutrophil activation, which combined with the products of arachidonic acid metabolism generated by MAC complex (C5b-9) stimulation (Salama et al., 1988), coagulation factor XIIa, and kallikrein leads to increased neutrophil adherence (Schapira et al., 1982; Wachfogel et al., 1989). This also results in free lysosomal enzyme release (Addonizio et al., 1982) and an increased capacity for neutrophil "respiratory burst" (Oeveren et al., 1985; Roccatello et al., 1990) in cardiac surgical patients.

Neutrophil-endothelial interaction is further promoted during cardiopulmonary bypass by the enhanced expression of neutrophil adherence molecules on the endothelial cell surface. These receptors upregulate in response to circulating inflammatory mediators released during cardiopulmonary bypass including C5a, leukotrienes (Hoover et al., 1984), and the cytokine interleukin-1 (IL-1) (Schleimer and Rutledge, 1986; Andersen et al., 1987).

The role of neutrophils in postcardiotomy stunned myocardium is supported by a recent study in which intracoronary administration of C5a resulted in a granulocyte-dependent reduction in coronary blood flow. This reduction in flow caused an imbalance between myocardial oxygen supply and demand and led to impaired ventricular function (Martin et al., 1988). Sequestration of leukocytes within the coronary vascular bed has been documented on initial reperfusion of the myocardium during cardiac surgery (Semb et al., 1988). Further investigation is required to evaluate the importance of inflammatory mediators and neutrophils in the generation of postoperative ventricular dysfunction.

IV. CLINICAL EVIDENCE OF STUNNED MYOCARDIUM IN CARDIAC SURGERY

The clinical manifestations of stunned myocardium are commonly encountered after cardiac surgery. Evidence for stunning is provided by documentation of reversible impairment of postischemic ventricular performance in clinical studies, and by the temporary requirement of myocardial support for some postoperative patients.

A. Reversible Postoperative Ventricular Dysfunction

Reversible impairment of systolic and diastolic ventricular function in both left and right ventricles has been demonstrated in clinical studies following cardiopulmonary bypass. This alteration of ventricular performance may have a profound effect in the early postoperative period, particularly in patients with preexisting impairment of ventricular function.

1. Systolic Ventricular Dysfunction

Depression of left ventricular contractility after removal of the aortic cross clamp has been recognized for many years in patients undergoing routine coronary artery surgery (Gold et al., 1979). However, the increased catecholamine levels associated with cardiopulmonary bypass (Tan et al., 1976) results in endogenous inotropic stimulation of the stunned myocardium. This tends to reduce the apparent occurrence of myocardial stunning (Becker et al., 1986) when assessed in the immediate postoperative period.

Serial postoperative assessment, utilizing radionuclide gated cardiac blood pool ejection fraction and regional wall motion as indicators of ventricular systolic function, demonstrates a reduction in ejection fraction 2–4 hours after uncomplicated coronary artery surgery in 46-90% of cases, despite unaltered systemic vascular resistance (Gray et al., 1979; Reduto et al., 1981; Roberts et al., 1981). The mean decline in ejection fraction was 12-17%, and in 92–100% of these patients ventricular performance returned to preoperative values by the seventh postoperative day. Similar reductions in regional wall motion occur in parallel with changes in ejection fraction (Roberts et al., 1981); both are shown in Figure 1.

The time course of the decrease in left ventricular ejection fraction following cardiac surgery was documented by Breisblatt (1990) in a compre-

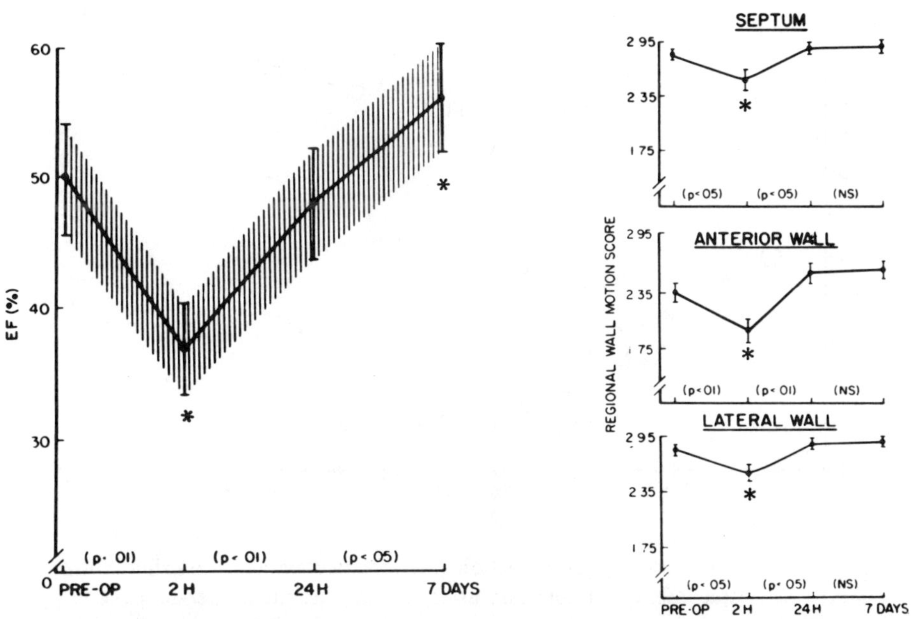

Figure 1 Schematic representation of ejection fraction and regional wall motion following uncomplicated coronary artery surgery. The *p* values relate to differences between two adjacent time periods. The asterisks show values significantly different from preoperative values. (From Roberts et al., 1981.)

hensive study using radionuclide ventriculography and serial monitoring of left ventricular ejection fraction with a nuclear probe. Left ventricular ejection fraction was depressed in the immediate postoperative period in 79% of patients undergoing uneventful coronary artery surgery. The mean preoperative left ventricular ejection fraction was 58%, which fell to 46% at 2 hours postoperatively. However, in 96% of patients, ventricular ejection fraction deteriorated further as time progressed, reaching a nadir of 37% at 4½ hours postoperatively. Recovery of left ventricular ejection fraction to 55% occurred by 8-10 hours, and full recovery was seen in all patients by 48 hours. A typical patient is depicted in Figure 2.

Analysis of ventricular performance using left ventricular stroke-work indices also reveals postoperative left ventricular dysfunction demonstrated by a reduction of stroke work index to less than 50% of the preoperative

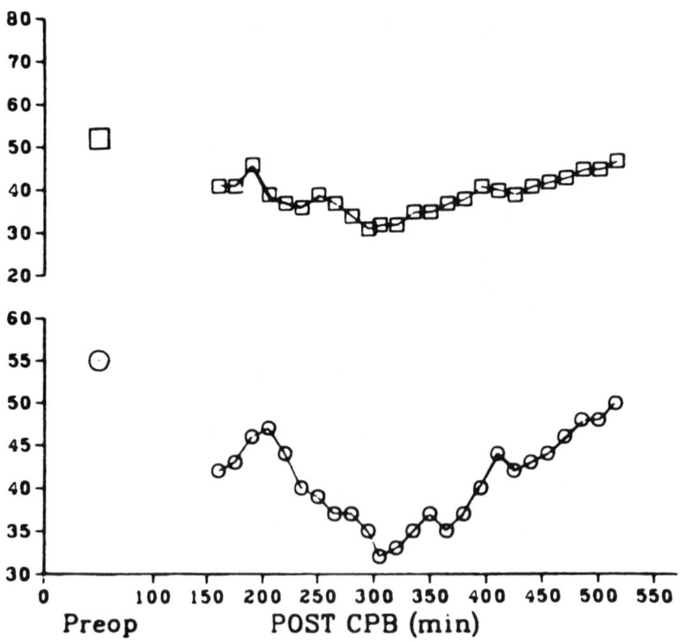

Figure 2 Serial biventricular ejection fractions in a patient requiring inotropes shortly after uncomplicated coronary artery surgery. Right (upper series) and left (lower series) ventricular ejection fractions were depressed in the early postoperative period, continued to worsen reaching a nadir at 5 hours, and improved thereafter reaching preoperative values by 8 hours postoperatively. CPB = cardiopulmonary bypass. (From Breisblatt et al., 1990.)

values in all patients 15 minutes after discontinuation of cardiopulmonary bypass (Mangano, 1985). However, the degree of depression and rate of recovery depends upon preoperative ventricular function. Ninety percent recovery occurs within 4 hours when preoperative ejection fraction is greater than 0.55, but only 60% recovery is achieved at 24 hours when preoperative ejection fraction is less than 0.45.

Transient depression of right ventricular systolic function has also been documented. At a mean time of 4 hours postcardiopulmonary bypass a decrease in RV ejection fraction (Breisblatt et al., 1990), RV stroke work index (Mangano, 1985), and an increase in RV end-systolic and end-diastolic volume indices (Stein et al., 1990) demonstrate postischemic right ventricular dysfunction following routine uneventful coronary artery surgery. The time course of right ventricular myocardial stunning parallels that of the left ventricle over the first 8-10 postoperative hours (Breisblatt et al., 1990). Systolic dysfunction responds readily to pharmacological therapy within 2 hours (Stein et al., 1990) and resolves completely within 24 hours.

However, in all the above studies the indicators of myocardial performance are altered by varying the ventricular preload and afterload. Recent series using relatively *load-insensitive* indicators of ventricular performance (stroke-work end-diastolic volume relationship and end-systolic pressure-volume relationship) have failed to show reduction in left ventricular systolic function following coronary artery surgery and cardiac valve replacement using cold potassium cardioplegic arrest (Fremes et al., 1985; Harpole et al., 1989; Sell et al., 1991). In these studies, the range of end-diastolic and end-systolic points was small and assessment of ventricular volume was problematic, which could therefore lead to inaccuracies of these theoretically superior techniques. The most recent study also evaluated left ventricular function very early after discontinuation of cardiopulmonary bypass; such early assessment could potentially fail to detect the late deterioration in postischemic ventricular function documented in other series (Sell et al., 1991).

2. Diastolic Ventricular Dysfunction

Intraoperative development of diastolic ventricular dysfunction has been demonstrated by perioperative transesophageal echocardiography (Wehlage et al., 1990) and postoperative radionuclide ventriculography (Fremes et al., 1985). Progressive deterioration in ventricular compliance occurs over the first 2-4 postoperative hours (Fig. 3), although diastolic function returns to normal within 18 hours after routine coronary revascularization (Rinder et al., 1988). The decrease in compliance with time could be related to a pericardial clot restricting ventricular filling or to an increased pulmonary vascular resistance causing right ventricular-left ventricular interaction, but it is most likely to represent accumulation of myocardial edema associated

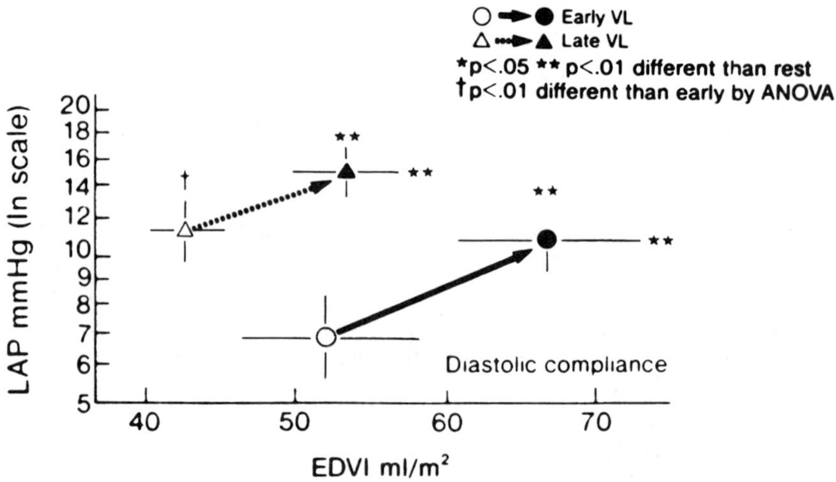

Figure 3 Diastolic pressure-volume relationships depicted before and after volume loading (VL), EARLY and LATE after cross clamp removal following routine coronary artery surgery. The relation between left atrial pressure (LAP) and end-diastolic volume index (EDVI) is monoexponential, and the natural logarithm (ln) of the LAP is plotted against the EDVI. Diastolic compliance was increased EARLY and returned to normal LATE. (From Fremes et al., 1985.)

with the ischemia/reperfusion injury. During the period of reduced ventricular diastolic performance, atrial contraction assumes a greater role in ventricular filling, as shown in Figure 4. This underscores the importance of sinus rhythm early after cardiac surgery and explains the increased morbidity associated with postoperative atrial dysrhythmia.

B. Postoperative Myocardial Support

The increased release of endogenous catecholamines following cardiopulmonary bypass reduces the clinical significance of minor degrees of stunned myocardium. However, more severe ventricular dysfunction, refractory to endogenous catecholamine stimulation, requires pharmacological or mechanical support in a number of patients undergoing open heart surgery. Temporary use of such support allows time for metabolic and functional recovery of reversibly injured myocytes and further emphasizes the reversible nature of a large proportion of postoperative ventricular dysfunction.

1. Pharmacological Support

The need for inotropic support of the myocardium following cardiac surgery is a relatively poor measure of postischemic ventricular dysfunction. It is dependent upon many variables including preference of the anesthetist and

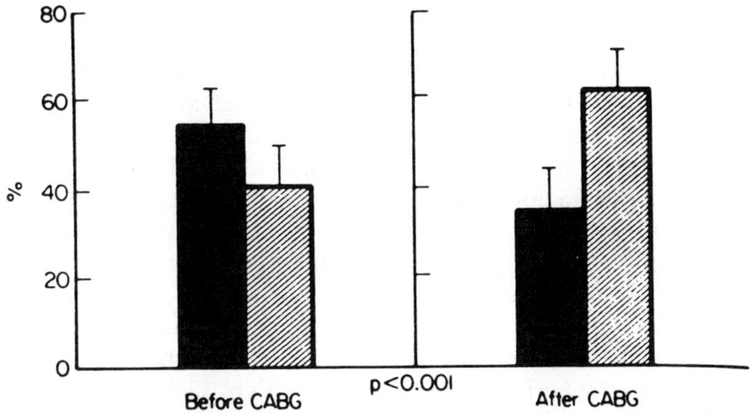

Figure 4 Participation (in %) of early diastolic filling and atrial contraction in left ventricular filling during coronary artery bypass grafting (CABG) as measured by transesophageal Doppler echocardiography. Results are given as mean and standard deviation with the p value reflecting the difference between the two time points. Black = early diastolic filling; hatch = atrial contraction. (From Wehlage et al., 1990.)

surgeon, the preoperative condition of the patient, the surgical procedure performed, and the adequacy of intraoperative myocardial protection. In a large series of adult patients undergoing cardiac surgery, inotropic stimulation of the myocardium was required to allow satisfactory weaning from cardiopulmonary bypass in only 3-5% of patients (McGee et al., 1980), although a further 15-50% of patients required support within the first 24 hours postoperatively (McGee et al., 1980; Breisblatt et al., 1990; Johnson et al., 1991). This high incidence of delayed inotrope requirement correlates with the initial progressive deterioration of postoperative ventricular performance demonstrated in clinical studies and may reflect gradual reduction of endogenous catecholamine release or an intrinsic impairment of ventricular function.

Administration of inotropes to patients with severely stunned myocardium following cardiopulmonary bypass improves ventricular systolic function. However, clinical reports suggest that use of such agents delays, but does not completely prevent, the nadir of depression of systolic ventricular function (Breisblatt et al., 1990). Inotrope use is only marginally predictive of less favorable long-term outcome following coronary artery bypass grafting, suggesting that their administration is predominantly for reversible ventricular dysfunction (Royster et al., 1991).

2. Mechanical Support

Patients with postischemic ventricular dysfunction refractory to management with pharmacological support require temporary mechanical assistance.

a. Intraaortic Balloon Pump. The role of the intraaortic balloon pump (IABP) and the incidence of its use after open heart operations is more clearly defined than for inotropes. Retrospective review of IABP use in major cardiac surgical institutions has revealed that 1-3% of patients require IABP counterpulsation to enable successful separation from cardiopulmonary bypass and a further 0.5-1% require delayed placement of the device within the first 48 postoperative hours (McGee et al., 1980; Lauwers et al., 1990). Sixty to eighty-six percent of patients with severe postoperative ventricular dysfunction can initially be supported satisfactorily with the IABP (Kuchar et al., 1987; Di Lello et al., 1988); 60% of these are weaned from the device and discharged home (Kuchar et al., 1987). Long-term results of these patients are good, with 85-90% remaining in NYHA functional class I or II at a mean postoperative period of 4 years (Kuchar et al., 1987). This demonstrates clearly the reversible nature of much of the immediate postoperative ventricular dysfunction.

b. Ventricular Assist Device. Use of ventricular assist devices (VAD) for postischemic ventricular dysfunction following cardiac surgery varies between institutions. This interinstitution variability is accounted for by the experience of individual units with the devices, which often reflects their threshold for insertion in patients with severe refractory postoperative ventricular dysfunction. The incidence of insertion varies between 0.1 and 1% of all cardiac surgical procedures requiring cardiopulmonary bypass (McGee et al., 1980). However, their use identifies a group of patients with extreme postischemic ventricular dysfunction whose survival is dependent upon mechanical support of reversibly injured myocardium during its recovery. A multicenter review of ventricular assist device use reveals that biventricular assistance is required in 33% of VAD patients, left ventricular assistance in 54%, and right ventricular assistance in 13% (Pae et al., 1991).

When analyzing the use of all ventricular assist devices for severe postoperative ventricular dysfunction, 41-50% of patients can be weaned from the device and 29-40% are discharged from hospital (Rose et al., 1989; Pennington et al., 1989). The combined registry experience reports a 2-year actuarial survival of hospital survivors of 92% for left VAD support, 88% for right VAD support, and 94% for biventricular support. Long-term follow-up of a large group of survivors of mechanical ventricular assistance demonstrated that only 17% had evidence of cardiac disability (New York Heart Association functional class III or IV) (Kanter et al., 1988) at an average follow-up of 29 months.

Illustration of the delayed recovery of severely stunned myocardium was recently documented by serial gated radionuclide ventriculograms in a patient requiring postoperative mechanical left ventricular assistance (Ballantyne et al., 1987). Preoperative left ventricular ejection fraction was 50%, but had fallen at 12 hours postoperatively to 6%. Following gradual improvement of ventricular function and discontinuation of myocardial support, the ejection fraction rose to 34% by postoperative day 17.

V. FACTORS INFLUENCING POSTOPERATIVE VENTRICULAR DYSFUNCTION

The susceptibility of the heart to postischemic ventricular dysfunction is dictated by the preoperative status of the ventricle, the intraoperative conditions during ischemia, and the characteristics of coronary reperfusion.

A. Preoperative Status

The intrinsic sensitivity of the myocardium to ischemia and reperfusion is influenced by many factors; one of the most important appears to be preoperative left ventricular performance. Serial monitoring of preoperative patients with reduced ejection fraction reveals more severe reversible depression of ventricular function, which persists longer than in patients with normal preoperative left ventricular ejection fractions (Mangano, 1985). The greater degree of myocardial stunning in these patients is associated with a higher postoperative mortality: mortality was 7.7% when the ejection fraction was less than 40% compared to 1.3% for patients with an ejection fraction greater than 60% undergoing coronary revascularization (Salomon et al., 1990). Preexisting myocardial energy depletion occurring in patients with unstable angina, complicated angioplasty (Stewart et al., 1990), myocardial infarction, or left ventricular failure (Hammermeister et al., 1990; Royster et al., 1991) further increases the incidence of clinically significant postischemic ventricular dysfunction. These conditions raise the need for postoperative myocardial support and result in higher postoperative mortality.

Myocardial maturity also influences the sensitivity of the myocardium to ischemia and reperfusion. Cardiac surgery in neonates (Durandy et al., 1988) and the elderly (Gersh et al., 1983) results in increased postoperative inotrope requirement.

B. Myocardial Conditions During Ischemia

Modification of perioperative myocardial injury may be achieved by altering the conditions of ischemia. The most critical factor influencing the severity of postischemic ventricular dysfunction is the length of ischemic time. In a number of clinical studies prolonged aortic cross clamping is associated with a significantly increased requirement for postoperative myocardial support.

Rapid induction of diastolic arrest, myocardial cooling to slow metabolic activity, and administration of anti-ischemic agents and buffers to attenuate the effects of myocardial ischemia (Hearse, 1988) allow prolongation of the time before which reversible myocardial damage occurs. These principles form the basis of the myocardial preservation regimens used by most cardiac surgeons. Although some disagreement exists about their relative importance, each of these therapeutic maneuvers can reduce postischemic ventricular dysfunction.

1. Hypothermia

Hypothermia protects myocardium by reducing the basal metabolic rate. Systemic hypothermia, cold cardioplegia administration, and topical cooling are used to reduce myocardial temperature during ischemia and to achieve uniform cooling of the heart. Maintaining myocardial temperature at 4-15 °C during crystalloid cardioplegic arrest results in significantly better postoperative ventricular function than temperatures of 15° or higher (Rosenfeldt, 1982). However, due to leftward shift of the oxygen dissociation curve and the temperature-dependent rheological properties of blood, the optimal temperature for blood cardioplegia is felt to be 20 °C (Rousou et al., 1988).

2. Cardioplegia

Numerous experimental and clinical studies have demonstrated that achieving satisfactory diastolic arrest of the heart by cardioplegia administration results in superior preservation of myocardial metabolism (Engleman et al., 1977), postischemic ventricular systolic and diastolic function (Ellis et al., 1979), and myocardial ultrastructure (Schaper et al., 1990) when compared to other forms of myocardial preservation. The ability of blood and fluorocarbons to deliver oxygen to the myocardium when incorporated into cardioplegia solutions results in further improvement of postischemic left ventricular function; these agents are associated with better preservation of myocardial high-energy phosphates (Magovern et al., 1982; Codd et al., 1985). Glutamate substrate enhancement of blood cardioplegia also improves the postischemic function of the preoperatively energy-depleted hearts, though no improvement was identified in the normal heart undergoing prolonged ischemia (Robertson et al., 1984; Rosenkranz and Buckberg, 1984). These cardioplegia regimens appear to reduce postischemic ventricular dysfunction, but their complex nature has inhibited wide acceptance.

3. Calcium Antagonists

Calcium channel blockers have also been used for myocellular protection during cardiac surgical ischemia. In patients undergoing coronary artery surgery, studies demonstrate improved postoperative left ventricular regional area ejection fraction following administration of intravenous nicardipine prior to aortic cross clamping (Lytle et al., 1987). In an experimental model of regional ischemia followed by superimposed global hypothermic cardioplegic ischemia, trifluoperazine, a calcium-calmodulin antagonist, also improved regional and global ventricular function and increased creatine phosphate content in the area of regional ischemia (Otani et al., 1989).

These studies provide evidence that prevention of intracellular calcium influx during ischemia and early reperfusion may have a role in limiting postischemic ventricular dysfunction following cardiopulmonary bypass.

C. Myocardial Conditions During Reperfusion

Reperfusion following ischemia is a critical stage during which reversible myocardial injury occurs. Manipulation of the conditions of reperfusion can reduce potentially detrimental effects on postoperative ventricular function.

1. Ventricular Decompression

Left ventricular decompression during ischemia and reperfusion reduces left ventricular wall tension and enhances preservation of endocardial blood flow. In clinical studies, improved ventricular function and a reduced myocardial oxygen consumption result from use of a left ventricular vent (Olinger and Boncheck, 1978; Kanter et al., 1982).

2. Normothermic Cardioplegia

Minimizing myocardial energy requirements while optimizing enzyme function during initial reperfusion also improves myocardial preservation. Administration of normothermic blood cardioplegia for 5 minutes prior to release of the aortic clamp improves postischemic ventricular function in experimental and clinical series (Lazar et al., 1979; Rosenkranz et al., 1983). The reason for this benefit is unclear, but may be related to the adequacy of free radical scavenging at initial reperfusion.

3. Free Radical Scavengers

Oxygen-derived free radicals are produced upon reperfusion of ischemic myocardium. Sources of these radicals include complement-activated polymorphonuclear leukocytes, endothelium, xanthine oxidase, mitochondria, catecholamine oxidation, and arachidonic acid metabolism.

In Langendorff and support animal models, administration of superoxide dismutase and catalase-enhanced cardioplegia during global myocardial ischemia and at initial reperfusion improves postischemic ventricular systolic function when compared to hearts protected by standard hypothermic cardioplegia (Shlafer et al., 1982a,b). Similar experiments using superoxide dismutase and mannitol as free radical-scavenging agents incorporated into hypothermic cardioplegia solutions demonstrate improved postischemic ventricular function and better preservation of sarcoplasmic reticular function (Stewart et al., 1983). Further research revealed that administration of free radical scavengers only at the time of reperfusion was equally effective in preserving postischemic ventricular function (Casale et al., 1983); this reaffirms the importance of reperfusion in generating oxygen-derived free radicals.

The influence of free radical scavengers on preserving postischemic ventricular systolic function in hearts with *preexisting* ischemia has recently been investigated in experimental models. Hearts subjected to normothermic reversible regional ischemia prior to hypothermic cardioplegic arrest were protected by superoxide dismutase and catalase (Johnson et al., 1987) or deferoxamine (Illes et al., 1989). Both regimens better preserved ventricular function in the previously stunned region when compared to those receiving standard cardioplegia solution.

These experiments suggest that oxygen free radicals play an important role in the etiology of postischemic ventricular dysfunction following cardiac surgery. Recently, a randomized controlled study of the use of allopurinol in coronary bypass surgery demonstrated significant reduction in postoperative inotropic or mechanical support and decreased mortality in pretreated patients (Johnson et al., 1991). However, mortality in the control group was high, and further clinical studies are therefore required to establish the role of antioxidants in myocardial protection.

4. Coenzyme Q_{10}

Coenzyme Q_{10} is a naturally occurring component of mitochondria which transports electrons between flavoproteins and cytochromes during oxidative phosphorylation. This coenzyme is a potent antioxidant against lipid peroxidation in the myocardial mitochondrial membrane in vitro; it therefore has a membrane-stabilizing effect (Greenburg and Frishman, 1990). Experimental and clinical studies utilizing Q_{10} in cardioplegia and intravenous infusions prior to reperfusion, as well as oral pretreatment before surgery, have demonstrated reduction in postischemic ventricular dysfunction (Nayler, 1980; Tanaka et al., 1982; Okamoto et al., 1986). This improvement in postoperative myocardial performance is believed to be the result of a reduction in myocardial stunning.

5. Leukocyte Depletion

The removal of activated neutrophils from the reperfusate may also enhance postischemic ventricular performance. In neonatal hearts following prolonged global ischemia, leukocyte depletion of coronary blood improved postischemic ventricular dysfunction when studied in a support animal preparation (Breda et al., 1989). The significance of these modifications in coronary reperfusion remains unclear and warrants further investigation.

VI. CONCLUSION

Despite improvements in operative technique and methods of myocardial protection, postoperative left ventricular dysfunction continues to be common in patients undergoing cardiopulmonary bypass. Although the mechanism for depression of ventricular performance in the early postoperative period is unclear, clinical and experimental results suggest that myocardial stunning following reversible ischemia/reperfusion injury plays a major role. An improved understanding of the numerous factors influencing postoperative ventricular dysfunction and their pathogenetic role in reversible myocardial injury will potentially enable cardiac surgeons to reduce postoperative morbidity and mortality in the future.

REFERENCES

Addonizio, V. P., Jr., Strauss, J. F., 3rd., Chang, L. F., Fisher, C. A., Colman, R. W., and Edmunds, L. H., Jr. (1982). Release of lysosomal hydrolases during simulated extracorporeal circulation. *J. Thorac. Cardiovasc. Surg. 84*: 28.

Andersen, L. W., Baek, L., Degn, H., Lehd, J., Krasnik, M., and Rasmussen, J. P. (1987). Presence of circulating endotoxins during cardiac operations. *J. Thorac. Cardiovasc. Surg. 93*: 115.

Ballantyne, C. M., Verani, M. S., Short, H. D., Hyatt, C., and Noon, G. P. (1987). Delayed recovery of severely "stunned" myocardium with the support of a left ventricular assist device after coronary artery bypass graft surgery. *J. Am. Coll. Cardiol. 10*: 710.

Becker, L. C., Levine, J. H., DiPaula, A. F., Guarnieri, T., and Aversano, T. (1986). Reversal of dysfunction in postischemic stunned myocardium by epinephrine and postextrasystolic potentiation. *J. Am. Coll. Cardiol. 7*: 580.

Braunwald, E., and Kloner, R. A. (1982). The stunned myocardium: Prolonged, post-ischemic ventricular dysfunction. *Circulation 66*: 1146.

Breda, M. A., Drinkwater, D. C., Laks, H., Bhuta, S., Corno, A. F., Davtyan, H. G., and Chang, P. (1989). Prevention of reperfusion injury in the neonatal heart with leukocyte-depleted blood. *J. Thorac. Cardiovasc. Surg. 97*: 654.

Breisblatt, W. M., Stein, K. L., Wolfe, C. J., Follansbee, W. P., Capozzi, J., Armitage, J. M., and Hardesty, R. L. (1990). Acute myocardial dysfunction and recovery: A common occurrence after coronary bypass surgery. *J. Am. Coll. Cardiol. 15*: 1261.

Brown, J. M., Grosso, M. A., Terada, L. S., Beehler, C. J., Toth, K. M., Whitman, G. J., Harken, A. H., and Repine, J. E. (1989). Erythrocytes decrease myocardial hydrogen peroxide levels and reperfusion injury. *Am. J. Physiol. 256*: H584.

Bulkley, B. H., and Hutchins, G. M. (1977). Myocardial consequences of coronary artery graft surgery. The paradox of necrosis in areas of revascularization. *Circulation 56*: 906.

Casale, A. S., Bulkley, B. H., Flaherty, J. T., Gott, V. L., and Gardner, J. T. (1983). Oxygen free-radical scavengers protect the arrested, globally ischaemic heart upon reperfusion. *Surgical Forum 34*: 313.

Chenoweth, D. E., Cooper, S. W., Hugli, T. E., Stewart, R. W., Blackstone, E. H. and Kirklin, J. W. (1981). Complement activation during cardiopulmonary bypass: Evidence for generation of C3a and C5a anaphylatoxins. *N. Engl. J. Med. 304*: 497.

Codd, J. E., Barner, H. B., Pennington, D. G., Merjavy, J. P., Kaiser, G. C., Devine, J. E. and Willman, V. L. (1985). Intraoperative myocardial protection: A comparison of blood and asanguineous cardioplegia. *Ann. Thorac. Surg. 39*: 125.

Czer, L., Hamer, A., Murphy, F., Bussell, J., Chaux, A., Bateman, T., Matloff, J. and Gray, R. J. (1983). Transient hemodynamic dysfunction after myocardial revascularization. Temperature dependence. *J. Thorac. Cardiovasc. Surg. 86*: 226.

Di Lello, F., Mullen, D. C., Flemma, R. J., Anderson, A. J., Kleinman, L. H., and Werner, P. H. (1988). Results of intraaortic balloon pumping after cardiac surgery: Experience with the Percor balloon catheter. *Ann. Thorac. Surg. 46*: 442.

Durandy, Y., Batisse, A., Bourel, P., and Lecompte, Y. (1988). [Postoperative inotropic treatment in cardiac surgery of the newborn infant and infant]. *Ann. Fr. Anesth. Reanim. 7*: 105.

Ellis, R. J., Gertz, E. W., Wisneski, J., and Ebert, P. A. (1979). Mild ventricular dysfunction following cold potassium cardioplegia. *Circulation 60(Suppl. 1)*: 147.

Engleman, R. M., Levitsky, S., O'Donoghue, M., and Auvil, J. (1977). Cardioplegia and myocardial preservation during cardiopulmonary bypass. *Circulation 58 (Suppl. 1)*: 107.

Fremes, S. E., Weisel, R. D., Mickle, D. A., Ivanov, J., Madonik, M. M., Seawright, S. J., Houle, S., McLaughlin, P. R., and Baird, R. J. (1985). Myocardial metabolism and ventricular function following cold potassium cardioplegia. *J. Thorac. Cardiovasc. Surg. 89*: 531.

Gardner, T. J., Brantigan, J. W., Perna, A. M., Bender, H. W., Brawley, R. K., and Gott, V. L. (1971). Intramyocardial gas tensions in the human heart during coronary artery-saphenous vein bypass. *J. Thorac. Cardiovasc. Surg. 62*: 844.

Gersh, B. J., Kronmal, R. A., Frye, R. L., Schaff, H. V., Ryan, T. J., Gosselin, A. J., Kaiser, G. C., and Killip, T., 3d. (1983). Coronary arteriography and coronary artery bypass surgery: morbidity and mortality in patients ages 65 years or older. A report from the Coronary Artery Surgery Study. *Circulation 67*: 483.

Gold, J. P., Roberts, A. J., Hoover, E. L., Blank, S., Gay, W. A., Jr., and Subramanian, V. A. (1979). Effects of prolonged aortic cross-clamping with potassium cardioplegia on myocardial contractility in man. *Surg. Forum. 30*: 252.

Gray, R., Maddahi, J., Berman, D., Raymond, M., Waxman, A., Ganz, W., Matloff, J., and Swan, H. J. (1979). Scintigraphic and hemodynamic demonstration of transient left ventricular dysfunction immediately after uncomplicated coronary artery bypass grafting. *J. Thorac. Cardiovasc. Surg. 77*: 504.

Greenburg, S., and Frishman, W. H. (1990). Co-enzyme Q10: A new drug for cardiovascular disease. *J. Clin. Pharmacol. 30*: 596.

Greene, P. S., Cameron, D. E., Mohlala, M. L., Dinatale, J. M., and Gardner, T. J. (1989). Systolic and diastolic left ventricular dysfunction due to mild hypothermia. *Circulation 80*: III44.

Hammermeister, K. E., Burchfiel, C., Johnson, R., and Grover, F. L. (1990). Identification of patients at greatest risk for developing major complications at cardiac surgery. *Circulation 82(Suppl. IV)*: IV-380.

Harpole, D. H., Rankin, J. S., Wolfe, W. G., Smith, L. R., Young, W. G., Clements, F. M., and Jones, R. H. (1989). Assessment of left ventricular functional preservation during isolated cardiac valve operations. *Circulation 80*: III1.

Hearse, D. J. (1977). Reperfusion of the ischemic myocardium. *J. Mol. Cell Cardiol. 9*: 605.

Hearse, D. J. (1988). The protection of the ischemic myocardium: Surgical success v. clinical failure. *Prog. Cardiovasc. Dis. 30*: 381.

Hoover, R. L., Karnovsky, M. J., Austen, K. F., Corey, E. J., and Lewis, R. A. (1984). Leukotriene B4 action on endothelium mediates augmented neutrophil/endothelial adhesion. *Proc. Natl. Acad. Sci. USA 81*: 2191.

Illes, R. W., Silverman, N. A., Krukenkamp, I. B., del Nido, P. J., and Levitsky, S. (1989). Amelioration of postischemic stunning by deferoxamine-blood cardioplegia. *Circulation 80*: III30.

Johnson, D. L., Horneffer, P. J., Dinatale, J. M. Jr., Gott, V. L., and Gardner, T. J. (1987). Free radical scavengers improve functional recovery of stunned myocardium in a model of surgical coronary revascularization. *Surgery 102*: 334.

Johnson, W. D., Kayser, K. L., Brenowitz, J. B., and Saedi, S. F. (1991). A randomized controlled trial of allopurinol in coronary bypass surgery. *Am. Heart J. 121*: 20.

Kanter, K. B., Glower, D. D., Schaff, H. V., and Gardner, T. J. (1981). Mechanism of defective oxygen extraction following global ischemia. *J. Surg. Res. 30*: 482.

Kanter, K. R., Ruzevich, S. A., Pennington, D. G., McBride, L. R., Swartz, M. T., and Willman, V. L. (1988). Follow-up of survivors of mechanical circulatory support. *J. Thorac. Cardiovasc. Surg. 96*: 72.

Kanter, K. R., Schaff, H. V., Gott, V. L., and Gardner, T. J. (1982). Reduced oxygen consumption with effective left ventricular venting during postischemic reperfusion. *Circulation 66*: I50.

Kirklin, J. K., Blackstone, E. H., and Kirklin, J. W. (1987). Cardiopulmonary bypass: Studies on its damaging effects. *Blood Purif. 5*: 168.

Kuchar, D. L., Campbell, T. J., and O'Rourke, M. F. (1987). Long-term survival after counterpulsation for medically refractory heart failure complicating myocardial infarction and cardiac surgery. *Eur. Heart J. 8*: 490.

Lauwers, E., Meese, G., Adriaensen, H., Amsel, B., and Van der Mast, M. (1990). Perioperative intra-aortic balloon counterpulsation in cardiosurgery: A retrospective study. *Acta Anaesthesiol. Belg. 41*: 41.

Lazar, H. L., Buckberg, G. D., Manganaro, A. J., Foglia, R. P., Becker, H., Mulder, D. G., and Maloney, J. V., Jr. (1979). Reversal of ischemic damage with secondary blood cardioplegia. *J. Thorac. Cardiovasc. Surg. 78*: 688.

Lytle, B. W., Loop, F. D., Cosgrove, D. M., Taylor, P. C., Goormastic, M., Peper, W., Gill, C. C., Golding, L. A., and Stewart, R. W. (1987). Fifteen hundred coronary reoperations. Results and determinants of early and late survival. *J. Thorac. Cardiovasc. Surg. 93*: 847.

Magovern, G. J. Jr., Flaherty, J. T., Gott, V. L., Bulkley, B. H., and Gardner, T. J. (1982). Optimal myocardial protection with fluosol cardioplegia. *Ann. Thorac. Surg. 34*: 249.

Mangano, D. T. (1985). Biventricular function after myocardial revascularization in humans: Deterioration and recovery patterns during the first 24 hours. *Anesthesiology 62*: 571.

Martin, S. E., Chenoweth, D. E., Engler, R. L., Roth, D. M., and Longhurst, J. C. (1988). C5a decreases regional coronary blood flow and myocardial function in pigs: Implications for a granulocyte mechanism. *Circ. Res. 63*: 483.

McGee, M. G., Zillgitt, S. L., Trono, R., Turner, S. A., Davis, G. L., Fuqua, J. M., Edelman, S. K., and Norman, J. C. (1980). Retrospective analyses of the need for mechanical circulatory support (intraaortic balloon pump/abdominal left ventricular assist device or partial artificial heart) after cardiopulmonary bypass. A 44 month study of 14,168 patients. *Am. J. Cardiol. 46*: 135.

Miller, D. D., Salinas, F., and Walsh, R. A. (1991). Simultaneous cardiac mechanics and phosphorus-31 NMR spectroscopy during global myocardial ischemia and reperfusion in the intact dog. *Magn. Reson. Med. 17*: 41.

Nayler, W. G. (1980). The use of coenzyme Q10 to protect ischemic heart muscle. In *Biomedical and Clinical Aspects of Coenzyme Q10,* Vol. 2 (Y. Yamamura, K. Folkers, and Y. Ito, eds.), Elsevier, Amsterdam, p. 409.

Okamoto, F., Allen, B. S., Buckberg, G. D., Leaf, J., and Bugyi, H. (1986). Reperfusate composition: supplemental role of intravenous and intracoronary coenzyme Q10 in avoiding reperfusion damage. *J. Thorac. Cardiovasc. Surg. 92*: 573.

Olinger, G. N., and Boncheck, L. I. (1978). Ventricular venting during coronary revascularization: Assessment of benefit by intraoperative ventricular function curves. *Ann. Thorac. Surg. 26*: 252.

Otani, H., Engleman, R. M., Rousou, J. A., Breyer, R. H., Clement, R., Prasad, R., Klar, J., and Das, D. K. (1989). Improvement of myocardial function by trifluoperazine, a calmodulin antagonist, after acute coronary artery occlusion and coronary revascularization. *J. Thorac. Cardiovasc. Surg. 97*: 267.

Pae, W. A., Miller, C. A., and Pierce, W. S. (1991). Ventricular assist devices for postcardiotomy cardiogenic shock: A combined registry experience. *J. Thorac. Cardiovasc. Surg.* (in press).

Pennington, D. G., McBride, L. R., Swartz, M. T., Kanter, K. R., Kaiser, G. C., Barner, H. B., Miller, L. W., Naunheim, K. S., Fiore, A. C., and Willman, V. L. (1989). Use of the Pierce-Donachy ventricular assist device in patients with cardiogenic shock after cardiac operations. *Ann. Thorac. Surg. 47*: 130.

Reduto, L. A., Lawrie, G. M., Reid, J. W., Whissenand, H. H., Noon, G. P., Kanon, D., DeBakey, M. E., and Miller, R. R. (1981). Sequential postoperative assessment of left ventricular performance with gated cardiac pool imaging following aortocoronary bypass surgery. *Am. Heart J. 101*: 59.

Rinder, C. S., Wheeler, L. R., and Alpern, W. D. (1988). Pulsed Doppler assessment of diastolic function before and after cardiopulmonary bypass. *Anesthesiology 69*: A2.

Roberts, A. J., Spies, S. M., Sanders, J. H., Moran, J. M., Wilkinson, C. J., Lichtenthal, P. R., White, R. L., and Michaelis, L. L. (1981). Serial assessment of left ventricular performance following coronary artery bypass grafting. Early postoperative results with myocardial protection afforded by multidose hypothermic potassium crystalloid cardioplegia. *J. Thorac. Cardiovasc. Surg. 81*: 69.

Robertson, J. M., Vinten Johansen, J., Buckberg, G. D., Rosenkranz, E. R., and Maloney, J. V. Jr. (1984). Safety of prolonged aortic clamping with blood cardioplegia. I Glutamate enrichment in normal hearts. *J. Thorac. Cardiovasc. Surg. 88*: 395.

Roccatello, D., Formica, M., Cavalli, G., Amprimo, M. C., Pignatelli, M. G., Costa, P., de Paulis, R., Quattrocchio, G., Molino, A., and Giordano, G. (1990). Changes in neutrophil oxidative potential in patients undergoing cardiopulmonary bypass with polypropylene hollow fiber oxygenators. *Artificial Organs 14*: 69.

Rose, D. M., Connolly, M., Cunningham, J. N., Jr., and Spencer, F. C. (1989). Technique and results with a roller pump left and right heart assist device. *Ann. Thorac. Surg. 47*: 124.

Rosenfeldt, F. L. (1982). The relationship between myocardial temperature and recovery after experimental cardioplegic arrest. *J. Thorac. Cardiovasc. Surg. 84*: 656.

Rosenkranz, E. R., and Buckberg, G. D. (1983). Myocardial protection during surgical coronary reperfusion. *J. Am. Coll. Cardiol. 1*: 1235.

Rosenkranz, E. R., Okamoto, F., Buckberg, G. D., Vinten Johansen, J., Robertson, J. M., and Bugyi, H. (1984). Safety of prolonged aortic clamping with blood cardioplegia. II Glutamate enrichment in energy-depleted hearts. *J. Thorac. Cardiovasc. Surg. 88*: 402.

Rousou, J. A., Engelman, R. M., Breyer, R. H., Otani, H., Lemeshow, S. and Das, D. K. (1988). The effect of temperature and hematocrit level of oxygenated cardioplegic solutions on myocardial preservation. *J. Thorac. Cardiovasc. Surg. 95*: 625.

Royster, R. L., Butterworth, J. F. 4th., Prough, D. S., Johnston, W. E., Thomas, J. L., Hogan, P. E., Case, L. D., and Gravlee, G. P. (1991). Preoperative and intraoperative predictors of inotropic support and long-term outcome in patients having coronary artery bypass grafting. *Anesth. Analg. 72*: 729.

Salama, A., Hugo, F., Heinrich, D., Hoge, R., Muller, R., Kiefel, V., Mueller Eckhardt, C. and Bhakdi, S. (1988). Deposition of terminal C5b-9 complement complexes on erythrocytes and leukocytes during cardiopulmonary bypass. *N. Engl. J. Med. 318*: 408.

Salomon, N. W., Page, U. S., Bigelow, J. C., Krause, A. H., Okies, J. E., and Metzdorff, M. T. (1990). Reoperative coronary surgery. Comparative analysis of 6591 patients undergoing primary bypass and 508 patients undergoing reoperative coronary artery bypass. *J. Thorac. Cardiovasc. Surg. 100*: 250.

Schaper, J., Hehrlein, F., Schlepper, M., and Thiedemann, K. U. (1977). Ultrastructural alterations during ischemia and reperfusion in human hearts during cardiac surgery. *J. Mol. Cell Cardiol. 9*: 175.

Schaper, J., Scheld, H. H., Schmidt, U., and Hehrlein, F. (1986). Ultrastructural study comparing the efficacy of five different methods of intraoperative myocardial protection in the human heart. *J. Thorac. Cardiovasc. Surg. 92*: 47.

Schaper, J., Hein, S., and Froede, R. (1990). Morphologic insights in clinical cardioplegia. *J. Moll. Cell Cardiol. 22 (Suppl. V)*: S41 (Abstract).

Schapira, M., Despland, E., Scott, C. F., Boxer, L. A., and Colman, R. W. (1982). Purified human plasma kallikrein aggregates human blood neutrophils. *J. Clin. Invest. 69*: 1199.

Schleimer, R. P., and Rutledge, B. K. (1986). Cultured human vascular endothelial cells acquire adhesiveness for neutrophils after stimulation with interleukin 1, endotoxin, and tumor-promoting phorbol diesters. *J. Immunol. 136*: 649.

Sell, T. L., Purut, C. M., Silva, R., and Jones, R. H. (1991). Recovery of myocardial function during coronary artery bypass grafting. Intraoperative assessment by pressure-volume loops. *J. Thorac. Cardiovasc. Surg. 101*: 681.

Semb, A. G., Vaage, J., and Sorlie, D. (1988). Coronary sequestration of granulocytes after release of the aortic cross clamp in open heart surgery. *J. Thorac. Cardiovasc. Surg. 610*: 610 (Abstract).

Shlafer, M., Kane, P. F., and Kirsh, M. M. (1982a). Superoxide dismutase plus catalase enhances the efficacy of hypothermic cardioplegia to protect the globally ischemic, reperfused heart. *J. Thorac. Cardiovasc. Surg. 83*: 830.

Shlafer, M., Kane, P. F., Wiggins, V. Y., and Kirsh, M. M. (1982b). Possible role for cytotoxic oxygen metabolites in the pathogenesis of cardiac ischemic injury. *Circulation 66*: I85.

Steenberg, C., Murphy, E., Levy, L., and London, R. E. (1987). Elevation in cytosolic free calcium concentration early in myocardial ischemia in perfused rat heart. *Circ. Res. 60*: 700.

Stein, K. L., Breisblatt, W., Wolfe, C., Gasior, T., and Hardesty, R. (1990). Depression and recovery of right ventricular function after cardiopulmonary bypass. *Crit. Care. Med. 18*: 1197.

Stewart, J. R., Blackwell, W. H., Crute, S. L., Loughlin, V., Greenfield, L. J., and Hess, M. L. (1983). Inhibition of surgically induced ischemia/reperfusion injury by oxygen free radical scavengers. *J. Thorac. Cardiovasc. Surg. 86*: 262.

Stewart, J. T., Ward, D. E., Pumphrey, C. W., Redwood, D. R., Parker, D. J., and Gray, H. H. (1990). Original articles: Major complications of coronary arteriography: The place of cardiac surgery. *Br. Heart J. 63*: 74.

Tan, C. K., Glisson, S. N., El Etr, A. A., and Ramakrishnaiah, K. B. (1976). Levels of circulating norepinephrine and epinephrine before, during, and after cardiopulmonary bypass in man. *J. Thorac. Cardiovasc. Surg. 71*: 928.

Tanaka, J., Tominaga, R., Yoshitoshi, M., Matsui, K., Komori, M., Sese, A., Yasui, H., and Tokunaga, K. (1982). Coenzyme Q10: the prophylactic effect on low cardiac output following cardiac valve replacement. *Ann. Thorac. Surg. 33*: 145.

van Oeveren, W., Kazatchkine, M. D., Descamps Latscha, B., Maillet, F., Fischer, E., Carpentier, A., and Wildevuur, C. R. (1985). Deleterious effects of cardiopulmonary bypass. A prospective study of bubble versus membrane oxygenation. *J. Thorac. Cardiovasc. Surg. 89*: 888.

van Vlies, B., van Royen, E. A., Visser, C. A., Meyne, N. G., van Buul, M. M., Peters, R. J., and Dunning, A. J. (1990). Frequency of myocardial indium-111 antimyosin uptake after uncomplicated coronary artery bypass grafting. *Am. J. Cardiol. 66*: 1191.

Wachfogel, Y. T., Harpel, P. C., Edmunds, L. H., Jr., and Colman, R. W. (1989). Formation of C1s-C1-inhibitor, kallikrein-C1-inhibitor, and plasma-alpha2-plasmin-inhibitor complexes during cardiopulmonary bypass. *Blood 73*: 468.

Wehlage, D. R., Bohrer, H., and Ruffmann, K. (1990). Impairment of left ventricular diastolic function during coronary artery bypass grafting. *Anaesthesia 45*: 549.

Weisel, R. D., Mickle, D. A., Finkle, C. D., Tumiati, L. C., Madonik, M. M., Ivanov, J., Burton, G. W., and Ingold, K. U. (1989). Myocardial free-radical injury after cardioplegia. *Circulation 80*: III14.

Westaby, S. (1987). Organ dysfunction after cardiopulmonary bypass. A systemic inflammatory reaction initiated by the extracorporeal circuit. *Intensive Care Med. 13*: 89.

22

Noninvasive Identification and Characterization of Blood Flow and Metabolic Alterations in Myocardial Stunning with Positron Emission Tomography

Heinrich R. Schelbert and Denis Buxton

UCLA School of Medicine, Los Angeles, California

I. INTRODUCTION

While the term myocardial stunning refers to an abnormal state of contractile function, it is also associated with metabolic alterations. As this particular condition is a dynamic process, changing patterns of abnormal substrate metabolism evolve as a function of time after the ischemic insult. These regional metabolic changes can be delineated noninvasively with positron emission tomography, or PET. This new imaging modality affords the evaluation and quantification of regional myocardial oxygen, fatty acid, and glucose metabolism as well as of regional myocardial blood flow. This chapter begins with a description of methodologic aspects of PET, then reviews findings with this noninvasive approach in the animal experimental setting, and subsequently discusses how these experimental observations pertain to patients with coronary artery disease.

II. TECHNICAL ASPECTS OF POSITRON EMISSION TOMOGRAPHY

A quantitative imaging capability and the availability of numerous physiological tracers are features unique to PET (Schelbert, 1991). The high temporal resolution of modern positron emission tomographs permits the noninvasive determination of the arterial input function of a positron emitting tracer and the myocardial tissue response to it. Both parameters are fundamental for the in vivo application of tracer kinetic principles for measurements of regional myocardial rates of substrate fluxes or of biochemical reaction rates. As only the activity concentrations of tracer label in blood and myocardium at any time after tracer administration can be measured, tracer kinetic models are predicated on a thorough understanding of the metabolic fate of the tracer label in tissue and its relation to the very physiological process to be studied. Biochemical validation studies have enabled the measurement and evaluation of regional myocardial oxidative metabolism and, by inference, of myocardial oxygen consumption, myocardial fatty acid metabolism, and exogenous glucose utilization. Moreover, regional myocardial blood flow can be evaluated and quantified with tracers including rubidium-82, N-13 ammonia, and 0-15 water.

A. Measurement of Oxidative Metabolism

Carbon-11-labeled acetate has been proved useful for measurements of regional myocardial oxidative metabolism (Buxton et al., 1988; Brown et al., 1988; Henes et al., 1989; Armbrecht et al., 1989, 1990). The tracer is administered intravenously, accumulates in myocardium in proportion to blood flow, and subsequently clears from myocardium in a biexponential fashion. While the slow clearance curve component appears to be related to incorporation of the tracer label into the myocardial glutamine pool (Ng et al., 1991), the rapid clearance curve component closely correlates with the release of C-11-labeled CO_2 from myocardium and, thus, with tricarboxylic acid (TCA) cycle activity. Because of the close linkage of the TCA cycle to oxidative phosphorylation, the clearance rate of C-11 activity from myocardium has been found to be a useful index of myocardial oxygen consumption. Because biexponential fitting of the myocardial C-11 activity time curve is frequently not possible, an index of oxidative metabolism is usually derived by monoexponential fitting of the initial downslope of the myocardial time activity curve (Henes et al., 1989; Armbrecht et al., 1989).

B. Measurement of Fatty Acid Metabolism

Carbon-11-labeled palmitate serves as a tracer of myocardial fatty acid metabolism (Schön et al., 1982; Schelbert et al., 1985). Because of back diffusion of nonmetabolized tracer from myocardium into blood and its effect on the noninvasively recorded myocardial time activity curve (Fox et al., 1985), this tracer has recently fallen into disrepute. Nevertheless, important information on myocardial fatty acid metabolism can be derived from the clearance curve morphology (Schwaiger et al., 1985; Grover-Mckay et al., 1986). Characteristic is the biexponential clearance pattern, which reflects the distribution of label between immediate oxidative breakdown and release of tracer label in the form of $^{11}CO_2$ and deposition of fatty acid in the endogenous myocardial lipid pool, consisting largely of phospholipids and di- and triglycerides. While the slope of the rapid clearance curve component may be of limited accuracy in describing rates of fluxes of fatty acid through β-oxidation and the TCA cycle, the relative sizes of the two curve components are probably more useful for delineating the distribution of fatty acid between oxidation and storage in myocardium.

C. Measurement of Glucose Utilization

Fluorine-18, 2-fluoro, 2-deoxyglucose traces the transmembranous exchange of glucose from blood into myocytes and the hexokinase mediated phosphorylation of glucose to glucose-6-phosphate as the initial metabolic step of exogenous glucose. Administered intravenously, the tracer accumulates in myocardium in proportion to the rate of the initial phosphorylation of glucose (Phelps et al., 1978). As the tracer becomes essentially trapped in myocardium, its regional myocardial concentrations reflect relative rates of regional glucose consumption. An extensively validated, largely unidirectional transport tracer kinetic model permits estimation of regional rates of glucose utilization in μmol glucose per minute per gram myocardium from serially acquired tomographic images (Ratib et al., 1982; Gambhir et al., 1989).

D. Measurement of Myocardial Blood Flow

N-13 ammonia and 0-15 water have thus far proved particularly useful for evaluating the relative distribution of blood flow as well as absolute measurements in ml blood/min/g myocardium (Schelbert et al., 1981; Bergmann et al., 1984, 1989; Hutchins et al., 1990; Araujo et al., 1991; Kuhle et al., 1991). Again, quantification of blood flow with these tracers is based on serial acquisition of images and appropriate tracer kinetic models.

III. ANIMAL EXPERIMENTAL STUDIES ON MYOCARDIAL STUNNING

A. Studies in Chronically Instrumented Animals

Noninvasive assessment of reperfused myocardium with PET has demonstrated prolonged metabolic abnormalities in stunned myocardium. Schwaiger et al. (1985) studied myocardial blood flow and metabolism with PET in chronically instrumented dogs following a 3-hour occlusion of the left anterior descending coronary artery. They demonstrated that myocardial F-18 deoxyglucose uptake was elevated 24 hours postreperfusion in postischemic myocardium relative to normal tissue (Fig. 1). The increased F-18 deoxyglucose uptake was accompanied by abnormalities in tissue kinetics of [1-^{11}C] palmitate. Clearance of activity from tissue following [1-^{11}C] palmitate administration was prolonged in ischemic tissue during coronary occlusion, consistent with decreased oxidation of fatty acids, and remained depressed 2 hours and 24 hours postreperfusion. The residual activity following the rapid clearance phase was also increased in ischemic tissue, consistent with a greater fraction of labeled palmitate being esterified to triglyceride. Increased accumulation of F-18 deoxyglucose and delayed clearance of [1-^{11}C] palmitate 24 hours postreperfusion were found to identify reversibly injured tissue that would eventually recover function with little necrosis, while the absence of blood flow and palmitate uptake were indicative of extensive necrosis.

F-18 deoxyglucose uptake remained elevated relative to blood flow at 1 week postreperfusion in postischemic tissue (Fig. 2). The myocardial clearance kinetics of [1-^{11}C] palmitate remained abnormal at this time, with a continued elevation of the fraction of label entering esterification. At 1 month postreperfusion, the metabolic abnormalities in postischemic tissue were no longer significant.

Increased F-18 deoxyglucose uptake in postischemic tissue postreperfusion could reflect either increased anaerobic glucose utilization in the reperfused tissue, or a switch in substrate preference leading to increased glucose oxidation. Invasive measurements of substrate utilization in dogs subjected to a 3-hour occlusion of the left anterior descending coronary artery demonstrated that, at 24 hours postreperfusion, increased glucose extraction reflected elevated anaerobic glucose metabolism (Fig. 3) (Schwaiger et al., 1989). Lactate release was greater from postischemic myocardium, and was derived almost exclusively from exogenous glucose; glycogen remained depleted in postischemic myocardium at this time while extraction of oxygen and of free fatty acid was depressed (Schwaiger et al., 1989).

B. Studies Using Shorter Occlusion Periods

The 3-hour coronary artery occlusions employed in the studies described above led to a mixture of reversibly and irreversibly injured tissue. Positron emission tomography has also allowed the demonstration of metabolic abnormalities in dogs subjected to shorter periods of ischemia in which necrosis was not produced (Buxton et al., 1989). Early (at 2 hours) postreperfusion, oxygen consumption as determined with [1-^{11}C] acetate was decreased approx-

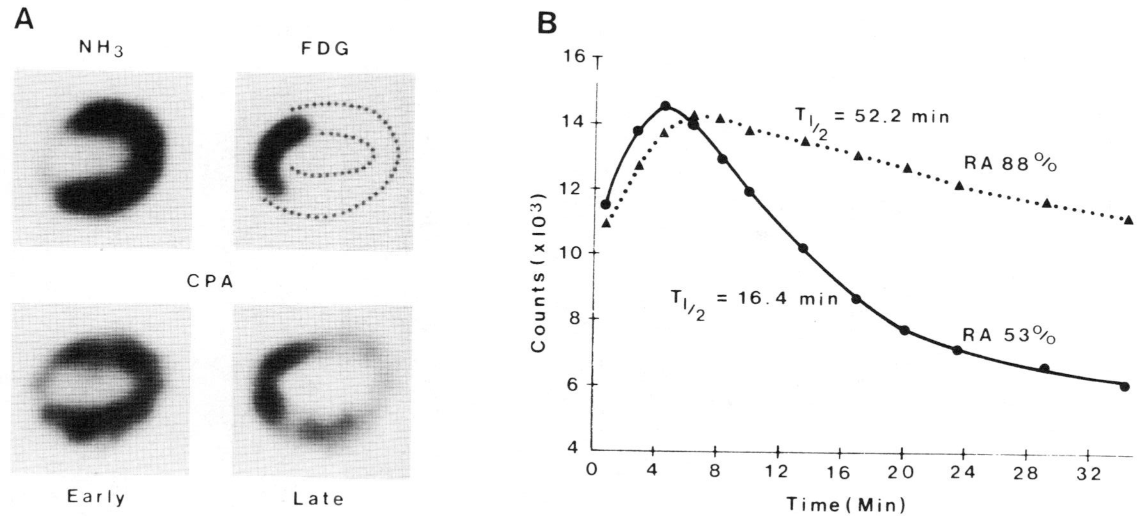

Figure 1 Abnormalities of substrate metabolism in reperfused canine myocardium. (A) Mid-left ventricular transaxial images were obtained in a dog 24 hours after occlusion (3 hours) and reperfusion of the LAD. The animal is on its right side, viewed from the tail; the anterior wall is to the left, septum to the bottom, and posterolateral wall to the right. Myocardial blood flow was assessed with intravenous N-13 ammonia (left top), and shows a residual defect in the reperfused anterior wall. Increased uptake of F-18 deoxyglucose was found in the reperfused tissue (right top). Initial uptake of [1-^{11}C] palmitate was depressed in the region, as seen in the image obtained early after injection of the tracer (bottom left), but clearance of tracer was slower from the reperfused tissue, so that in the late image (bottom right) activity was higher in the reperfused region. (B) Tissue time activity curves for normal (solid line) and reperfused (dotted line) tissue following intravenous administration of [1-^{11}C] palmitate. In reperfused tissue, the clearance half-time and residual activity (RA) at 20 min postinjection were increased. (Reproduced from Schwaiger et al., 1985, with permission of the authors and the *Journal of the American College of Cardiology*.)

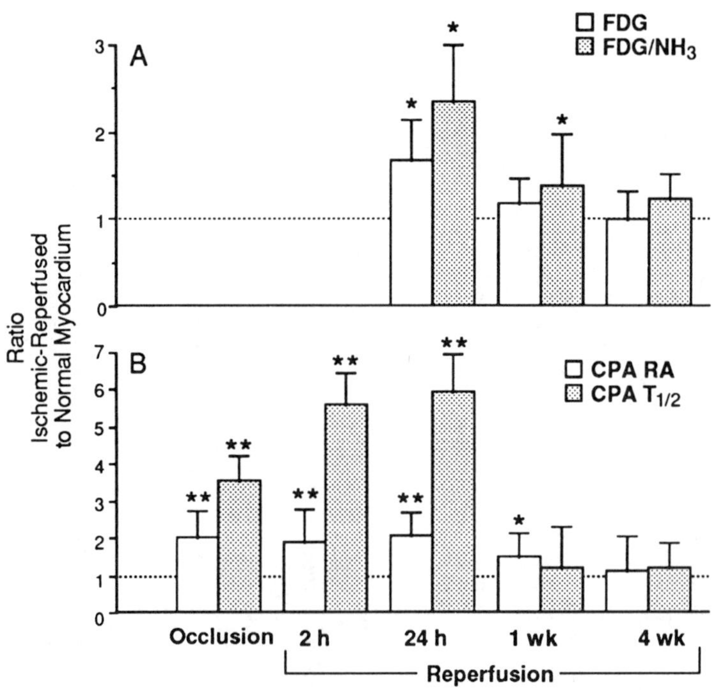

Figure 2 Glucose (A) and fatty acid (B) metabolism during occlusion and reperfusion in chronically instrumented dogs subjected to a 3-hour LAD occlusion. Data are expressed as the ratio of ischemic/reperfused to control myocardium. F-18 deoxyglucose uptake is also normalized to N-13 ammonia uptake (FDG/NH_3). [1-^{11}C] palmitate kinetics are represented by the clearance half-time ($T_{1/2}$) of [1-^{11}C] palmitic acid during the first 20 minutes after injection, and residual activity (RA) at 20 minutes after injection, $^{*}p < 0.05$; $^{**}p < 0.005$ vs. normal tissue. (Adapted from Schwaiger et al., 1989, with permission of the authors and the *Journal of the American College of Cardiology*.)

imately 30% in stunned myocardium previously subjected to a 20-minute intracoronary balloon occlusion (Buxton et al., 1989), while glucose metabolism was not increased in stunned relative to normal myocardium. By 24 hours postreperfusion, the average oxygen consumption in stunned myocardium was no longer significantly depressed. However, in a subset of dogs, a persistent decrease in oxygen consumption was observed which was associated with a more severe impairment in regional wall motion as determined with two-dimensional echocardiography and, further, with increased F-18 deoxyglucose uptake. These results are consistent with increased anaerobic glucose metabolism to compensate for persistent depression of oxidative

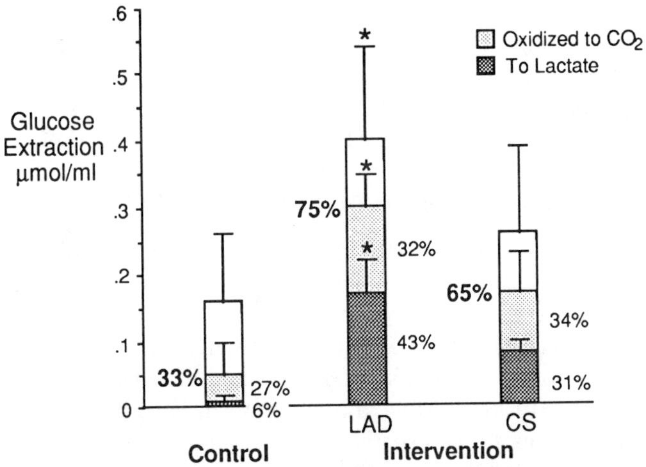

Figure 3 Metabolic fate of exogenous glucose in reperfused myocardium 24 hours after a 3-hour LAD occlusion. The bars represent glucose extraction, the hatched portions and percentage values in light type represent the fraction of the exogenous glucose oxidized to CO_2 and converted to lactate. The percentages in bold type represent the fraction of exogenous glucose entering glycolysis. Control values represent data from 4 dogs, intervention from 9 dogs. $^*p < 0.05$ vs. coronary sinus (CS) values. (Adapted from Schwaiger et al., 1989, with permission of the *Journal of the American College of Cardiology*.)

metabolism at 24 hours postreperfusion in dogs with a greater degree of ischemic injury.

Stunning without necrosis has also been obtained by 1 hour of graded stenosis in canine myocardium to produce akinesia (Heyndrickx et al., 1990; Wyns et al., 1988). Decreased oxygen consumption, demonstrated with [1-^{11}C] acetate, and slower clearance of [1-^{11}C] palmitate were found in stunned myocardium early (<8 h) postreperfusion (Wyns et al., 1988). Pacing or inotropic drugs increased clearance of [1-^{11}C] acetate in stunned myocardium, indicating that the postischemic tissue retained the ability to increase oxygen consumption in response to increased demand (Heyndrickx et al., 1990; Wyns et al., 1988). Similar findings were also obtained in dogs subjected to a 20-minute left anterior descending coronary artery occlusion (Hashimoto et al., 1989).

The findings of decreased oxygen consumption in stunned myocardium using PET are in agreement with several studies using direct measurement of regional MVO_2 by the Fick principle (Myears, 1987; Liedtke et al., 1988; Armbrecht et al., 1990). It should be noted, however, that a number of studies have found MVO_2 to be increased relative to the depressed mechanical function in reperfused myocardium, as reviewed by Zimmer and Bache in Chapter 3 of this volume. Thus, changes in MVO_2 in reperfused myocardium are likely to be highly dependent on the experimental model used. Different models may introduce many variables, including variable degrees of dysfunction and temporal differences between reperfusion and sampling of MVO_2.

C. Quantitative PET Studies in Stunned Myocardium

Earlier studies of stunned myocardium with PET were limited in spatial and temporal resolution by the tomograph capabilities, which hampered quantitative studies. In recent studies using chronically instrumented dogs subjected to a 3-hour intracoronary balloon occlusions of the left anterior descending coronary artery (Buxton et al., 1990a,b; Buxton and Schelbert, 1992), quantitative measurements of blood flow and metabolism have been made employing modern, high temporal and spatial resolution tomographs, allowing the area at risk to be divided into reversibly injured and infarct-containing sectors based on postmortem triphenyltetrazolium chloride (TTC) staining.

Blood flow returned to normal rapidly following reperfusion in the reversibly injured, stunned myocardium, but remained depressed in the sectors containing a mixture of reversibly and irreversibly injured tissue. Oxygen consumption, measured with [1-^{11}C] acetate, was depressed approximately 30% in stunned sectors, and recovered only slowly, remaining slightly depressed even 1 month postreperfusion. This depression of MVO_2 despite normalization of blood flow indicates decreased oxygen extraction in postischemic tissue (Buxton et al., 1990b). The recovery of MVO_2 paralleled functional improvement.

Glucose uptake, measured with F-18 deoxyglucose, was also depressed in stunned tissue early (at 3 hours) postreperfusion (Buxton and Schelbert, 1992). However, at 24 hours postreperfusion F-18 deoxyglucose uptake was higher in stunned myocardium relative to normal tissue. Relative increases in glucose metabolism in stunned tissue were found only when the glucose metabolic rate was low (Fig. 4). Similar results were obtained in dogs subjected to a 20-minute occlusion of the left anterior descending coronary artery (Vaghaiwalla-Mody et al., 1990). This suggests that the regulation of glucose metabolism by plasma substrates and hormones is altered in stunned tissue. In normal tissue, an inverse relationship was found between glucose metabolic rate and the plasma free fatty acid concentration, while in stunned tissue this relationship was not significant, suggesting that glucose metabolism in stunned tissue may be less susceptible to suppression by fatty acid (Buxton and Schelbert, 1992). Abnormal palmitate kinetics were also found in this study in reperfused tissue, with decreased palmitate clearance and increased esterification of tracer (Buxton et al., 1990a).

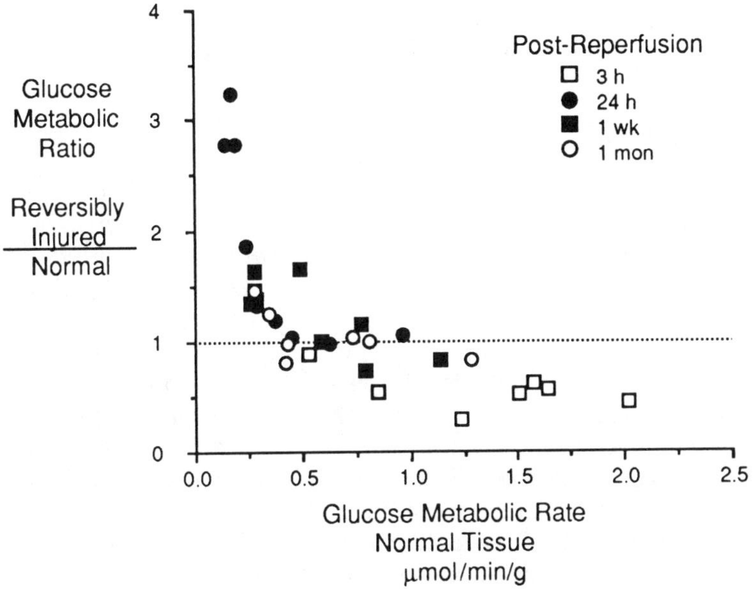

Figure 4 Relative glucose metabolic rate in reversibly injured tissue as a function of glucose metabolic rate in normal tissue at 3 hours, 24 hours, 1 week, and 1 month postreperfusion in dogs subjected to a 3-hour LAD occlusion. (Reproduced from Buxton and Schelbert, 1991, with permission of the *American Journal of Physiology.*)

Thus, animal studies with PET have demonstrated that stunned myocardium is characterized by decreased oxidative metabolism and a decrease in the ability of fatty acids to suppress glucose metabolism. This leads to relative increases in glucose utilization in reperfused tissue relative to normal myocardium, but only when glucose metabolic rates are low in normal myocardium. Twenty-four hours postreperfusion, the relative increase in glucose metabolism in stunned myocardium reflects increased anaerobic metabolism; it is unclear at present whether sustained increases in anaerobic glucose metabolism are found at later times.

IV. OBSERVATIONS IN HUMAN MYOCARDIAL STUNNING

The findings in animal experiments form a base for the study of myocardial stunning in human myocardium. Stunning refers to the functional sequelae after transient episodes of myocardial ischemia. Defined as an imbalance between demand and supply, ischemia can result from an acute but transient increase in demand in excess of supply, as, for example, during physical stress associated with an inadequate increase in supply of blood and oxygen (demand-induced ischemia).

A. Findings After Demand-Induced Ischemia

Kloner et al. (1991) recently reported transient wall motion abnormalities on two-dimensional echocardiography that persisted for at least 30 minutes after exercise stress-induced ischemia in patients with coronary artery disease. The segmental increase in F-18 deoxyglucose as observed by Camici et al. (1986) in coronary artery disease after supine bicycle exercise coincides temporarily with this transient impairment of contractile function and thus most likely represents a metabolic "fingerprint" of myocardial stunning after demand-induced myocardial ischemia. Repeated imaging of blood flow with rubidium-82 before, during, and after exercise revealed transient segmental flow defects. F-18 deoxyglucose was administered in these patients after resolution of the exercise-induced flow defects, which usually occurred within 15-20 minutes following cessation of exercise. Of note is that exercise-induced electrocardiographic abnormalities resolved more slowly than the flow defects and thus were present at the time of tracer injection. The investigators concluded that the enhanced postexercise glucose uptake might represent restoration of depleted glycogen pools and subsequently supported this conclusion by findings in isolated heart experiments (Camici and Bailey, 1984). On the other hand, it is also possible that other mechanisms, as, for example, a segmental augmentation of anaerobic glycolysis observed in animals after low-flow ischemia, might have accounted for this finding (Schwaiger et al., 1989). No comparisons were made with regional wall motion and its time course following exercise.

Similar observations were recently reported by Krivokapich et al. (1991) (Fig. 5). The same group of investigators also used inotropic stimulation with dobutamine as an alternative to exercise stress, which produced similar alterations (Krivokapich et al., unpublished data). Relative to normal myocardium, increases in blood flow were attenuated in territories supplied by significantly stenosed coronary arteries. Fluorine-18 deoxyglucose, administered in these studies at the end of a second dobutamine infusion, which achieved heart rate and rate pressure response similar to that during the stress study for blood flow, revealed segmental increases in glucose utilization in segments with dobutamine-induced flow deficits.

Acute stress-induced ischemia produces similar segmental increases in glucose utilization and thus may be difficult to distinguish from the metabolic pattern observed in stunned myocardium. In the study by Camici et al. (1986), for example, F-18 deoxyglucose was administered in eight patients after su-

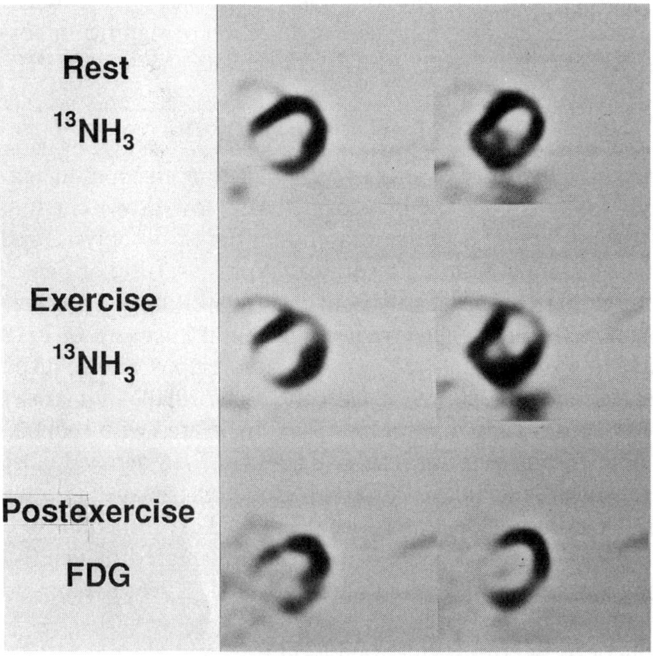

Figure 5 Metabolic consequences of demand-induced myocardial stunning in a patient with significant circumflex coronary artery disease. Myocardial blood flow was evaluated with intravenous N-13 ammonia at baseline (Rest $^{13}NH_3$) and again during supine bicycle exercise (Exercise $^{13}NH_3$) followed by evaluation of regional myocardial glucose utilization with intravenous F-18 deoxyglucose (postexercise FDG). Two transaxial tomographic images of the left ventricular myocardium are shown from left to right. Note the relatively homogeneous distribution of blood flow at baseline (top) and the stress-induced flow defect in the anterior wall (center panel). Following the exercise stress, glucose utilization is selectively enhanced in the postischemic territory of the left anterior descending coronary artery (lower panel). (Reproduced with permission of the *American Heart Journal* from Krivokapich et al., 1991.)

pine bicycle exercise. In contrast to injection of tracer after exercise, if F-18 deoxyglucose were given during exercise, its uptake might be uniform so that tracer uptake in acutely ischemic segments would be increased only if compared to the acutely reduced blood flow. Because of higher substrate demands in normal myocardium during exercise, glucose utilization would be increased. As contractile work and, thus, substrate demand in normal myocardium declined after exercise, F-18 deoxyglucose uptake would decline accordingly but persist in postischemically stunned myocardium. The approach further might prove useful for defining the metabolic consequences of an attenuated flow response to exercise stress and enhance the detection of significant coronary artery disease as suggested recently by Krivokapich and coworkers (1991).

B. Myocardial Stunning After Low-Flow Ischemia

As mentioned earlier, the majority of studies with PET in both experimental animals as well as in humans have been performed after low-flow ischemia: i.e., in patients after an acute myocardial infarction, after thrombolysis, and after interventional revascularization via surgical bypass grafting or percutaneous coronary angioplasty. Initial studies in early postinfarction patients without prior coronary thrombolysis revealed segmental increases in F-18 deoxyglucose uptake in a substantial fraction of infarct regions with reduced blood flow (Schwaiger et al., 1986, 1987; Czernin et al., 1990). In a subset of patients, hypoperfused myocardial regions were associated with reduced [1-^{11}C] palmitate uptake, but in instances of augmented F-18 deoxyglucose uptake, clearance of tracer label in the "infarct region" was delayed relative to that in remote myocardium. Consistent with the animal experimental findings, this delayed tracer clearance probably reflected increased deposition of fatty acid in the endogenous lipid pool (Schwaiger et al., 1986; Rosamond et al., 1987).

Concordant reductions in both segmental blood flow and glucose utilization accurately identify necrosis and subsequent scar tissue formation in clinical infarct regions as contractile function in such segments remained invariably depressed when reexamined 10-14 weeks later (Schwaiger et al., 1986). In contrast, different mechanisms might account for the augmented glucose utilization in infarct regions with blood flow metabolism mismatches. Such mechanisms are likely to include (1) a critical ischemic injury; (2) myocardial hibernation; and (3) myocardial stunning. The latter mechanism most likely existed in those myocardial segments that recovered contractile function spontaneously when reexamined several weeks after the acute myocardial infarction (Schwaiger et al., 1986; Czernin et al., 1991). The relatively high incidence of a blood flow-metabolism mismatch in patients with recent myocardial infarctions (Marshall et al., 1983; Hashimoto et al., 1988) suggests further that possibly as a result of persistently low segmental blood flow, the initial ischemic injury in a substantial portion of clinical infarct regions proceeded into a state of "myocardial hibernation." Another possibility, as suggested in preliminary reports by Nienaber et al. (1989) and Czernin et al. (1991), is that myocardial stunning may persist for prolonged periods in some segments while contractile function remains depressed and glucose utilization elevated despite an improvement, though only moderate, in segmental myocardial blood flow. As a third possibility, metabolic activity may have persisted early after the acute event because of some residual blood flow. However, because the magnitude of residual blood flow was insufficient to maintain metabolic activity for prolonged time periods, it is possible that ischemia progressed to necrosis and scar tissue formation. The conversion of an initial blood flow-metabolism mismatch to a blood flow-metabolism match as demonstrated by Schwaiger et al. (1986) supports the latter possibility. Equally important is the observation of a strong statistical association between blood flow-metabolism mismatches and residual antegrade blood flow through the infarct vessel (Schwaiger et al., 1987), again supporting the possibility that a significant fraction of blood flow-metabolism mismatches early after an acute myocardial infarction did in fact represent myocardial stunning.

While these initial observations were made in patients without thrombolysis or acute interventional revascularization, more recent studies in patients after revascularization therapy described findings characteristic of myocardial stunning. For example, preliminary observations demonstrated the classis disparity between blood flow and oxygen consumption as initially reported in animal experimental studies (Stahl et al., 1988; Nicklas and Gips, 1989). Serial investigations with ^{15}O water and [1-^{11}C] acetate in patients within 24 hours and at 48 hours after successful thrombolysis and again at hospital discharge revealed normal flows in reperfused "infarct" regions but markedly depressed oxidative metabolism, which had significantly improved at the time of hospital discharge (Henes et al., 1989). Similarly, Pierard et al. (1990) observed blood-flow metabolism mismatches in 11 of 17 patients (65%) at 9 days after thrombolysis. Consistent with animal experimental observations in stunned myocardium (Hashimoto et al., 1989), inotropic stimulation with intravenous dobutamine produced a transient improvement in contractile function in myocardial regions with blood flow-metabolism mismatches but not in infarct regions without augmented glucose utilization. Parenthetically, these observations raised the question of whether myocardial stunning can be equally well detected via a positive response of contractile function to inotropic stimulation. This issue clearly needs further investigation.

Serial studies with PET have further explored the time course of metabolic and functional recovery of "myocardial stunning" in postinfarction patients. Compared to 3.4 days after an acute myocardial infarction, blood flow had significantly improved in infarct regions exhibiting flow-metabolism mismatches during the early postinfarction period but not in segments with flow-metabolism matches when examined 97 days later (Czernin et al., 1991). Associated with this improvement were increases in segmental oxidative metabolism and in segmental wall motion. Interestingly, some blood flow-metabolism matches noted during the early postinfarction period revealed, on follow-up, augmented glucose utilization rates and thus had converted to mismatches. This occurred, however, without an improvement in regional blood flow or contractile function. These observations suggest that (1) depending on the severity of the transient ischemic injury, segmental blood flow, glucose utilization, oxidative metabolism, and contractile function may be altered to various extents in stunned myocardium; (2) the recovery from myocardial stunning may be highly variable; and (3) blood flow-metabolism mismatches after interventional revascularization generally do indicate the presence of stunned myocardium. In some instances, however, stunning may also result in blood flow-metabolism matches, presumably because of a more severe ischemic injury.

C. Chronic Coronary Artery Disease

The situation in patients with chronic coronary artery disease appears to be more complex. While blood flow-metabolism mismatches generally indicate the presence of potentially reversible contractile dysfunction and have been equated with "myocardial hibernation," it is also possible that a substantial fraction of such myocardial segments reflect "myocardial stunning" rather than hibernation. It is important to emphasize that 61% of dysfunctional myocardial regions in which contractile function improved after surgical revascularization exhibited normal blood flow and glucose metabolism prior to bypass grafting (Tillisch et al., 1986). It is possible that the impairment of contractile function in these segments resulted from "stunning" rather than from "hibernation" (Figs. 6,7). As another possibility, "stunning" may, in some instances, be superimposed on myocardial hibernation. Given the fact that contractile function fails to fully recover after revascularization in the majority of myocardial regions, it is further possible that in dysfunctional regions, "hibernating myocardium" and "stunned myocardium" coexist with myocardial fibrosis. Furthermore, the impairment of contractile function in many patients with chronic coronary artery disease may not result from a single transient ischemic episode but from repeated, symptomatic, or silent ischemic episodes and thus may reflect more "repetitive stunning."

Much of the difficulty in clearly defining the nature of chronic reversible segmental dysfunction (or "myocardial hibernation") is due to the lack of an appropriate experimental animal model. Studies in isolated heart preparations with moderate short-term reductions in myocardial blood flow have suggested that contractile function promptly returns upon restitution of blood flow (Marban, 1991). It remains, however, questionable whether such flow reductions of only 30 minutes can in fact be equated with myocardial hibernation. On the other hand, moderate flow reductions for as long as 5 hours in

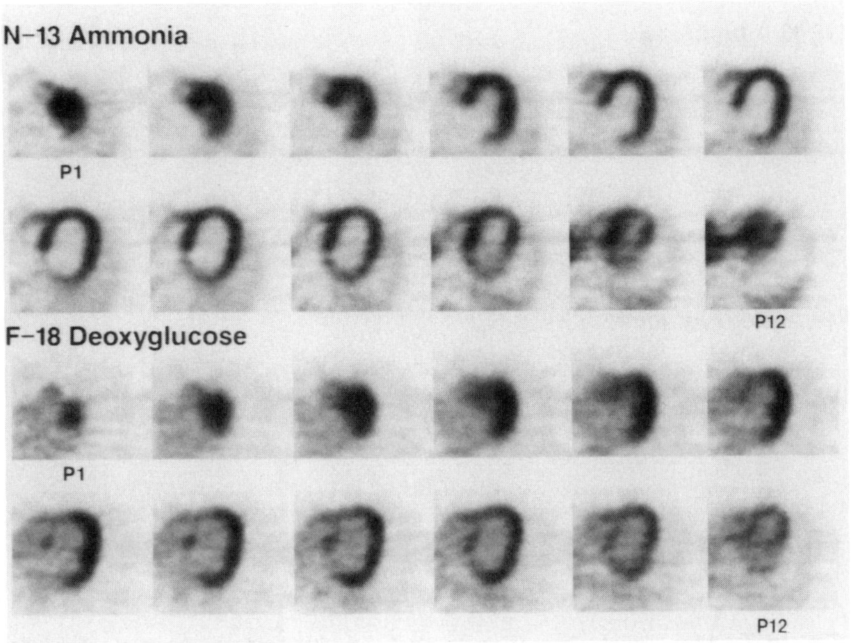

Figure 6 Myocardial stunning in coronary artery disease. The upper two rows depict 12 contiguous transaxial images of myocardial blood flow (N-13 ammonia) and the lower panel the corresponding images of exogenous glucose utilization (F-18 deoxyglucose). Images are shown from top (P1) to bottom (P12). Note the relatively homogeneous blood flow but the strikingly enhanced glucose utilization in the anterolateral and lateral wall. The images demonstrate a blood flow-metabolism mismatch. In this patient with left circumflex disease and mild hypokinesis of the lateral wall but normal blood flow, the augmented glucose utilization most likely represented stunning.

the canine myocardium were followed by considerable delays in functional recovery (Matsuzaki et al., 1983). Of interest in this context are recent observations in patients with blood flow-metabolism mismatches who underwent coronary angioplasty. For the group as a whole, segmental blood flow promptly improved after angioplasty while wall motion abnormalities remained initially unchanged (Nienaber et al., 1991). On late follow-up no further significant improvement in myocardial blood flow was noted, while wall motion had significantly improved (Figs. 8,9). When patients were categorized into those with stable and unstable angina, a different pattern emerged. Wall motion in stable angina patients appeared to improve in parallel with myocardial blood flow. In contrast, in patients with unstable angina, wall motion ab-

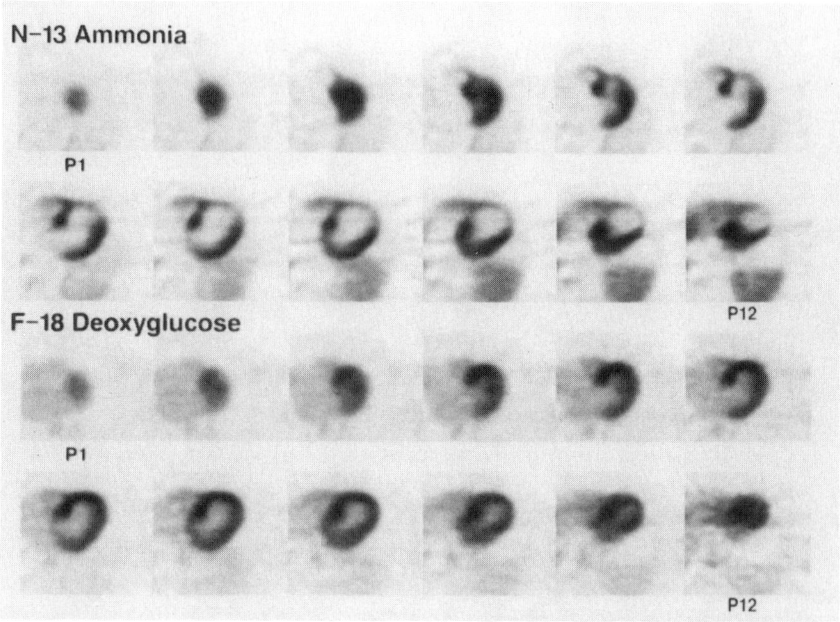

Figure 7 Myocardial hibernation in a patient with chronic coronary artery disease. The transaxial images of myocardial blood flow and of glucose utilization are arranged in the same fashion as in Figure 6. Unlike in the patient shown in Figure 6, blood flow is decreased in the anterolateral and lateral walls while glucose utilization is preserved, resulting in a blood flow-metabolism mismatch. Also unlike the patient in Figure 6, blood flow is reduced in the dysfunctional lateral wall.

Figure 9 Recovery of regional contractile function after angioplasty. Serially, two- and four-chamber views of the heart were obtained by two-dimensional echocardiography in the same patient shown in Figure 8. The numbers indicate the severity of wall motion abnormality (normal = 3, mild hypokinesis = 2, severe hypokinesis = 1, akinesis = 0, dyskinesis = -1). Note the severely impaired systolic wall motion in the territory of the left anterior descending coronary artery prior to angioplasty. Three days after angioplasty, wall blood flow and glucose utilization had largely returned to normal (see Fig. 8), wall motion remained essentially unchanged. However, when reexamined 2 weeks later, contractile function of the anterior wall has largely normalized. The striking temporal disparity between improvement in blood flow and wall motion is consistent with myocardial stunning. (Reproduced from Nienaber et al., 1991, with permission of the authors and the *Journal of the American College of Cardiology*.)

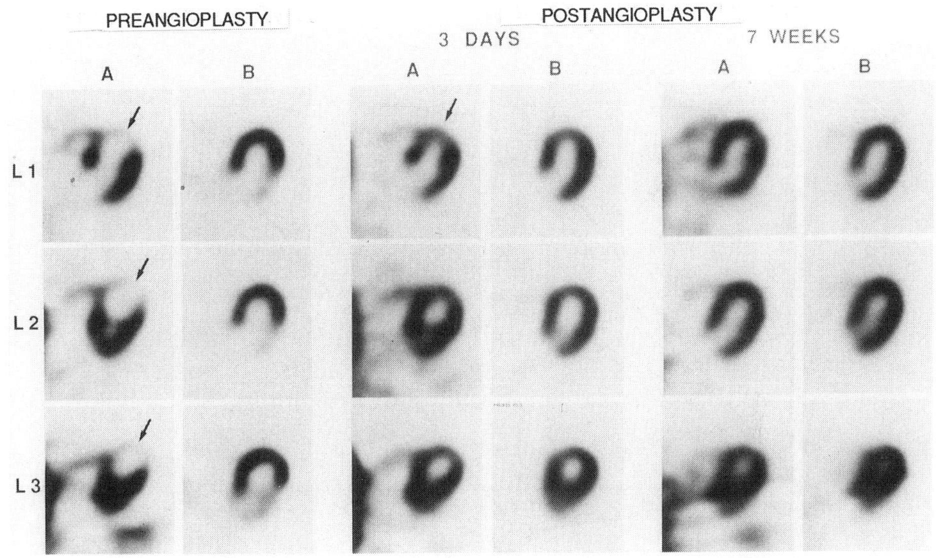

Figure 8 Serial changes in myocardial blood flow (A) and glucose utilization (B) in a patient with unstable angina before and after successful angioplasty of a subtotal occlusion of the proximal left anterior descending coronary artery. Note the strikingly reduced blood flow in the anterior wall (as seen in the three contiguous transaxial images) and the augmented glucose uptake. Both have normalized three days after angioplasty and remain normal when reexamined at 2 months.

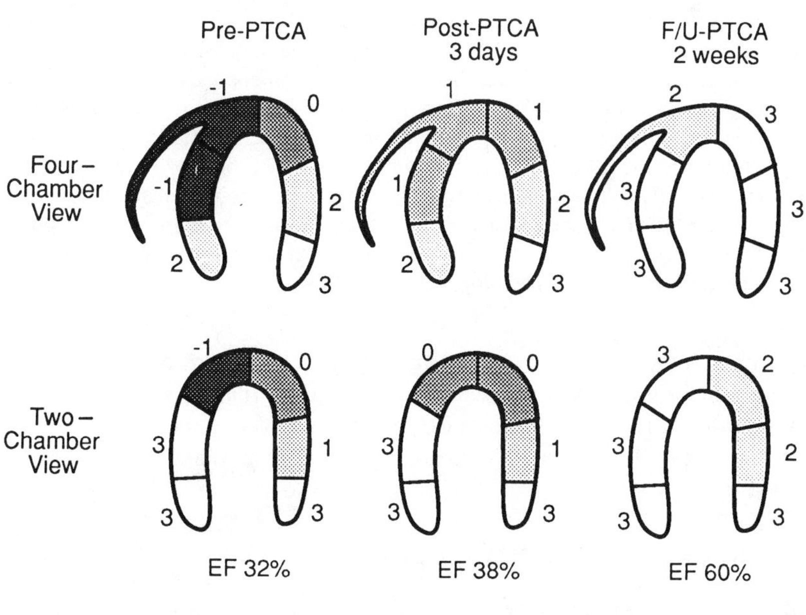

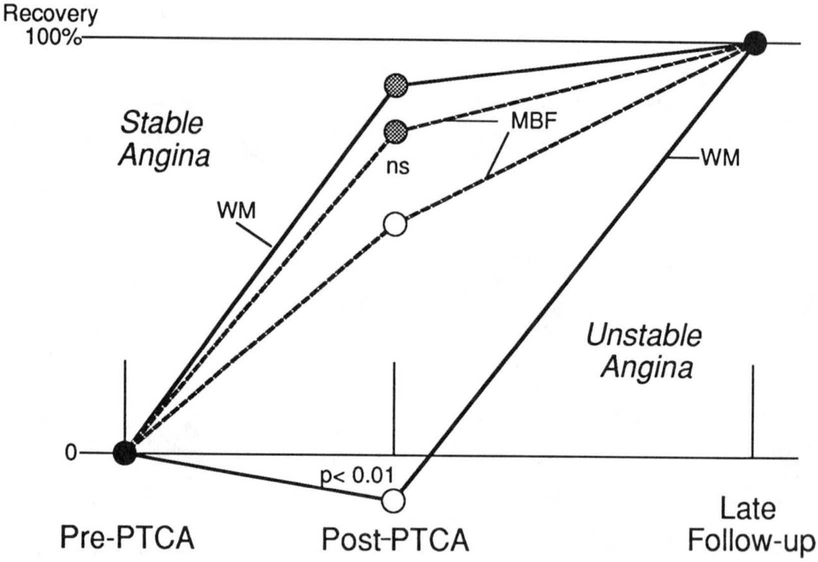

Figure 10 Serial changes in myocardial blood flow and systolic wall motion after angioplasty in 12 coronary artery disease patients with blood flow-metabolism mismatches. Patients were subgrouped into those who presented with stable angina and those who presented with unstable angina. The amount of improvement in both blood flow and wall motion as noted at the time of the late follow-up study (at 68 days after angioplasty) was defined as 100% and compared to the change observed at 48 hours after angioplasty. In patients with stable angina, blood flow and contractile function appeared to have recovered in parallel as compared to patients with unstable angina, in whom wall motion abnormalities initially persisted unchanged despite an early striking improvement in blood flow. Thus, it appears that stunning may have been the pervading mechanism explaining the wall motion abnormalities in the unstable angina patient. On the other hand, it should be emphasized that both the extent and severity of blood flow abnormalities and blood flow-metabolism mismatches were significantly larger in patients with unstable than in patients with stable angina. (Adapted from Nienaber et al., 1991, with permission of the authors and the *Journal of the American College of Cardiology*.)

normalities remained initially unchanged despite a prompt and significant improvement in segmental myocardial blood flow. It is thus possible that disparate rates of recovery of blood flow and contractile function in the latter group did in fact represent myocardial stunning in patients with unstable angina (Fig. 10).

V. SUMMARY AND CONCLUSIONS

Positron emission tomography permits the noninvasive assessment of metabolic consequences of myocardial stunning. Experimental animal as well as clinical investigations have demonstrated a relative or absolute augmentation of exogenous glucose utilization as the dominant feature of substrate metabolism in viable, postischemic myocardium. While the augmented glucose utilization is associated in animal models with an increase in anaerobic glycolysis despite adequate oxygen supply, it remains unclear whether the same applies to human myocardial stunning. Animal studies have further pointed out the dynamic nature of metabolic abnormalities in stunned myocardium. Observations in human myocardium are consistent with these findings. Thus, abnormally increased glucose utilization in the presence of adequate coronary flow usually indicates myocardial stunning. However, because of the dynamic nature of myocardial stunning, glucose utilization and oxidative metabolism may be severely depressed, especially early after reperfusion. Thus, in some instances, such as early after an acute infarction, even blood flow-metabolism mismatches may exist in stunned myocardium. Generally, however, either normal blood flow and glucose metabolism, or preserved or even enhanced glucose utilization together with adequate coronary blood flow, identifies dysfunctional myocardium as stunned.

ACKNOWLEDGMENTS

Our laboratory is operated for the U.S. Department of Energy by the University of California under Contract #DE-AC03-76-SF00012. This work was supported in part by the Director of the Office of Energy Research, Office of Health and Environmental Research, Washington, D.C., by Research Grants #HL 29845 and #HL 33177, National Institutes of Health, Bethesda, MD, and by an Investigative Group Award by the Greater Los Angeles Affiliate of the American Heart Association, Los Angeles, CA.

The authors are grateful to Eileen Rosenfeld for her skillful assistance in preparing this manuscript and to Wendy Wilson for preparation of the illustrations.

REFERENCES

Araujo, L., Lammertsma, A., Rhodes, C., McFalls, E., Iida, H., Rechavia, E., Galassi, A., De Silva, R., Jones, T., and Maseri, A. (1991). Noninvasive quantification of regional myocardial blood flow in coronary artery disease with oxygen-15-labeled carbon dioxide inhalation and positron emission tomiography. *Circulation 83*: 875.

Armbrecht, J. J., Buxton, D. B., Brunken, R. C., Phelps, M. E., and Schelbert, H. R. (1989). Regional myocardial oxygen consumption determined noninvasively in humans with [1-^{11}C] acetate and dynamic positron tomography. *Circulation 80*: 863.

Armbrecht, J. J., Buxton, D. B., and Schelbert, H. R. (1990). Validation of [1-^{11}C] acetate as a tracer for noninvasive assessment of oxidative metabolism with positron emission tomography in normal, ischemic, post-ischemic and hyperemic canine myocardium. *Circulation 81*: 1594.

Bergmann, S. R., Fox, K. A. A., Rand, A. L., McElvany, K. D., Welch, M. J., Markham, J., and Sobel, B. E. (1984). Quantification of regional myocardial blood flow in vivo with $H_2{}^{15}O$. *Circulation 70*: 724.

Bergmann, S. R., Herrero, P., Markham, J., Weinheimer, C. J., and Walsh, M. N. (1989). Noninvasive quantitation of myocardial blood flow in human subjects with oxygen-15-labeled water and positron emission tomography. *J. Am. Coll. Cardiol. 14*: 639.

Brown, M. A., Myears, D. W., and Bergmann, S. R. (1988). Noninvasive assessment of canine myocardial oxidative metabolism with ^{11}C-acetate and positron emission tomography. *J. Am. Coll. Cardiol. 12*: 1054.

Buxton, D. B., Schwaiger, M., Nguyen, A., Phelps, M. E., and Schelbert, H. R. (1988). Radiolabeled acetate as a tracer of myocardial tricarboxylic acid cycle flux. *Circ. Res. 63*: 628.

Buxton, D. B., Schwaiger, M., Vaghaiwalla-Mody, F., Krivokapich, J., Nienaber, C., Armbrecht, J., Luxen, A., Ratib, O., Phelps, M. E., and Schelbert, H. R. (1989). Regional abnormality of oxygen consumption in reperfused myocardium assessed with [1-^{11}C] acetate and positron emission tomography. *Am. J. Cardiac. Imaging* 276.

Buxton, D. B., Vaghaiwalla-Mody, F., Phelps, M. E., and Schelbert, H. R. (1990a). Quantitative measurement of sustained metabolic abnormalities in reperfused canine myocardium. *J. Nucl. Med. 31*: 795.

Buxton, D. B., Vaghaiwalla-Mody, F., Krivokapich, J., Hansen, H. W., Phelps, M. E., and Schelbert, H. R. (1990b). Oxygen utilization and blood flow in reperfused canine myocardium. *Circulation 82* (Suppl. III) 480 (Abstract).

Buxton, D. B., and Schelbert, H. R. (1992). Measurement of regional glucose metabolic rates in reperfused myocardium. *Am. J. Physiol.* (in press).

Camici, P., and Bailey, I. A. (1984). Time course of myocardial glycogen repletion following acute transient ischemia. *Circulation 70* (Suppl II): 85(Abstract).

Camici, P., Araujo, L. I., Spinks, T., Lammertsma, A. A., Kaski, J. C., Shea, M. J., Selwyn, A. P., Jones, T., and Maseri, A. (1986). Increased uptake of ^{18}F-fluorodeoxyglucose in postischemic myocardium of patients with exercise-induced angina. *Circulation 74*: 81.

Czernin, J., Porenta, G., Brunken, R., Chan, S., Kuhle, W., Phelps, M., and Schelbert, H. (1990). Oxidative and glycolytic metabolic tissue characterization in patients with acute infarction using dynamic PET. *J. Nucl. Med. 31*: 774.

Czernin, J., Porenta, G., Brunken, R., Bennet, R., Tillisch, J., Phelps, M. E., and Schelbert, H. R. (1991). Metabolic and functional fate of viable myocardium by PET early after acute infarction. *J. Am. Coll. Cardiol. 17*: 120A (Abstract).

Fox, K. A. A., Abendschein, D. R., Ambos, H. D., Sobel, B. E., and Bergmann, S. R. (1985). Efflux of metabolized and nonmetabolized fatty acid from canine myocardium. Implications for quantifying myocardial metabolism tomographically. *Circ. Res. 57*: 232.

Gambhir, S. S., Schwaiger, M., Huang, S. C., Krivokapich, J., Schelbert, H. R., Nienaber, C. A., and Phelps M. E. (1989). Simple noninvasive quantification method for measuring myocardial glucose utilization in humans employing positron emission tomography and fluorine-18 deoxyglucose. *J. Nucl. Med. 30*: 359.

Grover-McKay, M., Schelbert, H. R., Schwaiger, M., Sochor, H., Guzy, P. M., Child, J. S., and Phelps, M. E. (1986). Identification of impaired metabolic reserve by atrial pacing in patients with significant coronary artery stenosis. *Circulation 74*: 281.

Hashimoto, T., Kambara, H., Fudo, T., Hayashi, M., Tamaki, S., Tokunaga, S., Tamaki, N., Yonekura, Y., Konishi, J., and Kawai, C. (1988). Non-Q wave versus Q wave myocardial infarction: Regional myocardial metabolism and blood flow assessed by positron emission tomography. *J. Am. Coll. Cardiol. 12*: 88.

Hashimoto, T., Nienaber, C. A., Buxton, D. B., Armbrecht, J. J., Krivokapich, J., Phelps, M. E., and Schelbert, H. R. (1989). Disparity between blood flow and oxygen consumption in reperfused canine myocardium. *Circulation 80* (Suppl. II): 241(Abstract).

Henes, C. G., Walsh, M. N., Sobel, B. E., and Geltman, E. M. (1989a). Assessment of myocardial oxidative metabolic reserve with positron emission tomography and carbon-11 acetate. *J. Nucl. Med. 30*: 1489.

Henes, C. G., Bergmann, S. R., Walch, M. N., and Geltman, E. M. (1989b). Recovery of myocardial perfusion and oxygen consumption after thrombolysis delineated with positron emission tomography (PET). *Circulation 80* (Suppl. II): II-312(Abstract).

Heyndrickx, G. R., Wijns, W., Vogelaers, D., Bol, A., Vanoverschelde, J. L., Labar, D., Vambutsele, R., and Melin, J. A. (1990). Oxidative metabolism in stunned myocardium is enhanced by inotropic interventions. *Circulation 80*: II-600(Abstract).

Hutchins, G., Schwaiger, M., Rosenspire, K., Krivokapich, J., Schelbert, H., and Kuhl, D. (1990). Noninvasive quantification of regional blood flow in the human heart using N-13 ammonia and dynamic positron emission tomographihc imaging. *J. Am. Coll. Cardiol. 15*: 1032.

Kloner, R. A., Allen, J., Cox, T. A., Zheng, Y., and Ruiz, C. E. (1991). Stunned left ventricular myocardium after exercise treadmill testing in coronary artery disease. *Am. J. Cardiol. 68*: 329.

Krivokapich, J., Huang, S-C., Ratib, O., and Schelbert, H. R. (1991). Noninvasive detection of functionally significant coronary artery stenoses with exercise and positron emission tomography. *Am. Heart J. 122*: 202.

Kuhle, W., Porenta, G., Buxton, D., Huang, S. C., Hansen, H., Phelps, M. E., and Schelbert, H. R. (1991). Quantification of regional myocardial blood flow using N-13 ammonia and reoriented dynamic PET imaging. *J. Nucl. Med. 32*: 909.

Liedtke, A. J., DeMaison, L., Eggleston, A. M., Cohen, L. M., and Nellis, S. H. (1988). Changes in substrate metabolism and effects of excess fatty acids in reperfused myocardium. *Circ. Res. 62*: 535.

Marban, E. (1991). Myocardial stunning and hibernation: The physiology behind the colloquiolisms. *Circulation 83*: 681.

Marshall, R. C., Tillisch, J. H., Phelps, M. E., Huang, S. C., Carson, R. C., Henze, E., and Schelbert, H. R. (1983). Identification and differentiation of resting myocardial ischemia and infarction in man with positron computed tomography. ^{18}F-labeled fluorodeoxyglucose and N-13 ammonia. *Circulation 67*: 766.

Matsuzaki, M., Gallagher, K. P., Kemper, W. S., White, F., and Ross, J., Jr. (1983). Sustained regional dysfunction produced by prolonged coronary stenosis: Gradual recovery after reperfusion. *Circulation 68*: 170.

Myears, D. W., Sobel, B. E., and Bergmann, S. R. (1987). Substrate use in ischemic and reperfused canine myocardium: Quantitative considerations. *Am. J. Physiol. 253*: H107.

Ng, C. K., Huang, S. C., Schelbert, H. R., and Buxton, D. B. (1991). Tracer kinetic modeling for delineating C-11 acetate as a tracer for myocardial oxidative metabolism. *J. Nucl. Med. 32*: 910.

Nicklas, J. M., and Gips, S. J. (1989). Decreased coronary flow reserve after transient myocardial ischemia in dogs. *J. Am. Coll. Cardiol. 13*: 195.

Nienaber, C., Kotler, T. S., Maddahi, J., Brunken, R., Lew, A. S., Ostrzega, E., Berman, D. S., and Schelbert, H. R. (1989). Metabolic and functional abnormalities one month after successful coronary thrombolysis: Persistence of stunned myocardium? *J. Nucl. Med. 30*: 837.

Nienaber, C. A., Brunken, R. C., Sherman, C. T., Yeatman, L., Gambhir, S. S., Krivokapich, J., Demer, L., Ratib, O., Child, J., Phelps, M. E., and Schelbert, H. R. (1991). Metabolic and functional recovery in ischemic human myocardium following coronary angioplasty. *J. Am. Coll. Cardiol. 18*: 966.

Phelps, M. E., Hoffman, E. J., Selin, C. E., Huang, S. C., Robinson, G., MacDonald, N., Schelbert, H., and Kuhl, D. E. (1978). Investigation of [^{18}F] 2-fluoro-2-deoxyglucose for the measure of myocardial glucose metabolism. *J. Nucl. Med. 19*: 1311.

Pierard, L., De Landsheere, C., Berthe, C., Rigo, P., and Kulbertus, H. (1990). Identification of viable myocardium by echocardiography during dobutamine infusion in patients with myocardial infarction after thrombolytic therapy: Comparison with positron emission tomgraphy. *J. Am. Coll. Cardiol. 15*: 1021.

Ratib, O., Phelps, M. E., Huang, S. C., Henze, E., Selin, C. E., and Schelbert, H. R. (1982). Positron tomography with deoxyglucose for estimating local myocardial glucose metabolism. *J. Nucl. Med. 23*: 577.

Rosamond, T. L., Abendschein, D. R., Sobel, B. E., Bergmann, S. R., and Fox, K. A. A. (1987). Metabolic fate of radiolabeled palmitate in ischemic canine myocardium: Implications for positron emission tomography. *J. Nucl. Med. 28*: 1322.

Schelbert, H. R., Phelps, M. E., Huang, S. C., MacDonald, N. S., Hansen, H., Selin, C., and Kuhl, D. E. (1981). N-13 ammonia as an indicator of myocardial blood flow. *Circulation 63*: 1259.

Schelbert, H. R., Henze, E., Schön, H. R., Keen, R., Hansen, H. W., Selin, C., Huang, S. C., Barrio, J. R., and Phelps, M. E. (1983). C-11 palmitate for the noninvasive evaluation of regional myocardial fatty acid metabolism with positron computed tomography. III. In vivo demonstration of the effects of substrate availability on myocardial metabolism. *Am. Heart J. 105*: 492.

Schelbert, H. R. (1991). Principles of positron emission tomography. In *Cardiac Imaging* (Marcus, M. L., Schelbert, H. R., Skorton, D. J., and Wolf, G. L., eds.), W. B. Saunders Publishers, Philadelphia, PA.

Schön, H. R., Schelbert, H. R., Najafi, A., Robinson, G., Huang, S. C., Barrio, J., and Phelps, M. E. (1982). C-11 labeled palmitic acid for the noninvasive evaluation of regional myocardial fatty acid metabolism with positron computed tomography. I. Kinetics of C-11 palmitic acid in normal myocardium. *Am. Heart J. 103*: 532.

Schwaiger, M., Schelbert, H. R., Ellison, D., Hansen, H., Yeatman, L., Vinten-Johansen, J., Selin, C., Barrio, J., and Phelps, M. E. (1985). Sustained regional abnormalities in cardiac metabolism after transient ischemia in the chronic dog model. *J. Am. Coll. Cardiol. 6*: 336.

Schwaiger, M., Brunken, R., Grover-McKay, M., Krivokapich, J., Child, J., Tillisch, J. H., Phelps, M. E., and Schelbert, H. R. (1986). Regional myocardial metabolism in patients with acute myocardial infarction assessed by positron emission tomography. *J. Am. Coll. Cardiol. 8*: 800.

Schwaiger, M., Brunken, R., Krivokapich, J., Child, J., Tillisch, J., Phelps, M. E., and Schelbert, H. R. (1987). Beneficial effect of residual antegrade flow on tissue viability as assessed by positron emission tomography in patients with myocardial infarction. *Eur. Heart J. 8*: 981.

Schwaiger, M., Neese, R. A., Araujo, L., Wyns, W., Wisneski, J. A., Sochor, H., Swank, S., Kulber, D., Selin, C., Phelps, M., Schelbert, H. R., Fishbein, M. C., Gertz, E. W., and Hansen, H. (1989). Sustained nonoxidative glucose utilization and depletion of glycogen in reperfused canine myocardium. *J. Am. Coll. Cardiol. 13*: 745.

Stahl, L. D., Weiss, H. R., and Becker, L. C. (1988). Myocardial oxygen consumption, oxygen supply/demand heterogeneity, and microvascular patency in regionally stunned myocardium. *Circulation 77*: 865.

Tillisch, J., Brunken, R., Marshall, R., Schwaiger, M., Mandelkern, M., Phelps, M., and Schelbert, H. R. (1986). Reversibility of cardiac wall motion abnormalities predicted by positron tomography. *N. Engl. J. Med. 314*: 884.

Vaghaiwalla-Mody, F., Buxton, D. B., Krivokapich, J., Hansen, H. A., Selin, C. E., and Schelbert, H. R. (1990). Attenuated response of glucose metabolism in reperfused canine myocardium to changes in substrate levels. *J. Am. Coll. Cardiol. 15*: 80A(Abstract).

Wyns, W., Vogelaers, D., Melin, J. A., Bol, A., Michel, C., Labar, D., and Heyndrickx, G. R. (1988). Diverging effects of pacing on palmitate and overall oxidative metabolism in canine stunned myocardium. *Circulation 78* (Suppl. II): 494(Abstract).

23

Stunned Myocardium Is Important for the Cardiovascular Surgeon

Gregory Louis Kay, Curtis Anthony Prejean, Jr., Pablo Zubiate, and Atsushi Aoki

Hospital of the Good Samaritan, Los Angeles, California

I. THE IMPORTANCE OF STUNNING TO THE CARDIOVASCULAR SURGEON

Every cardiac surgeon has seen the patient who leaves the operating room requiring full mechanical and pharmacological circulatory support yet miraculously recovers over the ensuing days and weeks and who, on examination prior to hospital discharge, has near-normal or normal ventricular function. The only explanation for this observation is myocardial stunning. Failure of a patient with good preoperative ventricular function to wean from cardiopulmonary bypass, or failure to wean from cardiopulmonary bypass without extreme pharmacological and/or mechanical support represents myocardial stunning produced by the cardiac surgeon due to inadequate myocardial protection. Kuchar et al. (1987) reported that patients with good preoperative left ventricular function who required postoperative intraaortic balloon support showed 85% survivorship 6 years after operation if the patient survived hospitalization. Thus, patients who survive the early period after injury have an excellent long-term prognosis. Avoiding myocardial injury is more effective then supporting failing myocardium. Once the myocardium is stunned, it may take a week or longer to recover. Time is the only cure. Myocardial protection is a function of operative techniques and preoperative management. Inadequate myocardial protection does not occur only in the operating room. Thrombolysis and angioplasty also lead to myocardial stunning (Wijns et al., 1986). Preoperative patient management and intraoperative techniques should be open to analysis and modification.

The cardiologist who "bails out" (reopens) an artery, which acutely closed during angioplasty—often with an indwelling catheter—may actually be creating problems. Reperfusion occurs under suboptimal circumstances: after significant delay; with residual proximal obstruction; in a working heart; with unmodified perfusate. This is a prescription for stunning. These bail-outs are generally temporary measures to get the patient to the operating room. If stunning of a significant sector of myocardium results, although subsequent revascularization may be technically successful, separation from bypass may be difficult. Controlled reperfusion reduces the occurrence of stunning. This could significantly reduce morbidity and shorten hospitalization. It may be that bail-outs are a poor choice for restoring function to an ischemic segment under certain circumstances. It may at times be better to send the patient to the operating room directly where the surgeon can reperfuse ischemic myocardium under optimal circumstances (Buckberg et al., 1986).

The cardiologist and cardiac surgeon must work together in planning for such contingencies. Each situation requires individualized treatment.

II. HOW CAN THE CARDIOVASCULAR SURGEON RECOGNIZE STUNNING?

Mechanical dysfunction, whether systolic or diastolic, can be seen in stunned myocardium and infarcted myocardium. Frequently the two co-exist. Distinguishing between stunned and infarcted may be impossible except by watching how much function returns over time. Recruitment of function with inotropes proves the muscle is stunned, but failure of recruitment is not diagnostic. Likewise, electrocardiographic changes such as Q-waves are not proof of myocardial necrosis (Bateman et al., 1983). Myocardial ATP levels are neither distinguishing nor clinically practical (Braunwald and Kloner, 1982; Ellis et al., 1983; Kloner et al., 1983; Rosenkranz et al., 1986). Late structural changes may well be helpful, but early structural changes are not consistent, and performing biopsy in this setting would be impractical (Kloner et al., 1983; Buckberg, 1986; Zhao et al., 1987). At present the only way to clinically distinguish necrosis from stunning is the reversibility of mechanical and electrical dysfunction over time.

Experience with thrombolysis in acute myocardial infarction underscores our inability to distinguish between myocardium that is stunned and myocardium that is dead. Ventricular function studies early after reperfusion (less than 1 week) underestimate the degree of myocardial salvage as late studies (at 1 or 2 months) inevitably show significantly improved function (Ghitis et al., 1991; Kereiakes et al., 1991). The return to normal function of severely stunned myocardium remains a time-dependent process.

III. SUPPORTIVE MEASURES

The patient who "limps" off cardiopulmonary bypass does not allow us to ask whether myocardial stunning should be treated. There is no choice but to treat in such circumstances. The question reduces to "What is the best way to treat myocardial stunning?" The answer is not known, but there are clues that may facilitate clinical decision making.

A. Mechanical Balloon Assist Devices

The most extreme ventricular support is a mechanical ventricular assist device such as intraaortic balloon assist devices, the pneumatic roller pump, and centrifugal pump ventricular assist devices. The utility of these devices is well documented once one accepts the assertion that the devices were required in the first place. Certainly all experienced cardiac surgeons have seen the dramatic return of function that occurs in many patients after several days of balloon-assisted support (Pennington et al., 1985; Coleman et al., 1989). Since mechanical support reduces the demands on the myocyte and does not try to squeeze more work out of already damaged cells, it is easy to accept that this form of support is safe for the myocardium. The primary drawbacks are mechanical complications such as arterial insufficiency, systemic thromboembolism, and the rigors of anticoagulation.

B. Pharmacological Stimulation

It is more difficult to decide whether pharmacological stimulation of failing, stunned myocardium is damaging to the myocyte. There are no definitive answers. There is ample evidence that stunned myocardium maintains its capacity to contract at essentially normal levels. This capacity is independent of myocardial cellular ATP content (Buckberg, 1986; Kloner et al., 1990). Postextrasystolic potentiation is one manifestation of this latent capacity (Becker et al., 1986). Inotropic agents such as dopamine, dobutamine, isoproterenol, epinephrine, and calcium have the ability to augment the function of stunned myocardium (Arnold et al., 1985; Becker et al., 1986). Concern that pushing stunned myocardium in this way may impair recovery or produce myocyte death has not been supported by short-term experiments (Arnold et al., 1985; Becker et al., 1986; Bolli et al., 1989). Calcium may be an exception (see Section III.C).

Triiodothyronine has been reported to improve recovery in a dog model of myocardial stunning when administered 10 minutes into the reperfusion period (Novitzky et al., 1991). Glucose, insulin, and potassium solution administered to patients on intraaortic balloon counterpulsation support seems to have been beneficial, resulting in a shorter period of balloon support dependency, improved cardiac output, and short-term clinical outcome (Coleman et al., 1989). These studies are, however, anecdotal.

C. Calcium and Calcium Channel Antagonists

The calcium antagonists verapamil, nifedipine, and diltiazem have all been shown to attenuate stunning (Kloner et al., 1990). Postischemic myocardium appears to be very susceptible to injury from calcium influx during the early reperfusion period (approximately 15–30 minutes) (Bolli, 1990; Abbott et al., 1991).

Of even greater concern for clinicians is evidence that a condition virtually indistinguishable from myocardial stunning can be produced by transient calcium overload without antecedent ischemia (Bolli, 1990). Thus, administration of large doses of calcium can, on its own, stun the myocardium.

These experimental findings are not incompatible with the augmentation of function seen in stunned myocardium after the administration of calcium. Most patients are hypocalcemic after cardiopulmonary bypass, and the empirical observation suggests that calcium administration at the end of cardiopulmonary bypass frequently results in improved contractility and blood pressure, at least temporarily. This is a favorite drug of many cardiac surgical groups in the early postoperative period, and indeed, in the right context and given in judicious doses, is quite useful. Moderation, especially in the early postischemic period, is required if adverse events are to be avoided. After stunning of the myocardium has occurred, calcium may be an effective inotrope; it simply may not be a very good choice, especially if high doses are required.

IV. ALLOPURINOL

Both allopurinol and its primary metabolite oxypurinol are inhibitors of xanthine oxidase. During ischemia, hypoxanthine and xanthine oxidase accumulate in the cell. With reperfusion, xanthine oxidase acts on molecular oxygen and hypoxanthine to form oxygen free radicals. Allopurinol seems to work by blocking free radical formation. Emerit et al. (1988) tested the hypothesis that free radicals generated following ischemia and reperfusion in cardiac operations can produce clastogenic (chromosomal-breaking) factors that result in chromosomal aberration. Fourteen patients were randomized. Seven patients were treated with allopurinol and seven were not. Though there was no significant difference between the preischemic clastogenic activity for the two groups, there was a significant difference in the postischemic clastogenic activity ($p < 0.01$). This model carefully avoided factors such as ionizing radiation that may have increased clastogenic activity. The reduced clastogenic activity in the allopurinol group indicates less free radical generation and a potential protective effect for allopurinol. No clinical correlation could be identified in this small study, but the evidence for reduction of free radical generation is strong.

In a trial with clinical end points reported from the United Kingdom and Poland, patients pretreated with allopurinol had significantly better left ventricular stroke work index and fewer episodes of arrhythmias in the early postoperative period compared to controls. Electron microscopic and enzyme leak analysis revealed no differences between the allopurinol-treated and the control group (Bochenek et al., 1990).

Another clinical study examined the clinical impact of allopurinol administration in a prospective, randomized format. Randomization produced groups evenly matched for surgical risk factors. The hospital mortality in the placebo group was 18% versus 4% in the allopurinol group. The ventricular function scores after operation and need for mechanical and pharmacological support favored allopurinol administration (Johnson et al., 1991).

These studies support the beneficial effect of allopurinol in clinical settings. There were no reported side effects in these studies. The optimum dosing regimen for allopurinol is not known, but there is evidence that allopurinol improves myocardial protection if given prior to the onset of ischemia. Protection is most likely by reduction of free radical generation and therefore reduction of stunning.

In general, the experience with allopurinol pretreatment supports the concept that myocardial stunning is important in the management of cardiac surgery patients on a day-to-day basis and that there are clinical treatments that can reduce the risk of stunning.

V. CONTROL OF CONDITIONS OF REPERFUSION

In a series of superb experimental articles Buckberg and colleagues detailed the benefits of altering the conditions of reperfusion. Experimental design intentionally paralleled clinical situations.

The conditions of reperfusion dictated the degree of functional recovery for noninfarcted segments and the measurable histochemical evidence of infarction (Buckberg, 1986). The factors that Buckberg found to be important for the reperfusate were: hypocalcemia (Allen et al., 1986a); hyperglycemia and hyperosmolarity (Okamoto et al., 1986a); the presence of erythrocytes and absence of leukocytes (Acar et al., 1991a,b; Julia et al., 1991; Kofsky et al., 1991a,b); and substrate enrichment (glutamate and aspartate). The method of reperfusion was critical with respect to: minimizing left ventricular work load during reperfusion (Allen et al., 1986c,d); reducing the pressure under which the reperfusate was delivered (Okamoto et al., 1986a,b); and the avoidance of excessive cardioplegia administration (Kofsky et al., 1991a,b). It was not possible to prioritize the various factors since it would appear that each modification improved ventricular function and no one modification was, by itself, sufficient. These were acute experimental models. Histochemical studies did show significantly greater areas of infarction in the control groups in almost all the studies. The improvement in function in groups in which the reperfusate conditions were modified was dramatic compared to control groups. Histological evidence of infarction also was reduced in the experimental groups; triphenyltetrazolium chloride staining fell from 43% to 11% of the left ventricle.

Virtually all of the techniques described by Buckberg can be used in everyday clinical practice. In a series of patients with acute myocardial infarction treated either medically (thrombolysis with or without angioplasty) or surgically, the surgical patients had fewer electrocardiographically determined infarctions and reperfusion arrhythmias. Surgical patients also showed improved segmental contractility at discharge compared to the medically treated patients and actually had earlier discharge from the hospital (Allen et al., 1986e).

There seems to be a very brief period of ischemia, on the order of 10 minutes (as suggested by dog studies), to establish reperfusion and avoid stunning. Restoration of perfusion after that time results in stunning unless the conditions of reperfusion are controlled.

VI. AVOIDANCE OF ISCHEMIA, AND SUBSEQUENT STUNNING DURING AORTIC CROSS CLAMPING—NORMOTHERMIC AEROBIC ARREST

In 1991, hypothermic hyperkalemic cardioplegia is the most commonly used method to protect the myocardium during aortic cross clamping. It is not, however, necessarily the best. Although hypothermia reduces cellular metabolism, ATP generation is reduced to a greater degree. This is likely due to decreased glucose utilization and relative tissue hypoxia. Calcium homeostasis is disturbed, further increasing energy consumption. These and other theoretical concerns challenge the conventional wisdom that ischemic, hypothermic arrest offers optimal protection during aortic cross clamping (Lichtenstein et al., 1990).

The concept of normothermic cardiac surgery is not new. It has not gained acceptance, however, because previous techniques did not reduce myocardial oxygen demand. In the past, normothermic blood was supplied to a fibrillating or beating heart. The oxygen demand of the beating or fibrillating heart exceeded the supply with these techniques, producing a relative ischemia. Electromechanical arrest of the working heart at normothermia decreases oxygen consumption by 90%, making normothermic aerobic preservation practical.

The benefits of normothermic antegrade continuous cardoplegia during aortic cross clamping have been reported (Lichtenstein et al., 1990). This technique is cumbersome, especially for valvular surgery. Since we had extensive experience with the technique of retrograde cardioplegia, we were comfortable combining this technique with that of normothermic aerobic arrest during aortic cross clamping. Diastolic arrest is easily achieved and maintained by continuous infusion of hyperkalemic, normothermic blood. We have used this technique for well over a year.

From April 1990 to March 1991, retrograde continuous warm blood cardioplegia was used for 358 patients undergoing myocardial revascularization and/or valve operation (aerobic group) and intermittent cold blood cardioplegia was used for 650 similar cases (ischemic group). These cases were divided into a low-risk group and a high-risk group based on evaluation of preoperative risk factors according to the method of Parsonnet (Parsonnet et al., 1989). While the use of inotropes in the postoperative period varies according to surgeon preference and is therefore a soft end point, the use of intraaortic balloon pumping (IABP) and failure to wean from cardiopulmonary bypass are hard end points. In this retrospective analysis there was no significant difference between the aerobic group and the ischemic group for either end point in the low-risk group. In the high-risk group, the requirement for IABP was significantly less in the aerobic group ($p = 0.034$). Further, all high-risk patients in the aerobic group could be weaned from cardiopulmonary bypass, whereas 6.7% of high-risk patients in the ischemic group could not ($p = 0.013$) (see Fig. 1). Although there appears to be no difference between the aerobic group and the ischemic group for low-risk patients, normothermic aerobic arrest appears to provide superior myocardial protection for patients classified as high risk as determined by failure to wean from cardiopulmonary bypass or the need of balloon pump support after bypass. The determination of high or low risk can be made prospectively.

During the same time period, 111 patients underwent valve surgery using aerobic arrest and 111 patients using ischemic arrest. Patient profiles for the two groups with respect to age, gender, ejection fraction, the nature of val-

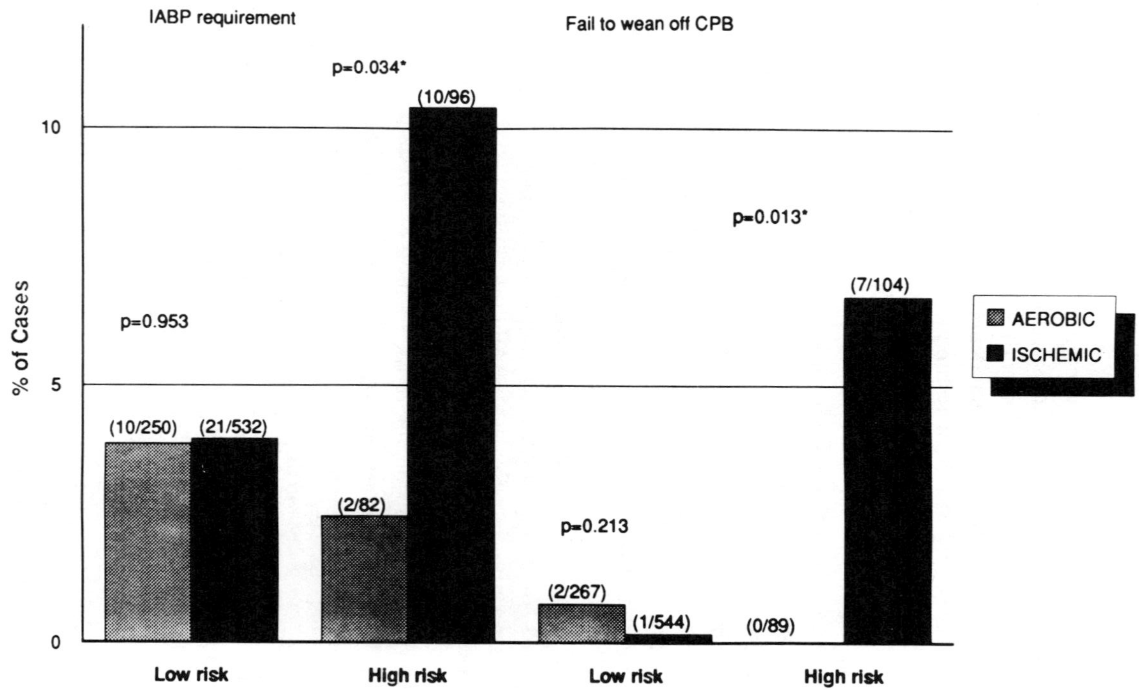

Figure 1 Need for mechanical assistance and failure to wean from cardiopulmonary bypass by risk group and cardioplegia technique. IABP = intraaortic balloon pump; CPB = cardiopulmonary bypass.

vular disease, procedure, bypass time, and cross clamp time were similar. To evaluate the influence of cardioplegia technique on cardiac rhythm, we analyzed the first rhythm after cross clamp removal, the occurrence of atrial fibrillation during hospitalization in patients whose preoperative rhythm was normal, and the need for permanent pacemaker placement before discharge (see Fig. 2). This analysis suggests that the complex factors that maintain normal sinus rhythm are better preserved using normothermic aerobic arrest than ischemic arrest and that this benefit may carry over to the late hospital period as a decreased incidence of atrial fibrillation.

Recovery time, defined as the period needed from cross clamp removal to effect termination of bypass, is an indication of myocardial recovery and therefore, we believe, of myocardial protection. In the same group of valve surgery patients the recovery time was briefer for the aerobic arrest group than for the ischemic arrest group for each type of valve procedure. While this result could be related to the rewarming period after whole body cooling or to other factors, the significant relationship between cross clamp time and recovery time in the ischemic arrest group suggests that cross clamp time is an important determinant of myocardial protection. There is no such correlation in the aerobic arrest group, suggesting that normothermic aerobic arrest effectively negates cross clamp time as a factor in myocardial recovery (see Fig. 3).

The continuous delivery of normothermic, hyperkalemic blood during the aortic cross clamp period induces electromechanical arrest and seems to avoid significant ischemia. Without ischemia there can be no reperfusion and stunning. Myocardial function does not appear to deteriorate with prolonged cross clamp periods using this form of protection. This is quite different from the findings with cold ischemic arrest.

VII. SUMMARY

Clinically, stunned myocardium can be defined as reperfused muscle that is temporarily unable to contract normally. There is no reliable, immediate method to distinguish reperfused myocardium that is stunned from reperfused myocardium that is necrotic, except by inference if inotropic agents augment performance. Stunning is a time-limited phenomenon, and even a very compromised ventricle, if supported long enough, is capable of complete recovery. Conditions of reperfusion are under control of the surgeon and cardiologist. Collaboration and reexamination of current clinical practices and assumptions is in order. There is clinical evidence to suggest that uncontrolled reperfusion, as can occur with thrombolysis or during unsuccessful angioplasty, may not be optimal. Allopurinol appears to improve clinical results in the cardiac surgery patient. There is good clinical evidence

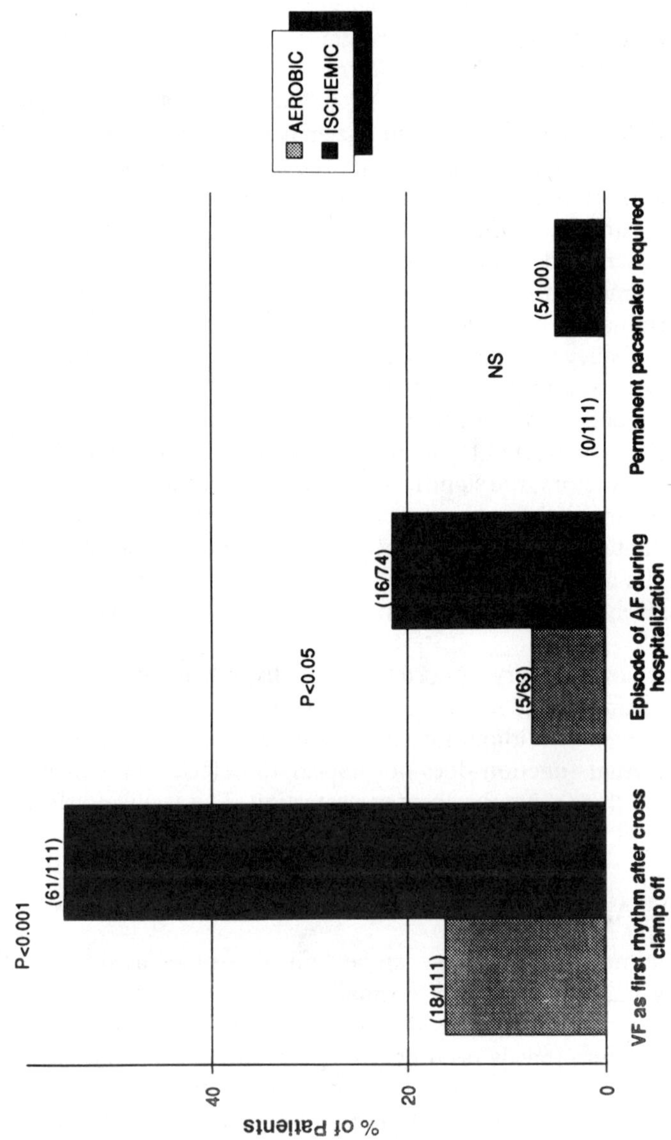

Figure 2 Effect of cardioplegia technique on cardiac rhythm. AF = atrial fibrillation; VF = ventricular fibrillation.

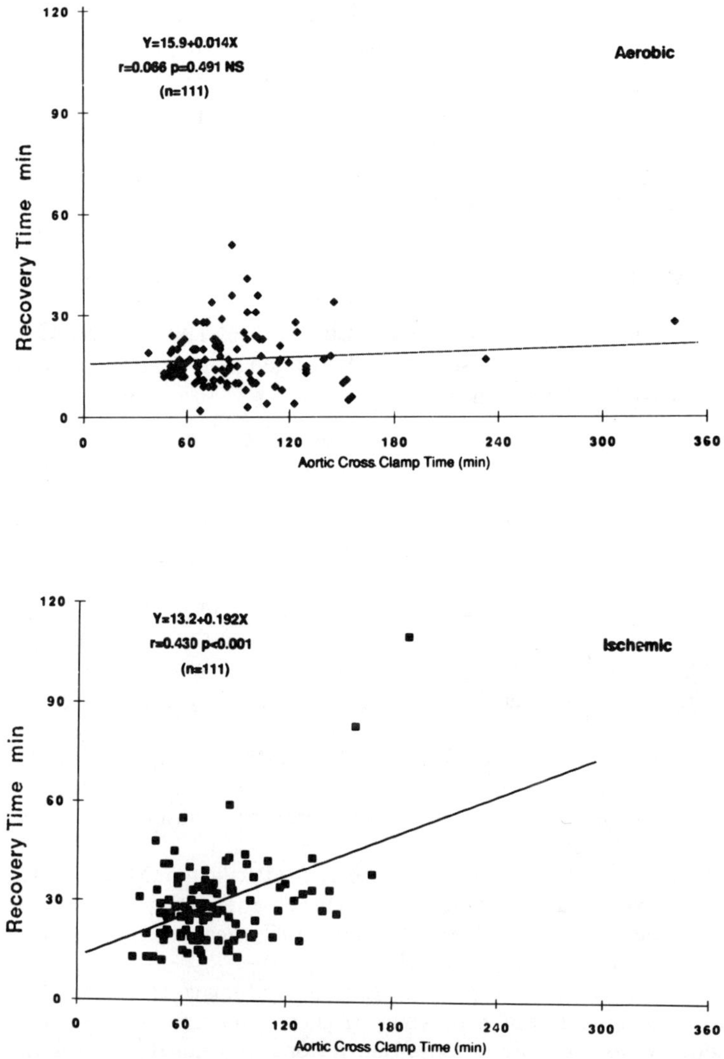

Figure 3 Recovery time as a function of cross clamp time—effect of cardioplegia technique for aerobic and ischemic arrest groups.

to suggest that the beneficial effects of allopurinol are due to decreasing free radical generation and therefore stunning. There are other agents with good experimental profiles which may offer similar clinical benefits, but there is no clinical experience yet with these agents. Finally, there is reason to challenge hypothermic, anaerobic arrest as the optimal method of protection during aortic cross clamping. There is reason to believe that a new technique, that of aerobic arrest, may provide superior results in some patient groups, particularly when a long cross clamping period is anticipated.

ACKNOWLEDGMENT

The authors were aided by a grant from the Los Angeles Thoracic and Cardiovascular Foundation and The Burton G. Bettingen Corporation in memory of Mr. Maynard J. Toll, Esquire.

REFERENCES

Abbott, A., Hill, R., Shears, L., Beamer, K., Gustafson, R., and Murray, G. (1991). Effects of calcium chloride administration on the postischemic isolated rat heart. *Ann. Thorac. Surg. 51*: 705.

Acar, C., Partington, M. T., and Buckberg, G. D. (1991a). Studies of controlled reperfusion after ischemia-reperfusate composition: Benefits of blood cardioplegia over fluosol DA cardioplegia during regional reperfusion—importance of including blood components in the initial reperfusate. *J. Thorac. Cardiovasc. Surg. 101*: 284.

Acar, C., Partington, M. T., and Buckberg, G. D. (1991b). Studies of controlled reperfusion after ischemia-reperfusate composition: detrimental effects of initial asanguineous cardioplegic washout after acute coronary occlusion. *J. Thorac. Cardiovasc. Surg. 101*: 294.

Allen, B. S., Okamoto, F., Buckberg, G. D., Acar, C., Partington, M. Bugyi, H., and Leaf, J. (1986a). Studies of controlled reperfusion after ischemia-reperfusate composition: Benefits of marked hypocalcemia and diltiazem on regional recovery. *J. Thorac. Cardiovasc. Surg. 92*: 564.

Allen, B. S., Okamoto, F., Buckberg, G. D., Leaf, J., and Bugyi, H. (1986b). Studies of controlled reperfusate after ischemia-effects of "duration" of reperfusate administration versus reperfusate "dose" on regional functional, biochemical, and histochemical recovery. *J. Thorac. Cardiovasc. Surg. 92*: 594.

Allen, B. S., Okamoto, F., Buckberg, G. D., Bugyi, H., and Leaf, J. (1986c). Studies of controlled reperfusion after ischemia-reperfusion conditions: Critical importance of total ventricular decompression during regional reperfusion. *J. Thorac. Cardiovasc. Surg. 92*: 605.

Allen, B. S., Okamoto, F., Buckberg, G. D., Bugyi, H., Young, H., Leaf, J., Beyersdorf, F., Sjostrand, F., and Maloney, J. V. (1986d). Studies of controlled reperfusion after ischemia-immediate functional recovery after six hours of regional ischemia by careful control of conditions of reperfusion and composition of reperfusate. *J. Thorac. Cardiovasc. Surg. 92*: 621.

Allen, B. S., Buckberg, G. D., Schwaiger, M., Yeatman, L., Tillisch, J. Kawata, N., Messenger, J., and Lee, C. (1986e). Studies of controlled reperfusion after ischemia-early recovery of regional wall motion in patients following surgical revascularization after 8 hours of acute coronary occlusion. *J. Thorac. Cardiovasc. Surg. 92*: 636.

Arnold, J. M. O., Braunwald, E., Sandor, T., and Kloner, R. A. (1985). Inotropic stimulation of reperfused myocardium: effects of infarct size and myocardial function. *J. Am. Coll. Cardiol. 6*: 1026.

Bateman, T. M., Czer, L. S. C., Gray, R. J., Maddahi, J., Raymond, M. J., Geft, I. L., Ganz, W., Shah, P. K., and Berman, D. S. (1983): Transient pathologic Q-waves during acute ischemic events: An electrocardiographic correlate of stunned but viable myocardium. *Am. Heart J. 6*: 1421.

Becker, L. C., Levine, J. H., DiPaula, A. F., Guarnieri, T., and Aversano, T. (1986). Reversal of dysfunction in postischemic stunned myocardium by epinephrine and postextrasystolic potentiation. *J. Am. Coll. Cardiol. 7*: 580.

Bochenek, A., Religa, Z., Spyt, T. J., Mistarz, K., Bochenek, A., Zembala, M., and Grzybek, H. (1990). Protective influence of pretreatment with Allopurinol on myocardial function in patients undergoing coronary artery surgery. *Eur. J. Cardio. Surg. 4*: 538.

Bolli, R., Patel, B. S., Hartley, C. J., Thornby, J. I., Jeroudi, M. O., and Roberts, R. (1989). Non-uniform transmural recovery of contractile function in stunned myocardium. *Am. J. Physiol. 257*: H375.

Bolli, R. (1990). Mechanism of myocardial "stunning." *Circulation 82*: 3.

Braunwald, E., and Kloner, R. A. (1982). The stunned myocardium: Prolonged, postischemic ventricular dysfunction. *Circulation 66*: 6.

Buckberg, G. D. (1986). Studies of controlled reperfusion after ischemia—When is cardiac muscle damaged irreversibly? *J. Thorac. Cardiovasc. Surg. 92*: 483.

Coleman, G. M., Gradinac, S., Taegtmeyer, H., Sweeney, M., and Frazier, O. H. (1989). Efficacy of metabolic support with glucose-insulin-potassium for left ventricular pump failure after aortocoronary bypass surgery. *Circulation 80*: I-91.

Ellis, S. G., Henschke, C. I., Sandor, T., Wynne, J., Braunwald, E., and Kloner, R. A. (1983). Time course of functional and biochemical recovery of myocardium salvaged by reperfusion. *J. Am. Coll. Cardiol. 1*: 1047.

Emerit, I., Fabiani, J. N., Ponzio, O., Murday, A., Lunel, F., and Carpentier, A. (1988). Clastogenic factor in ischemia-reperfusion injury during open-heart surgery: Protective effect of allopurinol. *Ann. Thorac. Surg. 46*: 619.

Ghitis, A., Flaker, G. C., Meinhardt, S., Grouws, M., Anderson, S. K., and Webel, R. R. (1991). Early angioplasty in patients with acute myocardial infarction complicated by hypotension. *Am. Heart J. 122*: 380.

Johnson, W. D., Kayser, K. L., Brenowitz, J. B., and Saedi, S. F. (1991). A randomized controlled trial of allopurinol in coronary bypass surgery. *Am. Heart J. 121*: 20.

Julia, P. L., Buckberg, G. D., Acar, D., Partington, M. T., and Sherman, M. P. (1991). Studies of controlled reperfusion after ischemia-reperfusate composition: Superiority of blood cardioplegia over crystalloid cardioplegia in limiting reperfusion damage—Importance of endogenous oxygen free radical scavengers in red blood cells. *J. Thorac. Cardiovasc. Surg. 101*: 303.

Kereiakes, D. J., Califf, R. M., George, B. S., Ellis, S., Samaha, J., Stuck, R., Martin, L. H., Young, S., and Topol, E. J. (1991). Coronary bypass surgery improves global and regional left ventricular function following thrombolytic therapy for acute myocardial linfarction. *Am. Heart J. 122*: 390.

Kloner, R. A., Ellis, S. G., Lange, R., and Braunwald, E. (1983). Studies of experimental coronary artery reperfusion: Effects of infarct size, myocardial function, biochemistry, ultrastructure, and microvascular damage. *Circulation 68*: I-8.

Kloner, R. A., Przyklenk, K., Rahimtoola, S. H., and Braunwald, E. (1990). Myocardial stunning and hibernation: Mechanisms and clinical implications. In *Heart Disease. Update* 11: 241.

Kofsky, E. R., Julia, P. L., Buckberg, G. D., Quillen, J. E., and Acar, C. (1991a). Studies of controlled reperfusion after ischemia-reperfusate composition: Effects of leukocyte depletion of blood and blood cardioplegic reperfusates after coronary occlusion. *J. Thorac. Cardiovasc. Surg. 101*: 350.

Kofsky, E. R., Julia, P. L., and Buckberg, G. D. (1991b). Overdose reperfusion of blood cardioplegic solution. A preventable cause of postischemic myocardial depression. *J. Thorac. Cardiovasc. Surg. 101*: 275.

Kuchar, D. L., Campbell, T. J., and O'Rourke, M. F. (1987). Long term survival after counterpulsation for medically refractory heart failure complicating myocardial infarction and cardiac surgery. *Eur. Heart J 8*: 490.

Lichtenstein, S. V., Salerno, T. A., and Slutsky, A. S. (1990). Warm continuous cardioplegia versus intermittent hypothermic protection during cardiopulmonary bypass. Pro: Warm continuous cardioplegia is preferable to intermittent hypothermic cardioplegia for myocardial protection during cardiopulmonary bypass. *J. Cardiothorac. Anesth. 42*: 279.

Novitzky, D., Matthews, N., Shawley, D., Cooper, D. K. C., and Zuhdi, N. (1991). Triiodothyronine in the recovery of stunned myocardium in dogs. *Ann. Thorac. Surg. 51*: 10.

Okamoto, F., Allen, B. S., Buckberg, G. D., Young, H., Bugyi, H., and Leaf, J. (1986a). Studies of controlled reperfusion after ischemia-reperfusate composition: interaction of marked hyperglycemia and marked hyperosmolarity in allowing immediate contractile recovery after four hours of regional ischemia. *J. Thorac. Cardiovasc. Surg. 92*: 583.

Okamoto, F., Allen, B. S., Buckberg, G. D., Bugyi, H., and Leaf, J. (1986b). Studies of controlled reperfusion after ischemia-reperfusion conditions: Importance of ensuring gentle versus sudden reperfusion during relief of coronary occlusion. *J. Thorac. Cardiovasc. Surg. 92*: 613.

Parsonnet, V., Dean, D., and Bernstein, A. D. (1989). A method of uniform stratification of risk for evaluating the results of surgery in acquired adult heart disease. *Circulation 79* (Suppl I-3):

Pennington, D. G., Bernhard, W. F., Golding, L. R., Berger, R. L., Khuri, S. F., and Watson, J. T. (1985). Long-term follow-up of postcardiotomy patients with profound cardiogenic shock treated with ventricular assist devices. *Circulation 72*: II-216.

Rosenkranz, E. L., Okamoto, F., Buckberg, G. D., Vinten-Johansen, J. Allen, B. S., Leaf, M. S., Bugyi, H., Young, H., and Barnard, R. J. (1986). Studies of controlled reperfusion after ischemia-biochemical studies: Failure of tissue adenosine triphosphate levels to predict recovery of contractile function after controlled reperfusion. *J. Thorac. Cardiovasc. Surg. 92*: 488.

Wijns, W., Serruys, P. W., Slager, C. J., Grimm, J., Krayenbuehl, H. P., Hugenholtz, P. G., and Hess, O. M. (1986). Effect of coronary occlusion during percutaneous transluminal angioplasty in humans on left ventricular chamber stiffness and regional diastolic pressure-radius relations. *J. Am. Coll. Cardiol. 7*: 455.

Zhao, M., Zhang, H., Robinson, T. F., Factor, S. M., Sonnenblick, E. H., and Eng, C. (1987). Profound structural alterations of the extracellular collagen matrix in postischemic "stunned" but viable myocardium. *J. Am. Coll. Cardiol. 10*: 1322.

24

Is Myocardial Stunning Important from a Clinical Standpoint?

Eugene Braunwald

Harvard Medical School and Brigham and Women's Hospital, Boston, Massachusetts

Before answering the question posed in the title of this chapter, it is useful to review the fundamental concepts underlying the pathogenesis of the myocardial ischemic syndromes—concepts that for many years appeared to be quite straightforward. A clear description of angina pectoris was first offered by Heberden (1771), and it was not long before Parry (1799) correctly attributed it to temporary deprivation of coronary blood flow, i.e., transient myocardial ischemia. Observations made during the nineteenth century and the first decade of the twentieth century culminated in the classic description of the relation between coronary artery occlusion and the clinical and pathological findings in acute myocardial infarction (Herrick, 1912). Since then, we have associated persistent, severe myocardial ischemia, as occurs with thrombotic occlusion of a coronary artery, with necrosis of the myocardium in the distribution of the occluded vessel.

In the decades that followed it was thought that myocardial dysfunction secondary to ischemic heart disease expressed itself in two principal ways: (1) myocardial infarction, associated with prolonged chest pain and persistent ventricular dysfunction and electrocardiographic changes; and (2) chronic stable angina pectoris, with brief discomfort and equally brief alterations in electrocardiographic and hemodynamic function. This notion was strengthened when Tennant and Wiggers (1935) demonstrated experimentally that transient coronary occlusion causes equally transient ischemic dysfunction. We now know that this formulation, while fundamentally correct, is incomplete and that these two expressions of myocardial ischemia represent the opposite ends of a clinical-physiological-pathological spectrum. In between are a number of other conditions, including unstable angina, as well as a frequently observed syndrome characterized by relatively severe but brief myocardial ischemia followed by prolonged myocardial dysfunction. This condition, which we have termed "stunning of the myocardium" (Braunwald and Kloner, 1982), was initially described in experimental laboratories at the Harvard Medical School (Heyndrickx et al., 1975; DeBoer et al., 1980; Ellis et al., 1983; Kloner et al., 1983a) but it is not simply a laboratory curiosity. Indeed, it may now be identified in many patients with myocardial ischemia (Patel et al., 1988; Kloner et al., 1983b, 1990; Myocardial stunning, 1991).

I. GLOBAL MYOCARDIAL STUNNING FOLLOWING CARDIAC SURGERY

Clinical evidence of myocardial stunning is perhaps most evident on a day-to-day basis in the operating and recovery rooms of hospitals where open-heart surgery is performed (Braunwald, 1990). Cardioplegic cardiac arrest (often with hypothermia), which is associated with severe, global ischemia, is now widely used to render the heart dry and motionless during the operation. When, upon completion of the procedure, the coronary arteries are reperfused with oxygenated blood, the recovery of contractile function may be quite slow (Reduto et al., 1981a; Ferrari et al., 1990). An experimental counterpart of this form of global stunning was described by Nayler et al. (1988), who produced ischemic arrest in the isolated Langendorff heart and observed slow recovery during reperfusion. Cardiovascular surgeons have learned how to manage patients who exhibit persistent left ventricular dysfunction after cardioplegia. First, output from the heart-lung machine is reduced slowly rather than abruptly, so that the load placed on the globally stunned myocardium is increased gradually as function returns. Fortunately, the stunned myocardium can be stimulated to contract more vigorously by treatment with positive inotropic agents, such as beta-adrenoceptor agonists (Mercier et al., 1982; Ellis et al., 1984; Becker et al., 1986) without increasing myocardial necrosis (Arnold et al., 1985). These drugs are used frequently, though cautiously, after cardiopulmonary bypass has been discontinued and for hours or even days thereafter as contractility returns. When stunning is unusually prolonged or severe, mechanical circulatory assistance—most often intraaortic balloon counterpulsation, but sometimes even the implantation of a left ventricular assist device (Ballantyne et al., 1987)—may be necessary to support the circulation during the hours or days required for myocardial function to recover.

Global myocardial stunning is also frequently manifest in the acutely transplanted heart, which is subject to the severe ischemia that accompanies prolonged cardioplegia. The measures described above for the nontransplanted globally ischemic heart may also be effective in this setting. A large majority of the hearts undergoing intraoperative cardioplegia ultimately regain normal function, especially if the underlying cardiac defect has been corrected.

However, the severe ischemia associated with unusually prolonged cardioplegia may cause patchy areas of myocardial necrosis—i.e., a mixture of noncontractile, irreversibly injured (infarcted) tissue and poorly contractile, reversibly injured (stunned) myocardium. This combination, if it involves sufficient myocardium, may cause severe, prolonged, and sometimes fatal cardiac dysfunction.

II. REGIONAL MYOCARDIAL STUNNING

It has been demonstrated experimentally that regional stunning may be exaggerated following cardioplegia when reflow occurs through a coronary artery with a residual, flow-limiting stenosis (Schroder et al., 1988; Farber et al., 1988). This observation has a number of clinical counterparts. First, if one artery remains severely obstructed after a coronary artery bypass operation, reflow through the myocardium perfused by this persistently narrowed vessel will be limited, possibly leading to severe, prolonged stunning of that segment. Such regional stunning may be prevented by assuring that no major coronary arteries have any severe residual obstruction, i.e., that revascularization is complete. A second clinical example of regional stunning is observed in patients with Prinzmetal's angina, who frequently also have atheromatous obstruction of the vessel that undergoes severe spasm. Although the spasm may cause total coronary occlusion, the residual narrowing after relief of the spasm can limit reflow and thereby intensify the stunning that would have occurred had the intense vasoconstriction taken place in an unobstructed vessel. A third example is apparent when thrombolytic therapy is compared with angioplasty in the treatment of acute myocardial infarction. When reperfusion by either technique occurs in a timely manner, it can salvage jeopardized myocardium. However, after thrombolysis alone, the patient is generally left with more severe residual obstruction than with angioplasty, and recovery of regional myocardial function is slower and less complete (O'Neill et al., 1980).

Stunning is not confined to systole but occurs in diastole as well, causing postischemic regional impairment of left ventricular relaxation and filling

(Charlat et al., 1989; Braunwald, 1991). Diastolic stunning has been described in the wake of transient occlusion during percutaneous transluminal coronary angioplasty carried out to relieve angina pectoris. Wijns et al. (1986) have reported that diastolic ventricular relaxation, as determined by ventriculography, was impaired during inflation of the angioplasty balloon, and that recovery was delayed after the balloon was deflated and myocardial perfusion was restored.

III. STUNNING AFTER THROMBOLYTIC THERAPY OF ACUTE MYOCARDIAL INFARCTION

In their earliest experience with thrombolytic therapy for patients with acute myocardial infarction, investigators were often surprised and disappointed when they measured left ventricular function relatively early, i.e., within hours or days after successful reperfusion, and found the degree of improvement nonimpressive. However, it is now appreciated that return of normal regional and global function is often quite gradual. An early study by Reduto (1981b) showed that successful thrombolysis with intracoronary streptokinase failed to improve global left ventricular function, as reflected in the ejection fraction, which averaged 44% prior to treatment and 46% 1 day after thrombolysis, but then rose to 55% by the tenth day after the procedure. Stack et al. (1983), Anderson et al. (1983), and Touchstone et al. (1989) used contrast angiography or two-dimensional echocardiography to show that regional myocardial function in the evolving infarct improved only slightly (or not at all) one day after successful thrombolysis but that considerable improvement had occurred during the next 10 days to 2 weeks. The report by Pfisterer et al. (1991) is especially interesting with respect to the duration of postthrombolytic myocardial stunning. Their patients underwent successful thrombolytic reperfusion but continued to exhibit depressed myocardial function as late as the ninth posttreatment day, when the radionuclide left ventricular ejection fraction averaged 40.9%; when measured 3-6 months later, this value had risen to 49.3%. Similar results of improvement of myocardial function beyond hospital discharge have been reported by Schmidt et al. (1989), Christian et al. (1990), and Otto et al. (1990). Gradual recovery of diastolic function (i.e., diastolic stunning) has also been described in studies of regional wall motion between 1 and 7 days after thrombolytic therapy in patients with acute myocardial infarction. Williamson et al. (1990) reported that diastolic filling improved, presumably owing to enhanced myocardial relaxation and reduced stiffness of the stunned myocardium in the peri-infarct area.

Taken together, these observations have important implications for the optimal time to assess left ventricular function in patients treated with thrombolysis for an evolving acute infarction. It is clear that assessment of myocardial function during the first 2 or 3 days after treatment may seriously underestimate recovery. Although most observers have relied on evaluations obtained after approximately 1 week (i.e., just prior to hospital discharge), some of the findings described above suggest that stunning may actually persist for longer periods and that total recovery may be delayed for several weeks or even months. While stunning tends to be more severe following thrombolysis than following angioplasty in patients with evolving infarction (O'Neill et al., 1980), very late recovery of ventricular function has been noted in patients with cardiogenic shock secondary to myocardial infarction who underwent emergency percutaneous transluminal coronary angioplasty (Zuber et al., 1989).

Even with successful treatment of evolving infarction by reperfusion with thrombolysis and/or angioplasty, myocardial necrosis is rarely prevented totally and the myocardium in the distribution of the infarct-related artery usually contains both reversibly and irreversibly injured tissue. How can one detect stunning and distinguish between these two types of injury? One useful approach is to "arouse" the stunned myocardium by means of inotropic stimulation using either postextrasystolic potentiation or infusion of a beta-adrenoreceptor agonist (Ellis et al., 1984; Arnold et al., 1985; Satler et al., 1986). Another is to demonstrate with positron emission tomography that poorly contracting myocardium exhibits abnormal uptake of ^{18}F-fluorodeoxyglucose and normal uptake of ^{82}Rb (Camici et al., 1986). Uptake of the former, which is an indicator of carbohydrate metabolism reflects the presence of ischemic, though viable, myocardium, while uptake of the latter reflects the presence of myocardial perfusion. A simpler, although less accurate, way of detecting myocardial stunning is to demonstrate a mismatch between regional perfusion and contractile function, as reflected in the uptake or redistribution of thallium-201 into an area of myocardium that exhibits reversible hypofunction (Moore et al., 1990). Sometimes reinjection of thallium-201 is necessary to demonstrate that the akinetic myocardium is perfused.

IV. MYOCARDIAL STUNNING IN UNSTABLE ANGINA AND CORONARY VASOSPASM

Episodes of intense myocardial ischemia occur, often repeatedly, in patients with unstable angina (Nixon et al., 1982), in patients with severe coronary spasm, as occurs in Prinzmetal's angina (Mathias et al., 1987), as well as in other conditions such as subarachnoid hemorrhage (Yuki et al., 1991). Although these episodes usually do not last long enough to cause necrosis, echocardiographic studies have shown that myocardial dysfunction may persist for hours after the disappearance of ischemia. Using serial left ventricular angiography, Renkin et al. (1990) showed that unstable angina associated with T-wave inversion in left precordial leads caused by obstruction of the left anterior descending coronary artery is usually accompanied by hypokinesis of the left ventricular anterior wall. Furthermore, angioplasty to augment perfusion of this vessel frequently restored contraction of the hypokinetic segment and resulted in a normal electrocardiogram, indicating that the ventricular dysfunction was caused by myocardial stunning (Renkin et al., 1990) and not permanent myocardial damage. Occasionally, myocardial stunning in unstable angina and Prinzmetal's angina is accompanied by transient Q-waves, a condition sometimes referred to as "electrical stunning" (Bashour et al., 1983; Bateman et al., 1983).

V. MYOCARDIAL STUNNING IN DEMAND ISCHEMIA

As summarized above, there is substantial evidence that myocardial stunning may occur in patients with ischemia secondary to severe reductions of myocardial oxygen supply ("supply ischemia"). However, stunning is also seen with an equally or perhaps even more common cause of myocardial ischemia—increased cardiac oxygen requirements in the presence of a restricted coronary blood supply ("demand ischemia"). Experimental evidence for stunning following this type of ischemia has been provided (Homans et al., 1986; Thaulow et al., 1989). As measured by ultrasonic crystals implanted into the myocardium of dogs with partial coronary stenosis, left ventricular function became impaired during treadmill exercise and recovered only gradually following exercise. Myocardial stunning has been demonstrated clearly on postexercise two-dimensional echocardiography in patients with coronary obstruction (Robertson et al., 1983; Kloner et al., 1991). The latter noted persistence of left ventricular wall motion abnormalities for 30 minutes after the cessation of exercise in 19 of 21 patients with angiographically documented obstructive coronary artery disease. Galli et al. (1991) have demonstrated transient prolonged postischemic ventricular dilation by ^{99m}TC MIBI scans in patients with coronary artery disease undergoing exercise.

VI. OTHER CLINICAL EXAMPLES OF MYOCARDIAL STUNNING

Hypertrophic cardiomyopathy has been reported to cause prolonged stunning (Fine et al., 1989; Pasternac, 1989). A number of factors may be responsible for myocardial ischemia in this condition, including compression of septal perforator branches by the hypertrophied ventricular septum, prolonged diastolic relaxation, luminal narrowing and thickening of small intramural coronary arteries, as well as other microcirculatory changes, all of which may impair coronary filling.

Dipyridamole-thallium imaging is now widely used to detect myocardial ischemia in patients suspected of having coronary artery disease. As myocardial blood flow is distributed away from poststenotic areas after the administration of dipyridamole, regional perfusion defects occur. The resulting ischemia, which is often silent, has been reported to lead to myocardial stunning severe enough to cause pulmonary edema (Lette et al., 1989). However, it is important to differentiate between myocardial stunning and silent ischemia. Ischemia is sometimes totally asymptomatic (Kellermann and Braunwald, 1990), and the ischemia that leads to myocardial stunning may or may not be associated with symptoms. The absence of discomfort during myocardial stunning should not lead to confusion of this condition with silent ischemia. The latter is most commonly evidenced by asymptomatic electrocardiographic ST-segment changes; the resolution of such changes, accompanied by persistent left ventricular dysfunction will allow recognition of the combination of silent myocardial ischemia and stunning. Frequent episodes of silent ischemia followed by stunning may contribute to ischemic cardiomyopathy (Kloner, 1991), which may improve when these episodes are prevented by coronary revascularization.

VII. CONCLUSIONS

As summarized here and elsewhere in this book, many clinical examples of myocardial stunning have been identified, and it is likely that more circumstances in which this phenomenon plays a role will come to light. Therefore, it is necessary for clinicians to understand the pathophysiology underlying this process and to be alert to its development. A variety of new and sensitive noninvasive methods to assess myocardial contractile function are now available. These include biplane esophageal echocardiography and rapid magnetic resonance imaging in which the myocardium is labeled or "tagged" by localized radio frequency pulses (Zerhouni et al., 1988). When these techniques are applied after a stress (such as atrial pacing), many other instances of myocardial stunning will undoubtedly be uncovered.

Regardless of whether stunning occurs in the cardiac surgical patient, the patient who has undergone thrombolytic therapy for acute myocardial infarction, or one who has experienced severe ischemia in the course of unstable angina or Prinzmetal's angina, it is important not to confuse the myocardial dysfunction due to *reversibly* injured myocardium with that due to myocardial necrosis. Aggressive methods to prevent stunning, to diminish its severity by pharmacological means or reperfusion, and when necessary to support the circulation while myocardial function recovers should prove enormously useful in clinical care.

As to the question of whether myocardial stunning is important from a clinical standpoint—my answer is a resounding yes, I certainly believe that it is. Indeed, I think that an awareness of this phenomenon, its manifestations, consequences, treatment, and prevention, is essential to optimal management of patients with ischemic heart disease.

REFERENCES

Anderson, J. L., Marshall, H. W., Bray, B. E,. Lutz, J. R., Frederick, P. R., Yanowitz, F. G., Datz, F. L., Klausner, S. C., and Hagan, A. D. (1983). A randomized trial of intracoronary streptokinase in the treatment of acute myocardial infarctions. *N. Engl. J. Med. 308*: 1313.

Arnold, J. M. O., Braunwald, E., Sandor, T., and Kloner, R. A. (1985). Inotropic stimulation of reperfused myocardium. Effects on infarct size and myocardial function. *J. Am. Coll. Cardiol. 6*: 1026.

Ballantyne, C. M., Verani, M. S., Short, H. D., Hyatt, C., and Noon, G. P. (1987). Delayed recovery of severely "stunned" myocardium with the support of a left ventricular device after coronary artery bypass graft surgery. *J. Am. Coll. Cardiol. 10*: 710.

Bashour, T. T., Kabbani, S. S., Brewster, H. P., Wald, S. H., Hanna, E. S., and Cheng, T. S. (1983). Transient Q waves and reversible cardiac failure during myocardial ischemia. Electrical and mechanical stunning of the heart. *Am. Heart J. 106*: 780.

Bateman, T. M., Czer, L. S. C., Gray, R. J., Maddahi, J., Raymond, M. J., Geft, I. L., Ganz, W., Shah, P. K., and Berman, D. S. (1983). Transient pathologic Q waves during acute ischemic events. An electrocardiographic correlate of stunned but viable myocardium. *Am. Heart J. 106*: 1421.

Becker, L. C., Levine, J. H., DiPaula, A. F., Guarnieri, T., and Aversano, T. (1986). Reversal of dysfunction in postischemic stunned myocardium by epinephrine and postextrasystolic potentiation. *J. Am. Coll. Cardiol. 7*: 580.

Braunwald, E., and Kloner, R. A. (1982). The stunned myocardium: Prolonged, postischemic ventricular dysfunction. *Circulation 66*: 1146.

Braunwald, E. (1990). The stunned myocardium: Newer insights into mechanisms and clinical applications (editorial). *J. Thorac. Cardiovasc. Surg. 100*: 310.

Braunwald, E. (1991). Stunning of the myocardium. *Cardiovasc. Drugs Ther. 5*: 849.

Camici, P., Araujo, L. I., Spinks, T., Lammertsma, A. A., Kaski, J. C., Shea, M. J., Selwyn, A. P., Jones, T., and Maseri, A. (1986). Increased uptake of ^{18}F-fluorodeoxyglucose in postischemic myocardium of patients with exercise-induced angina. *Circulation 74*: 81.

Charlat, M. L., O'Neill, P. G., Hartley, C. J., Roberts, R., and Bolli, R. (1989). Prolonged abnormalities of left ventricular diastolic wall thinning in the "stunned" myocardium in conscious dogs: Time course and relation to systolic function. *J. Am. Coll. Cardiol. 13*: 185.

Christian, T. F., Behrenbeck, T., Pellikka, P. A., Huber, K. C., Chesebro, J. H., and Gibbons, R. J. (1990). Mismatch of left ventricular function and infarct size demonstrated by Technetium-99m isonitrile imaging after reperfusion therapy for acute myocardial infarction: Identification of myocardial stunning and hyperkinesia. *J. Am. Coll. Cardiol. 16*: 1632.

DeBoer, L. W. V., Ingwall, J. S., Kloner, R. A., and Braunwald, E. (1980). Prolonged derangements of canine myocardial purine metabolism after a brief coronary artery occlusion not associated with anatomic evidence of necrosis. *Proc. Natl. Acad. Sci. USA 77*: 5471.

Ellis, S. G., Henschke, C. I., Sandor, T., Wynne, J., Braunwald, E., and Kloner, R. A. (1983). Time course of functional and biochemical recovery of myocardium salvaged by reperfusion. *J. Am. Coll. Cardiol. 1*: 1047.

Ellis, S. G., Wynne, J., Braunwald, E., Henschke, C. I., Sandor, T., and Kloner, R. (1984). Response of reperfusion-salvaged, stunned myocardium to inotropic stimulation. *Am. Heart J. 107*: 13.

Farber, N. E., Pieper, G. M., and Gross, G. J. (1988). Postischemic recovery in the stunned myocardium after reperfusion in the presence or absence of a flow-limiting coronary artery stenosis. *Am. Heart J. 116*: 407.

Ferrari, R., Alfieri, O., Curello, S., Ceconi, C., Cargnoni, A., Marzollo, P., Pardini, A., Caradonna, E., and Visioli, O. (1990). Occurrence of oxidative stress during reperfusion of the human heart. *Circulation 81*: 201.

Fine, D. G., Clements, I. P., and Callahan, M. J. (1989). Myocardial stunning in hypertrophic cardiomyopathy: Recovery predicted by single photon emission computed tomographic thallium-201 scintigraphy. *J. Am. Coll. Cardiol. 13*: 1415.

Galli, M., Giubbini, R., and Tavazzi, L. (1991). Transient prolonged postischemic ventricular dilatation documented by ^{99m}Tc MIBI scan. *Chest 99*: 1536.

Heberden, W. (1771). Some account for a disorder of the breast. *Med. Trans.* (published by the College of Physicians in London) *2*: 59.

Herrick, J. B. (1912). Certain classical features of sudden obstruction of the coronary arteries. *JAMA 59*: 2015.

Heyndrickx, G. R., Millard, R. W., McRitchie, R. J., Maroko, P. R., and Vatner, S. F. (1975). Regional myocardial function and electrophysiological alterations after brief coronary artery occlusion in conscious dogs. *J. Clin. Invest. 56*: 978.

Homans, D. C., Sublett, E., Dai, X-Z., and Bache, R. J. (1986). Persistence of regional left ventricular dysfunction after exercise-induced myocardial ischemia. *J. Clin. Invest. 77*: 66.

Kellermann, J. J., and Braunwald, E., eds. (1990). *Silent Myocardial Ischemia: A Critical Appraisal.* Karger, Basel.

Kloner, R. A., Ellis, S. G., Lang, R., and Braunwald, E. (1983a). Studies of experimental coronary artery reperfusion: Effects on infarct size, myocardial function, biochemistry, ultrastructure, and microvascular damage. *Circulation 68*(Suppl. I): 8.

Kloner, R. A., Ellis, S. G., Carlson, N. V., and Braunwald, E. (1983b). Coronary reperfusion for the treatment of acute myocardial infarction. Postischemic ventricular dysfunction. *Cardiology 70*: 233.

Kloner, R. A., Przyklenk, K., Rahimtoola, S. H., and Braunwald, E. (1990). Myocardial stunning and hibernation: Mechanisms and clinical implications. In *Heart Disease: Update* (E. Braunwald, ed.), W. B. Saunders, Philadelphia.

Kloner, R. A. (1991). Ischemic cardiomyopathy: A manifestation of stunned myocardium? *Heart Failure 7*: 5.

Kloner, R. A., Allen, J., Cox, T. A., Zheng, Y., and Ruiz, C. E. (1991). Stunned left ventricular myocardium following exercise treadmill testing in coronary artery disease. *Am. J. Cardiol. 68*: 329.

Lette, J., Gagnon, A., and Waters, D. (1989). Acute pulmonary edema caused by prolonged myocardial stunning after dipyridamole-thallium imaging. *Am. J. Med. 87*: 461.

Mathias, P., Kerin, N. Z., Blevins, R. D., Cascade, P., and Rubenfire, M. (1987). Coronary vasospasm as a cause of stunned myocardium. *Am. Heart J. 113*: 383.

Mercier, J. C., Lando, U., Kanmatsuse, K., Ninomiya, K., Meerbaum, S., Fishbein, M. C., Swan, H. J., and Ganz, W. (1982). Divergent effects of inotropic stimulation on the ischemic and severely depressed reperfused myocardium. *Circulation 66*: 397.

Moore, C. A., Cannon, J., Watson, D. D., Kaul, S., and Beller, G. A. (1990). Thallium 201 kinetics in stunned myocardium characterized by severe postischemic systolic dysfunction. *Circulation 81*: 1622.

Myocardial stunning (editorial). (1991). *Lancet 337*: 585.

Nayler, W. G., Elz, J. S., and Buckley, D. J. (1988). The stunned myocardium. Effect of electrical and mechanical arrest and osmolality. *Am. J. Physiol. 254*: H60.

Nixon, J. V., Brown, C. N., and Smitherman, T. C. (1982). Identification of transient and persistent segmental wall motion abnormalities in patients with unstable angina by two-dimensional echocardiography. *Circulation 65*: 1497.

O'Neill, W., Timmis, G., Bourdillon, P., Lai, P., Ganghadarhan, V., Walton, J. Jr., Ramos, R., Laufer, N., Gordon, S., Schork, M. A., and Pitt, B. (1980). A prospective randomized clinical trial of intracoronary streptokinase versus coronary angioplasty therapy of acute myocardial infarction. *N. Engl. J. Med. 314*: 812.

Otto, C. M., Stratton, J. R., Maynard, C., Althouse, A., Johannessen, K-A., and Kennedy, J. (1990). Echocardiographic evaluation of segmental wall motion early and late after thrombolytic therapy in acute myocardial infarction. The Western Washington tissue plasminogen activator emergency room trial. *Am. J. Cardiol. 65*: 132.

Parry, C. H. (1799). *An Inquiry into the Symptoms and Causes of the Syncope Anginosa, Commonly Called Angina Pectoris*. R. Crutwell, Bath.

Pasternac, A. (1989). Myocardial stunning in hypertrophic cardiomyopathy? *J. Am. Coll. Cardiol. 13*: 1419.

Patel, B., Kloner, R. A., Przyklenk, K., and Braunwald, E. (1988). Postischemic myocardial "stunning": A clinically relevant phenomenon. *Ann. Intern. Med. 108*: 626.

Pfisterer, M., Zuber, M., Wenzel, R., and Burkart, F. (1991). Prolonged myocardial stunning after thrombolysis: Can left ventricular function be assessed definitely at hospital discharge? *Eur. Heart J. 12*: 214.

Reduto, L. A., Lawrie, G. M., Reid, J. W., Whissenand, H. H., Noon, G. P., Kanon, D., DeBakey, M. E., and Miller, R. R. (1981a). Sequential postoperative assessment of left ventricular performance with gated cardiac blood pool imaging following aortocoronary bypass surgery. *Am. Heart J. 101*: 59.

Reduto, L. A., Freund, G. C., Gaetal, J. M., Smalling, R. W., Lewis, B., and Gould, K. L. (1981b). Coronary artery reperfusion in acute myocardial infarction: Beneficial effects of intracoronary streptokinase on left ventricular salvage and performance. *Am. Heart J. 102*: 1168.

Renkin, J., Wijns, W., Ladha, Z., and Col, J. (1990). Reversal of segmental hypokinesis by coronary angioplasty in patients with unstable angina, persistent T wave inversion, and left anterior descending coronary artery stenosis. *Circulation 82*: 913.

Robertson, W. S., Feigenbaum, H., Armstrong, W. F., Dillon, J. C., O'Donnell, J., and McHenry, P. W. (1983). Exercise echocardiography: A clinically practical addition in the evaluation of coronary artery disease. *J. Am. Coll. Cardiol. 2*: 1085.

Satler, L. F., Kent, K. M., Fox, L. M., Goldstein, H. A., Green, C. E., Rogers, W. J., Pallas, R. S., Del Negro, A. A., Pearle, D. L., and Rackley, C. E. (1986). The assessment of contractile reserve after thrombolytic therapy for acute myocardial infarction. *Am. Heart J. 111*: 821.

Schmidt, W. G., Sheehan, F. H., von Essen, R., Uebis, R., and Effert, S. (1989). Evolution of left ventricular function after intracoronary thrombolysis for acute myocardial infarction. *Am. J. Cardiol. 63*: 497.

Schroder, E. S., Sirna, S. J., Kieso, R. A., and Kerber, R. E. (1988). Sensitization of reperfused myocardium to subsequent coronary flow reductions. An extension of the concept of myocardial stunning. *Circulation 78*: 717.

Stack, R. S., Phillips, H. R., III., Grierson, D. S., Behar, V. S., Kong, Y., Peter, R. H., Swain, J. L., and Greenfield, J. C., Jr. (1983). Functional improvement of jeopardized myocardium following intracoronary streptokinase infusion in acute myocardial infarction. *J. Clin. Invest. 72*: 84.

Tennant, R., and Wiggers, C. J. (1935). The effect of coronary occlusion on myocardial contraction. *Am. J. Physiol. 112*: 351.

Thaulow, E., Guth, B. D., Heusch, G., Gilpin, E., Schulz, R., Kroeger, K., and Ross, J., Jr. (1989). Characteristics of regional myocardial stunning after exercise in dogs with chronic coronary stenosis. *Am. J. Physiol. 257*: H113.

Touchstone, D. A., Beller, G. A., Nygaard, T. W., Tedesco, C., and Kaul, S. (1989). Effects of successful intravenous reperfusion therapy on regional myocardial function and geometry in humans. A tomographic assessment using two-dimensional echocardiography. *J. Am. Coll. Cardiol. 13*: 506.

Wijns, W., Serruys, P. W., Slager, C. J., Grimm, J., Krayenbuehl, H. P., Hugenholtz, P. G., and Hess, O. M. (1986). Effect of coronary occlusion during percutaneous transluminal angioplasty in humans on left ventricular chamber stiffness and regional diastolic pressure-radius relations. *J. Am. Coll. Cardiol. 7*: 455.

Williamson, B. D., Lim, M. J., and Buda, A. J. (1990). Transient left ventricular filling abnormalities (diastolic stunning) after acute myocardial infarction. *Am. J. Cardiol. 66*: 897.

Yuki, K., Kodama, Y., Onda, J., Emoto, K., Morimoto, T., and Uozumi, T. (1991). Coronary vasospasm following subarachnoid hemorrhage as a cause of stunned myocardium. *J. Neurosurg 75*: 308.

Zerhouni, E. A., Parish, D. M., Rogers, W. J., Yang, A., and Shapiro, E. P. (1988): Human heart tagging with MR imaging. A method of noninvasive assessment of myocardial motion. *Radiology 169*: 59.

Zuber, M., Pfisterer, M., Kiowski, W., Schmitt, H. E., Ritz, R., and Burkart, F. (1989). Emergency coronary dilatation in acute myocardial infarct with contraindications to thrombolytic therapy: Salvage of the myocardium by early intervention. *Schweiz. Rundsch. Med. 78*: 863.

Index

About the Editors

ROBERT A. KLONER is Director of Research at the Heart Institute of the Hospital of the Good Samaritan, Los Angeles, California, and Professor of Medicine in the Section of Cardiology, University of Southern California, Los Angeles. The author or coauthor of over 300 professional papers and book chapters, he serves on the editorial boards of nine cardiovascular journals, is a Fellow of the American College of Cardiology and the Council on Clinical Cardiology of the American Heart Association, and a member of the American Association of Pathologists, the American Physiological Society, and the American Society for Clinical Investigation, among other organizations. Dr. Kloner received an Established Investigator Award from the American Heart Association (1981-1986). Dr. Kloner received the Ph.D. degree (1974) in experimental pathology and the M.D. degree (1975) from Northwestern University, Chicago, Illinois.

KARIN PRZYKLENK is Assistant Director of Research and Director of Cardiac Function at the Heart Institute of the Hospital of the Good Samaritan, Los Angeles, California, and Associate Professor of Research Medicine, University of Southern California, Los Angeles. A member of the American Heart Association, and the American Section of the International Society for Heart Research, she is the author of numerous professional papers that reflect her research interest in the acute and chronic consequences of coronary artery occlusion/reperfusion on myocyte morphology, recovery of contractile function, coronary blood flow, and high energy phosphate content. Dr. Przyklenk received the Ph.D. degree (1982) in biophysics from the University of Western Ontario, London, Ontario, Canada.